# Integrated Holistic Yoga Movement

Volume 2 in Therapeutic Yoga Teaching, Clinical Service, and Practice

# ALSO BY CHRISTIANE BREMS, PhD, ABPP, ERYT500, C-IAYT

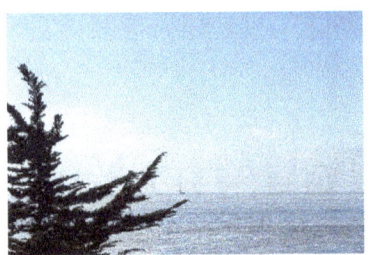

*Integrated Holistic Yoga Psychology (Volume 1 in Therapeutic Yoga Teaching, Clinical Service, and Practice)*

*Therapeutic Breathwork: Clinical Research and Practice in Healthcare and Yoga*

*Comprehensive Guide to Child Psychotherapy and Counseling* (4th edition)

*Basic Skills in Psychotherapy and Counseling*

*Instructor's Manual for "Basic Skills in Psychotherapy and Counseling"*

*Dealing with Challenges in Psychotherapy and Counseling*

*Psychotherapy: Processes and Techniques*

*The Child Therapist: Personal Traits and Markers of Effectiveness*

*Between Two People: Exercises Toward Intimacy (with Johnson & Fortman)*

# Integrated Holistic Yoga Movement

*Volume 2 in* THERAPEUTIC YOGA TEACHING, CLINICAL SERVICE, AND PRACTICE

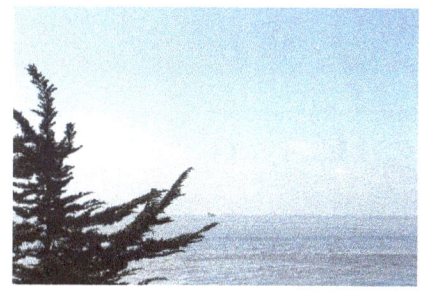

*Christiane Brems, PhD, ABPP, ERYT500, C-IAYT*

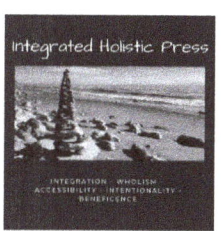

**Integrated Holistic Yoga Movement:
Volume 2 in Therapeutic Yoga Teaching, Clinical Service, and Practice**

**Copyright © 2025** by Christiane Brems, PhD, ABPP, ERYT500, C-IAYT
**Integrated Holistic Press**
**Goleta, California**

All rights reserved. No part of this publication may be reproduced, stored in a retrieval system, or transmitted in any form or by any means, electronic, mechanical, photocopying, recording, or otherwise, without the prior written permission of the publisher and copyright holder.

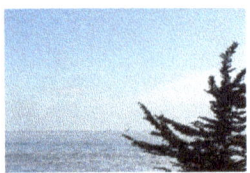

**US Library of Congress Cataloging-in-Publication Data:**

| | |
|---|---|
| **Title**: | *Integrated Holistic Yoga Movement: Volume 2 in Therapeutic Yoga Teaching, Clinical Service, and Practice* |
| **Author**: | Christiane Brems, PhD, ABPP, ERYT500, C-IAYT |
| **Format**: | Softcover |
| **ISBN**: | 979-8-9928567-2-9 |
| **Publication Date**: | 2025 |
| **Disclaimers**: | The information provided in this book is not intended to substitute for medical, movement, breathing, or other practice advice of qualified healthcare providers. This book is not intended to diagnose or treat any medical or mental health conditions, but rather serves to describe an approach to integrated holistic movement, breathing, and inner yoga practices. Readers are advised to consult with their qualified healthcare providers if they have questions about the appropriateness of any of the strategies offered in this book for themselves or their students or clients. The publisher and the author is not liable for any injuries, damages, or negative consequences allegedly arising from any actions, movements, applications, or preparations by anyone reading or otherwise perusing the information in this book. |
| | References and websites provided throughout this book are strictly for informational purposes and do not constitute an endorsement of any websites or other named sources. Readers should also be aware that website addresses listed in this book may change. The information and references included in this book were up to date at the time of its writing but given that medical evidence progresses quickly, they may not be up to date by the time of reading. |
| **Cover Image**: | Layers of Tree Limbs near the Pacific Ocean by Christiane Brems |

## Dedication

This book is dedicated to all movers and yogis everywhere.

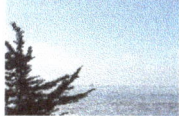

May your movements and actions support your health and wellbeing
and provide you a sense of agency and personal empowerment.

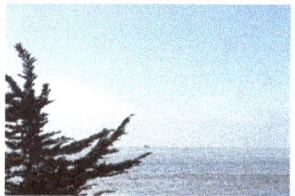

May your movements and actions reflect awareness, wisdom,
compassion, lovingkindness, joy, and balance.

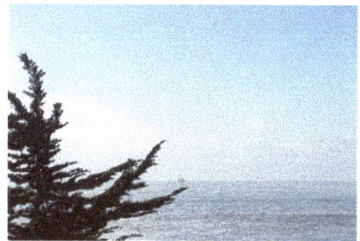

May your movements and actions reverberate into your communities,
creating wise and thriving collectives that serve the greater good
for the entire web of life and the planet that supports it.

# Foreword

*"If you close your eyes and feel carefully, you won't feel a 'body.' Body is only a word, the idea or concept level. What you will actually feel are areas of hardness and softness, of pressure, heaviness, and textures such as rough and smooth. This is the earth element. You will also feel areas of warmth and coolness. This is the fire or temperature element. You feel areas of vibrations and stillness. This is the air or vibratory element. And you will feel cohesion and fluidity. This is the water element: you only need to blink your eyes or swallow to sense it."*
Jack Kornfield, 2009, The Wise Heart, p. 119

> *"Movement is the song of the body, [breath, and mind]."*
> Vanda Scaravelli
> [bracketed material added]

The capacity for movement is a precious gift, a life-giving and health-preserving necessity, a way to be in community for the sake of pleasure, joy, combat, food security, self-protection, and the protection of loved ones. We need movement to live and stay healthy. We are evolved to move, and movement has contributed to the profound and revolutionary evolution of our human brain. The intimate link between motion and cognition, between movement and emotion, between action and wellbeing is not just metaphorical – it is deeply biological.

Consider the sea squirt, a marine invertebrate born with a primitive brain and spinal cord, allowing it to swim through the ocean in search of a home. Once it anchors to a rock and no longer needs to move, it digests its own brain. In the absence of movement, its nervous system becomes superfluous. This evolutionary tale invites reflection: the brain, even in its most basic forms, appears to exist in service of movement. In humans, our capacity for dynamic, intentional motion – walking upright, grasping, gesturing, dancing – has contributed to the very structure and complexity of our unique nervous system. From the cerebellum's fine-tuned coordination to the motor cortex's role in planning and executing voluntary action, our brains (and bodies) are sculpted by the demands of movement. To move is to think and to love; engaging with the world through action means cultivating the very structures that just may define our humanity.

Yoga practice in general, and this series of three books in particular, is offered as a way to begin to learn about ourselves and others: our places in the world and our impacts on the greater web of life. It is an invitation to become aware, curious, and mindful; to gain greater understanding about how, what, and why we act, think, and feel the way we do; to live with compassion, open-heartedly, gratefully, joyfully, and peacefully. Becoming mindful about how we move through life, how we take action and express our capacity to move, breathe, think, feel and relate is the very essence of embarking on a journey of self-discovery. Recognizing the nuances and joys of moving in the world, moving with the rhythm of life, flowing with grace in communities and relationships, and recognizing the ripple effects of every small movement and action – that is the power of yoga. The power of a yoga that is about creating change in the world, about creating a web of life that can sustain itself with grace, wisdom, joy, and health.

Move gratefully, joyfully, and compassionately. Many hugs,

*Chris Brems*

# Content Overview of the Series
# Therapeutic Yoga Teaching, Clinical Service, and Practice

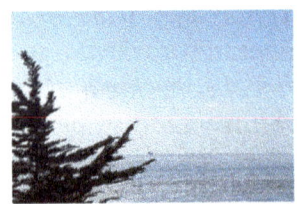

## Volume 1 – Integrated Holistic Yoga Psychology

Section 1: Integrated Holistic Yoga History and Psychology

Section 2: Integrated Holistic Yoga Pedagogy and Practice Principles

## Volume 2 – Integrated Holistic Yoga Movement

Section 1: Integrated Holistic Yoga Anatomy and Physiology

Section 2: Integrated Holistic Yoga Approaches to Asana

## Volume 3 – Integrated Holistic Introspective Yoga Practices

Section 1: Integrated Holistic Yoga Approaches to Pranayama

Section 2: Integrated Holistic Yoga Approaches to Inner Practices

# Introduction to the Series
## Therapeutic Yoga Teaching, Clinical Service, and Practice

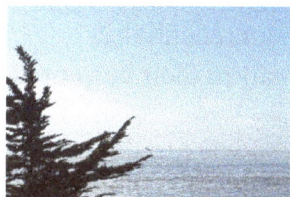

The three-volume series "*Therapeutic Yoga Teaching, Clinical Service, and Practice*" offers an integrated holistic approach to the teaching, clinical service provision, and practice of therapeutic yoga. Integrated holistic yoga is defined by its focus on intentionality, beneficence, accessibility, wholism, and integration. It carefully reviews, weaves together, and scientifically and practically grounds therapeutic yoga practices and lifestyles in the traditional eight limbs of yoga. It simultaneously contextualizes all offered yoga principles and practices within the wholism of the five layers of human experience postulated by ancient wisdom and supported by modern science. It explores and honors interrelationships among body, vitality (energy and affect), mind (emotions and thoughts), wisdom and self-discovery, and relationships within families and communities, in support of personal and collective healing and thriving.

## Therapeutic Yoga Contents Covered in the Series

In three comprehensive volumes, the series "*Therapeutic Yoga Teaching, Clinical Service, and Practice*" elucidates the principles of therapeutic yoga guided by a strong commitment to wholism and integration, as well as accessibility, intentionality, and beneficence.

- Volume 1, *Integrated Holistic Yoga Psychology*, explores neurophysiological and psychological mechanisms underlying physical, energetic, emotional, cognitive, and relational patterns and habits, combining ancient wisdom about human nature with modern scientific findings. Relying on yoga psychology – ancient and modern, it dives deeply into mind and emotion, exploring the development and transformation of physical, mental, and emotional habits, based on the cultivation of compassion, awareness, and insight to serve personal and collective healing and thriving.
- Volume 2, *Integrated Holistic Yoga Movement*, reviews anatomical and physiological science as relevant to the teaching of yoga movements and forms, integrating ancient wisdom with modern anatomical and kinesiological research. A multitude of movement teaching principles and practice strategies are offered for supporting enhanced health and wellbeing through therapeutic yoga classes, yoga-therapeutically informed healthcare, and individually-tailored personal practices.
- Volume 3, *Integrated Holistic Introspective Yoga Practices*, offers scientifically-based and ancient yogic approaches to breathwork, sense-guarding, concentration, and meditation practices. It offers scientific insights that guide applied inner practices (including mindfulness). Offered practices lead practitioners toward the cultivation of compassion, awareness, purpose, and wisdom, with deliberate implications for personal and collective wellbeing.

## Therapeutic Yoga Audiences for the Series

The series *"Therapeutic Yoga Teaching, Clinical Service, and Practice"* is written for
- yoga teacher and therapeutic yoga training programs
- individuals seeking yoga teacher credentials,
- yoga teachers who seek to transform their current teaching to become more therapeutic and person-centered,
- dedicated yoga practitioners who want to deepen and tailor their personal practice, and
- healthcare providers seeking to integrate yoga therapeutics into their clinical practice.

The series is an excellent resource for yoga teacher training programs, carefully designed to exceed educational contents and standards required by Yoga Alliance, the association that registers yoga schools, programs, and teachers internationally. It augments current yoga teachers' training by offering a unique therapeutic lens that allows yoga professionals to broaden their yoga teaching skills and understanding to serve populations of students and clients in community health settings and healthcare systems. The volumes in the series are an invaluable resource for healthcare practitioners who hope to integrate therapeutic yoga strategies into their extant clinical practice. They provide an in-depth exploration of how therapeutic yoga can serve patients in healthcare and mental health care and how it can be infused in clinical service delivery. The series is also appropriate for advanced yoga practitioners who seek to refine their yoga practice to be more person-centered, relevant to their unique biopsychosociocultural context, and tailored to their specific physical, vital, emotional, mental, behavioral, and relational needs.

## Therapeutic Yoga Approach and Lineage of the Series

The series *"Therapeutic Yoga Teaching, Clinical Service, and Practice"* offers historically-respectful, science-informed guidance for therapeutic yoga practices and interventions development across all limbs of yoga – from *asana*; *pranayama*; mindfulness, concentration, and meditation; to ethical and committed lifestyle practices – emerging from a respectful context of tradition and science. The series focuses on yoga therapeutics, highlighting yoga as a transformative lifestyle and healing practice that is available to and appropriate for all humans.

The series is unique due to its embrace of the integrated holistic yoga (IHY) paradigm that is defined by accessibility, intentionality, beneficence, wholism, and integration. This unique approach to the teaching, clinical offering, and personal practice of yoga was developed by the author to create a system of yoga therapeutics that offer yoga to the very populations who can most benefit from, but often have limited access to, the practice.

The integrated holistic yoga approach offers a vision that honors the deep cultural traditions of transformative practices, such as yoga and Buddhism, that date back thousands of years. It integrates modern neuroscience with ancient psychologies and practices; it demonstrates the profound wisdoms from the original teachings that we are relearning and rediscovering every day, with research increasingly supporting their usefulness. The integrated holistic framework underlying all practices offered in the series embraces inclusiveness, access, diversity, health, wellbeing, and resilience for everyone. It is a practice of and for community; it honors interdependence and coregulation. Integrated holistic work embraces an honoring of traditional yogic practices – practices (grounded in the eight limbs of yoga) that are physical only to prepare practitioners for more important interior practices (such as concentration and meditation) and interpersonal applications of a thoughtful and deliberate code of ethics, lifestyle, and discipline.

The integrated holistic approach combines body, emotion, mind, spirit, and community through a comprehensive lifestyle with implications for individual and collective wellbeing. It promotes self-compassion, introspection, and community that lead to insights that alter human physiology and anatomy and – perhaps more importantly – emotions, cognitions, behaviors, and relationships. Integrated holistic practices are accessible to anyone who can breathe without assistance, almost anywhere, for little to no cost. They motivate practitioners to adhere to a complete practice that honors all human needs and experiences, more so than a unidimensional posture practice - freed from Western stereotypes that tend to limit who engages with yoga or other types of transformative work. The following central principles of IHY are interwoven throughout all volumes in the series and guide all teachings and practices.

- *Integrated Holistic Yoga is a practice of intentionality* – commitment to making the world a better place; to living and practicing with intention, purpose, and meaning; to helping all beings develop meaningful goals and life purpose
- *Integrated Holistic Yoga is a practice of beneficence* – commitment to facilitating mechanisms of change that do no harm and lead to positive health and mental health outcomes individually and collectively
- *Integrated Holistic Yoga is a practice of accessibility* – commitment to creating communities of healing that honor and practice diversity, inclusion, equity, advocacy, engaged action, and personal as well collective empowerment and evolution
- *Integrated Holistic Yoga is a practice of wholeness* – commitment to honor human complexity, biopsychosociocultural contexts, interconnection, and community
- *Integrated Holistic Yoga is a practice of integration* – commitment to offering a diversity of integrated practices, carefully tailored to individual and collective needs of each human being, interweaving science and soul, as well as interdependence and coregulation

In sum, the three-volume series *"Therapeutic Yoga Teaching, Clinical Service, and Practice"*
- uses an integrated holistic model that covers a multitude of yoga practices for body, breath, mind, and relationships;
- focuses on preparing yoga professionals who offer therapeutic applications of yoga, especially in healthcare settings; and
- is a perfect and unique accompaniment for therapeutic yoga teacher training, personal yoga practice, and self-study to adapt clinical services or standard yoga teaching to become therapeutic, person-centered, and individually tailored.

Please enjoy the three volumes in this series and the journey into self-discovery and thriving that may result. I wish you and your students, clients, and patients the wisdom, awareness, compassion, and joy that is inherent in an integrated holistic practice of yoga. May you and yours discover a practice that leads to coping, healing, and thriving – individually and collectively.

Gratefully,

*Chris Brems*

# Acknowledgements

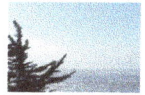

No book is ever a solitary effort. All books arise out of a particular context and set of experiences, causes, and conditions. This book is no exception – I am forever grateful to all the individuals and collectives that have contributed to the emergence of this book during the many decades of my life.

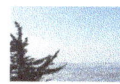 *To My Wise and Beautiful Colleagues and Yoga Role Models:*

My deepest gratitude to the amazing human beings who shared the practice of yoga via the pictures offered in this volume. Your openness of heart and deeply compassionate embrace of integrated holistic yoga leaps off every photograph. Your willingness to allow your photos to be included in this volume reflects your boundless generosity and altruistic joy. Thank you for your profound commitment to making yoga accessible, intentional, beneficent, whole, and integrated. You are guiding lights in this world.

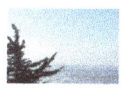 *To My Wise and Compassionate Teachers:*

Deep appreciation and ever-lasting gratitude also goes to my many teachers and guides on the path to self-discovery. Your collective depth of knowledge and commitment left indelible marks on my work and my life. All of you remain in my heart and continue to move me. You have shaped me as a human being, teacher, clinician, colleague, and partner. I am filled with gratitude to each and every one of you.

Klaus, my very first yoga teacher when I was just a wide-eyed youth – you started me on this journey and I cannot thank you enough. You helped me move with grace into an awkward adolescent body. I may have forgotten your last name (it was after all 50 years ago), but your impact on my life is as palpable today as it was back then. Lynne Minton – you are an eye-opening inspiration, a yogi in the truest sense of the word, and a wonderful mentor as I started my journey into teaching yoga. Monica Devine, Sarahjoy Marsh, Judith Hansen Lasater, and Christopher Wallis – you inspired me and moved me in the most meaningful ways.

Marty Rossman – you gave me the gift of guided imagery; Patrick McKeown – you shared your profound wisdom and belief in the Buteyko method; Stephen Porges – you imparted your insights into polyvagal theory; Yongey Mingyur Rinpoche, Joseph Goldstein, and Lama Tillmann Borghardt – your Buddhist teachings have deeply inspired and transformed me although I have not (yet) met some of you in person.

My commitment to diversity, equity, and accessibility was shared, shaped, and nourished by two beloved (late) colleagues – indigenous psychologist Robert Morgan and Yupik healer Rita Blumenstein (once an elder on the International Council of 13 Grandmothers). Your impact on the world and your deep commitment to creating change through understanding, love, and compassion still deeply move me and always will.

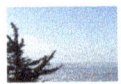 ### *To My Wise and Resilient Students and Clients:*

I am forever grateful to you, my students and clients, who may have taught and changed me most of all. I am grateful to you for sharing your wisdom, insights, vulnerabilities, faith, courage, hearts, and experiences. Nothing in life taught me more than being a part of your journeys and witnessing your resilience, compassion, joy, and learning as we have moved and reflected together. I have learned more from you than I could have ever hoped for. I am filled with the deepest gratitude and love for all of you. You have enriched my life in endless ways that will be with me always.

To my *Breast Cancer Resource Center* 'students' (well, you are really my teachers as much as I am yours) who have shared the journey through cancer – my weekly time and movement with you has been nothing short of miraculous. You have shown the strongest spirit, deepest capacity for mutual compassion and caring, and most remarkable resilience in the wake of intense suffering.

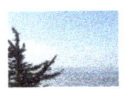 ### *To My Wise and Loving Family:*

I am filled with gratitude and love for all of my German family, especially my father Bernard Brems, my sister Gabriele Strubel, and brother-in-law Floh Strubel. You are my roots. We may be thousands of miles apart; yet whenever we meet, whenever we talk or walk together, whenever we are in one another's thoughts, the distance is gone. We are connected in spirit – always. I am deeply thankful for your presence in my life – Ich danke Euch allen von ganzem Herzen.

Finally, I am most profoundly and eternally grateful for my intrepid, compassionate, patient (beyond belief), supportive, loving, funny (thanks for the strong core muscles), and unwavering partner, Mark Johnson. You are the love of my life, my best friend, my most trusted human being, and my inspiration. During the immeasurable movements of having walked, hiked, kayaked, swum, run, and done yoga together, you have helped shape my way of being and moving in the world more than anyone. You constantly rekindle my faith and my joy; you help me feel whole. The greatest miracle in my life was crossing paths with you some 40 years ago and having moved, played, enjoyed, and suffered together ever since.

*Thank you all!*
*Chris*

# Integrated Holistic Yoga Movement
## Volume 2 in Therapeutic Yoga Teaching, Clinical Service, and Practice

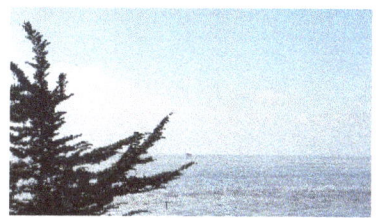

### SECTION 1 INTRODUCTION ........................................................................................... 3
- Yoga Anatomy and Physiology Overview ................................................................ 3
- Anatomy and Physiology Learning Objectives ....................................................... 5
- Anatomy and Physiology Recommended Readings ............................................... 6

### CHAPTER 1: KEY CONCEPTS OF INTEGRATED HOLISTIC MOVEMENT ............... 7
- Understanding the Essential Nature of Movement ................................................ 7
  - *Benefits of Integrated Holistic Movement* ......................................................... 8
  - *The Miracle of Coordinated Movement* ............................................................. 9
  - *Biopsychosociocultural Individuality* ............................................................... 10
  - *Physical Resilience and Adaptability Through Movement* .............................. 14
  - *Implications for Yoga Asana* ............................................................................. 18
- Understanding Anatomical Language and Associated Concepts ........................ 19
  - *Directions of Body Movement* ........................................................................... 19
  - *Planes of Movement* ........................................................................................... 22
  - *Anatomical Directions* ....................................................................................... 23

### CHAPTER 2: KEY CONCEPTS OF INTEGRATED HOLISTIC PHYSIOLOGY ........... 25
- Interdependence of Physical Structures and Systems .......................................... 25
- Human Physiology – Key Knowledge for Yoga .................................................... 27
  - *Types of Tissue in The Human Body* ................................................................. 28
  - *Organ Systems with Relevance for Yoga* .......................................................... 30
- What's Ahead ........................................................................................................... 46

### CHAPTER 3: KEY CONCEPTS OF INTEGRATED HOLISTIC ANATOMY ................ 47
- Connective Tissues .................................................................................................. 47
  - *Connective Tissues with Great Tensile Strength* ............................................. 48
- Bones – Connective Tissue with Greater Compressive Strength ........................ 55
  - *Functions of Bones* ............................................................................................. 56
  - *Characteristics of Bones* .................................................................................... 56

*Overview of Bones and Their Bioindividuality* ............................................................................. 59
*Joints – Articulations of Bones* ....................................................................................................... 62
MUSCLES .................................................................................................................................................. 68
*Muscle Functions* ............................................................................................................................. 69
*Muscle Types and Muscles as Neuromuscular Tissue* .................................................................... 72
*Skeletal Muscle* ................................................................................................................................ 75
ONE MORE NOTE ABOUT ANATOMY TRAINS ......................................................................................... 84
*Superficial Front Line* ..................................................................................................................... 85
*Superficial Back Line* ....................................................................................................................... 85
*Deep Front Line* ............................................................................................................................... 85
*Lateral Line* ...................................................................................................................................... 86
*Spiral Line* ........................................................................................................................................ 86
WHAT'S AHEAD ...................................................................................................................................... 86

# CHAPTER 4: ANATOMY OF THE AXIAL REGION OF THE BODY ........................... 87

HEAD ....................................................................................................................................................... 87
BONES AND JOINTS OF THE HEAD ........................................................................................................... 87
*Bones of the Head* ............................................................................................................................ 87
*Joints of the Head* ............................................................................................................................ 88
*Bony Landmarks on the Head* ......................................................................................................... 89
MUSCLES OF THE HEAD, FACE, AND NECK ............................................................................................ 89
VERTEBRAL COLUMN AND THORAX ....................................................................................................... 91
BONES OF THE VERTEBRAL COLUMN AND THORAX .............................................................................. 91
*Overview of the Vertebral Column, Thorax, and Vertebrae* ......................................................... 92
*Anatomy of the Vertebrae* ............................................................................................................... 94
JOINTS AND LIGAMENTS OF THE VERTEBRAL COLUMN AND THORAX ................................................. 97
*Vertebral Body Joints* ...................................................................................................................... 97
*Facet Joints* ...................................................................................................................................... 97
*Specialized Joints Between the Vertebrae* ..................................................................................... 98
*Sternochondral Joints* ..................................................................................................................... 99
*Ligaments Across the Joints of the Vertebral Column and Thorax* ............................................. 99
MUSCLES ALONG THE VERTEBRAL COLUMN AND THORAX ................................................................ 101
*Muscles of the Back* ....................................................................................................................... 101
*Muscles of the Core* ....................................................................................................................... 107
KINESIOLOGY OF THE SPINE .................................................................................................................. 110
*Spinal Curves in the Sagittal Plane* .............................................................................................. 112
*Scoliosis or Spinal Curves in the Frontal Plane* .......................................................................... 118
*Ranges and Directions of Motion across Spinal Sections* ........................................................... 121
WHAT'S AHEAD .................................................................................................................................... 127

# CHAPTER 5: ANATOMY OF THE LOWER APPENDICULAR REGION ................... 129

PELVIC GIRDLE AND THIGHS ................................................................................................................ 129
BONES OF THE PELVIC GIRDLE AND THIGHS ........................................................................................ 129
*Hip Bones* ....................................................................................................................................... 130
*Sacrum and Coccyx* ....................................................................................................................... 130
*Femur* ............................................................................................................................................. 131
JOINTS AND LIGAMENTS OF THE PELVIC GIRDLE AND THIGHS ........................................................... 131

  *Pubic Symphysis* ............................................................................................................. *131*
  *Acetabulofemoral Joint* .................................................................................................. *132*
  *Sacroiliac Joints* ............................................................................................................. *133*
 Muscles of the Pelvic Girdle and Thighs ............................................................................ 134
  *Hip Flexors, Spinal Flexors, and Lateral Flexors* ......................................................... *135*
  *Deep Gluteal Muscles* .................................................................................................... *136*
  *Superficial Gluteal Muscles* ........................................................................................... *137*
  *Hamstrings* ..................................................................................................................... *139*
  *Adductors* ....................................................................................................................... *140*
  *Quadriceps Femoris* ...................................................................................................... *141*
  *Muscles of the Pelvic Floor* ........................................................................................... *142*
 Kinesiology of the Pelvic Girdle and Thighs ...................................................................... 143
  *Understanding Movement in the Acetabulum* ............................................................... *144*
  *Understanding Movement in the Sacroiliac Region* ...................................................... *146*
  *Understanding the Lumbar-Sacral Rhythm* .................................................................. *148*
 Lower Legs, Ankles, and Feet ............................................................................................. 149
 Bones of the Legs, Ankles, and Feet ................................................................................... 150
  *Bones of the Legs* .......................................................................................................... *150*
  *Bones of the Ankles and Feet* ........................................................................................ *151*
 Joints and Ligaments of the Legs, Ankles, and Feet .......................................................... 152
  *Knees* ............................................................................................................................. *152*
  *Ankles* ............................................................................................................................ *154*
  *Feet (Including Arches)* ................................................................................................. *156*
 Muscles of the Lower Legs, Ankles, and Feet .................................................................... 159
  *Muscles Acting on the Knee and Ankle* ........................................................................ *159*
  *Muscles Acting Primarily on the Ankle* ........................................................................ *160*
  *Muscles Acting on the Ankle and Feet* ......................................................................... *160*
  *Intrinsic Muscles of the Foot* ........................................................................................ *161*
 Kinesiology of the Knee, Ankle, and Feet .......................................................................... 162
  *Understanding Movement in the Knee* ......................................................................... *162*
  *Understanding Movement in the Ankle* ........................................................................ *165*
  *Understanding Movement in the Foot* .......................................................................... *166*
 What's Ahead ....................................................................................................................... 168

## CHAPTER 6: ANATOMY OF UPPER APPENDICULAR REGION ................................ 169

 Pectoral Girdle and Upper Arms .......................................................................................... 169
 Bones of the Pectoral Girdle and Upper Arms .................................................................... 169
  *Scapulae* ......................................................................................................................... *170*
  *Clavicles* ........................................................................................................................ *171*
  *Humerus of the Upper Arm* ........................................................................................... *172*
 Joints of the Shoulder Girdle ............................................................................................... 173
  *Scapulothoracic Junction* .............................................................................................. *174*
  *Acromioclavicular Joint* ................................................................................................ *174*
  *Sternoclavicular Joint* ................................................................................................... *174*
  *Glenohumeral (Shoulder) Joint* ..................................................................................... *175*
 Muscles of the Arms and Shoulder Girdle .......................................................................... 176
  *Muscles that Stabilize the Scapulae on the Back Body* ................................................ *176*

*Muscles that Stabilize the Arms and Scapulae on the Front Body* .................................... *178*
*Rotator Cuff Muscles* .................................................................................................... *179*
*Muscles Connecting the Arms and Shoulder Joints* ..................................................... *181*
KINESIOLOGY OF THE PECTORAL GIRDLE .............................................................................. 182
*Scapular Stabilization Through Anterior-Posterior Balance* ........................................ *182*
*Glenohumeral or Scapulohumeral Rhythm* ................................................................. *183*
*Stability and Load Management in the Glenohumeral Joint* ........................................ *184*
FOREARMS, WRISTS, AND HANDS ........................................................................................ 185
BONES OF THE FOREARMS, WRISTS, AND HANDS .................................................................. 185
JOINTS OF THE FOREARMS, WRISTS, AND HANDS .................................................................. 187
MUSCLES OF THE FOREARMS, WRISTS, AND HANDS .............................................................. 188
*Muscles Around the Elbow* .......................................................................................... *188*
*Muscles of the Wrists and Forearms* ............................................................................ *188*
*Intrinsic Muscles of the Hands* ..................................................................................... *190*
KINESIOLOGY OF THE FOREARMS, WRISTS, AND HANDS ....................................................... 190
*Journey of Force During Load-Bearing in Inversions and Half-Inversions* ................. *191*
WHAT'S AHEAD .................................................................................................................. 192

## SECTION 2 INTRODUCTION .............................................................................. 195

YOGA ASANA AND MOVEMENT OVERVIEW ......................................................................... 195
YOGA ASANA AND MOVEMENT LEARNING OBJECTIVES ...................................................... 196
YOGA ASANA AND MOVEMENT RECOMMENDED READINGS ................................................ 197

## CHAPTER 7: PRINCIPLES OF INTEGRATED HOLISTIC YOGA ASANA AND MOVEMENT .................................................................................................................. 199

INTENTION AND PURPOSE RELATED TO TEACHING YOGA ASANA AND MOVEMENT ............. 199
BENEFICENCE RELATED TO TEACHING YOGA ASANA AND MOVEMENT .............................. 200
*Benefits of Integrated Holistic Shapes and Movement* ................................................ *200*
*Contraindications For Particular Shapes and Movements* .......................................... *201*
*Potential Risks or Challenges of Some Shapes or Movements* .................................... *202*
PRACTICE PRINCIPLES FOR TEACHING OF YOGA ASANA AND MOVEMENT .......................... 203
*Sequencing with Focus on Yoga Asana and Movement* ............................................... *203*
*Optimization of Opportunities for Physical Safety* ...................................................... *211*
*General Movement and Alignment Principles and Cues* .............................................. *212*
TROUBLESHOOTING PHYSICAL DISCOMFORT AND PHYSICAL RESISTANCE .......................... 219
*Working with Physical Pain, Discomfort, and Soreness* .............................................. *219*
*Working with Physical Resistance* ............................................................................... *222*
BIOMECHANICS RELATED TO TEACHING SHAPES AND MOVEMENT ..................................... 225
*Understanding Force and Load* ................................................................................... *225*
*Understanding Open- Versus Closed-Chain Movement* .............................................. *237*
*Understanding and Making Use of Reflexes* ................................................................ *239*
WHAT'S AHEAD .................................................................................................................. 248

## CHAPTER 8: UPRIGHT STANDING SHAPES ................................................... 251

ANATOMICAL FOCI FOR UPRIGHT STANDING SHAPES .......................................................... 251
*Understanding and Recruiting the Natural Spine* ........................................................ *251*
*Recruiting Core Stabilization and Engagement* .......................................................... *256*

  *Assembling Standing Shapes from the Bottom Up* .................................................................... 257
  *Creating Tailored Foundations for Standing Shapes* ............................................................... 260
 ANALYSIS AND EXPERIENCE OF SAMPLE UPRIGHT STANDING SHAPES ............................... 264
  *Mountain or Tadasana* ................................................................................................................. 265
  *Warrior 1 Lunge or Virabhadrasana I Lunge* ........................................................................ 271
  *Warrior 3 or Virabhadrasana III* .............................................................................................. 275
  *Eagle or Garudasana* .................................................................................................................. 279
  *Warrior 2 or Virabhadrasana II* ................................................................................................ 283
  *Side Angle or Utthita Parsvakonasana* .................................................................................... 289
  *Triangle or Utthita Trikonasana* ............................................................................................... 294
  *Tree or Vrksasana* ....................................................................................................................... 299

## CHAPTER 9: ARM STANDING .................................................................................................... 305
 ANATOMICAL FOCI FOR ARM STANDING ................................................................................... 305
  *Understanding the Journey of Force through the Arms* ...................................................... 305
  *Understanding and Recruiting the Shoulder Girdle* ............................................................ 306
  *Core/Trunk Engagement and Stabilization* ............................................................................ 315
 ANALYSIS AND EXPERIENCE OF SAMPLE ARM STANDING SHAPES .......................................... 320
  *Table Top or Bharmanasana* ..................................................................................................... 322
  *Downward Facing Dog or Adho Mukha Svanasana* ............................................................ 327
  *Plank or Phalakasana* ................................................................................................................. 333
  *Side Plank or Vasisthasana* ....................................................................................................... 337

## CHAPTER 10: UPRIGHT SEATS ................................................................................................. 341
 ANATOMICAL FOCI FOR UPRIGHT SEATS ................................................................................... 341
  *Natural Spine* ................................................................................................................................ 341
  *Core Stabilization* ........................................................................................................................ 342
  *Pelvic Girdle – Structures and Relationships* ....................................................................... 342
  *Tailored Foundations for Different Seated Shapes* ............................................................. 345
 ANALYSIS AND EXPERIENCE OF SAMPLE UPRIGHT SEATS ........................................................ 348
  *Easy Seat or Sukhasana* .............................................................................................................. 350
  *Bound Angle Seat or Baddha Konasana* ................................................................................. 355
  *Hero or Virasana and Diamond or Vajrasana* ...................................................................... 359
  *Staff or Dandasana* ..................................................................................................................... 363
  *Cow Face Seat or Gomukhasana* .............................................................................................. 367

## CHAPTER 11: TWISTS OR ROTATIONS .................................................................................. 371
 ANATOMICAL FOCI IN TWISTS OR ROTATIONS .......................................................................... 371
  *Natural Spine and Pelvis* ............................................................................................................ 372
  *Anatomical Principles for Sacroiliac Joint Health in Twists* ............................................. 373
  *Protecting the Sacroiliac Joints in Twists* ............................................................................. 375
  *A Few Final Asides About Twists* ............................................................................................. 377
 ANALYSIS AND EXPERIENCE OF SAMPLE TWISTS AND ROTATIONS ......................................... 379
  *Standing Twists from Mountain or Tadasana* ...................................................................... 381
  *Seated Twists or Parivrtta Sukhasana* .................................................................................... 385
  *Revolve-Around-the-Belly Twist or Jathara Parivartanasana* .......................................... 390
  *Supported Prone Twist (with Belly on a Bolster)* ................................................................ 395

## CHAPTER 12: FORWARD FOLDS ... 399

### Anatomical Foci for Forward Folds ... 399
*Natural Spine and Spinal Flexion versus Extension in Forward Folds* ... 400
*Natural Pelvis with Healthful Movement in the Hip Joints* ... 403
*Core Stabilization* ... 408

### Analysis and Experience of Sample Forward Folds ... 409
*General Concepts about Forward Folding* ... 411
*Standing Forward Fold or Uttanasana* ... 414
*Wide-Legged Standing Forward Fold or Prasarita Padottanasana* ... 418
*Seated Forward Fold or Paschimottanasana* ... 422
*Wide-Legged Seated Forward Fold or Upavistha Konasana* ... 425
*Head-of-Knee Shape or Janu Sirsasana* ... 429
*Child or Balasana* ... 432

## CHAPTER 13: BACKBENDS OR HEART OPENERS ... 437

### Anatomical Foci for Backbends or Heart Openers ... 437
*Overview of Relevant Body Regions* ... 437
*Neck and Head Regions* ... 439
*Thoracic Region* ... 441
*Pelvic Region* ... 445
*Abdominals and More* ... 447
*Mind* ... 447

### Analysis and Experience of Sample Backbends or Heart Openers ... 449
*General Concepts about Backbends or Heart Openers* ... 450
*Camel or Ustrasana* ... 454
*Cobra or Bhujangasana* ... 457
*Locust or Salabhasana* ... 461
*Bridge or Setu Bandha Sarvangasana* ... 464

## CHAPTER 14: INVERSIONS AND PARTIAL INVERSIONS ... 469

### Helpful Anatomical Foci by Type of Inversion ... 469
### Analysis and Experience of Sample Inversions ... 471
*General Concepts about Inversions* ... 472
*Handstand and Half Handstand* ... 475
*Headless Headstands* ... 481
*Candlestick Shoulderstand and Supported Lifted Bridge* ... 489

## CHAPTER 15: RESTING AND RESTORATIVE SHAPES ... 493

### Benefits of Restorative Practices ... 493
*Cautions and Contraindications* ... 494
### Anatomical, Energetic, and Psychological Foci for Restorative Practices ... 495
### Tips for Cueing for Restoratives ... 496
*Cueing Tips for Grounding, Expansion, and Stability* ... 497
### Images of Resting and Restorative Shapes ... 498
*Restorative Seats* ... 498
*Restorative Forward Folds* ... 499

| | |
|---|---|
| *Restorative Twists* | *500* |
| *Restorative Backbends* | *500* |
| *Restorative Inversions* | *501* |
| CORPSE OR SAVASANA | *502* |
| *Key Teaching Invitations* | *502* |
| *Savasana Positioning Options* | *503* |
| *Instructions for Settling into the Ritual that is Savasana* | *505* |//

**CLOSING COMMENTS** ............................................................................................. **509**
**BIBLIOGRAPHY AND CITATIONS** ...................................................................... **511**
**INDEX** ............................................................................................................................. **517**

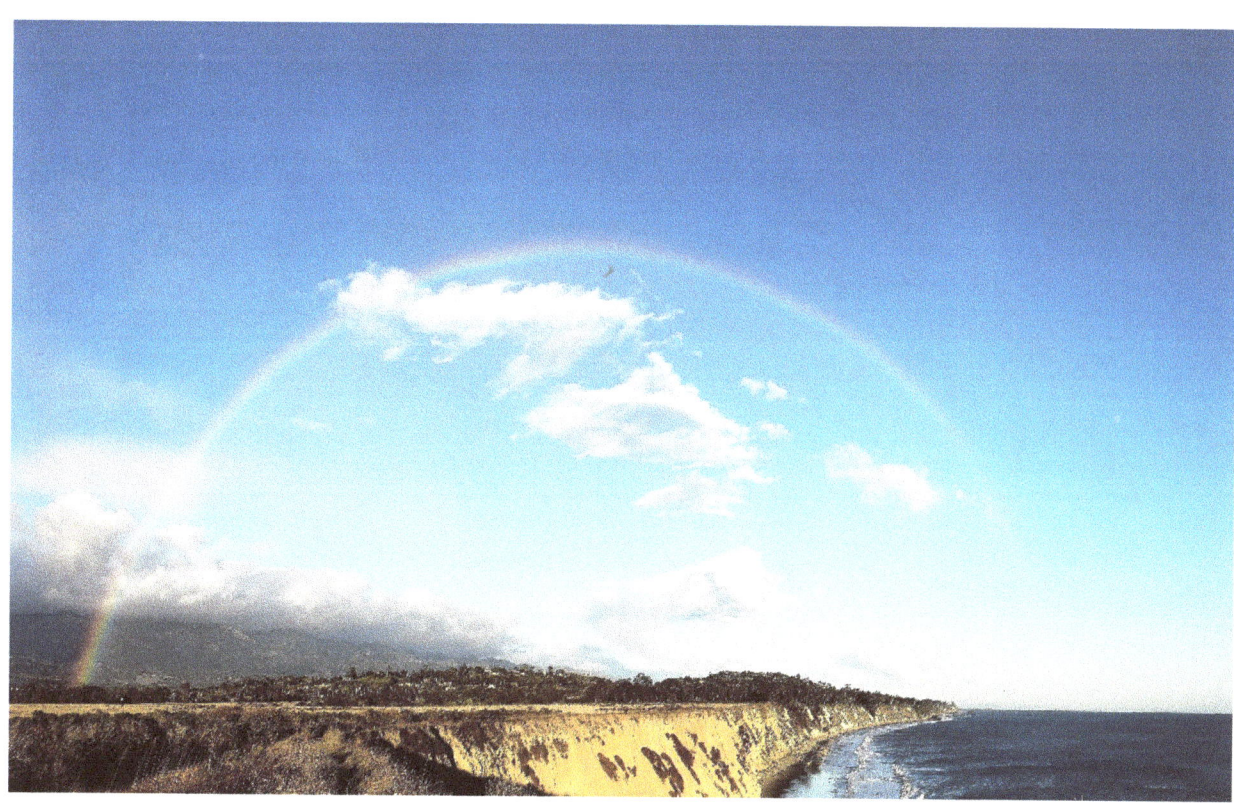

# Section 1:

# Integrated Holistic Yoga Anatomy and Physiology

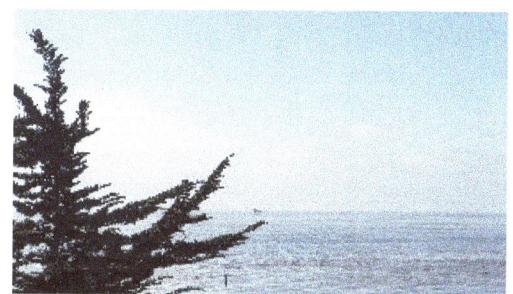

# Section 1 Introduction

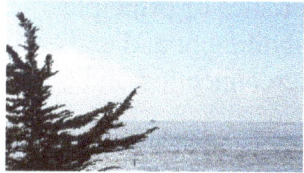

## Yoga Anatomy and Physiology Overview

The definition of integrated holistic yoga anatomy and movement used in this volume is based in the same integrated holistic yoga lineage and principles defined in *Integrated Holistic Yoga Psychology*, Volume 1 in the 3-part series. From this perspective, all yogic interventions and practices address the integration of all limbs of yoga and the wholism of all human layers of experience. All interventions and practices are offered with an emphasis on accessibility, intentionality, and beneficence. All work and interventions related to movement, anatomy, kinesiology, and physiology (including yoga *asana* and *pranayama*, as well as other healthful physical lifestyle practices) honor all layers of human experience and emphasize diverse and integrated approaches to the use of movement-oriented strategies and tools. Each human being is understood in a greater context that helped shape their experience, development, and growth. This context is complex in nature, being reflective of the biopsychosociocultural influences in play in each human being's development of self; experiences within their family, community, and world; experiences in relationships and interpersonal encounters of all types; and aspirations about their own contributions to the greater web of life.

> Integrated Holistic Yoga – A Definition and Commitment
>
> - *A practice of integration* – embracing the eight traditional practices (limbs) of yoga, for ways to glean a deeper understanding of our students or clients, interweaving of science and soul, and interdependence and coregulation
>
> - *A practice of wholeness* – addressing the layered experiences of consciousness, biopsychosociocultural context, interconnection, and community in all their complexity
>
> - *A practice of intentionality* – promising to make the world a better place; living with intention; committing to basic ethical values and practices
>
> - *A practice for accessibility* – creating affiliation, solidarity, and belonging; promoting social justice, engaged action, and personal as well collective empowerment
>
> - *A practice of beneficence* – creating access to the health and mental health benefits of yoga via several mechanisms of change; pledging first to do no harm

Given the commitment to integration, wholism, intentionality, accessibility, and beneficence, integrated holistic anatomy and movement (including yoga *asana*) are defined for purposes of this volume by the following characteristics or principles:
- Movement always arises from embodiment and embeddedness
- Movement reflects our human interconnection and interdependence within our layers of experience and our relationships
- Understanding movement means honoring each human being's biopsychosociocultural context
- Guiding movement requires attunement to each human being's
  - bioindividuality (*annamaya kosha*)
  - vital and affective individuality (*pranamaya kosha*)
  - mental and emotional individuality (*manomaya kosha*)
  - relational and intuitive individuality (*vijnanamaya kosha*)

With this integrated holistic understanding as the backdrop, Section 1 of this volume focuses on human physiology and anatomy with the intention of helping yoga professionals develop a sufficiently detailed and complex understanding of the body and its embeddedness in vitality, mind, community, and relationship to offer movement practices that deeply honor each student's or client's physical, vital, mental, emotional, behavioral, and relational reality. As such, Section 1 of *Integrated Holistic Yoga Movement* sets out to identify and successfully apply to yoga the main anatomical structures of the body, including gaining facility with identifying and defining ligaments, tendons, fascia, and other connective tissue; muscles (types, movement principles, muscle actions, major groups, cautions and effects); bones (axial and appendicular skeleton, quality and features, functions, cautions and effects), and joints (types, actions, major joints, cautions and effects). This section emphasizes familiarity with and use of anatomical terminology to identify planes of movement, types and directions of movement, and anatomical language for location and direction of body parts. Implications for applying this language in the context of teaching yogic movement, whether in yoga classes or in therapeutic yoga applications in clinical practice, are discussed to facilitate accuracy in cueing for students and clients as well as in communications with other healthcare providers involved in their care.

Using proper anatomical language, yoga professionals and practitioners are invited to explore and apply practically the kinesiology that supports healthful movement, optimal alignment, and safe transitions into and out of yoga shapes, with focus on general applications and principles rather than specific alignment rules for identified yoga postures (this will be covered in Section 2). Section 1 emphasizes critical thinking about how to teach *asana* and other yoga-based mindful movement safely based on anatomical and kinesiological knowledge and principles, rather than based on rote memorization of alignment instructions. Yoga professionals learn to define, explain, and apply principles of coordinated movement with emphasis on understanding physiology, anatomy, and kinesiology of each individual student in a yoga class or client during therapeutic yoga services, acknowledging and working with the reality that all bodies are different, biological unique, and diverse in need. Collaboration with other healthcare providers is stressed to ensure that yoga professionals understand the specifics of each student or client and create a healthful and optimal yoga practice for everyone they serve.

## Anatomy and Physiology Learning Objectives

1. Identify and use in teaching anatomical terminology, including
   a. planes of movement
   b. types and directions of movement
   c. anatomical language for location and direction of body parts

2. Understand and be able to identify the major systems and organs or glands of human physiology and their intersection with yoga practices, including effects, cautions, and contraindications
   a. circulatory system; effect on heart rate, flow of blood and lymph
   b. digestive system; mindful eating, effects of twisting
   c. endocrine system; homeostasis and allostasis
   d. excretory system; removal of toxins
   e. immune system; enhanced immunity and lymph flow
   f. muscular system; strength, flexibility, tone
   g. nervous system; resilience, emotional balance, behavioral regulation
   h. respiratory system; lung capacity, breath control, endurance
   i. skeletal system; bone mass, joint health, ligament and tendon resilience

3. Understand, identify, and successfully apply to yoga the main anatomical structures of the body, including facility with demonstrating and defining
   a. ligaments, tendons, fascia, and other connective tissue
   b. muscles (types, movement principles, action, major groups, cautions and effects)
   c. bones (axial and appendicular skeleton, quality and features, functions, cautions and effects)
   d. joints (types, actions, major joints, cautions and effects)

4. Understand and apply to yoga movement practice the various sections of the body, including being able to define, describe, and apply anatomy (muscles, bones, and connective tissues) and kinesiology principles associated with the:
   a. head region of the body
   b. axial region of the body
   c. lower appendicular region of the body
   d. Upper appendicular region of the body

5. Understand and apply to yoga movement practice the basic principles of kinesiology, including being able to define, describe, and apply
   a. coordinated movement
   b. reflexes
   c. reciprocal muscle inhibition and proprioceptive neuromuscular facilitation
   d. contraindications, recognize misalignments and offer commensurate variations/adaptations

## Anatomy and Physiology Recommended Readings

Biel, A., & Dorn, R. (2019). *Trail guide to the body: A hands-on guide to locating muscles, bones, and more* (6th ed.). Books of Discovery.
Clark, B. (2016). *Your body, your yoga*. Wild Strawberry Productions.
Clark, B. (2018). *Your spine, your yoga: Developing stability and mobility for your spine*. Wild Strawberry Productions.
Coulter, D. (2001). *Anatomy of Hatha yoga*. Body and Breath.
Lasater, J. H. (2020). *Yoga myths*. Shambhala.
Lasater, J. H. (2009). *Yogabody: Anatomy, kinesiology, and asana*. Rodmell.
Myers, T. W. (2022). *Anatomy trains* (4th ed.). Elsevier.
Rountree, S. (2020). *The professional yoga teacher's handbook*. Bloomsbury.

> *"A recognized fact which goes back to the earliest times is that every living organism is not the sum of a multitude of unitary processes but is - by virtue of interrelationships and of higher and lower levels of control - an unbroken unity."*
>
> *Walter Hess*
> Nobel Prize Winner for Work on the Brain, 1949

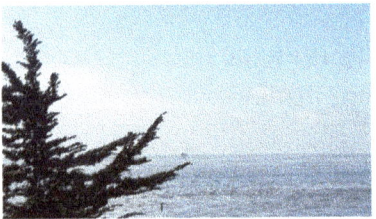

# Chapter 1: Key Concepts of Integrated Holistic Movement

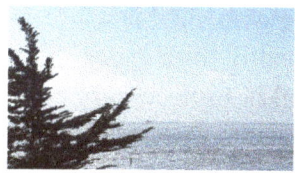

Movement is a basic need that is different from physical activity or exercise – though these are often conflated. Movement refers to all motion in the body. It is not exercise; it is not a privilege; it is not something we should need to 'make time for'; it is a human right essential to health and wellness and needs to be varied and frequent (Stults-Kolehmainen, 2023). Humans are wired to move – movement connects us to one another; movement is essential to healthy development.

In fact, movement has been essential to human evolution and is linked directly to the development of the complexity of the human brain (Scaer, 2012). Even infants, or perhaps especially infants, create connection and attunement through movement. Even before they can exert conscious control over movement, infants' reflexes are such that they actively engage interaction with adults. They can mimic facial expressions and reach out. Movement and its connection to cognitive, emotional, and social growth and development cannot be overstated and has been well-documented (Brems & Rasmussen, 2019; Haidt, 2024; Scaer, 2012). These aspects of movement as connections and a means of learning and growing for children (Nery et al., 2023) remain active throughout the lifespan (McGonigal, 2019). Movement remains an essential aspect of quality of life for seniors, who live healthier lives if they maintain an active lifestyle that allows then to remain physically strong and flexible, as well as emotionally and socially connected. One only needs to look at the lifestyles in the so-called Blue Zones to see the impact of movement on health and wellbeing (Buettner, 2023).

## Understanding the Essential Nature of Movement

As a society, we are in a state of movement deprivation having fallen prey to technologies that supposedly save us time, but really only save us movement (Bowman, 2017). In fact, the evolution of time-saving technologies can be linked directly to the development of inactivity (Woessner et al., 2021). Modern life and the ubiquitous access to electronic devices and enticing solitary activities, such as gaming and social media, has created a state of movement deprivation, especially for children and adolescents (Haidt, 2024; Stults-Kolehmainen, 2023) . It is almost as though we have collectively gone on a movement fast. Sedentary lifestyles have become the default in our society and Western culture where many factors exist that are linked to lack of movement (Beltrán-Carrillo et al., 2022; Martins et al., 2021). Whole aspects of our lives are set up to save us time when they really are simply saving us movement – not a great idea.
- We slump over our devices
- We drive everywhere
- We buy chopped vegetables
- We sit on soft furniture
- We wear shoes
- We pave our walkways

- We control the temperature in our environment
- We avoid stairs
- We park as close as possible to the gym
- We prefer interactions in virtual reality to engagement with others in reality
- We perceive movement as optional or unnecessary
- We do not have access to environments that encourage or even allow movement
- We want to save time and, in the process, reduce activity level

Our ecologies and neighborhoods are set up in such a way that they discourage movement and any movement that remains is often repetitive and unbalanced. Bringing movement back in the form of going to the gym is not an optimal solution. Instead, movement needs to become a human default again (Bantham et al., 2021); it needs to be an integral way of being in the world. Exercise tends to be repetitive, specific, and targeted rather than varied, non-local, and open-ended. As such, it – unlike natural movement – can create pattern locks that may result in vigor in portions of our physical body, while other aspects of our body are literally sedentary and movement deprived. It is as though we are putting parts of our bodies in a cast and allowing them to atrophy while we challenge other parts of our bodies to move and become strong. Thus, exercise can result in movements that carve patterns and ruts (in Sanskrit, *samskaras*) into our anatomy and physiology, creating overuse or repetitive stress injuries (Bell et al., 2018; Sun et al., 2024).

We need to reconceptualize movement as something that activates and energizes the entirety of our body, vitality, mind and emotions (Ratey, 2008, 2014). This is an important consideration as we are teaching *asana*, other yoga-based movement, and even *pranayama*. We need to make sure that our movement practices are integrated and holistic; that they help us move all our parts and that they reverberate into all of our layers of experience, or *koshas*. Yoga *asana* taught integratedly and holistically teaches us how to take movement off the mat and into daily life in a functional matter. It is not enough to move on a yoga mat; we also need to move in integrated and holistic ways when we are sitting, standing, walking, and lying down in day-to-day life. We need to reclaim movement in our daily routines, moving away from strategies that extinguish movement and toward ways of being in our lives that integrate movement as the nourishment that it is for all of our layers of experience.

## *Benefits of Integrated Holistic Movement*

Evolutionarily, movement contributed to the development of our brains (Lieberman, 2021; Mitchell, 2019). It is wired into our dopamine system and is joyful and rewarding in and of itself (McGonigal, 2019). Movement releases endorphins (which can facilitate a state of euphoria or joy), endocannabinoids (which help us feel connected to others as well as compassionate and engaged), and oxytocin (which supports depth of relationships and lovingkindness). These are important hormones for human survival and have clear evolutionary purposes. As hunters and gatherers, we had to move to eat and support ourselves and our communities. Our physiology had to evolve in such a way that movement in and of itself was rewarding enough to be sustained; it then had to result in nervous system states of ventral vagal connection so that we were literally and figuratively moved to share the results of our hunting and gathering with our communities.

Movement of skeletal muscles is healing for a variety of scientifically well-documented reasons. Movement (especially during muscular contraction) results in the release of myokines – hormones and proteins that reduce inflammation and enhance immunity (Bičíková et al., 2021; Gustafson et al., 2021), positively affect mood and mental health (Schuch et al., 2018, 2019), enhance emotional regulation (Chekroud et al., 2018; van Geest et al., 2021), enhance learning and memory (Singh et al., 2025), and increase energy and vitality (Rodrigues et al., 2022). In other words, through movement and the resultant contraction of our skeletal muscles, we communicate positively with all our tissues, including our organs and brains. Through myokine actions, we heal, repair, restore, invigorate, create joy, move into connection with one another, and make meaning. Through ongoing movement throughout our lifespan, we promote healthful aging (Bowman, 2018). Such movement is not about exercise. It is truly about optimizing how often, how much, how strongly, how persistently, how complexly, and how variedly we moved our bodies in every moment.

Movement is profoundly linked to mind and vitality (Rodrigues et al., 2022; Rozanski, 2023; Schuch et al., 2018, 2019). Specifically, movements, instincts, and sensory perceptions are deeply intertwined with arousal, emotional regulation, and mental processes to help us adapt, survive, and thrive in complex environments. There is a reciprocal relationship between these layers of experience that highlights the importance of embodied intelligence in shaping human experience and decision-making and vice versa. Mind and mindset can affect how we move; in turn, how we move can change our mind, emotions, and heart. Physical action, movement, and embodied experience are integral to how humans think, learn, and make decisions (Grafton, 2020).

Thus, in the integrated holistic paradigm, we think of wholesome movement as movement that:
- Supports overall health, wellness, and resilience – immune, digestive, cardiovascular, pulmonary, hormonal and tissue health
- Promotes physical health and fitness – strength, balance, mobility, stability, coordination (not just for expending calories)
- Is key to functional capacity and daily living skills – sitting, squatting, walking, lifting, carrying, cleaning
- Enhances good posture and endurance
- Integrates safety without suggesting fragility
- Invites connection and community
- Contributes to the experience of joy and exhilaration

### *The Miracle of Coordinated Movement*

Movement (including holding our day-to-day-posture) is the coordinated dance of muscles, connective tissue, epithelial tissues, nervous system control, and gravity with effects all the way down to our DNA. Muscles, bones and other connective tissues, and epithelial tissues interact in miraculously coordinated ways to support life and movement. This happens via nervous system control and always in the context of the force of gravity. It also happens in collaboration with all *koshas* – always involving breathing, thought, affect and emotion, relationship and community. In other words, movement is not simply about muscles despite the fact that in yoga *asana*, muscles are mentioned most often in cueing; it is not even simply about the physical body.

Movement engages us physically, mentally, emotionally, behaviorally, and relationally. Movement is about joy and connection – about engaging our ventral vagal nervous system response and about reclaiming our health. Movement engages us with our life, connecting us to all our *koshas* in their ever-widening layers. Movement connects us to community, to our interdependence, and to our co-arising and co-creating humanity. It has the power to create profound changes in the way we are in the world – in our bodies, vitality, thoughts, emotions, actions, relationships, and communities. It is no surprise that research has revealed yoga *asana's* profound impact on practitioners' health and wellbeing beyond the physical, including enhanced (self-)compassion and sense of connection (Kishida et al., 2018, 2019). Yoga as an integrated practice can become even more meaningful if teachers and other yoga services providers recognize the strong embeddedness of the yoga-based (and other) movement practices in all other limbs of yoga, in all *koshas*, and in the overall biopsychosociocultural context.

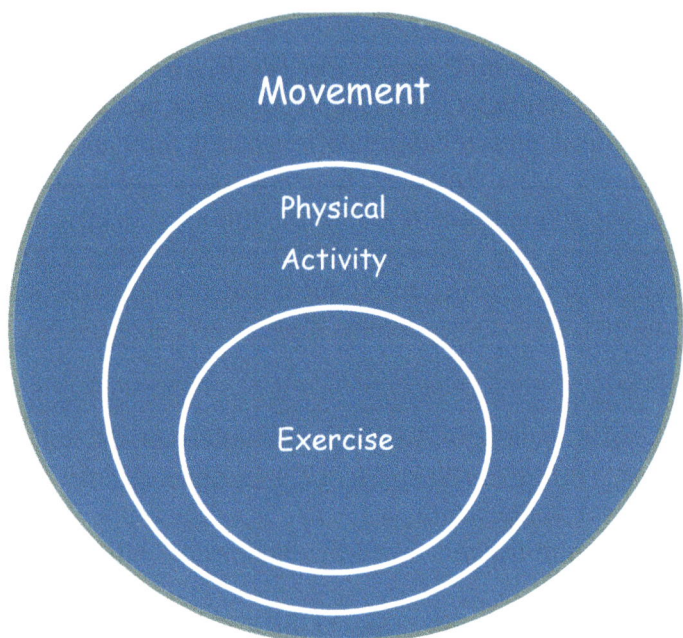

All movement happens in the context of our biopsychosociocultural background. Movement and attitudes about movement are heavily influenced by various personal and environmental factors (beyond muscles, gravity, connective tissue, and nervous system control in the sense of sensory and motor signals). They are influenced by (likely among many other factors) our context, developmental history, cultural beliefs, lifetime of movement-related experiences, and access to movement from a sociopolitical and sociocultural perspective (such as access to spaces that invite movement; (Ball et al., 2015; Kegler et al., 2022). Movement reflects our biopsychosociocultural individuality and embeddedness.

### *Biopsychosociocultural Individuality*

A key consideration in learning and applying anatomy and physiology (i.e., the sciences of movement and living), is the understanding that there are large individual variations in how anatomy and physiology are expressed and how movement and physical activity, including yoga *asana*, are embraced (Clark, 2016, 2018; Myers, 2022; Porter, 2013). In other words, how people perceive and engage with movement of all types is affected by many highly individual and collective factors that may challenge them to engage in movement, to work at their own edges of comfort in with regard to movements and physical activity, and how open they are to trying new ways to move and engage with their vitality. Biology, psychology, social context, and cultural values are key elements that need to be considered as movement practices are offered. A brief discussion is offered for each of these dimensions to raise awareness about the many barriers and facilitators that may be present in people's lives and that help explain their perceptions and level of engagement with physical activity, movement, and yoga *asana* practices.

*Biological Factors of Uniqueness*

We are enormously bioindividual, unfathomably unique. This makes understanding anatomy and physiology a central key to teaching yoga *asana* well – we cannot teach to the average body; we cannot just teach *Norm* or *Norma*. We must teach the bodies in front of us. That means alignment cues have to be tempered with bioindividuality cues, with the acknowledgment that each shape and movement needs to be created and perceived from the inside out, not formed from the outside in - with keen attention to individual edges and boundaries (White, 2007).

Anatomical charts and models show average bodies; we do not exist that way in nature. Each human being has *different bones, different joints, different structures* (Clark, 2016, 2018). Just as we differ in blood pressure, weight, height, skin tone, age, backgrounds, culture, education, we differ in bone shapes, joint cavity depth, location of body structures, angles of bony protrusions, and so much more. Many *physiological variables* have to be factored in when we ask people to move. Blood pressure, blood sugar, digestive symptoms, bone health, and hormonal states are just a few examples that can alter how we move and function. Following are additional examples of possible influences and considerations that can affect how and what we offer during yoga *asana* practice.

- We may be tighter or more flexible depending on hormones (Clark, 2016, 2018; Coulter, 2001). Some examples include:
  - estrogen (e.g., higher estrogen levels have been associated with increased flexibility, even laxity in ligaments; lower estrogen levels may be related to less muscle mass and bone loss; this has implications for aging)
  - relaxin (e.g., relaxes all ligaments in the pelvis, maybe throughout the body; this can lead to injury from overstretching)
  - other hormonal effects of the menstrual cycle on thermoregulation, water retention, energy, etc.
- We may get light-headed from postural orthostatic tachycardia syndrome, or orthostatic hypotension. We may not safely go upside down because of high blood pressure, glaucoma, or vitreous detachment.
- Blood sugar levels may affect physical capacity and even concentration.
- Bone health may affect necessary load distribution (e.g., creating the need for providing more padding under the back for individuals with osteoporosis).
- Level of hydration (overly hydrated or poorly hydrated) affects flexibility or mobility (Clark, 2016, 2018). For example:
  - lack of water in the extracellular matrix causes stiffness; this can be due to lack of adequate fluid intake or due to lack of movement; lack of movement reduces hyaluronic

acid in the extracellular matrix which, in turn, reduces hydration in our tissues; aging results in fewer fibroblasts in our tissues – as these are the water-loving proteins in our body, fewer of them means less hydration
    - dehydrated tissue is more prone to trapping toxins and metabolic waste products, as well as bacteria
    - too much water in our tissues reduces mobility as well; too much hydration can happen due to inflammation or certain hormones
- *Acute or chronic injuries* can influence what is or is not possible for an individual and may necessitate props and creativity to make the physical practice accessible (Bydon, 2021; Coulter, 2001; Krentzman, 2016). Specifically, inflammation (and hence swelling) post-injury or post-stress (including emotional or psychological stress) can result in decreased mobility, especially in the fascia (via the myofibroblasts in the fascia contracting).
- *Sleep and restedness* – chronic or acute disturbances – can affect how we move and how our energy can be used (Walker, 2018). Relatedly, time of day for the practice can make a big difference with regard to energy level and what type of practice may be most auspicious.
- *Nutritional patterns* and status can affect how well we can function physically, related to movement, energy, and stamina (e.g., 81-year-old client who suddenly started feeling weak during practice; could have mistaken this for "normal aging" – turns out she failed to eat breakfast prior to session; once she took time to eat and we pushed our time back a bit, she was fine again; this was a general huge lesson to her).
- *Nervous system regulation and polyvagal state* (*gunas, samskaras*) or our state of exhaustion or fatigue versus alertness or energy level affect the practice and may strongly affect physical (and psychological) needs (Brems, 2024b; Schwartz, 2024).

Check out this video for more about the anatomy of the individual as opposed to the anatomy of the textbook: *"Picture or Person? Learn Integral Anatomy with Gil Hedley"* on YouTube – https://youtu.be/qr4dqWLeSWc

*Psychological Factors of Uniqueness*

Emotional and mental factors can profoundly affect how students or clients show up on the mat and how they approach *asana* and the other limbs of yoga. Just as there are idiosyncratic anatomical and physiological factors that affect the shapes we can invite clients to embody or the movements in which we can invite them to engage, there are a plethora of psychological issues that can set boundaries and edges around what is possible or auspicious emotionally and mentally. The *how* and *what* of the practice can be affected by many factors that need to be attended to, including but not limited to:

- *Affective and arousal state* – Polyvagal states or *gunas* have a great influence on the types of movements we crave, need, or avoid.
- *Emotional influences* – Experience and context of trauma, patterns of fear (e.g., elders terrified of balancing postures; anyone afraid of going upside down), and emotional predilections (e.g., *kleshas*) can limit movement choices and predispose us to certain movement preferences or aversions; even ego plays a large role, leading us to make movement choices informed by expectations rather than discernment.
- *Mental influences* – Mental habits, prior practice patterns, beliefs, attitudes, and stories about movement can influence how we do or do not choose to move. Coping styles and resilience

(including *vrittis* and *samskaras*) can keep us locked in movement and activity patterns and styles that may have been useful at one point in life, but no longer serve.
- *Cognitive capacity* – Access to jargon, intelligence, educational level, and language skills can become barriers or facilitators for seeking out physical activity and movement as they may enhance or limit our capacity to understand how movement can help and how it may hinder.

## Social and Socioeconomic Factors of Uniqueness

Many social and sociopolitical factors are present in people's lives that affect their relationship with their bodies and with movement. Current social and socioeconomic circumstances often limit access to healthful movement. A few examples include:
- *Use of modern conveniences*: Our environment has evolved such that is no longer encourages and supports spontaneous movement. In fact, if anything, it discourages movement and supports inactivity and passivity. Elevators have replaced stairs; kitchen gadgets have replaced hand-driven food preparation; cars have replaced legs and bikes. Movement has become equated with exercise and often exercise is dreaded as yet another burden of modern life. We would be better off losing some of our modern conveniences and skipping the gym (Bowman, 2017).
- *Quality of environments of care*: Types of yoga spaces available, availability of props, cost of the practice, insurance reimbursement options, and interaction or coordination of care with other care providers can create barriers to accessing movement and physical activity, including yoga (Brems et al., 2015).
- *Environmental factors*, such as temperature, climate, altitude of our location, and terrain can have profound effects on motivation to move (McKeown, 2015).
- *Quality of air and noise levels:* Modern life has created many restrictions on access to safe and enjoyable outdoor spaces, especially for urban livers, that would support movement and physical activity. Noise levels, pollution, and temperatures in spaces where movement, including yoga, might occur can hinder or facilitate desire to move and practice.
- *Neighborhood safety and crime:* Lack of access to outdoor life in neighborhoods that invite movement in safe and welcoming environments (e.g., can a person of color go jogging in safety in a neighborhood?) get in the way of movement as a matter of course. Even perceptions of lack of safety or emotional and physical accessibility of movement or yoga spaces can prevent people from seeking out such helpful practices and activities (Bondy, 2020; Johnson, 2021)

## Cultural Factors of Uniqueness

Cultural and familial factors may influence how students relate to movement and physical activity, both positively and negatively, via any number of cultural beliefs or attitudes, including but not limited to:
- *Stereotypes about yoga:* Yoga is only for the select few (e.g., "guys don't do yoga…"; only flexible people can do yoga, etc.) – who, what, how, why, when (Heyman, 2019, 2021; Justice et al., 2016; Razmjou et al., 2017; Sulenes et al., 2015; Vladagina et al., 2016).
- *Stereotypes about exercise in general:* If movement is framed as exercise and exercise is just another burden of modern life, then motivation may be low; yet, exercise is only one small aspect of physical activity, which in turn is only one aspect of movement (Bowman, 2017).

- *Attitudes about movement and physicality:* Family and cultural values may affect attitudes about the meaning and value of physical activity, exercise, and movement.
- *Attitudes about psychological and physical intervention for health and mental health concerns:* Family and cultural values may affect attitudes about the meaning and value of meditation, breath and energy work, guided imagery, and other emotional or psychological interventions that are part of yoga.
- *Attitudes about spirituality:* Misperceptions of yoga as a religion that may be incompatible with personal religious or spiritual beliefs.

> *Movement is the key to health.*
>
> *Immobility and sedentary lifestyles are like junk food for the human anatomy:*
> *they impair the ability to stay mobile and healthy.*
>
> *Who we are and our biopsychosociocultural contexts affect how we move and load:*
>
> *Biopsychosociocultural individuality*

## *Physical Resilience and Adaptability Through Movement*

The capacity to thrive under challenge is a fundamental characteristic of all human tissue. Fundamental to the body's resilience and function is movement, including yoga *asana*. In fact, movement is not optional and needs to be as varied as possible. Movement expresses the profound interconnection of all physical structures and systems in the body, as well as their linkage to all other layers of experience. In the current context, our attention is on the creation of physical resilience. Physical resilience and antifragility (i.e., not just rebounding from challenge, but thriving from challenge) always are understood in the context of interconnection and interdependence (Taleb, 2019).

We can consider a large array of movement dynamics that can create variety and complexity. The more dimensions we consider, the more we realize the incredible variation we can create via movement, thus bringing more joy, resilience, and health to our existence (individually and collectively). A few movement factors yoga professionals can consider as they develop yoga *asana* sequences and interventions include, but are not limited to the following:

- *Frequency*, including regularity and quantity
- *Distribution* (i.e., across the whole body or local)
- *Temperature* (e.g., move rather than turning up the heat in our homes)
- *Geography* (e.g., what shapes do we take on; in which planes of movement do we move; how do we move the different body parts)
- *Quality* and type
- Interactions with the *environment* (e.g., barefoot versus shoes; looking only up closely or in the distance)
- *Pressure* (i.e., how and where do we load our various body parts)

- *Posture* (e.g., how do lifestyle contribute to posture; how do actions, especially those that reflect *samskaras*, affect posture)

Human tissues and cellular health in all organ systems (cardiovascular, digestive, immune, etc.) are entirely dependent on optimal movement and stress (or challenge) to stay healthy, maintain resilience, and thrive (Mitchell, 2019). Optimal challenge to tissues via physical activity and movement can be seen as an application of Yerkes-Dodson's law of optimal performance, which posits that optimal levels of physiological, mental, emotional, or cognitive arousal and stress are needed for best possible performance. This law reminds us that we need some amount of physical stress to thrive in our bodies – too little is as harmful as too much. That is, we need just the right amount of challenge to build resilience and resourcefulness:

- *Too little stress* does not challenge us to perform at our best and, in terms of human tissues, can lead to atrophy:
  - human jaws are atrophying because we chew less than we used to
  - myopia is rampant because all the indoor time places less stress on eyes to adjust from near vision to far vision
  - always wearing shoes with high arches leads to weakening of the natural arches for the feet
  - sedentariness leads to cardiovascular inefficiencies
  - too much rest after injury results in poor healing with too much tissue atrophy
- *Too much stress* overtaxes our physical (or emotional, mental, and behavioral) resources and can lead to deteriorating performance or, in terms of tissues, to injury and degeneration:
  - sudden excessive overload may lead to tears in ligaments or tendons
  - repetitive stress from computer work may lead to carpal tunnel syndrome
  - habitual asymmetrical activities may lead to muscular, even bone density or structural imbalance
  - habitual body postures may reshape bones and fascia (e.g., tech-neck)
- *Optimal stress* leads to physical resilience, tissue health, and tissue recovery (including post-injury) at a minimum. Ideally, it even leads to antifragility, allowing tissue to emerge from stress stronger and healthier than before:
  - occasional fasting (creating the stress called hunger) leads to enhanced autophagy
  - being exposed to germs and other immune challenges leads to better immune functioning
  - working at the edge of physical strength enhances muscular strength
  - weight-bearing increases bone density
  - endurance activities increase resilience and cardiovascular health

The optimal physical stress window may be vastly different from person to person based on life and childhood experiences (Badenoch, 2018; Dana, 2018; Levine, 1997) and may vary within individuals based on a variety of present-moment factors, such as hormonal levels, injury, biorhythms, and more (Clark, 2016, 2018). As yoga professionals, we need to help people cultivate sufficient interoception and awareness to monitor their own optimal stress window, knowing when sensation turns to pain and when and how to work at their edge with awareness (Coulter, 2001; Schwartz, 2024). Once individuals have sufficient awareness, they can be encouraged to work at the edge of their physical, emotional, mental, and psychological resilience to invite ongoing growth, evolution, and change.

Working at the edge means paying attention to physical, energetic, mental, and emotional sensation. For example:
- Physical sensation that is dull can help build resilience
- Physical sensation that is sharp or burning signals pain and may be outside the window of tolerance
- Energetic challenge may signal the need for ease or relinquishment of over-effort
- Confusion may suggest the need for greater concentration or more accessible guidance from the teacher
- Emotional hesitation may signal the need to stop or may signal an opportunity to grow

Creating varied loads and stress is essential to physical health overall. It creates *antifragility* – the capacity not just to recover but to *thrive* and improve as a result of being exposed to circumstances that result in stress, emerging strengthened and more resilient. This may apply not only physically, but also emotionally and cognitively. Antifragility points to the reality that we are not subject to wear-and-tear (as are machines), but instead are evolved for "wear-and-repair" (Clark, 2016). Optimal loading of and resultant stress on tissue makes it stronger and denser; optimal stress creates enhanced performance (as long as there is rest and recovery), and resistance work can prevent or delay the onset of cognitive decline (Cavalcante et al., 2023). Physical (and likely emotional and psychological) antifragility or thriving can arise from many factors, including but not necessarily limited to (Mitchell, 2019):
- Use (including loading and movement)
- Mechanical stresses such as force and load (other than gravity; e.g., exercise)
- Posture
- Gravity
- Temperature (higher temperatures make it more pliable)
- Hormones in general (e.g., pregnancy via relaxin)

Tissue over time takes on the shape we assume most commonly – even bones can change shape (e.g., tech-neck, forward head, uneven wear); that is, form and function are intimately related. This fact (that form follows function) helps and hurts. Repetitive unhealthy patterns (*samskaras*) will show up in the form of pathology; healthful movement, on the other hand, becomes a prevention and treatment opportunity (Clark, 2016; Mitchell, 2019; Porter, 2013). Through healthful movement:
- Bone remodels – e.g., compression makes bone more resilient, not shorter
- Tensile tissue (ligaments, tendons, fascia, joint cartilage, aponeuroses) increases its capacity for tolerance – to strengthen them, engage in progressive overload (not just force or magnitude, but also rate and direction); load makes tissue more resilient, not longer

> *Most of our pain is due to a lack of a deeper truth.*
> *The opposite of pain is not pleasure, but clarity.*
> (Stephen Levine, 2002, Turning Toward the Mystery, p. 99)

Because of humans' resilience and capacity to make auspicious use of optimal stress, we need to transcend the notion of wear and tear and think instead of wear and repair:
- Tissue takes whatever shape it has because of the function it serves; tissues adapt to the loads placed on them.
- We can use this principle to train and strengthen the body via progressive overload and via tensile loading of various types.

Similarly, given human tissue adaptability, when injured, we might want to forget about RICE (Rest, Ice, Compress, Elevate). Instead, we may choose to TAME the fire of injury via **T**emperature (applying ice or heat as appropriate), **A**nalgesics (using means for dealing with pain and inflammation, such as meditation, breathing, aspirin, topical pain relievers, NSAIDs, etc.), **M**obilization, and **E**xercise. TAME uses healthy loading and gentle mobilization to heal injury. Beyond working with injury, healthy loading can restructure fascia, bone, and muscular architecture. There are several types of loading that happen in response to applied force:
- *Compressive loading* (compression) – squeezing or pushing the object together
- *Tensile loading* (tension) – stretch the object apart
- *Bending* – curving the object
- *Torsion* – twisting or rotating the object
- *Shear* – sliding surfaces parallel to each other

Thus, *movement = health* as the following examples might show (and as several examples above have already demonstrated):
- When skeletal muscle moves, the resultant compression squeezes arterioles in the muscle tissue, causing them to open and pulling blood into the working areas (muscle and associated connective tissue).
- Blood moving into the working areas brings with it more oxygen, fueling the cells and pushing out metabolic waste.
- Movement enhances circulation and thus nourishes and cleanses our tissues. Without movement, tissues can starve and store toxins. Varied movement is key to ensure that all skeletal muscles move; if movement is missing, cell and tissue health will suffer (e.g., flaccid fin syndrome in captive orcas).

> **Mechanotransduction**
> *"The process by which cells sense and then translate mechanical signals (compression, tension, fluid shear) created by their physical environment into biochemical signals, allowing cells to adjust their structure and function accordingly."*
> (Bowman, 2017)
>
> For example, stretching results in muscle growth; load or strain results in greater bone density; pressure or vibration results in perception of touch.

Lack of loading or unhealthy loading creates less fascial organization, resilience, and mobility. Conversely, healthful loading supports fascial organization, increases muscular strength and resilience, and supports bone density. Fascia, bones, and muscles organize along the lines of

loading and movement. That means if there is no movement, then there is no organization and less health. To reiterate, lack of movement (immobility), lack of loading, and non-optimal stress arising from poor diet, inflammation, trauma (e.g., accidents, overloading, overtraining), or lack of hydration interfere with the health of our tissues. Here are a couple of examples:
- No loading or lack of movement leads to no orientation in the fascia (as might occur in excessive rest after injury); this kind of fascia is like fuzz or felt and becomes increasingly immobile; these adhesions interfere with freedom of movement and contribute to unhealthy physical patterns
- Lack of movement (immobility), poor diet, inflammation, trauma (e.g., accidents, overloading, overtraining), and lack of hydration creates fuzzy, adhesive fascia that restricts mobility

## *Implications for Yoga Asana*

The upshot of human adaptability or antifragility and of human needs for optimal load and stress is this: Do not scare people away from yoga with fragility language – find a balance between giving cautions and contraindications versus creating fear or worry. Given our adaptability and antifragility as well as our needs for optimal movement, load, and stress, it is important to think about how we, as yoga professionals, talk about anatomy and physiology as related to yoga *asana* practice. We need to acknowledge risks without creating fragility; we need to talk about benefits without exaggerating. A few suggestions are as follows and are offered only as food for more thought and thoughtfulness.
- Do not scare people away from yoga with fragility language
- Find a balance between giving cautions and contraindications versus creating fear or worry
- Some common body patterns related to modern life deserve to be addressed, but do it as a way of addressing them proactively, not as a way of worrying or giving up
- Individually tailored cautions are legitimate
- Educate, do not frighten – create discerning self-agency and self-empowerment
- Embed cueing and demonstration in all layers of experience, attending to the physical, vital, emotional, mental, and cultural factors that are present

---

**Integrated Holistic Yoga Asana
is not about stretching or flexibility**

Within the student's *koshas* and biopsychosociocultural context,
integrated holistic yoga *asana* is about creating

stability & mobility
strength & endurance
balance & coordination
balance in arousal and vitality
management of energy budgets
emotional resilience & mental health
functional capacity & long-term health
and perhaps most of all – joy & connection

Although we will soon move on to the nitty-gritty of anatomy and physiology of movement, the hope is that the larger context continues to accompany the reader: movement principles are embedded in a greater whole; in a profoundly biological, psychological, social/socioeconomic, cultural, familial, and relational matrix. As yoga professionals, we need to know anatomy and physiology; however, we always remember that this not enough. We work with whole (or wholistic) beings and their development and continued evolution in an interpersonal matrix and biopsychosociocultural context. It is certainly important to know muscles, bones, and other anatomical structures individually; however, anatomy does not come alive until it is put into motion and until it is understood as a well-coordinated dance across all layers of experience. This dance is by its very definition and biology a joyful and beneficial endeavor. We will now move on to begin the exploration of our physical bodies – never forgetting they are embedded in all layers of experience and a complex biopsychosociocultural context.

## Understanding Anatomical Language and Associated Concepts

Before exploring anatomy and physiology, it is important to become familiar with movement-related language. To understand movement, a few anatomical definitions are in order. Following is an overview of *directions of movements*, *planes of movements*, and *anatomical directions*. As a preview, directions of movement refer to the general types of motion that occur at joints, describing how body parts move in space, such as bending, straightening, or rotating. Planes of movement refer to imaginary two-dimensional surfaces that divide the body and describe the direction in which movement occurs, such as forward-backward, side-to-side, or rotational. Anatomical directions are standardized terms used to describe the location of one body part relative to another, providing consistent spatial orientation regardless of body position. These concepts are completely intertwined and often one dimension is explained through language borrowed from another dimension. This reality makes organization of the material difficult. Here the choice is to start with defining *directions* of movement. There will be references to the other dimensions; thus, it will be helpful – for full understanding of the material – to read over all three sections and then to review them again. All three dimensions are important to understand for teaching yoga *asana* and to communicate with other professionals. Yoga professionals need familiarity with this language if they work with clients who are also receiving healthcare or mental healthcare and whose providers may want to give guidance to yoga clinicians about contraindications and helpful or contraindicated movements.

### *Directions of Body Movement*

Planes of movement and anatomical directions interact to define and categorize the directions of movement by describing how a body part moves relative to specific reference points or axes (Coulter, 2001). The discussion starts with a summary of the various directional movements of the body, showing how the planes and directions come together to create directional movements, such flexion, adduction, and others. For more information check out the *Trail Guide of the Human Body* (Biel & Dorn, 2019) or similar anatomical textbooks. Online resources abound as well. It may help to review the images in Figure 1.1 first and then to peruse the table that provides definitions and references to the primary planes of movement in which body movements occur.

| Direction | Definition | 1º Plane of Movement |
|---|---|---|
| *Flexion* | Reducing an angle at the joint; in joints that can move forward and backward, flexion is a movement that goes in the anterior direction in most cases (e.g., forward bend in neck or trunk) | Generally occurs in the sagittal plane |
| *Extension* | Straightening or increasing an angle at the joint; in joints that can move forward and backward, extension is a movement in the posterior direction in most cases (e.g., a backbend in the spine); hyperextension means straightening past 180º and is generally unhealthy for the joint | Generally occurs in the sagittal plane |
| *Adduction* | Bringing a body part across the midline (e.g., moving the right leg across the midline to bring the toes to the floor on the body's left side); bringing digits toward the centerline of the hand or foot | Generally occurs in the frontal plane |
| *Abduction* | Bringing a limb away from the midline (e.g., raising an arm out sideways); bringing digits away from the midline of the hand or foot | Generally occurs in the frontal plane |
| *Lateral flexion* | A side bending movement of the spine, leaning the torso to the right or to the left | Generally occurs in the frontal plane |
| *External Rotation* | Moving the bone along its long axis away from the midline or another anatomical reference point; also called lateral rotation | Generally occurs in the transverse plane |
| *Internal Rotation* | Moving the bone along its long axis toward the midline or another anatomical reference point; also called medial rotation | Generally occurs in the transverse plane |
| *Axial Rotation* | A twisting or rotational motion in the spine either to the right or to the left; axial rotation may occur in the spine overall or in specific sections along the length of the spine (e.g., cervical, thoracic) | Generally occurs in the transverse plane |
| *Supination* | Movements occurring in the elbow vis-à-vis the hands and in the ankle vis-à-vis the feet: turning the hand up (as if to carry a tray on it) or turning the sole of the foot up (e.g., in Butterfly when the feet are opened up; or a movement that happens suddenly from tripping and causes a sprained ankle); in the foot this is also called inversion | Generally occur in the transverse plane given the rotation away from the midline |
| *Pronation* | Movements occurring in the elbow vis-à-vis the hands and in the ankle vis-à-vis the feet: turning hands down (e.g., in Staff when hands are at the side, turned down to the floor) or turning the sole of the foot down (as in a foot with a collapsed inner arch); in the foot this is also called eversion | Generally occur in the transverse plane given the rotation toward the centerline |
| *Dorsiflexion* | Flexion at the ankle as the foot/toes moves closer to the tibia | Generally occurs in the sagittal plane |
| *Plantar flexion* | Pointing the toes; in essence, extension at the ankle as the angle between foot and shin increases; flexion of the plantar region of the foot as the angle between tarsals and phalanges decreases – hint: "plant" the foot | Generally occurs in the sagittal plane |

| Plantar extension | Flexing the toes of a pointed foot; this action stretches the plantar fascia (hence the reference to the plantar region of the foot) | Generally occurs in the sagittal plane |
|---|---|---|
| Circumduction | The combination of flexion, extension, abduction and adduction in a sequence in a ball-and socket joint (e.g., making a shoulder or hip circle) | Occurs in all planes of movement |

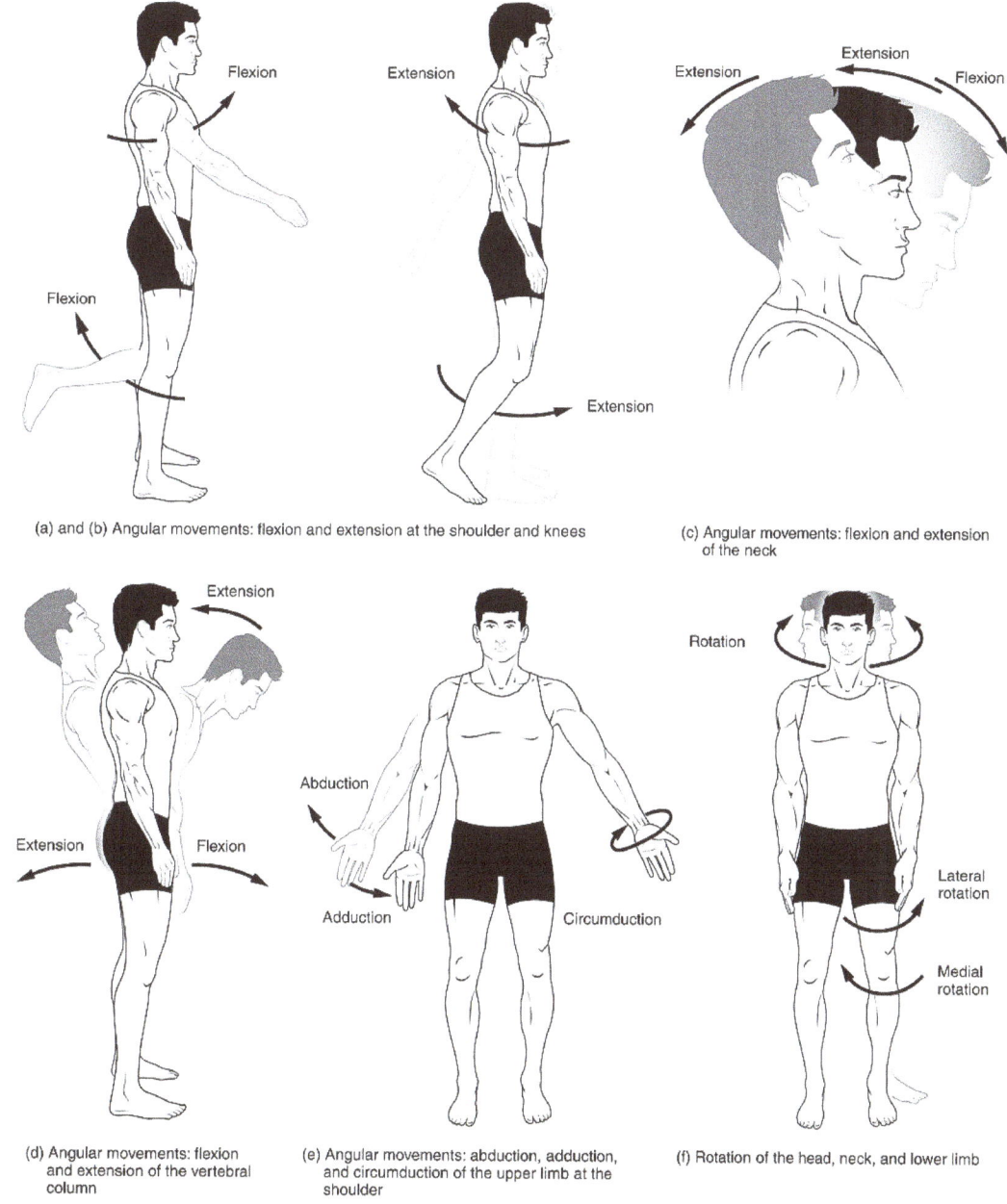

**Figure 1.1** Directions of body movements. (Data source: Tonye Ogele; https://en.m.wikipedia.org/wiki/File:Body_Movements_I.jpg; Creative Commons Attribution 3.0)

## Planes of Movement

Movement happens in particular orientations in space (Biel & Dorn, 2019), namely in two-dimensional planes called sagittal, frontal, and transverse. Why is knowing about planes of movement important for yoga professionals? Muscles contract more efficiently in the plane of movement in which they lie. Imagine the biceps in yoga pushups; bicep lie in and work most effectively in the sagittal plan. If the arms are held parallel to the body when in a pushup position, the biceps work well as they are in the sagittal plane. If the arms are out to the side (i.e., in abduction) during a pushup, they are now in the frontal plane, work less efficiently, and may be more prone to injury, especially among individuals who are perhaps somewhat deconditioned.

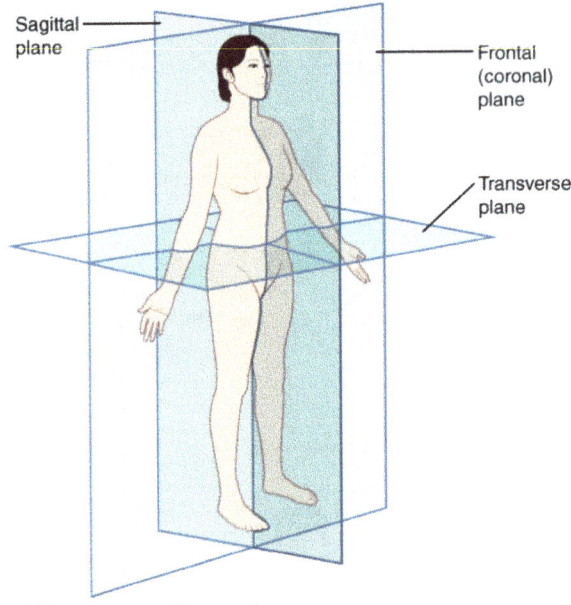

**Figure 1.2** Planes of movement. (Data source: Connexions; https://commons.wikimedia.org/wiki/File:Planes_of_Body.jpg; Creative Commons Attribution 3.0)

### Sagittal Plane

The sagittal plane is also known as the longitudinal (and the anteroposterior) plane. This plane of movement runs perpendicular to the ground and divides the body into its right side and left sides anywhere along the length of the body (facing the body from the front). The midsagittal or median plane, also known as the *midline* in yoga *asana*, runs exactly down the middle of the body dividing it into two equal (right and left) parts, passing through the navel and the spine (shown in Figure 1.2). Movement in the sagittal plane parallels the sagittal plane (i.e., is anterior and posterior movement). Thus, movements in the sagittal plane move a body part either forward or backward. Generally speaking, flexion and extension happen in this plane of movement.

### Frontal Plane

The frontal plane is also known as the coronal (or the mediolateral) plane. This plane of movement runs perpendicular to the ground and divides the body into front (anterior or ventral) and back (posterior or dorsal) portions when viewed from the side. The midfrontal or median coronal plane, also known as the *center line* in yoga *asana*, runs exactly down the middle of the body, dividing it into equal anterior and posterior halves, passing through the shoulders and hips (see Figure 1.2). Movement in the frontal plane parallels the frontal plane (i.e., is side-to-side movement). Movements in the frontal plane move a body part either outward or inward in the sagittal plane (e.g., arm moving out to the side or across the front or back of the body). Generally speaking, abduction, adduction, and lateral flexion or extension occur in this plane of movement.

## *Transverse Plane*

The transverse plane is also known as the horizontal (axial or transaxial) plane. This plane of movement runs parallel to the ground and divides the body into upper (superior) and lower (inferior) portions when viewed from above or below. The midtransverse or median horizontal plane runs exactly through the middle of the body, dividing it into superior and inferior halves, passing through the body near the navel and the lower ribs (shown in Figure 1.2). Movement in the transverse plane is rotational movement. This means movements in the transverse plane involve rotating a body part either toward or away from the midline of the body. Generally speaking, internal and external rotation, as well as axial rotation, occur in this plane of movement. Rotation can happen in the superior or inferior body as well as in the appendicular aspects of the body (e.g., rotation of an arm or leg).

## *Anatomical Directions*

To describe the location of one body part relative to another, providing consistent spatial orientation regardless of body position, it is important to know appropriate language for such anatomical directions. Yoga teachers and clinicians need to be facile with anatomical directional language to help them give clear, precise, and universally understood cues that support safety and alignment. This shared vocabulary minimizes ambiguity, especially in healthcare-based or other therapeutic settings; it enables yoga professionals to offer nuanced verbal adjustments, describe subtle positional changes, and guide clients through complex shapes more effectively. Additionally, facility with this language helps in communicating with other professionals (e.g., physiotherapists or bodyworkers), enhancing transdisciplinary understanding and care. Following are key terms to describe anatomical positioning; Figures 1.3 and 1.4 provide visual representations. This listing is likely not all-inclusive but offers definitions of the most commonly used terms in therapeutic yoga settings.
- *Midline* in the sagittal plane – runs from top of skull, between the eyes, sternum, naval, between the legs to the feet (aka median plane) to divide the body into a right and left half
- *Center line* in the frontal plane – line that runs from the top of the skull, opening of the ear, shoulder, hip, ankle; it can use a plumb line to visualize the midline from the side (aka coronal plane) to divide the body into an anterior and posterior half
- *Posterior* – refers to any position behind the center line of the frontal plane or another anatomical reference point (e.g., the hamstrings are posterior to the femur)
- *Anterior* – refers to any position forward of the frontal plane or another anatomical reference point (e.g., the quadriceps are anterior to the femur)
- *Lateral* – refers to distance from the center of the body; it means farther away outward from the midline as compared to another anatomical reference point (e.g., the trochanter is more lateral than the acetabulum)

- *Medial* – also refers to distance from the center of the body; it means closer in toward the midline as compared to another anatomical reference point (e.g., the big toe is more medial than the little toe)
- *Proximal* – indicates that something is closer in proximity to an anatomical landmark than another body part; refers to all structures of the body but is most commonly used to refer to the limbs (e.g., the thumb is more proximal to the pointer finger than the little finger) – helpful hint: proximal refers to proximity
- *Distal* – farther in proximity to an anatomical landmark than another body part; refers to all structures of the body but is most commonly used to refer to limbs (e.g., the foot is more distal to the hip joint then the knee) – helpful hint: distal refers to distance
- *Cranial* – higher up on the torso; closer to the head or skull; another essentially synonymous term that is used in this context is *cephalic* (which means related to the head); relatedly, the word *rostral* refers to an area on the head; specifically, it means toward the nasal or oral regions of the head
- *Caudal* – lower down on the torso; closer to the buttocks or tailbone
- *Superior* – higher up in the body as relative to another anatomical structure (e.g., the shoulder joint is superior to the elbow joint)
- *Inferior* – lower down in the body as relative to another anatomical structure (e.g., the knee joint is inferior to the hip joint)
- *Superficial* – more toward the body's outside (e.g., skin is more superficial than muscle)
- *Deep* – more toward the inside of the body (e.g., the transverse abdominis is deeper than the rectus abdominis)

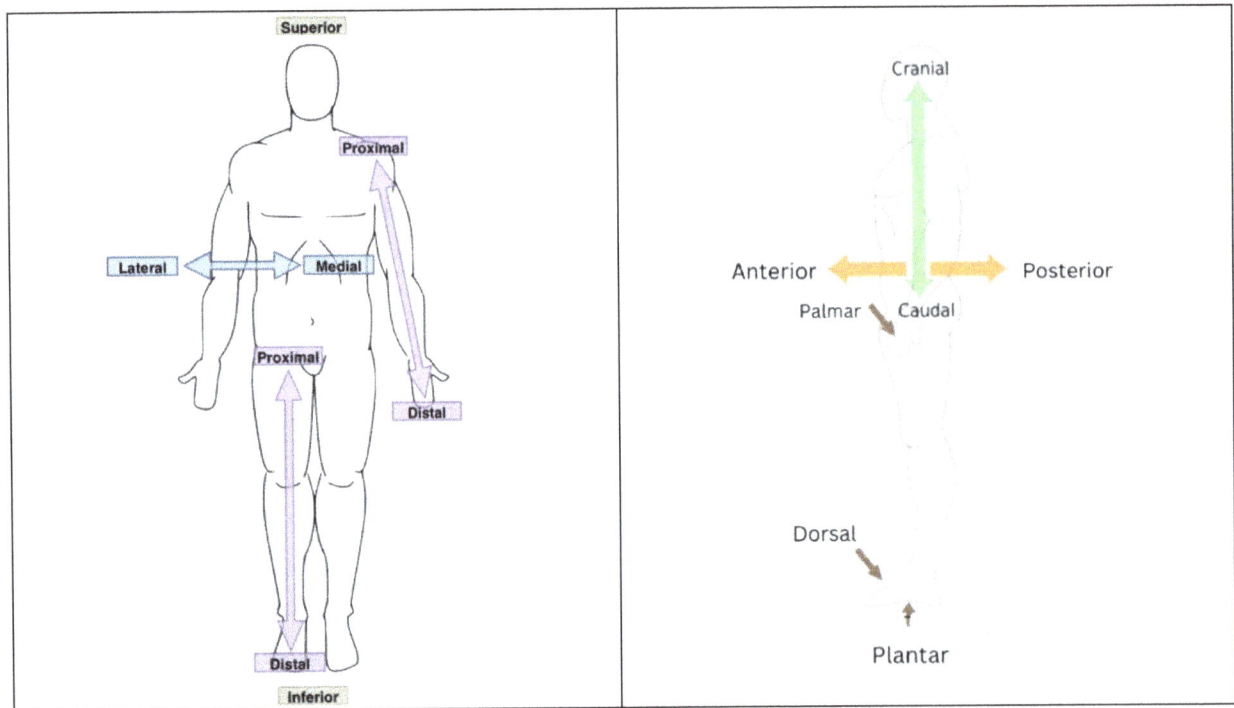

**Figure 1.3** Anatomical directions – frontal view. (Data sources: Osteomyoamare; https://commons.wikimedia.org/wiki/File:Anatomical_Directions.png

**Figure 1.4** Anatomical directions – sagittal view. Osteomyoamare; https://commons.wikimedia.org/wiki/File:Anatomical_Directions_2.png; Creative Commons Attribution 3.0)

# Chapter 2: Key Concepts of Integrated Holistic Physiology

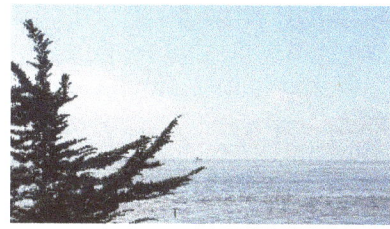

Consistent with the integrated holistic paradigm, all bodily systems interact and are fully connected to one another, reverberating collectively into all human layers of experience. Anatomy or physical structures are related to personal and collective psychological factors, reflect social and socioeconomic circumstances, and may reveal cultural and familial influences. Everything in one anatomical structure or physical system connects to all other systems and structures. Although we will explore anatomical structures related to the teaching of yoga *asana*, it is important to remember throughout that discussion, that humans are an interactive whole, a *Gestalt* – a whole that is greater than the sum of its parts. Because of humans' wholism, the discussion of structures starts by first taking a closer looks at how all structures interdepend and then interact. From that backdrop of wholism, we then move into an overview of the general structures, kinesiology basics, and then individual body sections (e.g., structures around the spine; structures related to the legs; structures related to the shoulder girdles).

## Interdependence of Physical Structures and Systems

Interdependence of physical structures and systems refers to the reality that as change is introduced into one physical system or anatomical structure, this shift reverberates through all other systems, structures, and layers of experiences. As we invite movement in a particular manner, there may be automatic shifts in breath and energy. As we affect the nervous system via gentle *asana*, we may create shifts in digestion or immunity. As we shift movement patterns in one part of the body, strong emotions may emerge and transform. To provide a few more examples of this interdependence, research has provided ample evidence that we can affect and transform:

- Endocrine health through strength-based movement
- Nervous system responses through shifting to more healthful respiratory patterns
- Gastrointestinal health through changes in our perceptions and mind states
- Psychological experiences and wellbeing through changes in nutrition and digestive health
- Cardiovascular health through changes in breathing patterns or aerobic exercise
- Immune health through nutrition and movement
- The examples are endless …

Additionally, movement, anatomy, kinesiology, and physiological systems – all heavily involved in yoga *asana* (and *pranayama*) – are not only in relationship with one another but also with all other aspects of the human experience and each person's biopsychosociocultural context. We cannot understand what we or others experience or perceive physically (anatomically) without considering how this experience or perception has been shaped by cultural, social, familial, and biological influences; nor can we fully appreciate how new ways of moving and experiencing the body may reverberate back into the individual's biopsychosociocultural context. To ignore human beings' profound interconnection (within their own organism and across their biopsychosociocultural contexts) can lead to a wide range of misunderstandings, including confusing symptoms and causes, choosing inauspicious cueing or guidance of movement, disempowerment, unwholesome interactions, misreading of reactions or responses in ourselves or our clients, and shifts in clients' or students' relationships in their life off the mat or outside the clinical office.

It is the profound interdependence across all experiences (or *koshas*) and contexts that makes yoga *asana* (and other movement practices) so powerful as they affect multiple systems and experiences each time we move, especially when embracing an integrated eight-limbs practice, informed by accessibility, beneficence, and intention (i.e., integrated holistic yoga). Changes in each layer of experience (i.e., in all *koshas*) reverberate into the biopsychosociocultural context and affect all aspects of interpersonal embeddedness. The profound interdependence of body parts, systems, and *koshas* with one another and the biopsychosociocultural environment is a central concept in understanding the function and resilience of our amazing bodies and psyches.

We are a continuous and interconnected physiological and anatomical system – divisions of anatomical structures and physiological systems are entirely artificial and simply helpful for communication. Differentiating structures and systems allows us to define, understand, and talk about them. Such *differentiation* was never meant to imply *separation*. Nothing within the body is separate; in fact, nothing within our overall human experience is separate. Each system is connected to all other systems; each physical expression and process is intimately linked to vitality (i.e., energy and arousal), mind (e.g., thoughts, opinions, attitudes, and emotions), and relationships (e.g., cultural or familial beliefs, strictures, understandings, and more).

Human brains do not think about or understand the body in terms of single muscles or structures. They understand action and movement and automatically recruit all necessary structures. There is a general misconception in anatomy of old that the body consists of separate body structures, often comparing the functioning of the body to that of a machine (with parts interchangeable). Modern anatomy understands instead, that the body is completely interconnected and interdependent, as demonstrated by the following examples:
- Our approximately 28 (women) to 36 (men) trillion cells all came from one cell (Hatton et al., 2023).
- Tom Myers (2022) says our bodies are more like a plant than a machine – all one entity, with many interdependent cells, not separate parts.
- There are often no clear boundaries between anatomical structures. For example, dissection shows that one cannot really discern with clarity where a tendon ends and where it becomes a muscle.
- When we move, we do not stretch or contract one muscle (although this is often how we use language). Instead, we move whole sections of the body and this movement affects breath and psyche.
- Where we feel stretch or pain may not be where the restrictions or causes of these sensations originate.

- Even our organs play a role in movement, affecting range of motion and being affected by motion. For example, moving organs in the abdominal cavity reverberates throughout the entire torso (e.g., sucking the belly in displaces organs upward or downward – with lasting effects if held long-term).

Fascia, connective tissue fibers (sheets, bands, gristly bits, fluids), and all the different types of tissues blend to make a continuous web of tissue throughout the body – this contributes to movement in one part of the body reverberating through all other parts. Fascia and connective tissues are completely interwoven with muscle tissue – we cannot always clearly differentiate where a tendon starts and a muscle ends (Clark, 2016; Myers, 2022). Neural tissue is also embedded in this connected matrix as nerves, just as blood vessels are integrated in connective, epithelial, and muscle tissue. The position of bones and posture depend much more on the alignment and structure of the soft (connective and muscle) tissue around them than the alignment of individual bones (which calls into question high-speed chiropractic adjustments of bone positioning – they often do not hold because soft tissue patterns pull them back). Holding the understanding of interconnection and resilience in mind, we can now move into an overview of human physiology, followed by a deeper dive into human anatomy. In all explorations, we will continuously look at the implications for the practice and guidance of yoga *asana*.

> *Facts have a half-life –*
> *we constantly have to learn new things*
> *and change our views as science and experience evolve.*
>
> *And sometimes we ignore or overlook facts others long recognized.*

## Human Physiology – Key Knowledge for Yoga

Physiology concerns itself with the functions of the body, assuring that the body can regulate itself, bring itself into balance, and achieve homeostasis. Death results when the body's physiology can no longer function in a manner that returns the entire body into balance. As noted previously, although discussions of the human being are always grounded in a review of specific systems or part, such *differentiation is not meant to imply separation*. Everything is connected to everything else, and all sequential and differentiated descriptions are merely a matter of need for clarity of communication and learning. To make this point in another way: the human body consists of 28 to 36 trillion cells (Hatton et al., 2023), *all grown from a single cell* – the ovum, the largest cell in the body, capable of conduction, contraction, absorption/secretion, and support (a precursor of the four types of cells in the body). We are a holistic single system, not a collection of separate parts. That said, and in the context provided, the first system that develops as the ovum begins to divide is the digestive system, followed by the circulatory system, and then the fascial system. Fascia, so key to understanding physical interdependence (as we will explore below), comes into being on the 14$^{th}$ day of embryonic development.

As cells divide, they organize themselves into tissues. If cells are like words, tissues are like sentences. Tissues are made up of more than 200 kinds of cells that bind to one another via specialized proteins. Tissues are made of similar morphology (shape) and function that arrange themselves in an orderly pattern (when healthy). At their simplest, tissues are membranes that cover or separate structures (e.g., organs, joint capsules) or line a body surface. Tissues at their most complex combine into organs.

## *Types of Tissue in The Human Body*

There are four types of tissues in the body, each type defined by its specific function or purpose. All types of tissues are relevant to the physical and vital practice of yoga *asana*, though some types of tissues receive more attention than others. The four types of tissue are nervous, epithelial, connective, and muscle tissues.

### *Nervous Tissue*

Nervous tissue is a specialized type of tissue in the human body that is primarily responsible for conduction and communication. It is composed of two main types of cells: neurons and neuroglia. Neurons are the fundamental units of this tissue and consist of three key structures—axon, dendrites, and cell body that work together to transmit electrochemical signals throughout the body. Neuroglia, also known as glial cells, support and protect neurons, ensuring their optimal function. Nervous tissue is highly responsive to internal and external stimuli, allowing the body to perceive, process, and react to various environmental and physiological changes. By propagating electrical impulses along nerves, nervous tissue plays a crucial role in coordinating movement, regulating organ function, and maintaining overall homeostasis.

For yoga professionals, understanding nervous tissue is essential because yoga practices directly influence the nervous system. Yoga *asana*, breathwork, and meditation engage and regulate nervous tissue, affecting the central and peripheral nervous systems. By comprehending how electrochemical signals govern movement, sensation, and autonomic functions, yoga teachers and therapists can better design sequences that promote nervous system balance. For example, they can use gentle movement, breath focus on the exhalation, and restorative yoga *asana* to stimulate the parasympathetic nervous system, reducing stress and enhancing recovery for individuals who tend to be stuck in sympathetic nervous system arousal. Conversely, dynamic movements and intentional engagement of the body can activate the sympathetic nervous system, fostering energy and focus for individuals who may be prone to dorsal collapse. Such tailored knowledge and strategic applications of specific yoga practices allows yoga professionals to tailor sequencing and cueing to meet the needs of students with varying nervous system responses, such as individuals with anxiety, chronic pain, or neurological conditions, ultimately enhancing the therapeutic potential of their teachings.

### *Epithelial Tissue*

Epithelial tissue is a vital component of the human body, forming protective sheets of cells that serve multiple functions, including secretion and absorption. These cell layers act as a barrier against harmful substances (such as toxins, bacteria, and viruses) while also regulating the movement of nutrients, fluids, and other essential compounds. Depending on their location and function, epithelial cells can be arranged in flat (squamous), cuboidal, or columnar sheets, existing in either single-layered (simple) or multi-layered (stratified) formations. This tissue type is found covering the external surface of the body, forming the outermost layer of skin, and lining internal passageways such as blood vessels, lymphatic vessels, and the digestive tract. Additionally, epithelial tissue plays a crucial role in glandular function, forming specialized structures that secrete essential substances such as hormones, stomach acid, saliva, and milk. By facilitating selective permeability, epithelial tissue ensures the proper exchange of materials while maintaining a crucial defense system for overall health and homeostasis.

For yoga professionals, understanding epithelial tissue is important because it highlights the body's intricate balance between protection, absorption, and secretion – three processes that are influenced by movement, breathwork, and overall lifestyle. Yoga practices can support epithelial tissue function by improving circulation, which enhances nutrient delivery and waste removal in organs lined with epithelial cells. Additionally, certain yoga techniques, such as deep breathing and twists, may stimulate the digestive tract's epithelial lining, promoting better absorption of nutrients and aiding detoxification. Furthermore, glandular epithelial tissues, responsible for hormone secretion, are influenced by stress levels, making yoga an effective tool for balancing endocrine function through relaxation and mindful movement. By recognizing the role of epithelial tissue in systemic health, yoga teachers and therapists can better understand how yoga practices support immune function, digestive health, and overall vitality, allowing them to guide students toward optimal wellbeing.

## *Connective Tissue*

Connective tissue is a fundamental tissue type in the human body that provides structural support, stability, and integration for all bodily systems. It consists of various cell combinations that bind organs and hold structures together, ensuring protection and cohesion throughout the body. There are multitudes of connective tissue types (as will be detailed below), including loose connective tissue (including adipose [fat] and reticular [supportive] tissues); dense connective tissues (including tendons and ligaments, as well as elastic tissues in arteries); specialized connective tissues (including several types of cartilage and bones); and fluid connective tissues (including blood and lymph). Connective tissues play crucial roles in maintaining the integrity of joints, muscles, and internal organs by creating a balance between movement and stability. Connective tissues are diverse in their function and composition, with loose connective tissue allowing flexibility while still providing support, and fibrous connective tissue offering a denser, more rigid framework that reinforces strength and endurance. Together, these tissues facilitate movement while maintaining structural integrity, allowing the body to function cohesively as a wholistic interdependent and resilient structure.

For yoga professionals, understanding connective tissue is essential because its many types directly influence mobility, stability, and overall movement patterns. Yoga *asana* and therapeutic techniques engage various connective tissues in different and deliberate ways. Some practices stretch loose connective tissue to increase resilience and flexibility; others strengthen fibrous connective tissues to enhance joint stability. Yoga practices such as slow, sustained stretching may target fascia, a specialized form of connective tissue, promoting hydration and resilience within the body. Understanding the various types of connective tissues helps yoga teachers and therapists adapt their instructions for clients with conditions such as hypermobility, arthritis, or injury recovery, ensuring that movement is supportive rather than strain-inducing. By integrating knowledge of connective tissues into their teaching, yoga professionals can create practices that promote and integrate freedom of movement with the stability necessary for long-term health. Because of its importance to the teaching of yoga *asana*, connective tissues are covered in much more detail below. Bones, ligaments, and tendons in particular, receive detailed attention in Chapters 4 through 6, in the context of specific regions of the body, namely, the axial skeleton, lower appendicular skeleton, and upper appendicular skeleton. Fascia and its role in anatomy trains (to be explained below) remains a central focus throughout.

## *Muscular Tissue*

Muscular tissue is a specialized type of tissue in the human body responsible for contraction, the fundamental mechanism behind movement. It makes up the muscles throughout the body and has the unique ability to respond to internal and external stimuli, allowing for voluntary movements, such as walking and stretching, as well as involuntary processes, such as the beating of the heart and digestion. Muscular tissue is the only tissue capable of contracting, and through this function, it generates force, facilitates movement, and supports posture. Whether it is skeletal muscle working to produce motion, smooth muscle regulating internal organ function, or cardiac muscle ensuring the continuous pumping of blood, muscular tissue is essential to diverse conscious and unconscious bodily actions.

For yoga professionals, understanding muscular tissue is crucial because it allows them to design practices that effectively engage, strengthen, and lengthen muscles while promoting functional movement. Yoga postures rely on muscular contractions to stabilize joints, control transitions between shapes, and develop strength and flexibility in a balanced way. By recognizing how muscles respond to stimuli, yoga teachers and therapists can guide students in refining body awareness, preventing injury, and improving neuromuscular coordination. Furthermore, specific techniques, such as eccentric muscle engagement in slow movements or isometric holds in static postures, can be used strategically to build endurance and enhance proprioception. Knowledge of muscular tissue helps yoga professionals adapt practices for individuals with muscle imbalances, weakness, or conditions such as muscular dystrophy or post-injury rehabilitation, ensuring that movement is safe and supportive of overall wellbeing. Because muscles (always in a greater context of other tissues) are of central importance in the teaching and therapeutic practices of yoga *asana*, muscle tissue are covered in thorough detail below. Specific groups of muscles are elucidated further in the context of the various body regions covered in Chapters 4 through 6.

## *Organ Systems with Relevance for Yoga*

Organs are complex structures made up of multiple types of tissues that perform a particular function; multiple organs that collaborate to carry out a particular body function are called organ systems. If cells are words, and tissues are sentences, organs and organ systems are short stories and long narratives. Below, the chapter outlines nine organ systems of particular relevance to yoga. Depending on source, fewer or more organ systems can be identified (e.g., adding the excretory system or collapsing some of the systems listed below into a single system).

Regardless of how many organ systems are listed, yoga likely intersects with all. Some systems are affected by yoga in terms of enhanced functionality; other are important to consider because they may present risks or bring along contraindications for the practice. Some systems have a bearing on the safety of yoga and the need for cautions, adaptations, and variations to create access to the practice for all – even those who evidence challenges in one or more of their organ systems. It is important to note that these nine organ systems, although covered in sequence, are intimately interconnected and co-regulating. They are never separate from one another and yoga's deliberate and planned effects on one system will likely reverberate into several, if not all. In other words, we may plan a practice to calm the nervous system, inviting a vagal brake on the sympathetic nervous system via a shift to a ventral vagal parasympathetic state. This practice will likely also have profound effects on digestion, immunity, and circulation. It will reverberate into all *koshas* – with effects reaching far beyond the physical into vitality, emotional regulation, cognitive functioning, executive control, and relational patterns. One more time: *differentiation does not imply separation.*

Clearly, we are interconnected beings and our various parts create an integrated and holistic whole that is always much greater than the sum of these parts. It is important to maintain an integrated holistic yoga lens while perusing the individual descriptions of the organ systems that follow. This lens reminds us in all interventions via yoga practice for these organ systems to work with intentionality, accessibility, and beneficence. The key to a wholesome yoga practice is to see and work with the whole person, deeply honoring their biopsychosociocultural individuality; and to understand that all anatomical and physiological descriptions are based on an *average normative* human being – this human being does not exist in reality (truly, not a single one of us is average, nor the norm).

## Circulatory System

The circulatory system, often called the body's transport system, includes the heart, blood, blood vessels, and the lymphatic system, which comprises lymph fluid, lymph nodes, and lymphatic vessels. This intricate network performs the essential task of circulating life-sustaining materials (including oxygen, nutrients, hormones, and immune cells) throughout the body while also collecting and managing waste products. The circulatory system can be deeply influenced through yoga-based practices, such as breathwork, mindful movement, and inner practices. Understanding how this system works helps yoga teachers and therapists make informed choices in sequencing and cueing that is sensitive to health or mental health conditions related to the circulatory system.

### Understanding the Circulatory System's Role

At its most basic level, the circulatory system exists to keep the body nourished and in balance. Every cell depends on a consistent flow of oxygen and nutrients to function properly, and the bloodstream delivers these essential materials from the lungs and digestive system to the tissues. Just as importantly, it removes waste products such as carbon dioxide and urea, the by-products of cellular metabolism. Beyond its transport functions, the circulatory system plays an integral role in temperature regulation, hormonal communication, and immune defense. Through the movement of blood and lymph, the system distributes heat to help regulate body temperature, carries hormones from glands to their target tissues, and supports immunity by circulating white blood cells and filtering pathogens through lymph nodes.

The lymphatic system, often overlooked, is particularly relevant in yoga due to its reliance on physical movement and breath for circulation. Unlike the cardiovascular system, which is powered by the heart, the lymphatic system depends on muscular contraction and diaphragmatic movement to move fluid. This makes yoga an ideal modality for supporting lymphatic health, especially through gentle motion and deep breathing.

### *Yoga's Potential Impacts on the Circulatory System*

Yoga can have a profound and multi-dimensional influence on the circulatory system, stimulating, soothing, and supporting flow of blood and lymph in subtle yet significant ways. Through *asana* and other yoga-based movement, blood flow is enhanced, particularly in areas of the body that tend to be compressed or rarely moved. Moving the body rhythmically, in tune with the breath, and mindfully can stimulate venous return and support oxygen delivery throughout the tissues. Holding shapes can enhance circulation by engaging muscles in subtle ways that create a natural pumping effect, especially in the lower limbs (in fact, the soleus muscles in the calf are figuratively referred to as the second heart). Inverted and half-inverted shapes, even gentle variations such as Legs-Up-the-Wall (*viparita karani*), offer restorative means to encourage venous and lymphatic return toward the heart. Twisting postures may assist the lymphatic system by alternately compressing and releasing various lymph node regions, especially in the abdomen and chest.

Slow, subtle, and nasal breathing have powerful effects as the diaphragm functions like a supportive pump for the lymphatic system and influences heart rate through vagus nerve stimulation. Breathing practices help reduce resting heart rate, improve heart rate variability, and regulate blood pressure, especially when paired with mindfulness and relaxation practices. Relatedly, the inner practices of yoga (such as sense guarding, concentration, and meditation) support the circulatory system by reducing stress. Chronic stress places the cardiovascular system under strain, contributing to high blood pressure, inflammation, and impaired immune function. Restorative shapes, meditative breathing, and guided relaxation (such as yoga nidra) support circulatory health by calming the mind and easing the physical effects of stress on the heart and vessels. Yoga offers a counterbalance through these practices as they shift the autonomic nervous system toward parasympathetic responsiveness, inviting a ventral vagal state of being.

### *Cautions, Contraindications, and Guidance for Yoga vis-à-vis the Circulatory System*

When working with the circulatory system through yoga, it is essential to recognize that although the practice offers tremendous support, certain cardiovascular conditions require thoughtfulness in approach. For individuals with high blood pressure, strong inversions, prolonged breath retentions, and forceful *pranayama* techniques may best be avoided, as they may elevate pressure within the cardiovascular system. Instead, grounding postures, gentle forward folds, and soft, rhythmic breathing can help regulate blood pressure and promote parasympathetic activation. Individuals experiencing orthostatic hypotension or postural orthostatic tachycardia syndrome (POTS) may be prone to dizziness or rapid heart rate with postural changes. Slow and mindful transitions are essential, particularly when moving from reclined to upright positions.

In the context of lymphatic health, especially for individuals living with lymphedema or at risk for it, it is key to prioritize gentle, rhythmic movement, and avoid practices that create excessive compression or prolonged holding in affected areas. Gentle motion and diaphragmatic breathing can support lymphatic flow and fluid balance, whereas overexertion, long inversions or half-inversions, or deep compression (e.g., passive twists) may exacerbate swelling or discomfort. Props, bolsters, and elevated limb support can be helpful, particularly in restorative or reclined positions. For circulatory and lymphatic concerns, therapeutic focus on breath awareness, gentle pacing, and interoception support self-regulation and resilience. Encouraging clients or students to maintain awareness of subtle shifts in breath, heart rate, and vitality or arousal throughout the practice supports physical and emotional safety as well as creating empowerment and agency.

## *Immune System*

Very much related and interactive with the circulatory system, the immune system serves as the body's vital defense network, distinguishing self from non-self and protecting against pathogens, toxins, and abnormal cell growth. It involves a wide array of tissues, cells, and signaling molecules spread across multiple body systems. While white blood cells, lymph nodes, and the thymus are central players, the immune system also includes bone marrow, spleen, mucosal barriers, and gut-associated lymphatic tissues. Its functions are deeply interwoven with the circulatory, lymphatic, and nervous systems. Yoga's capacity to regulate stress, support lymphatic circulation, and cultivate systemic balance makes it a potent contributor to immune system resilience. For yoga teachers and therapists, understanding the immune system's mechanisms and vulnerabilities can help shape practices that support immune health and respond compassionately to states of depletion, inflammation, or dysregulation.

### *Understanding the Immune System's Role*

The immune system is essentially a guardian of the body's integrity, constantly surveying inner environments for threats and activating appropriate responses. It performs this work through a complex coordination of innate and adaptive defenses. The innate immune system is always on guard, using barriers such as the skin and mucous membranes, along with immune cells (including macrophages and natural killer cells), to respond quickly to invaders. The adaptive immune system offers more specific and long-lasting protection, relying on lymphocytes (T-cells and B-cells) to recognize and remember pathogens for future defense.

The protective function of the immune system extends beyond infection control. The immune system plays critical roles in wound healing, tissue regeneration, inflammation regulation, even mood and energy levels. It is influenced by circadian rhythms, sleep quality, nutrition, and stress. Prolonged activation of the stress response (through the hypothalamic-pituitary-adrenal axis and sympathetic nervous system) can dysregulate immune function, increasing inflammation and/or suppressing immune responsiveness. This interplay between mind, body, and immunity creates a clear entry point for the integrated practices of yoga.

*Yoga's Potential Impacts on the Immune System*

Yoga supports immune health primarily by helping regulate the nervous and endocrine systems, improving lymphatic circulation, reducing systemic inflammation, and promoting rest and recovery. Because the lymphatic system is one of the primary transport routes for immune cells and plays a key role in detoxification, yoga-based movement, especially when gentle, rhythmic, and breath-guided, can encourage circulation of lymph and support immune surveillance. Practices that include dynamic movement, shakes and wiggles, gentle folding or rotation, and mild inversions help facilitate lymphatic movement through the thoracic duct and abdominal lymphatic reservoirs.

Breathwork, mindfulness, and restorative practices shift the autonomic nervous system toward a ventral vagal parasympathetic state, putting the vagal brake on sympathetic arousal and decreasing stress hormone output and inflammation. This parasympathetic shift supports digestive health, which is closely linked to immune function due to the abundance of immune cells and microbiota in the gastrointestinal tract. Meditation and focused concentration practices reduce psychological stress, which can otherwise impair immune regulation and resilience.

Yoga may be especially beneficial for individuals living with chronic inflammatory conditions, autoimmune disorders, or stress-related immune dysregulation. Although not curative, these practices help recalibrate the nervous system, reduce reactivity, and support sustainable energy and wellbeing. Practicing in ways that foster interoception, neuroception, agency, and compassion can strengthen both emotional and physiological immune boundaries.

*Cautions, Contraindications, and Guidance for Yoga vis-à-vis the Immune System*

Although yoga can offer powerful support for immune health, it is important to recognize the nuances of immune dysregulation when guiding yoga practices. During active illness or states of immune compromise (such as following chemotherapy, with autoimmune flare-ups, or in the context of long COVID or chronic fatigue syndrome), practitioners may benefit most from deeply restorative practices focused on breath awareness, gentle movement, and rest. Overexertion, heat-inducing sequences, or fast-paced flows can place additional strain on already taxed systems, potentially leading to symptom flare-ups or delayed recovery.

In autoimmune conditions or inflammatory syndromes, yoga professionals prioritize clients' self-regulation and pacing, offering options that allow for responsiveness to daily energy fluctuations. Practices that emphasize mindful awareness, rather than performance or endurance, help avoid exacerbating underlying inflammation. For individuals with allergies, asthma, or environmental sensitivities (i.e., conditions linked to immune reactivity) attention to environmental setup (such as fragrance-free rooms and fresh air) is helpful, as is cueing that honors optimal breathing.

## Nervous System

The nervous system is a complex network of specialized cells (i.e., neurons) that transmit signals throughout the body. It is the primary communication and control system of the body. It comprises the brain, spinal cord, peripheral nerves, and sense organs, all working together to regulate behavior, control movement, receive and interpret sensory information, and maintain internal balance. This intricate system integrates signals from the external environment and internal world, guiding moment-to-moment responsiveness (or reactivity) while also shaping long-term patterns of perception, emotion, and behavior. Essential to the nervous system are the sensory organs (e.g., eyes, ears, nose, tongue, skin and all other receptors for interception, neuroception, and proprioception) that receive and transmit the signals through which the brain interprets the external and internal world. These organs help orient us and influence the degree of arousal or calm we experience. In essence, the nervous system allows the body to perceive, interpret, and respond to its surroundings and internal state, enabling coordination and regulation of all bodily functions. Although the nervous system thrives on input, too much or too little stimulation, especially when mismatched with internal needs, can dysregulate arousal, affect, emotion, attention, cognition, and behavior.

The nervous system mediates self-awareness, attention, and embodied experience – all central to the practice of yoga. Thus, the nervous system and yoga are partners in the process of the humans' state of mind, wellbeing, thriving, development, and transformation. Whether through breath regulation, mindful movement, or deep stillness, yoga affects how the nervous system functions and how humans experience themselves, others, and the world. For yoga teachers and therapists, understanding the role and sensitivity of the nervous system is vital for creating safe, effective, and healing practices and spaces, especially when working with diverse populations or neurological conditions.

### *Understanding the Nervous System's Role*

Broadly viewed, the nervous system governs all conscious and unconscious activity, from reflexes and muscle movement to complex thought and emotional processing. It has the following functions:
- *Receiving sensory information*: detecting stimuli from internal and external environments through sensory receptors (e.g., touch, taste, sight, sound, smell)
- *Processing and integrating information*: analyzing sensory inputs in the brain and spinal cord to make decisions and generate appropriate responses; includes functions such as thought, memory, learning, and emotions
- *Responding to information*: initiating actions by sending signals to muscles and glands (effectors); results in voluntary movements, involuntary actions (like breathing and digestion), and secretion of hormones
- *Maintaining homeostasis*: regulating and allostatically adapting internal body conditions such as temperature, heart rate, blood pressure, and more

The nervous system is broadly divided into the central nervous system (CNS; i.e., brain and spinal cord, which act as the control center that processes information and directs action) and the peripheral nervous system (PNS; which extends throughout the body via motor and sensory nerves, relaying sensory information to the CNS and carrying motor commands from the CNS to muscles and glands). The PNS is further divided into the somatic nervous system (responsible for voluntary movement) and autonomic nervous system (responsible for regulating involuntary functions like heart rate, respiration, digestion, and immune responses). The ANS is further divided into the sympathetic nervous system, which mobilizes the body in response to stress or threat (a state preparing the organism for fight or flight), and the parasympathetic nervous system, which supports rest, digestion, and healing (a ventral vagal state of ease, healing, and social engagement) or a last resort state of managing life threat via physical collapse and emotional distancing or dissociation (a dorsal vagal state of collapse).

### *Yoga's Potential Impacts on the Nervous System*

Yoga deeply influences the nervous system on structural and functional levels. While a short overview is offered here, the depth and profoundness of the relationship between yoga and the nervous system would actually deserve a whole book in and of itself. An ample literature exists delineating this relationship (Brems, 2024a, 2024b, 2024c, 2025). To give a few examples:

- Physical movement (*asana*) increases proprioception and interoception - inner sensory experiences that inform the brain about the body's position and internal state. *Asana* sequences that are rhythmic, balanced, and breath-guided can help regulate the sensory and motor systems and support a shift toward greater autonomic stability. Gentle backbends and lateral movements stimulate spinal nerves and energize the system, whereas forward folds and restorative shapes may soothe and down-regulate sympathetic activity.
- Breathing practices (*pranayama*) directly influence the autonomic nervous system. Slower breathing rates, longer exhalations, and nasal breathing stimulate the vagus nerve, which enhances parasympathetic tone and supports emotional regulation. Practices such as alternate nostril breathing, bumble bee breath, and gentle work with breath pauses can help balance nervous system activity, improve vagal tone, and build tolerance for stillness and sensation.
- Inner practices (i.e., sense guarding, concentration, and meditation) encourage the nervous system to settle into peacefulness and ease by reducing external sensory input and supporting a state of focused calm. Over time, such practices reshape neural pathways, support neuroplasticity, and can help reduce habitual reactivity and emotional volatility. This is particularly relevant for individuals living with anxiety, depression, trauma, or chronic stress, as yoga offers a non-pharmacological means to shift internal states and improve regulation.

From a behavioral and psychological perspective, yoga fosters self-awareness, agency, and emotional resilience, as practitioners learn to observe and respond to internal cues without immediate reactivity. This growing capacity for emotional regulation is a direct reflection of a more balanced nervous system and has wide-reaching effects on cognition, mood, and interpersonal connection.

### *Cautions, Contraindications, and Guidance for Yoga vis-à-vis the Nervous System*

Although yoga offers profound support for the nervous system, certain neurological and sensory conditions require nuanced, individualized approaches. For example, individuals with glaucoma or vitreous detachment should avoid practices involving downward pressure in the head, such as strong inversions or intense forward folds, as these may elevate intraocular pressure. Similarly, those with inner ear or balance challenges may struggle with rapid directional changes or unstable postures, and may benefit from using a wall or chair for support, especially during standing or balancing shapes.

Practitioners with nerve compression issues (e.g., sciatica, thoracic outlet syndrome, or carpal tunnel syndrome) require careful attention to alignment, transitions, and prop use to avoid exacerbating nerve irritation. For individuals with neurodegenerative conditions (e.g., Parkinson's disease, multiple sclerosis, or dementia), yoga spaces and practice are adapted to support and optimize access to cognitive clarity, physical stability, and emotional safety. Practices are slow-paced and repetitive, emphasizing predictable structure, grounding, and simplicity in cueing. Visual or tactile cues, and chairs, walls, or other supports can enhance safety, create intentionality, avoid harm, and communicate accessibility. Encouraging a non-judgmental, process-oriented attitude is essential, as students with neurological conditions may have fluctuating abilities and experience frustration.

Across all conditions, it is important to remember that the nervous system thrives in environments that are safe, attuned, and appropriately stimulating. Too much stimulation (e.g., fast movement, intense music, strong lighting) can overwhelm the system, while under-stimulation may lead to disengagement or collapse. The key is to cocreate a space where students feel seen, respected, and in control of their experience.

Yoga teachers and therapists can support nervous system health by fostering attunement, choice, and co-regulation in their classes. Practices that build awareness of nervous system states (e.g., polyvagal states, arousal, affect or hedonic tone) help students become familiar with their patterns and responses. Emphasizing interoception, neuroception, proprioception, and exteroception is key. Over time, awareness and familiarity lead to enhanced self-regulation and resilience. Through mindful movement, breath, and attention, yoga becomes a (re-)training ground for the nervous system, offering pathways into to balance, vitality, and presence.

## *Digestive System*

Related very strongly to the immune and nervous systems, the digestive system, or gastrointestinal (GI) system, is responsible for breakdown, absorption, and assimilation of nutrients, as well as elimination of waste. This system includes the mouth, esophagus, stomach, small and large intestines, liver, gallbladder, and pancreas, each organ contributing to the conversion of food into usable energy and building blocks for the body. Beyond its mechanical and chemical functions, the digestive system plays a vital role in immune function and is in constant communication with the nervous system through what is now well-recognized as the gut-brain axis. Through breathwork, movement, and nervous system regulation, yoga can profoundly support the health of the digestive system. Understanding this system's function allows yoga teachers and therapists to guide practices that enhance digestive efficiency, reduce stress-related gastrointestinal dysfunction, and offer yoga therapeutics that may help ameliorate digestive disorders.

### *Understanding the Digestive System's Role*

The primary role of the digestive system is to process food and convert it into nutrients usable for energy, growth, and cellular repair. This process begins with ingestion of food and water; it continues through a complex process of mechanical and enzymatic breakdown in the stomach and small intestine, absorption of nutrients into the bloodstream, and elimination of indigestible matter through the large intestine. Further, a significant portion of the body's immune function is located in the GI tract, especially within the gut-associated lymphoid tissue, making digestive health essential to systemic immunity.

The digestive system is also home to a vast network of nerves and immune cells. This *enteric nervous system*, referred to as a second brain, communicates constantly with the central nervous system with reciprocal effects. Functionally, digestion is closely linked with the autonomic nervous system. It helps to recall that the parasympathetic branch of the ANS is often described as "rest and digest" state. It is necessary for healthful digestion, whereas sympathetic dominance, often secondary to chronic stress, anxiety, or other forms of human suffering and experiences of danger, can impair gastrointestinal function. Chronic sympathetic arousal or dorsal collapse can contribute to many GI symptoms, including – but not limited to – bloating, constipation, diarrhea, acid reflux, and irritable bowel syndrome.

### *Yoga's Potential Impacts on the Digestive System*

Yoga-based practices can significantly influence digestive health by supporting parasympathetic tone, improving circulation to digestive organs, and facilitating healthy abdominal motility. Breath-centered movement can stimulate peristalsis, the rhythmic muscular contractions of the intestinal walls, aiding digestion and elimination. Shapes that compress, twist, or lengthen the abdominal cavity can offer gentle mechanical stimulation to abdominal organs, potentially improving circulation and inter-organ communication. Twisting, when approached mindfully, encourages alternating compression and decompression of the abdominal region, which may support motility, fascial cleansing and rehydration, and lymphatic drainage in and around the digestive tract. Forward folds and gentle core engagement can provide proprioceptive, interoceptive, and neuroceptive feedback that may enhance vagal tone and overall regulation of digestive function.

*Pranayama* and other breathwork have particularly strong relevance to digestive (and lymphatic) health. Diaphragmatic breathing increases movement in the thoracic and abdominal cavities, gently massaging the heart and abdominal organs, supporting intestinal motility as well as venous and lymphatic return. Slow, nasal, and coherent (i.e., optimally functional) breathing is known to increase vagal tone and reduce sympathetic dominance, offering a valuable approach to mitigating stress-induced digestive issues. The same benefits can arise from other yoga practices that similarly engage interoception and mindfulness, including body scans, breath awareness, and meditative stillness, all of which help restore autonomic balance and support GI function. In the context of chronic inflammation or disorders such as irritable bowel syndrome (IBS), yoga has shown promise as an adjunctive therapy, especially when practices emphasize compassionate awareness and gentle self- and emotional regulation rather than exertion or effort. Grounded, predictable sequencing and supportive internal focusing so prevalent in mindfully embodied yoga practices may reduce stress-related GI sensitivity.

### *Cautions, Contraindications, and Guidance for Yoga vis-à-vis the Digestive System*

Although yoga can provide meaningful support for digestive health, certain digestive conditions require care and careful person-centered tailoring. For example, individuals with inflammatory bowel diseases such as Crohn's disease or ulcerative colitis may benefit from gentle, restorative yoga during flare-ups, while avoiding deep abdominal compression, excessive heat, or intense twisting. Students experiencing acid reflux or gastroesophageal reflux disease (GERD) may need to avoid or vary up positions that compress the stomach or involve inversion (after eating).

In cases of abdominal surgeries, hernias, or gastrointestinal malignancies, pressure in the abdominal cavity needs to be carefully managed. Similarly, excessive intra-abdominal pressure from forceful breathing techniques (e.g., *kapalabhati* or *bhastrika*) may not be appropriate for individuals with certain GI conditions, especially when inflammation or weakness in the abdominal wall is present. To ensure that yoga optimizes digestive health, teachers and therapists prioritize nervous system regulation over physical intensity. Careful pacing allows for recovery between shapes, breath remains natural and easeful, and practitioners are encouraged to monitor subtle cues from their bodies related to discomfort, peristalsis, or fatigue.

## *Endocrine System*

Deeply interactive with the circulatory, digestive, immune, and nervous systems, the endocrine system is a complex network of glands that regulate metabolism, growth and development, reproduction, mood, and physiological homeostasis through secretion of hormones. Key components include the hypothalamus, pituitary gland, thyroid, parathyroid glands, adrenal glands, pancreas, ovaries (in biologically female bodies), and testes (in biologically male bodies). These glands release hormones into the bloodstream to signal distant target organs, playing a crucial role in communication and coordination throughout the body. The endocrine system is highly responsive to stress and deeply interconnected with the nervous and immune systems, and thus is significantly influenced by yoga-based practices. Breath regulation, mindful movement, and contemplative practices can help modulate endocrine activity by supporting autonomic balance and systemic regulation. An informed understanding of hormonal actions enables yoga professionals to design practices that are appropriately paced, supportive of hormonal health, and sensitive to endocrine-related conditions.

### *Understanding the Endocrine System's Role*

The endocrine system governs long-term processes in the body through the gradual release of hormones, the chemical messengers that regulate all types of cellular activity. The hypothalamus and pituitary gland function as the central command centers, intimately linking the nervous system with the endocrine system and coordinating hormonal signals that affect peripheral glands. For example, the pituitary stimulates the thyroid to regulate metabolism, the adrenal glands to manage stress responses, and the reproductive organs to control fertility and sexual development.

Unlike the immediate electrical impulses of the nervous system, endocrine messages operate on a slower timeline, initiating systemic changes that unfold over minutes to hours and regulate circadian rhythms, energy availability, hydration, reproductive cycles, and immune readiness. Feedback loops are essential to this system's integrity; when hormonal levels deviate from a desired range, inhibitory signals are sent to reduce or increase glandular output accordingly. As already noted, the endocrine system is tightly interwoven with the autonomic nervous system, especially the hypothalamic-pituitary-adrenal (HPA) axis, which helps govern the body's response to stress. Chronic activation of the HPA axis can lead to dysregulation in cortisol secretion, with downstream effects on metabolism, immune function, and mental health. Similarly, conditions such as hypothyroidism, polycystic ovarian syndrome (PCOS), diabetes mellitus, and adrenal insufficiency require careful management of stress and lifestyle factors, including physical activity and relaxation.

*Yoga's Potential Impacts on the Endocrine System*

Yoga has the capacity to influence the endocrine system *directly*, through physical stimulation of glands, and *indirectly*, through autonomic regulation. *Asana* that gently compresses or otherwise affects areas near key glands (e.g., the throat for the thyroid, abdomen for the pancreas, or low back for the adrenals) may support circulation and interoceptive and neuroceptive feedback in these regions. However, the most consistent and research-supported benefit of yoga for the endocrine system comes through its regulation of stress. Optimal functional nasal diaphragmatic breathing and practices such as meditation or yoga *nidra*, help attenuate hyperactivity of the HPA axis by increasing vagal tone and putting the vagal brake on sympathetic arousal. Supporting parasympathetic ventral vagal states leads to reductions in circulating stress hormones (e.g., cortisol and epinephrine) and helps rebalance hormonal rhythms disrupted by chronic stress, acute or complex trauma, disturbed sleep, or chronic pain.

Mindful movement and somatic awareness may improve hormonal balance by enhancing perceptions of safety and facilitating allostatic recalibration. For example, regular yoga practice has shown promise in regulating blood glucose in individuals with diabetes, supporting menstrual regularity for individuals with polycystic ovarian syndrome, and improving symptoms of perimenopause and menopause. The endocrine system also governs fluid and electrolyte balance through hormones such as aldosterone and antidiuretic hormone (ADH), and yoga practices that include hydration awareness, breath retention, or controlled sweating may influence these parameters. Such practices are best approached with caution and clear intention, particularly in hot environments or in populations with endocrine vulnerabilities.

*Cautions, Contraindications, and Guidance for Yoga vis-à-vis the Endocrine System*

Individuals with endocrine disorders such as diabetes, Addison's disease, Cushing's syndrome, hyper- or hypothyroidism, or reproductive hormone imbalances typically thrive with practices that minimize physiological stress while supporting systemic regulation. For example, individuals with adrenal insufficiency may experience fatigue or blood pressure fluctuations and benefit most from restorative or gentle breath-guided practices rather than dynamic movement or excessive effort. Individuals with thyroid disorders may need to be aware of their temperature sensitivity, being prone to overheating or intolerance to cold. Individuals with blood sugar irregularities, including diabetes or hypoglycemia, benefit from slow transitions, ongoing cueing related to interoceptive awareness of hydration and blood sugar level cues, and supportive environments that express compassion and inner awareness. Individuals struggling with perimenopausal changes may benefit from sequences that emphasize grounding, nervous system downregulation, and awareness of cyclical changes in energy and mood (Baginski, 2020; Lasater, 2017). Overall, yoga best supports endocrine health by promoting consistency, self-awareness, and practices that foster stability in internal rhythms, whether related to energy, mood, metabolism, or reproductive cycles.

## Respiratory System

The respiratory system is responsible for human vitality, brining oxygen into all tissues and cells as well as balancing carbon dioxide and other body chemistry. The system includes the nose, throat, larynx, trachea, bronchi, lungs, and respiratory muscles (most centrally the diaphragm). Closely interconnected with the circulatory system, the respiratory system ensures that every cell receives oxygen needed for energy production, maintains pH balance, and facilitates speech, smell, and immune protection (Brems, 2024b).

The respiratory system takes on central importance in yoga, through which breath and breathing has both direct and indirect effects on physiological as well as mental and emotional regulation. Understanding the functions of the respiratory system, and how they may be affected by yoga practices, enables yoga professionals to guide students with attunement and patient-centered approaches that carefully consider clients' health and mental health conditions related to breathing, energy, and nervous system balance.

### Understanding the Respiratory System's Role

Most centrally, the respiratory system enables gas exchange, supplying oxygen to the tissues and balancing carbon dioxide as well as pH via internal and external respiration. It contributes to vocalization, immune defense, and olfaction. It is a key player in posture, spinal stability, and the regulation of intra-abdominal pressure. Crucially, the respiratory system is both voluntary and involuntary, meaning it operates autonomically but can be consciously modulated. Human capacity to make conscious changes to breath and breathing facilitates powerful interface between breath and body as well as breath and mind. Through conscious breathing, yoga practitioners can influence their states of arousal, emotional reactivity, and even patterns of thought and behavior.

### Yoga's Potential Impacts on the Respiratory System

Yoga's influence on the respiratory system is multifold. At a physical level, *asana* and other yoga-based movement mobilize the rib basket, spine, and diaphragm (among other functions), affecting respiratory efficiency and pattern locks related to breath and breathing. For example, heart-opening shapes may facilitate inhalation, whereas forward folds and gentle twists may be engaged to support longer, smoother exhalations. Proprioceptive, neuroceptive, and interoceptive awareness are key to more healthful breathing and its up- and downstream effect on body and mind. Deliberate physical and vital practices can affect respiratory muscle tone, diaphragmatic movement, and lung capacity, with profound effect on autonomic nervous system regulation. Regular practice can lead to improved oxygen uptake in tissues along with enhanced carbon dioxide tolerance and more efficient energy metabolism.

Yoga offers powerful support for respiratory regulation, especially under stress. Chronic stress and anxiety often lead to dysfunctional breathing patterns (e.g., shallow chest breathing, breath holding, or rapid, irregular rhythms) or vice versa. Yoga's optimal functional breathing, combined with awareness and compassion, supports a shift toward parasympathetic states and enhanced vagal tone. In therapeutic settings, subtle and gentle breathing and movement practices can help manage symptoms of asthma, COPD, hyperventilation syndrome, and anxiety-related breath dysfunction. Equally affected are related mental health conditions, such as anxiety, panic, and trauma-related conditions.

*Cautions, Contraindications, and Guidance for Yoga vis-à-vis the Respiratory System*

Although yoga offers profound support for respiratory function, caution must be exercised when working with individuals who have compromised respiratory health (e.g., asthma, chronic bronchitis, or COPD). For such individuals, rapid or forceful breathing techniques are contraindicated. Instead, practices emphasize breath awareness and optimal functional breathing, defined by nasal and diaphragmatic breathing with a slow rate, low volume, subtle rhythm, smooth texture, and quiet sound. Individuals with severe allergies, nasal polyps, or recent respiratory infections may experience irritation or congestion but also symptom relief during practice. Caution and vigilance are key in these cases.

Care is also taken with individuals prone to dorsal vagal collapse and/or stress apnea in response to stress, trauma, or panic. For them, subtle breathing practices can aggravate chronic under-breathing. Interoceptive and neuroceptive cueing that invites breath awareness without breath control is a great place to start with anyone who presents with respiratory challenges either due to physical or mental health conditions. Awareness is followed by focus on developing optimal functional breathing that is nasal, diaphragmatic, subtle, smooth, and quiet, and that invites a sense of agency and resilience. Props may be used to support upright, open posture and promote unrestricted breath flow. By respecting the unique biopsychosociocultural individuality of each human being yoga can affect the respiratory system in ways that create access to ease, vitality, and thriving one breath at a time. For a very detailed analysis of the respiratory system and yoga, see Brems (2024b).

*Skeletal System*

Intimately linked to the muscular and myofascial systems (covered below), the skeletal system provides the framework that supports the body's shape, protects vital organs, facilitates movement via joints and muscular attachments. On average, the skeletal system includes 206 bones in the adult human body, as well as the joints, cartilage, and supporting ligaments that connect them. Bones further serve as reservoirs for essential minerals (e.g., calcium, phosphorus) and are dynamic tissues that house bone marrow and produce red blood cells, white blood cells, and platelets.

In the context of yoga, the skeletal system is literally and metaphorically foundational. Shapes and movements offered in yoga *asana* are made possible through the architecture of bones and joints; humans' internal senses of grounding, expansions, and stability are deeply connected to the interplay between skeletal structure and muscular systems to create movement and alignment, including posture in daily living. Understanding the skeletal system allows yoga teachers and therapists to make informed decisions about load, alignment, and auspicious variations for yogic practices, especially in the context of skeletal conditions, including – but not limited – to osteoporosis, disc-related pathologies, arthritis, scoliosis, and injury recovery.

### Understanding the Skeletal System's Role

The primary roles of the skeletal system include structural support, movement in conjunction with the muscular and myofascial systems, organ protection, hematopoiesis (blood cell formation), and mineral storage. Bones are not static; they are constantly remodeling in response to mechanical forces and systemic signals. Osteoblasts build new bone tissue, while osteoclasts resorb it, maintaining a balance that is sensitive to both weight-bearing activity and hormonal inputs (particularly from the parathyroid glands, adrenal glands, and ovaries/testes).

Joints, the places where bones articulate, vary in type and degree of mobility. Synovial joints (such as the hip, knee, and shoulder) are freely movable and surrounded by joint capsules containing synovial fluid, which nourishes cartilage and reduces friction. Cartilage itself provides shock absorption and smooth movement surfaces. Ligaments connect bone to bone and provide passive joint stability, while tendons connect muscle to bone and transmit muscular force to create movement. Yoga *asana* engages the skeletal system directly, through load-bearing shapes and alignment cues, and indirectly, by supporting systems that maintain bone health, such as the endocrine system (e.g., sex hormones that influence bone density), muscular system (e.g., through active support), and nervous system (e.g., through interoception and neuroception and through autonomic nervous systems states). A nuanced understanding of skeletal variability, including differences in bone shapes and joint architecture, is crucial for creating inclusive and safe practices. Thus, the anatomy of the skeletal system is covered in great detail in later chapters.

### Yoga's Potential Impacts on the Skeletal System

Yoga can be highly beneficial for the skeletal system when practiced with awareness of load, alignment, and adaptability. Weight-bearing yoga *asana* can stimulate osteogenesis (i.e., the formation of new bone) by applying mechanical stressors that prompt remodeling. Standing postures and balances support bone health and strength, particularly in hips, spine, and legs, common sites for osteoporosis-related fractures. Joint mobility and cartilage nourishment are enhanced through movements that gently take joints through their available range of motion. Synovial fluid is secreted in response to movement, supporting lubrication and maintaining joint health. Gentle repetition and smooth transitions through *asana* may be particularly effective for joint health without overstressing surrounding connective tissue.

Bone health is influenced by hormonal balance and systemic inflammation. Thus, yoga's impact on the nervous and endocrine systems, particularly in reducing stress and supporting hormonal regulation, indirectly supports skeletal integrity. Practices that promote rest, vagal tone, and stable circadian rhythms may be especially important for populations at risk for bone loss, such as postmenopausal and andropausal individuals. Importantly, yoga offers a unique opportunity to explore skeletal awareness through proprioception and interoception. Cultivating a relationship with alignment not as a fixed ideal but as a dynamic relationship between structure, sensation, and function helps practitioners embrace their unique skeletal architecture (e.g., variations in femoral neck angles, spinal curvature, or hip socket depth; more of this below). Such understandings help reduce injury and empower new learning that can translate into agency and functional movement off the mat.

### *Cautions, Contraindications, and Guidance for Yoga vis-à-vis the Skeletal System*

When working with the skeletal system, intentionality, accessibility, and beneficence are essential, especially in populations with diagnosed skeletal conditions or acute or injuries. Individuals with osteoporosis or osteopenia may be at increased risk for fractures, especially in the spine, hips, and wrists. *Asana* is adapted to these individuals' needs by adding more cushioning and avoiding higher-risk movements involving deep flexion or extension, or spinal rounding under load. Instead, gentle extension, weight-bearing in a controlled range, and postures that encourage axial elongation are generally safe and beneficial. Similarly, for individuals with arthritis, practices may need to be varied according to flare cycles. During acute phases, rest and gentle range of motion may be appropriate, whereas during periods of remission, low-impact movement and gradual strengthening may support healthful joint function. Props and bolsters can be used to reduce load and offer joint support as needed.

Structural differences such as scoliosis, hypermobility, or joint replacements require thoughtful and creative variations. In the cases of hypermobility, muscular engagement and stability cues are essential. For individuals with joint replacements, care needs to be taken not to challenge safe directions and ranges of motion. Ideally, medical clearance is accompanied with clear guidance about contraindication and students are empowered to make auspicious choices for themselves. Cueing focuses on encouraging interoception, neuroception, and proprioception to honor functional range, skeletal diversity, and risk reduction. Yoga taught from this perspective optimizes inner work, not outer alignment or perfection, exploring alignment choices that feel supportive and sustainable for each unique skeletal system.

### *Muscular and Myofascial Systems*

The muscular system, responsible for producing movement, maintaining posture, and generating heat, traditionally refers to the body's skeletal (also, less relevant to yoga, smooth and cardiac) muscles and their associated tendons. However, in the context of yoga and modern movement science, the muscular system cannot be fully understood in isolation from the broader network of tendons, ligaments, fascia, and other connective tissues. These structures form a continuous, interwoven matrix that supports and responds to movement, load, and perception throughout the entire body. Within this expanded lens, supported by wholistic models (e.g., Thomas Myers' *Anatomy Trains)* and principles of biotensegrity, muscles, tendons, ligaments, and fascia function less as isolated levers and pulleys and more as dynamic participants in a responsive, elastic, and interconnected system. For yoga teachers and therapists, appreciating this whole-system view enriches the understanding of muscular effort, flexibility, and balance, while also deepening insight into subtle sensations, postural patterns, and healing practices. This wholistic systems view is applied throughout this volume and addressed in additional detail below, in a variety of contexts.

## Understanding the Muscular and Myofascial Systems' Role

At its core, the muscular system moves and stabilizes the body through coordinated contraction and release of skeletal muscles. These muscles exert force on bones via tendons to create movement at joints; they play a vital role in stabilizing the skeleton during both movement and rest; and they contribute to postural alignment and stability. Some muscles act as large prime movers, while others serve as fine-tuned stabilizers or synergists, contributing to balance, coordination, and proprioception. However, it is not just the muscle fibers that enable motion, it is the entire myofascial web. Fascia envelops and integrates every muscle, transmitting force and information throughout the body. Tension and tone in one region can influence movement patterns in another through fascial lines, which often correspond with traditional yoga postures and alignment patterns.

Ligaments, which connect bone to bone, contribute to postural integrity and joint stability. Together, muscles, tendons, fascia, and ligaments form a continuous, adaptable system that structures how we move, hold ourselves, and experience our bodies. Clearly, these systems are key to auspicious yoga practices and thus their anatomy and implications are explored in great detail in several chapters below.

## Yoga's Potential Impacts on the Muscular and Myofascial System

Yoga supports the muscular and myofascial systems in complex and powerful ways. Through conscious movement, yoga *asana* engages a spectrum of muscular actions, from strength to posture to stabilization, and invites a balance between effort and ease. Shapes such as Warrior 2 or Plank build strength in major muscle groups, while balance postures such as Tree or Half Moon recruit deep stabilizers. Flow sequences (e.g., *kriyas* and Sun Salutations) support functional endurance and neuromuscular coordination. Many yoga shapes challenge and improve active mobility (i.e., the ability to control movement through a healthful range of motion), which supports joint health and functional movement. *Asana* practices that incorporate eccentric loading (such as lowering slowly into a shape) and isometric are particularly helpful to improving strength and tissue resilience.

Importantly, yoga engages the entire myofascial web through multi-directional movement, tension, rotation, elongation, and compression. Rather than isolating muscles, yoga invites integrated patterns of movement that stimulate entire chains of muscles, fascia, and other connective tissues. Mobilization and wholesome alignment help hydrate fascia, improve glide between tissue layers, and support adaptability and responsiveness across all organ system.

Therapeutically, yoga can be used to retrain imbalances in muscular patterning, support recovery from injury, and improve postural dynamics. Rather than focusing on strengthening or stretching isolated muscles, a biotensegrity-informed approach to yoga tends to assess and influence whole-body integration. Movement cues based on fascial lines or functional patterns can help reawaken underused areas and redistribute effort across the system.

*Cautions, Contraindications, and Guidance for Yoga vis-à-vis the Muscular and Myofascial Systems*

Although yoga *asana* is generally beneficial for the muscular and fascial systems, certain cautions apply, especially related to fascial and connective tissue layers that surround and interpenetrate muscles. As covered in detail in relevant chapters, especially in Chapter 7, overstretching or passive end-range loading, particularly when students are not warmed up or force themselves into shapes based on outer aesthetics (rather than inner experience), can lead to microtears, instability, or long-term dysfunction. Fascia responds best to gradual, hydrated, and variable movement, qualities that yoga *asana* can provide when approached mindfully.

Individuals with acute or chronic musculoskeletal injuries, such as tendonitis, strains, or ligament sprains, benefit from slow progressions, attentiveness to sensation, and alignment cues that support functional recruitment as opposed to maximal range. In hypermobile bodies, the goal may be less about deepening flexibility and more about cultivating controlled movement, strength, and proprioceptive feedback. Yoga teachers and therapists also are aware of fascial sensitivity or areas of chronic tension that may hold emotional charge or are influenced by ego-drivenness. Releasing or working with such issues requires sensitivity and skill.

Neuromuscular conditions, such as Parkinson's disease, multiple sclerosis, or muscle dystrophies, may present with rigidity, weakness, tremor, or fatigue. For such individuals, yoga *asana* and *pranayama* can offer gentle ways to promote motor coordination, interoception, neuroception, and nervous system regulation. For such individuals, sequences are paced slowly, with attention to safety, support, and rest. Prop use and individualized variations are essential.

## What's Ahead

Having explored the physiology of the human body in some detail, it is now time to turn to integrated holistic anatomy. The discussion starts with a general overview of the key anatomical structures that are important to the practice, teaching, and therapeutic offering of yoga *asana*. Chapter 3 provides an overview of connective tissues, bones, joints, ligaments, muscles, and tendons. It closes with a brief review of the concept of anatomy trains or myofascial channels. Once this structural overview has been accomplished, Chapters 4, 5, and 6 provide additional detail about the key structural regions of the human body – namely, the axial, lower appendicular, and upper appendicular skeletons. Each chapter provides detail about the various structures of each respective region and closes with a closer look at understanding movement principles within it. Section 2 of the volume then applies all of this information to the teaching and clinical use of yoga *asana*.

*The human body is designed to live off nature. It is also designed to move. When it does very little of those two things, it fails to function properly and you pay the price.*
Beau Norton

# Chapter 3: Key Concepts of Integrated Holistic Anatomy

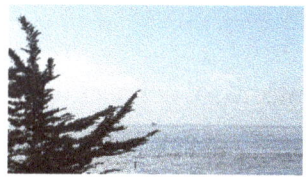

To repeat a central premise of integrated holistic yoga movement yet again, humans (all animals, really) exist within a continuous interconnected biotensegrity system. Any divisions or classification systems for biological structures are entirely artificial. Our brain does not think about or understand bodies (well, all *koshas*) in terms of single muscles or structures; it understands action and movement and automatically recruits and coordinates all necessary structures and layers of experience. This chapter covers human anatomy from a general overview perspective. Its focus on anatomy is not to be understood as a yogic focus on biology and the physical experience of what it means to be human - not even when strictly teaching or offering *asana* practices. Everything in human anatomy is intricately interwoven and interrelated with physiology, vitality, mind, emotions, relationships, and even our collective and communal or cultural embeddedness. As descriptions and implications of anatomy for yoga *asana* are offered, it is important always to hold this greater wholism in mind and to remember that a human being's entire experience and context comes to the mat.

The anatomical structures of interest to yoga that are emphasized in this chapter include connective tissues with tensile strength (e.g., tendons, ligaments, fascia), connective tissues with compressive strength (i.e., bones), joints (the articulation points of bones), and muscles. Their separate discussion does in no way imply their separation.

## Connective Tissues

In learning more about various connective tissues, it is helpful to recall that all of them come from the same stem cells. As noted previously, types of connective tissue vary widely and include fascia, ligaments, tendons, cartilage, bones, adipose tissue (fat), blood, and lymph. In other words, some connective tissues are fibrous sheets, bands, or gristly bits; some are fluids. Given their variety, it comes as no surprise that connective tissue is the most widely distributed and abundant tissue in the body. Via connective tissue, everything in the body is connected to everything else – nothing is separate. Connective tissue is the very essence of wholism.

Connective tissues are elastic and viscous; they are affected and built up by movement. Depending on our movement habits, we may build up symmetry and healthfulness or asymmetries and suffering. Connective tissues (especially fascia) line and protect the entirety of our insides. Any places where there is no connective tissues can be considered our "outsides", including (perhaps counterintuitively) the alimentary canal (i.e., food tube from mouth to anus) and respiratory channels (e.g., bronchi, trachea). Our discussion starts with connective tissues with great tensile strength and from there moves to connective tissues with compressive strength.

## Connective Tissues with Great Tensile Strength

### Fascia

The primary function of fascia is stabilization, connection, protection, and shape (organization). Fascia is the great stabilizer and organizer; it is a connective tissue that holds everything together – muscles, bones, joints, ligaments, tendons, organs – everything. There is superficial fascia (close to the body surface right under the skin) and deep fascia (e.g., wrapping organs). Fascia is essentially inseparable from the rest of the body, *links* all the structures of the body, *separates* structures to allow movement with minimal friction and to provide some shock absorption (e.g., nerves gliding within fascial structures, organ compartmentalization), and protects nerves, blood vessels, and muscle fibers. It transmits force via an uninterrupted, web-like organization that reaches throughout the body. It is the primary conductor of tensegrity and anatomy trains.

Fascia is essentially a large net that wraps everything and thus holds our shape (fascia, not skin, is this meta-membrane that holds our shape for us). There are four types of fasciae (see Figure 1.5):

- *Superficial* - the outermost layer, located directly beneath the skin and fatty tissue; a loose and web-like layer that helps connect the skin to the underlying muscles and stores fat
- *Deep* – deeper, denser, and more fibrous than superficial fascia, it surrounds muscles, bones, tendons, nerves, and blood vessels; it separates muscles into groups, provides support to muscles, and transmits forces of muscle contraction
- *Visceral* – surrounds and supports internal organs, such as the heart, lungs, and intestines; helps to hold organs in place and protects them from injury
- *Parietal* – lines the walls of body cavities (e.g., thoracic cavity and abdominal cavity), providing structural support and separating them from surrounding organs and tissues

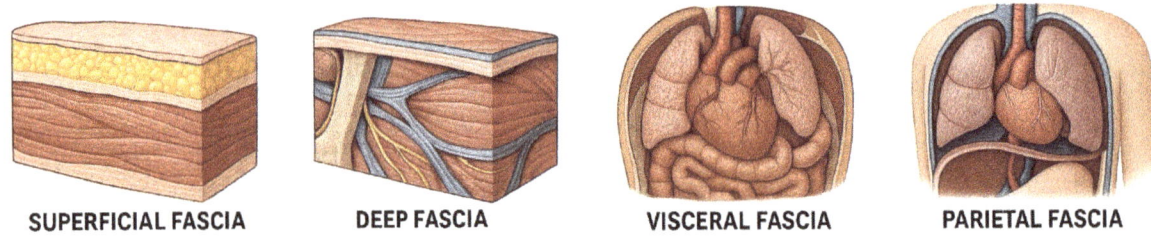

**Figure 1.5** Types of fascia. (Data source: Image generated by the author with support from AI).

### Fascia and Muscle

Fascia and muscle are essentially inseparable in form and function. While muscles generate force, fascia organizes, transmits, and modulates that force throughout the body. Understanding their relationship is essential for appreciating how movement occurs; namely, not as isolated action at joints, but as coordinated behavior across a continuous myofascial network. Fascia wraps not only entire muscles, but every muscle fiber within each individual muscle, ultimately transforming into the tendon through which muscles attach to bones (or, more accurately, attach to the periosteum of the bones which, in turn, is also made of fascia). In fact, 30% of every muscle is actually fascia (aka myofascia). These layers of fascia within and around muscle interconnect with tendons, ligaments, joint capsules, and neighboring fascial structures, forming a unified, load-sharing system. This continuity allows for lateral force transmission across adjacent muscles and along distant chains of tissues, not just from start to finish of a single muscle. In this way, fascia coordinates muscles into functional units (also known as anatomy trains – more about this later) rather than isolated movers.

Fascia is richly innervated with mechanoreceptors and sensory neurons, more so than muscle tissue itself. These receptors detect tension, pressure, vibration, pain, and stretch, feeding the central nervous system with vital proprioceptive and interoceptive information. This makes fascia a key player in movement coordination, balance, stability, and sensory awareness, helping increase physical adaptability and control. Fascia is also a dynamic tissue that responds to sustained patterns of stress, not unlike muscle tissue. It can thicken and stiffen with repetitive strain or immobility; it can increase or decrease in elasticity, and it can remodel itself based on habitual movement patterns. Some contractions and pain that are attributed to muscles are actually due to myofibroblasts in the fascia that are contracted due to physiological or psychological stress. They contract to stabilize the area in the face of stress and once this happens, myofibroblasts (cells involved in tissue repair and remodeling) multiply. As they multiply, pain can intensify, creating a vicious cycle. Interestingly, greater concentrations of myofibroblasts are found in painful tissue, especially as related to low back pain. Similarly, people with low back pain have many more myofibroblasts than people without such pain. It is unclear as to the direction of this relationship – in other words, it is difficult to discern whether individuals with more myofibroblasts are more prone to pain or whether pain increase the number of myofibroblasts.

### *Fascia and the Skeleton*

Fascia is integral to the way the musculoskeletal system maintains its internal coherence, and this includes the bones themselves. The outer surface of every bone is covered by a dense fascial layer known as the periosteum. The periosteum is a richly innervated and vascularized membrane that plays a critical role in bone nourishment, repair, and sensory feedback. The periosteum is continuous with the fascial sheaths of muscles and tendons that anchor into the bone, creating a seamless mechanical and sensory interface between bone and soft tissue. In addition to the periosteum, deeper fascial layers interweave through the trabecular matrix and marrow spaces of bones (more about this below), participating in the internal organization of osseous (or bony) tissue. Fascia's connection to bone is not a passive one; it contributes to distribution of mechanical load, transmission of force, and maintenance of spatial relationships within the skeletal system. In this way, fascia serves as both a boundary and a bridge, linking the solid framework of the skeleton with the dynamic movement of the body as a whole.

### *Fascia and the Nervous System*

Fascia, being the continuous, responsive connective tissue network that it is, also contributes significantly to the structural and functional integrity of the nervous system. Beginning at the level of the meninges (i.e., the specialized fascial layers that surround the brain and spinal cord), the fascial system in the brain and along the spinal cord includes the dura mater, arachnoid mater, and innermost pia mater, which adheres directly to neural tissue and anchors inferiorly near the coccyx. This uninterrupted fascial continuity provides mechanical support and protection for the central nervous system. Beyond the brain and spinal cord, fascia extends to enwrap peripheral nerves as they branch from the spinal column. Each peripheral nerve is composed of numerous axons, bundled together with vascular and fascial elements, collectively referred to as neurofascia. Integrated at the macroscopic meningeal layers and the microscopic wrappings around individual nerve fibers, fascia is an integral part and plays an important role in the overall organization, resilience, and potential adaptability of the nervous system's architecture and functions.

### *Fascia and the Organ Systems*

Fascia plays a central role in supporting and compartmentalizing the internal organs of the thoracic, abdominal, and pelvic cavities. Each organ is enwrapped by and infused in layers of visceral fascia that suspend, protect, and integrate the organ into the surrounding anatomical context (e.g., anchoring organs to the anterior longitudinal ligament of the spine). This visceral fascial integration includes the individual sheaths that directly encase an organ and the broader connective structures, such as mesenteries, ligaments, and membranes lining the abdominal cavity, all of which help connect organs to one another and the body wall and support the transmission of forces and maintain spatial relationships among the abdominal organs. This fascial fabric is richly vascularized and innervated, and thus serves not only structural functions but also contributes to proprioception, fluid dynamics, and communication across organ systems. Coordinated movement of organs during respiration, digestion, and elimination is made possible in part by the adaptability and glide capacity of the fascial network, which allows for differential movement between adjacent structures while maintaining overall coherence and support.

> *Fascia connects everything and can even be the sources of other structures:*
> - **Tendons** are the continuation of the fascia wrapping the individual muscle fibers (or myofibrils) in our muscles. There is no specific point where the muscles' fascia becomes a tendon; there is a diffuse myotendinous junction where this transition occurs.
> - **Ligaments,** also a continuation of fascia, are in series with the muscle-to-tendon transitions, working not in parallel so much as in conjunction.
> - **Fascia of tendons and ligaments** become the periosteum of bones and then penetrate deep inside the bone.

### *Fascia's Features and Importance*

This overview of fascia and its relationships to various human systems demonstrates that fascia is a most appropriate context for understanding movement, posture, and stability because it connects every structure in the body to everything else. Fascia is defined as a viscoelastic tissue that glues and weaves cells together. Fascial fibers are made of elastin, collagen, and reticulin (an immature form of collagen) and run between cells in a mucus-like extracellular ground substance of glycosaminoglycans (GAGs). Fascia contains a plethora of sensory receptors, contributing (significantly) to mechanoreception (e.g., pressure, tension, stretch, vibration, being stroked), proprioception (i.e., orientation in space), interoception (i.e., sensing the body from within, somatic mindfulness), nociception (i.e., pain perception; implicated in referred pain), and even neuroception (i.e., the perception of safety versus threat) via the autonomic nervous system.

As noted above, fascia has myofibroblasts that can contract, either due to physical stress or injury, or even in response to emotional or psychological stress. Such contraction in the fascia may limit range of motion more so than muscle tissue. If myofibroblasts stay chronically contracted (i.e., remain in an ongoing state of stress), tissues around it will remodel themselves to the shortened, contracted state over time. Relatedly, fascia provides a sliding surface between muscles and if it is damaged (e.g., due to injury or dehydration or inadequate nutrition (more below), adhesions are developed that limit movement between muscles fibers, and even between whole muscles. Because we are a connected whole, mobility limitations caused by adhesions are typically not only felt locally (where they are happening), but reverberate throughout the entire myofascial meridian connected to the fascia in question. One significant downside of such adhesions and the effect on movement patterns is related to head placement.

> Fascinatingly, healthy movement, facilitated by healthy fascia and healthy surrounding anatomy trains, holds the head still during action (see YouTube video of cheetah running https://www.youtube.com/watch?v=THA_5cqAfCQ). If fascial and related adhesions develop, unhealthy movement patterns develop and the head gets pulled out of alignment.

Fascia is a *biomechanical auto-regulating system* (Tom Myers in a workshop environment) and health in the fascia supports health to the rest of the body (e.g., research has demonstrated that as fascia heals, an irregular menstrual cycle may naturally reregulate). Fascia is either healthily mobile or unhealthily sticky. Unhealthy fascia can be caused by immobility, sedentary lifestyles, inflammation, injury/strain, poor nutritional status, over-exercise or excessive strain, movement pattern locks, and dehydration. Unhealthy fascia forms adhesions and becomes rigid (felt-like, rather than lattice-like) and can limit movement and adaptability. Fascia stays healthy via nutrition, hydration, and movement. Nutrition reaches fascia via capillaries that leak food, oxygen, and neuropeptides (messenger molecules). Adequate hydration creates well-lubricated fascia that moves freely.

Movement is key in any of these processes, creating the environment so that available nutrients and fluids can enter and leave the fascia as needed to maintain health. Movement helps organize fascia into a double lattice organization rife with collagen fibrils that absorb water and stay hydrated. In that sense, fascia acts like a sponge: squeezing releases water and releasing the squeeze allows new water to enter. Movement not only hydrates the fascia, but also cleanses and nourishes fascial tissue by removing detritus and toxins (including metabolites and cytokines). Movement of fascia even exerts a mechanical force on our DNA and thus has epigenetic influences on genetic expression.

### *Fascia and Integrated Holistic Yoga Movement*

With lack of movement, fascia becomes felt-like, losing mobility, resilience, and its double lattice orientation. The more varied the movement, the more resilient the fascia. Therefore, it is helpful to move not only linearly, but to incorporate spirals, cross-crawl movement, and shearing actions (all of which are actions that are incorporated into yoga *asana* practices) to adequately engage, stimulate, and hydrate fascia. Immobility traps toxins in fascial cells and in the extracellular ground substance. When we begin to move again, these toxins are released. For example, deep massage or a yoga class focused on twisting can make people feel 'liverish' – the liver gets overwhelmed with toxins temporarily; it is important to integrate more movement until such a reaction no longer occurs. At the other extreme, over-exercise without rest, only squeezes fluid out and dehydrates fascia. The ongoing strain prevents rehydration and can cause fascia to become immobile and more injury prone. Relevant to teaching *asana*, over-stretching can be problematic for individuals who are hypermobile – the very people who are often drawn to yoga. For them, focus needs to be on strengthening and slow, controlled transitions between shapes and movements to support fascial tensioning without overlengthening.

## Tendons

Tendons are dense, fibrous connective tissues that anchor muscle to bone. They are vital to joint mobility and mechanical precision, acting as anatomical bridges that translate the force of muscle contraction into skeletal movement. Each muscle typically attaches to two bones via tendons: the *origin* is the fixed or less mobile attachment point (usually proximal to the body's center), and the *insertion* is the more mobile attachment point (usually the distal bone further away from the body's center). When a muscle contracts, the tendon transmits force from the region of the muscle's origin to the region of the muscle's insertion, generating motion across the joint that lies between origin and insertion. Unlike muscles, which actively generate force, tendons transmit that force, ensuring efficient and coordinated movement across joints. Tendons are composed primarily of collagen fibers arranged in parallel bundles, aligned in the direction of tensile stress. This architecture allows them to withstand high loads during muscle contraction while minimizing excess elongation.

The structural relationship between tendon, muscle, and bone is continuous. Specifically, at their origin, tendon fibers blend seamlessly with the muscle's connective tissue layers (epimysium and perimysium) at the musculotendinous junction. At their insertion points, tendons merge with the periosteum (connective tissue surrounding bone), creating a structural continuum from muscle to skeleton. In some anatomical texts, tendons are even described as a specialized extension of the periosteum, adapted for load transmission across muscle groups. It is noteworthy in a yoga *asana* movement context to understand that the area where tendon transitions into bone, at the enthesis, is biomechanically complex and considered more vulnerable to strain or injury, particularly under repetitive or excessive load.

Tendons contribute to joint mobility not by stretching significantly, but by providing tensioned precision. They have limited elasticity, which enhances the accuracy and responsiveness of skeletal movement. Rather than introducing slack or range, tendons help direct the exact amount of motion dictated by muscle contraction. Their carefully calibrated (and appropriately limited) elasticity supports flexion and extension without compromising joint stability. It serves to reduce energy loss during force transmission and minimizes excessive joint motion, enhancing proprioceptive control. Although tendons themselves are relatively inelastic, they function in coordination with myofascia, which can contribute to tissue flexibility through mechanisms like myofibroblast contraction and multidirectional force dispersion.

## Tendons and Integrated Holistic Movement

Tendons (samples are shown in Figures 1.6 and 1.7) have less blood supply than muscle tissue, which limits their healing capacity. However, they are more vascularized than ligaments and generally heal faster when injured. Still, healing is slower than in richly perfused tissue, and repetitive microtrauma or poorly managed stress can lead to chronic issues such as tendinopathy. Tendons can tolerate minor elongation (typically up to 4% strain), but beyond approximately 10%, structural damage may occur. Such injury is usually classified as a strain or partial tear.

Given the structural and vascular realities of tendons and their limitations on healing, a few cautions and considerations are helpful when offering yoga *asana* and other yoga-based movement.

- Monitor sensation at the origin and insertion points of muscles. Pain at these sites may indicate stress on the tendon. Stretching should produce sensation primarily in the muscle belly, not at attachment points.
- Avoid bouncing, aggressive end-range loading, or holding extended joint positions under strong force, especially in vulnerable joints.
- Tendon strain is more likely if a muscle is overloaded in a stretched position or repeatedly used without adequate recovery.
- Although care is essential, some stress on tendons is beneficial. Emerging research suggests that optimal loading of tendons can stimulate collagen remodeling and enhance recoil capacity, supporting tissue resilience and injury prevention. The key is progressive, well-distributed, and varied load over time.

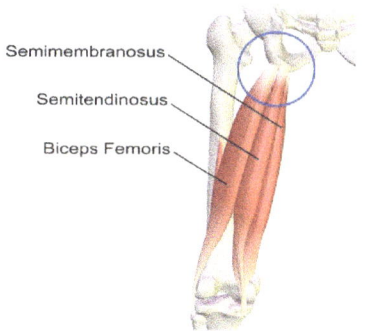
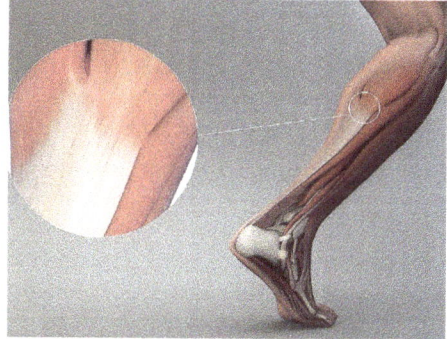

**Figure 1.6** Hamstrings with tendons (origin circled at the ischial tuberosity). (Data source: Paul Hermans; https://upload.wikimedia.org/wikipedia/commons/2/2b/Opgespannen_hamstrings_%28cropped%29.jpg; Creative Commons Attribution 4.0)

**Figure 1.7** Magnified view of a tendon. (Data source: Scientific Animations; https://upload.wikimedia.org/wikipedia/commons/e/ea/Magnified_view_of_a_Tendon.jpg; Creative Commons Attribution 4.0)

## Ligaments

Ligaments are dense bands of connective tissue that link bone to bone, providing stability at joints and contributing to controlled range of motion. While tendons transmit the force of muscular contraction, ligaments restrain and stabilize, guiding movement and preventing excess or aberrant motion. They are especially crucial at synovial joints, where mobility and structural integrity must be carefully balanced.

When observing a ligament, it is helpful to ask: What motion is this structure meant to resist or support? Each ligament is oriented to control specific vectors of stress, contributing to a joint's overall functional stability.

### *Form: Multidirectional Design for Multiplanar Demand*

Ligaments are composed of collagen and elastin fibers; however, unlike tendons, these fibers are not aligned in one consistent direction. Instead, they are arranged multidirectionally, adapted to handle the complex forces acting on a joint from various angles. The ratio of elastin to collagen determines a ligament's pliability – some are more supple, allowing for controlled give, while others are stiff and resist movement.
- With age, elastin content decreases and ligaments become less pliable, reducing adaptability and increasing vulnerability to strain.
- Some ligaments, such as the ligamentum flavum in the spine, are more elastic than others by design. However, even these do not behave like rubber bands – they do not fully recoil to original length once overstretched.

### *Function: More Than Passive Restraints*

Ligaments are not passive end-range limiters. They are deeply integrated into the myofascial and skeletal system and work in concert with muscles, tendons, and joint capsules. When a joint requires increased range, such as during sustained practice or developmental movement, ligaments can release low-level contracture to allow for that motion. Still, ligaments are not the primary determinants of mobility. Joint stability and flexibility arise from the collaborative behavior of contiguous tissues: dynamic control of muscle, directional tension of fascia, transmission of force by tendons, and restraining influence of ligaments together define a joint's capacity for safe movement.

### *Ligaments and Integrated Holistic Movement*

Ligaments (samples are shown in Figures 1.8 and 1.9) respond to load over time, developing resilience and structural tolerance. However, they do not and cannot adapt by becoming significantly longer. A ligament can distend (lengthen) under sufficient force, but it does not return fully to its original shape if overstretched. In other words, a sprained ligament (overstretched or torn) will never again be quite the same. It may contribute to a new range of motion, but often with reduced stability. Spraining a ligament trades stability for mobility – not a great trade. It is noteworthy in a yoga *asana* context that ligaments are more vulnerable to sprain when tissues are warmed or hypermobile, especially in high-heat environments.

Given the structural and vascular realities of ligaments and their limitations on healing, a few cautions and considerations are helpful offering yoga *asana* and other yoga-based movement.
- Avoid end-range loading that is forceful or repeated, especially in heated environments; ligaments are more susceptible to overstretch in warmth.
- Never cue for a "stretch in the joint" as this risks placing strain directly on ligamentous structures. Instead, direct attention to muscle lengthening and myofascial sensation.

- Do not assume that greater range of motion equals healthier tissue. Ligamentous overlengthening is not functional flexibility; it is micro-injury.
- Do not overpower conscious control and support in joints – that is, never force a range of motion passively.
- Optimal loading over time can build resilience in ligamentous tissue, but that must be done with slow progression and deep respect for anatomical limits.

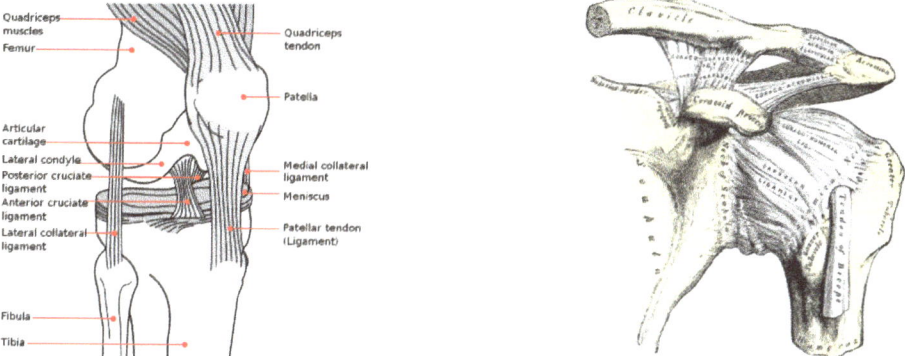

**Figure 1.8** Knee anatomy. (Data source: Mysid; https://commons.wikimedia.org/wiki/File:Knee_diagram.svg; public domain)

**Figure 1.9** Shoulder anatomy. (Data source: Henry Gray, 1918; https://commons.wikimedia.org/wiki/File:Gray326.png; public domain)

## Bones – Connective Tissue with Greater Compressive Strength

Bone, or osseous tissue, is a specialized form of connective tissue with exceptional compressive strength. It is the densest, hardest, and most rigid of the connective tissues in the body, yet it remains remarkably dynamic and responsive to load and demand. Its structural integrity is largely due to its mineralized matrix, primarily composed of calcium hydroxyapatite, which gives bone its rigidity, while its functional adaptability stems from its living cellular makeup. Unlike other connective tissues that are more tensile or elastic (including fascia, tendons, and ligaments), bones are uniquely designed to withstand gravitational pressure and support compressive loads. Figure 1.10 shows the relaxed bony skeleton of a human.

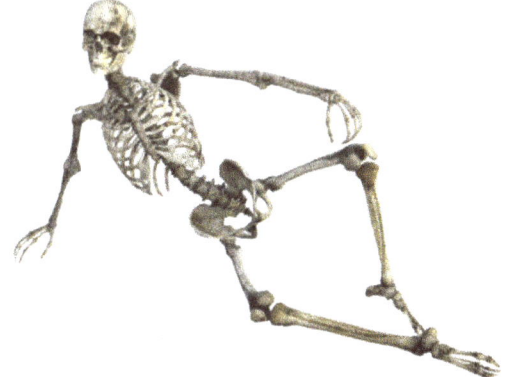

**Figure 1.10** Relaxing skeleton. (Data source: TheDigitalArtist; https://commons.wikimedia.org/wiki/File:Skeleton_relaxing.png; public domain)

Bones are constantly remodeled throughout life in response to mechanical stimuli, a principle described by Wolff's Law, which states that bone develops along lines of mechanical stress. This means that weight-bearing activities not only preserve bone density but also shape and strengthen bones in a functionally specific way. Consequently, bones exhibit significant bioindividuality, as each individual's movement habits, posture, and loading patterns leave lasting impressions on skeletal structure, health, and function. Bones never operate in isolation. They are deeply interconnected with muscles, tendons, ligaments, and fascia, forming a continuous, interdependent, co-regulating, co-moving, co-stabilizing interconnected system that functions as a unified whole. This interdependence allows for stability, mobility, and adaptability in response to both internal forces and external demands.

## *Functions of Bones*

Although the function of bones is most commonly associated with structural support and movement, their roles are much more diverse than and, in fact, vital across multiple physiological systems. They serve as:
- *Levers for movement*: Acting as rigid attachment points for muscles, bones, in conjunction with joints, convert muscular contractions into directed movement.
- *Structural support*: Providing a framework for the body, bones support regions such as the head, neck, and upper limbs.
- *Protection*: Encasing delicate internal organs, bones protect critical structures such as the brain (skull), heart and lungs (rib basket), and pituitary gland (sella turcica).
- *Mineral reservoirs*: Serving as dynamic stores, bones store and provide calcium, potassium, magnesium, and other minerals that are continuously exchanged with the bloodstream.
- *Blood cell production*: Within the bone marrow, bones generate millions of blood cells per minute, including red blood cells (lifespan ~120 days), white blood cells (hours to days), and platelets (1–2 days).
- *Adaptation to gravity*: The skeletal system allows the body to function efficiently in a gravitational field. Proper alignment of bones and joints enables force to travel effectively through the system, reducing unnecessary strain and optimizing balance and stability.

## *Characteristics of Bones*

### *Types of Bones*

Bones have two main components or types of osseus tissue (see Figure 1.11): compact and trabecular, each serving distinct structural and metabolic purposes. Depending on location and function of a particular bone, the proportion of types of bone varies widely. Specifically, the more weight bearing demands are made on the bone, the higher proportion of compact bone. Blood vessels flow in the bone's inner spaces to provide nutrients to the bone and receive and distribute the blood cells made in the bone marrow.
- *Compact bone* (or cortical bone): Dense, strong, and smooth in appearance, compact bone forms the outer layer of most bones. It consists of collagen fibers mineralized with calcium salts and contains minimal porosity (5–30%), allowing it to bear significant weight and resist bending forces.

- *Trabecular bone* (or cancellous or spongy bone): Found primarily in the interior of bones, trabecular bone has a lattice-like structure that makes it lighter while maintaining strength. The spaces within this matrix house bone marrow and allow for the flow of blood vessels that nourish the tissue and support hematopoiesis (blood cell production).

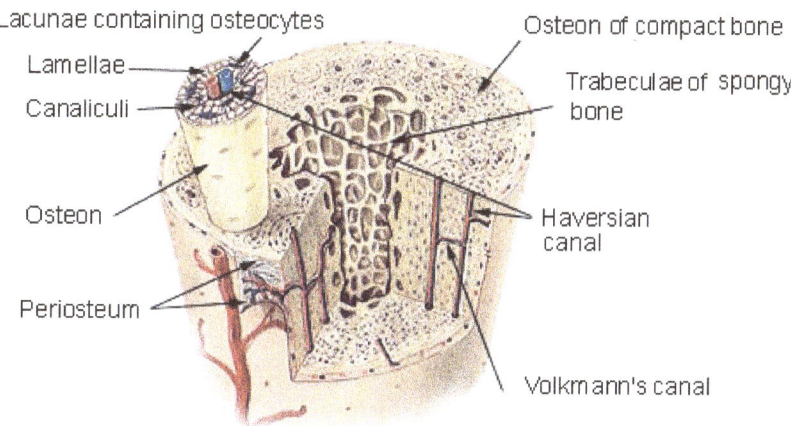

**Figure 1.11** Bone anatomy. (Data source: SEER; https://commons.wikimedia.org/wiki/File:Illu_compact_spongy_bone.jpg; public domain)

## Bone Remodeling, Adaptation, and Health

Bone is highly responsive to its mechanical environment; it has tremendous plasticity and capacity for remodeling, changing shape (over time) according to (repetitive) stresses put on it. This adaptive process can be advantageous and beneficial, but it can also have disadvantages. Poor postural habits, excessive load, or misalignment can lead to degenerative changes, whereas thoughtful movement and alignment practices can promote skeletal health and resilience. The bone remodeling process happens across the entire human life span, and relies on two main types of cells:

- *Osteoblasts* build new bone by secreting collagen fibers and glycoproteins that bind with calcium salts to form the mineralized matrix.
- *Osteoclasts* break down old or damaged bone, enabling repair and reshaping in response to injury, disuse, or increased demand.

Bones are embedded in and continuous with fascial tissue, underscoring their role in an integrated biomechanical system. This connection also supports bone health in that bone is nourished via the periosteum, a vascularized fascial covering. The periosteum is a fibrous, vascular membrane that surrounds bones and connects them to tendons and muscles. It plays a vital role in nourishing bone and transmitting mechanical load. The periosteum is continuous with the endosteum, the inner lining of compact bone, creating a seamless fascial interface from the external muscle layers to the interior of the skeletal structure. This fascial continuity reinforces the idea that bones are not isolated mechanical levers but key collaborative elements in the human biotensegrity that is a dynamic, interconnected system.

## Bone Classifications and Key Features

Bones can be categorized based on shapes and functions (see Figure 1.12):
- *Long bones* (e.g., femur, humerus, tibia): facilitate movement and support body weight; primarily found in the limbs
- *Short bones* (e.g., tarsals, carpals): provide stability and fine-tuned movement; commonly found in the wrists and ankles
- *Flat bones* (e.g., scapula, sternum, cranial bones): Protect internal organs and offer broad surfaces for muscle attachments
- *Irregular bones* (e.g., vertebrae): serve specialized functions and have complex shapes suited to their specialization
- *Sesamoid bones* (e.g., patella): form within tendons to protect them from stress and enhance their mechanical leverage across joints

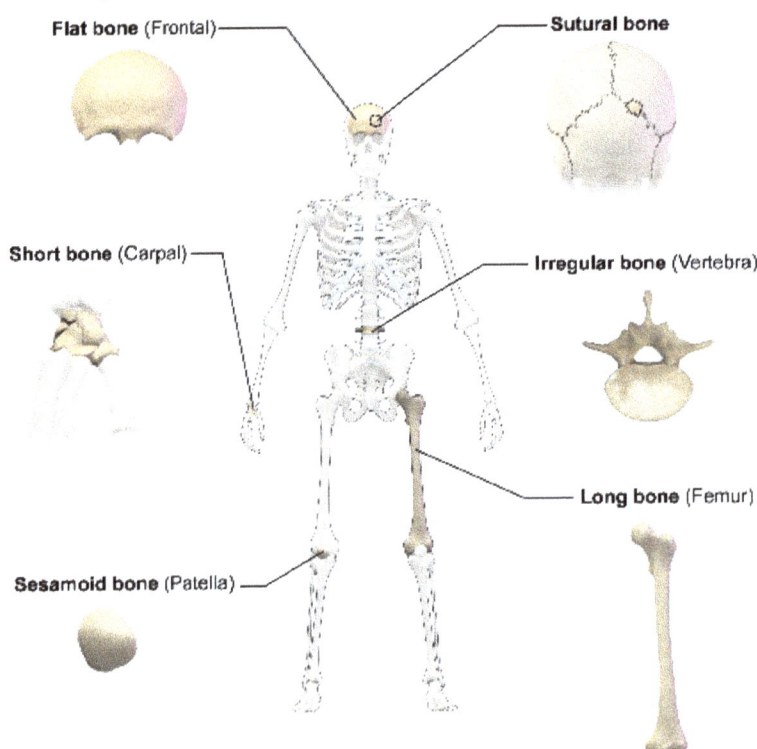

**Figure 1.12** Classification of bones. (Data source: BruceBlaus; https://commons.wikimedia.org/wiki/File:Blausen_0229_ClassificationofBones.png; Creative Commons Attribution 3.0)

Bones have several key anatomical features that serve specific functions:
- *Foramina*: These openings in bone allow passage for nerves and blood vessels.
- *Fossae and depressions*: These indentations may accommodate articulating bones or soft tissues.
- *Bony prominences*: These projections, such as tubercles, condyles, trochanters, spines, and crests, serve as attachment points for tendons and ligaments and can profoundly influence joint mechanics and range of motion:
  - processes, condyles, or tuberosity serve as attachment points for tendons, ligaments, and other connective tissue

○ ridges, spines, or crests, (e.g., trochanter of the femur) serve as attachment points for tendons, ligaments, and other connective tissue; they affect ranges of motion and pushing past bony limits created by these bony features can result in wear-and-tear injuries

## *Overview of Bones and Their Bioindividuality*

At birth, human babies have approximately 270 bones. As children grow, many of these bones fuse together, particularly in the skull, spine, and pelvis. By adulthood, most individuals have around 206 bones, but this number is an average, not an absolute. The precise number can vary from person to person due to differences in development, genetics, or evolutionary remnants. These differences are generally not pathological; they simply reflect the diversity of human form. A few common examples of normal bone number variations include, but by no means are limited to, the following:

- *Accessory ribs*: Some people are born with an extra rib, most commonly a cervical rib extending from the seventh cervical vertebra. This occurs in roughly 0.5–1% of the population and may be asymptomatic or, in some cases, contribute to thoracic outlet syndrome, if the extra bone compresses nearby nerves or blood vessels.
- *Sacral vertebrae*: The sacrum is typically formed by the fusion of five vertebrae, but in some individuals, one additional vertebra may fuse with the sacrum (called sacralization), or the lowest lumbar vertebra may remain unfused (lumbarization), affecting both structure and movement patterns in the low back.
- *Coccyx variation*: The coccyx usually consists of three to five small bones, and the exact number may vary. These bones may be partially fused or completely separate.
- *Supernumerary bones*: Extra bones, known as accessory or supernumerary bones, can appear in the hands (e.g., extra carpal bones) or feet (e.g., *os trigonum*, an additional bone behind the ankle). These extra bones are generally harmless though they can contribute to pain or restricted movement.
- *Missing bones*: Conversely, some individuals may naturally lack a bone, such as a congenitally absent vertebra or a missing third molar (technically a bone-like structure, though not part of the skeleton). This does not necessarily lead to dysfunction and is simply part of that person's unique skeletal blueprint.

## *Bioindividuality of Bones and Integrated Holistic Yoga Movement*

In addition to differences in the number of bones, subtle to significant variations in the shapes, sizes, and angles of bones are common and can have crucial implications for movement, joint function, and range of motion. Just like variation in number of bones, these shape-based differences are not abnormalities; they are normal variations within human anatomy, influenced by genetics, developmental patterns, habitual movement, and even cultural and environmental factors. Shape, size, and angle variations affect joint congruence, leverage, muscle recruitment, and mobility. Understanding them supports safer and more individualized approaches to movement practices like yoga *asana*, where anatomical uniqueness can guide how a person expresses a shape. A few common examples of normal shape, size, and angle variations include, but by no means are limited to, the following:

- *Femoral neck angle* (neck-shaft angle): The angle between shaft (the long, main part of the femur) and neck of the femur varies between individuals. The average angle is around 125°, but it can range from 110° to 140°. Angle variations can greatly affect movement patterns and ranges of motion in shapes that require hip adduction, abduction, and/or rotation (e.g., Butterfly or Pigeon). Yoga professionals need to take care not to cue and never to force outer alignments that are not accessible to individuals with specific variation in the angle of their femoral neck.
    o A smaller angle (*coxa vara*) can increase hip stability but may reduce range in abduction.
    o A larger angle (*coxa valga*) may allow more lateral movement but can reduce stability and increase risk of dislocation.
- *Femoral anteversion/retroversion*: This shape differentiation refers to the rotation of the femoral neck relative to the shaft. In anteversion, the femoral neck twists forward, which can result in inward rotation of the hip and femur. In retroversion, the neck angles backward, contributing to outward rotation. These rotational differences can significantly affect a person's available range of motion in shapes such as Warrior 2 or certain seated shapes and should not be 'corrected' to a presumed 'normal' position or range of motion.
- *Pelvic inlet shape*: Pelvis shapes differ across individuals and, broadly, across biological sexes. Some pelvises are wider and shallower (more typical in women), while others are narrower and taller (more typical in men), affecting spinal curvature, hip alignment, and weight transfer through the sacroiliac joints. These differences can show up in foundational placement of the legs and feet in standing shapes, especially asymmetrical shapes, such as Lunge, Warrior, and side-angle shapes. Yoga professionals therefore take care not to require particular foot placements in these positions (e.g., avoid cues about paralleling feet to an outer referent or cues about how far apart the feet should be), instead allowing students to place the feet (width-wise and length-wise) to reflect their natural anatomy.
- *Acetabular depth and orientation*: The depth and angle of hip sockets vary, affecting the degree to which the femur can flex, abduct, or externally rotate. A deeper socket increases stability but may limit range or motion; a shallower socket allows for greater mobility but can increase susceptibility to joint wear. Individuals with greater range of motion may be inadvertently encouraged by yoga teacher to 'abuse' their mobility in an effort to seek a particular idealized outer alignment of a shape.
- *Tibial torsion*: The tibia can exhibit internal or external torsion, where the distal end of the tibia (near the ankle) rotates relative to the proximal end (near the knee). This affects foot placement in standing postures and walking gait. This alignment cannot be fixed through cueing or shaming; it is structural. Yoga teachers best refrain from absolutes with regard to foot placement.
- *Scapular and clavicular variation*: The size, curve, and orientation of the clavicle and scapula influence shoulder mechanics, including how far and easily one can abduct or flex the arm overhead. These structures are rarely symmetrical side to side. Yoga professionals honor individual variability by not prescribing certain ranges of motion, especially in the context of using props or passive movement. For example, raising the arms with a strap in hand and then lowering them behind the back requires great sensitivity to range of motion and flexible hand placement on the strap. Better yet, instead of using a strap, a resistance band is used to create a natural adjustment to individuals' anatomy.
- *Humeral torsion*: Like the femur, the humerus can twist along its length. This impacts internal and external rotation of the shoulder and affects expressions of shapes such as

Downward Facing Dog or Cow Face. Offering a variety of movements in the arms and placements for the hands with invitations for interoception and proprioception are key to helping students or clients find their authentic embodiment of such shapes.

Bone variability, whether in number, shape, size, or angles, underscores the principle of bioindividuality among humans. Although anatomical texts and images offer useful normative averages, they do not and cannot capture the wide range of natural variation. Understanding this great uniqueness in how humans are structured is especially relevant in yoga *asana*, other movement practices, and clinical settings, where a teacher or clinician cannot assume identical structure and function across different bodies. Respecting human structural and functional differences helps support individualized and person-tailored movement strategies and prevents forcing bodies into unsuitable alignments or ranges of motion. It invites yoga teachers, clinicians, and practitioners to shift away from rigid alignment models in posture practice and toward functional movement patterns that honor each body's structure and capacity.

## *Normative Overview of the Bones in the Human Body*

Having elucidated human skeletal variation, a few normative skeletal averages are offered nevertheless. Specifically, the human skeleton (shown in Figures 1.13 and 1.14) is typically divided into three distinct portions: axial skeleton, upper appendicular skeleton, and lower appendicular skeleton. Additionally, there are six bones in the ears, called ossicles, that are not covered in this volume. An overview of the three primary divisions of the skeleton is provided here; a detailed analysis follows in Chapters 4 to 6. Implications are covered in Section 2 of this volume, in the context of yoga-based movement.

- The axial skeleton has an average of 74 bones and consists of the following structures – all covered in detail in Chapter 4:
  - cranium (frontal, temporal, occipital, and parietal bones)
  - face (e.g., mandible, sphenoid bone [behind the eyes])
  - spine – vertebrae (C1-7; T1-12; L1-5; S1-S5 [fused]; coccyx [3-5 fused vertebrae])
  - rib basket (12 rib pairs and sternum)
- The lower appendicular skeleton has an average of 62 bones, 52 (or so) of which are in the feet, and consists of the following structures – all covered in detail in Chapter 5:
  - pelvic girdle
  - leg bones
  - feet
- The upper appendicular skeleton has an average of 64 bones, 54 (or so) of which are in the hands, and consists of the following structures – all covered in detail in Chapter 6.
  - shoulder girdle
  - arm bones
  - hands

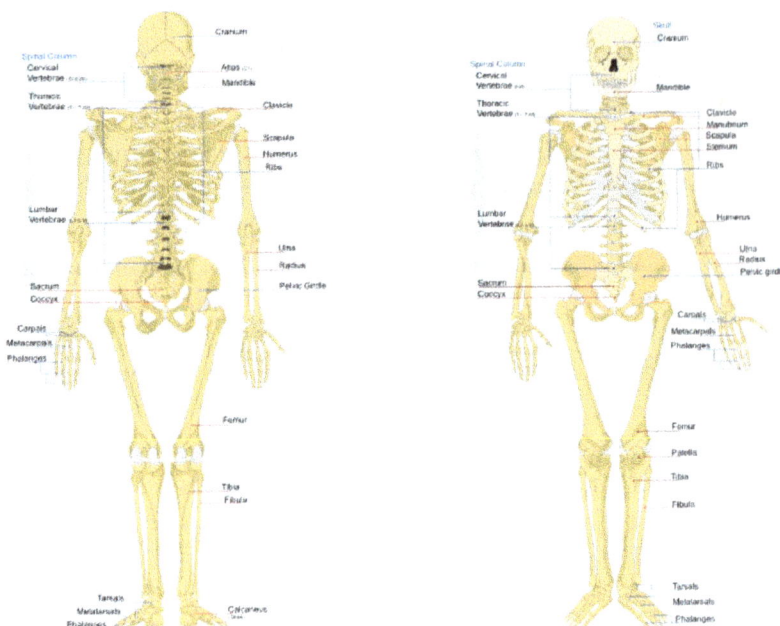

**Figure 1.13** Human skeleton: Back. (Data source: LadyofHats; https://commons.wikimedia.org/wiki/File:Human_skeleton_back_en.svg; public domain)

**Figure 1.14** Human skeleton: Front. (Data source: LadyofHats; https://commons.wikimedia.org/wiki/File:Human_skeleton_front_en.svg; public domain)

## Joints – Articulations of Bones

Joints (aka arthroses) are the connections or *articulations* between bones. The articulating surfaces of joints protect and connect bones via a range of special features and structures. Joints are the bridge between two bones and are either movable (e.g., knee, elbow), semi-rigid (e.g., pubic symphysis), or completely rigid (e.g., the skull sutures). Not surprisingly, and as alluded to above, joint depths and shapes have tremendous bioindividuality, meaning that most joints do not conform to what is depicted in anatomy books or this volume. The same joint in ten different people will like have ten variations in shape, function, and range of motion.

Notably, joints have no direct blood supply. Their nourishment comes from the periosteum of adjacent bones. Nourishment moves into the joints mostly via movement in the joint. This, of course, is one of the many reasons why yoga *asana* – any movement, really – is so healthful for joints. Joints have to balance stability versus mobility. It is important to understand which joint emphasizes which aspect. Active joints have to stabilize during movement, a feat accomplishes via collaboration of joint capsules, ligaments, tendons, and muscles, all of which contribute to the stiffening or stabilization of a joint when it is in action. A very accessible way to notice this collaboration is to sit on the floor with legs outstretched (i.e., in Staff shape). From here, relax the legs and palpate the patella (or knee cap) of the knee. It will likely move quite freely. Now engage the quadricep muscles of the upper thighs by pressing the legs into the earth and flexing the ankle so the toes move toward the hips (dorsiflexion). From this braced position once again palpate the patella and note the profound change as it has now stabilized along with the entire knee joint.

## Types of Joints by Structure

Joints can be classified by their structural composition, which determines how they connect and move. The three primary structural types are fibrous joints, cartilaginous joints, and synovial joints, each defined by the type of tissue that links the bones.

### Fibrous Joints

Fibrous joints, also known as synarthroses, are highly stable articulations where bones are connected by dense fibrous connective tissue. They allow little to no movement, which is why anatomists often classify them as immovable. However, kinesiologists acknowledge that some fibrous joints permit minimal motion that may still hold biomechanical significance, especially in areas such as the sacroiliac (SI) joints. Despite their limited mobility, fibrous joints often play critical roles in stability, force transmission, and structural integrity across the skeleton.

There are three subtypes of fibrous joints:
- *Sutures*, found between skull bones, which may ossify with age (see Figure 1.15)
- *Syndesmoses*, such as the interosseous membrane between the radius and ulna or tibia and fibula
- *Gomphoses*, peg-in-socket joints like the connection between teeth and the alveolar bones

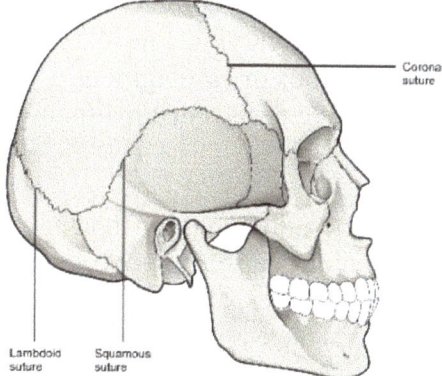

**Figure 1.15** Skull sutures. (Data source: OpenStax; https://commons.wikimedia.org/wiki/File:901_Skull_Sutures.jpg; Creative Commons Attribution 3.0)

### Cartilaginous Joints

*Cartilaginous joints, or amphiarthroses*, are stable connections where bones are united by cartilage – either hyaline cartilage or fibrocartilage (see Figures 1.16 and 1.17). These joints allow for limited movement, balancing stability with flexibility in regions that need to absorb and transmit force. A cartilaginous disc or pad provides shock absorption and load distribution, while surrounding ligaments add further reinforcement. Common examples include the pubic symphysis and the intervertebral joints of the spine. Although movement at cartilaginous joints is minimal, their structural design supports essential functions in shock absorption, axial alignment, and the transmission of forces through the spine and pelvis.

Cartilaginous joints are divided into two subtypes:
- *Synchondroses* are formed by hyaline cartilage and are often temporary, such as the epiphyseal (growth) plates in developing long bones. Some, like the joint between the first rib and the manubrium, are permanent but still relatively rigid.
- *Symphyses* involve fibrocartilage, which provides greater resistance to compression. These are permanent and slightly movable joints, such as the pubic symphysis and the intervertebral discs.

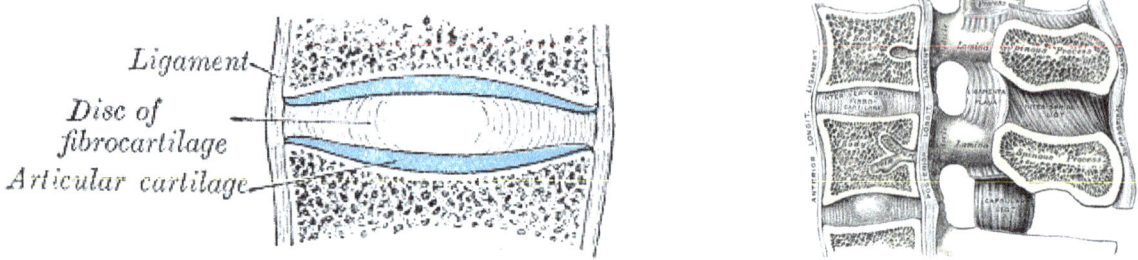

**Figure 1.16** Ligament and cartilage anatomy. (Data source: Henry Vandyke Carter; https://commons.wikimedia.org/wiki/File:Gray298.png ; public domain)

**Figure 1.17** Lumbar vertebrae and ligaments. (Data source: Henry Vandyke Carter; https://commons.wikimedia.org/wiki/File:Gray301.png; public domain)

## *Synovial Joints*

*Synovial joints, also known as diarthroses*, are the most mobile and structurally complex type of joint in the body. They allow for a wide range of movement, with mobility varying considerably depending on the specific joint. Although less inherently stable than fibrous or cartilaginous joints, synovial joints are supported by an integrated system of connective tissues that maintain relative stability during motion.

Each synovial joint contains a joint cavity between the articulating bones, allowing for freer movement than in other joint types. The joint is enclosed by a ligamentous capsule composed of two layers: an outer fibrous layer that blends with the periosteum of the bones, and an inner synovial membrane that produces synovial fluid. This viscous fluid fills the cavity and lubricates the joint, reducing friction and nourishing the articular cartilage. The ends of the bones are covered with hyaline (articular) cartilage, a tough, smooth, and dense tissue that ensures virtually frictionless movement when healthy. Joint health in synovial structures relies heavily on fluid dynamics. During compression, synovial fluid is expelled from the joint space; after the compressive load is removed, movement such as gentle shaking helps reintroduce fluid into the joint. This rehydration is especially important in older bodies, in which inadequate return of fluid can lead to drying and degeneration of the cartilage. Practices that encourage joint decompression and gentle motion are essential for preserving synovial joint function over time.

Surrounding the joint capsule, ligaments provide varying levels of passive stabilization, whereas muscles and tendons contribute dynamic support (see Figures 1.18 and 1.19). Ideally, the muscles on either side of the joint are balanced in strength and tone. Imbalances can lead to uneven compressive forces, increasing the risk of articular cartilage wear, especially in joints such as the hips and knees. Over time, chronic muscular imbalances may contribute to degenerative changes in joint structure. Additional features of synovial joints include:

- Bursae, fluid-filled sacs located in areas of high friction, such as the elbows, knees, and beneath the deltoid muscle at the shoulder
- Tendon sheaths, which protect tendons that pass through confined or high-friction pathways

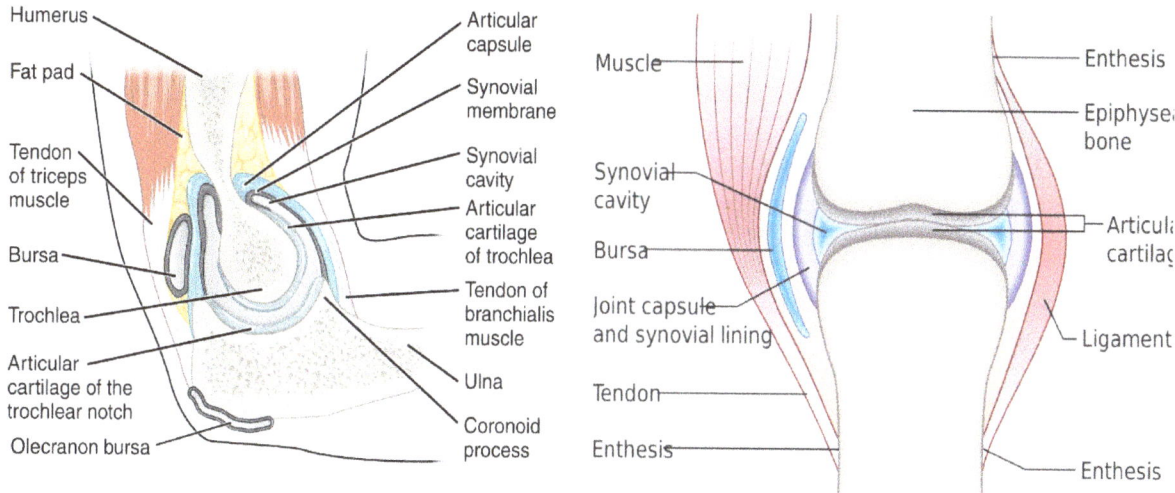

**Figure 1.18** Synovial joint anatomy - elbow. (Data source: OpenStax College; https://commons.wikimedia.org/wiki/File:915_Elbow_Joint.jpg; Creative Commons Attribution 3.0)

**Figure 1.19** Synovial joint anatomy - knee. (Data source: Madhero88; https://commons.wikimedia.org/wiki/File:Joint_white-bone.svg; Creative Commons Attribution 3.0)

## Types of Synovial Joints by Function

While joints can be structurally classified as fibrous, cartilaginous, or synovial, they can also be categorized by their function, that is, by the type and degree of movement they allow. Although structure and function are closely related, they are not synonymous. Structural features influence, but do not entirely dictate, a joint's mobility versus stability. Understanding joint function (beyond structure) provides additional insight, especially when considering movement practices like yoga *asana*, where range, direction, and control of motion are all relevant. Among all joint types, synovial joints are the most functionally significant for yoga *asana* and movement-based disciplines due to their wide range of motion and dynamic adaptability.

Synovial joints can be functionally classified by the number of axes around which they permit movement (see Figure 1.20 for images of all of the following types of synovial joints):
- *Gliding joints* – These articulations allow one bone to slide alongside another with minimal rotation. Movement typically occurs in a single plane. Examples include the anterior sacroiliac (SI) joints and the facet joints between vertebrae (excluding the intervertebral disc joints, which are cartilaginous).
- *Uniaxial joints* – In these articulations, movement is restricted to one axis. These joints can function as either hinges or pivots.
   - *Hinge joints* allow flexion and extension (e.g., elbow joint between the humerus and ulna)
   - *Pivot joints* allow rotational movement around a central axis (e.g., proximal radioulnar joint, where the radius rotates around the ulna)

- *Biaxial joints* – These articulations allow for movement in two perpendicular directions, namely, flexion/extension and abduction/adduction. However, they do not allow rotation. A good example are the metacarpophalangeal joints in the fingers (where the metacarpal meets the phalanx).
- *Multiaxial joints* – These joints allow movement in multiple directions, including rotation. There are two subtypes, ball-and-socket and saddle joints.
    - *Ball-and-socket joints* permit movement in all planes allowing for circumduction as well as all other movements (e.g., hip and shoulder joints)
    - *Saddle joints* permit movement in several directions with more control than a gliding joint, but less range than a ball-and-socket joint (e.g., the carpometacarpal joint of the thumb)

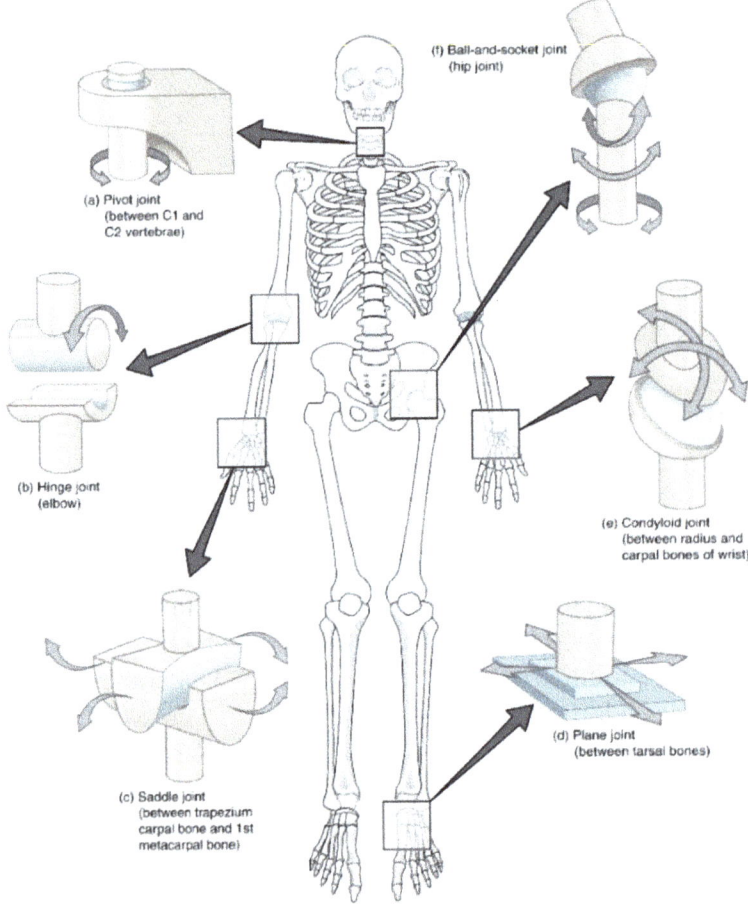

**Figure 1.20** Synovial joints. (Data source: OpenStax; https://commons.wikimedia.org/wiki/File:909_Types_of_Synovial_Joints.jpg; Creative Commons Attribution 3.0)

*Range of Motion in Joints and Integrated Holistic Yoga Movement*

Joint structures and functions are further related to range of motion, another aspect of joint movement or activation that deserves careful attention and needs to be appreciated for its individual diversity. The notions of active and passive range of motion along with range of control, as defined below, have profound implications for yoga *asana* and type of cueing and assisting that is offered to students or clients.

### Active Range of Motion

This type of range refers to movement that is voluntarily initiated and controlled by the individual using their own muscular effort. It demonstrates the strength, coordination, and motor control available at a joint without external assistance. In yoga *asana*, this is the range an individual accesses when entering, holding, or transitioning through shapes without physical support.

### Passive Range of Motion

This range of motion describes joint movement that is performed by an external force (rather than by an individual's own muscles), such as by another person, use of a yoga prop, use of another limb to move a particular body part, or gravity. Range of motion is achieved without the active engagement of the muscles around the particular joint(s) that are being moved. Passive range is typically greater than active range, but does not ensure or imply that a joint is stable or safely usable in that range. A common example is a yoga teacher providing a hands-on adjustment to deepen a shape, a maneuver that carries risks if not done with awareness of the individual's anatomical limits, tissue readiness, or other consideration and preexisting conditions.

### Range of Control

Range of control refers to the portion of a joint's range of motion that the individual can actively stabilize and control under load or during movement under their own muscular power. It highlights the dynamic relationship between mobility and stability that varies across regions of the body (e.g., hips tend to be more stable, shoulders more mobile). To find healthful range of control:
- It is important to identify hypermobile joints (excess range with limited control) versus hypomobile joints (limited range due to stiffness or restriction).
- It is helpful to recognize and/or utilize accessory movements, small and often unnoticed motions in adjacent joints that must occur to allow larger movements to happen (e.g., during shoulder flexion, the sternoclavicular joint must rotate slightly to accommodate full arm elevation).
- It is crucial to cultivate a range of control in yoga *asana* and other movement practices that honors and protects joints and supports long-term joint health.

Less so in current times, but with some frequency in the past, yoga teachers have encouraged and taught passive ranges of motions (e.g., inviting students to pull themselves into 'deeper' versions of twists by using torque from their hands and arms) and have even forced passive range of motion in their students through hands-on adjustments (e.g., pressing students' low back more deeply into a seated forward fold). Such actions are not without significant risks and need to be used only with wise discernment and clear purpose. This issue is revisited in the next section of this volume and was also addressed in the Yoga Pedagogy section of Volume 1. A review of the latter will serve well.

## Muscles

Muscle mass makes up approximately 23% of body mass in biological women and 40% in biological men. This muscle mass is comprised of approximately 639 muscles that are an integrated part of the body's deeply connected structures that contribute to biotensegrity. Given the discussion of bioindividuality related to number of bones, it is clear now that when we read *639 muscles*, it is necessary to think again. Interestingly, Clark (2016) argues (and many agree) that we could say that *there is a single muscular structure that runs through the entire body* because of all the fascial connections from muscle to muscle, from muscle to bone, from muscle to tendons and ligaments. Alternatively, it can be argued that there are many more than 639 muscles because of bioindividuality that leads to some people having two muscles where others have one, or having three muscles where others have two. In other words, the precise number of 639 exists only in textbooks. Figure 1.21 depicts the major muscles in the human body.

As noted, all muscles are interconnected via fascia, ligaments, and tendons – humans have movement systems or myofascial chains, not individual muscles. These myofascial structures, or anatomy trains, promote an *anatomy of connection* (as opposed to an anatomy of separation or isolation). The biotensegrity structure that is the human body has cell matrix adhesions, which means that all structures within that tensegrity transmit force to each other because *the whole system is connected*. All cells across all structures talk to each other, influence each other, interdepend, and co-regulate. This connection clarifies that muscles do not simply have origins and insertions (see section about tendons above); they have connections beyond their tendinous ends, an integration that is highly bioindividual. This connection is, of course, also attributable to the myofascia that wraps each muscle fiber as well as the muscle overall.

Muscles are also highly bioindividual in the sense of the origin and insertion of each muscle and in its length compared across individuals. One person's bicep is not the same as another person's bicep. For example, in one individual, the bicep may be relatively short with insertions that are much closer together along the length of the humerus than for another person. Thus, we cannot assume that what works in yoga or in life for one person will work for another because the very shape and length of the same muscle in two bodies may differ profoundly. Such bioindividuality deeply affects how different humans express yoga shapes in their individual bodies – no two people will embody the same yoga position in the same outer shape and inner experience. Skillful yoga professionals reflect this reality in their cueing, in how they demonstrate and offer yoga shapes during a practice, and in how they encourage students to embody their own reality.

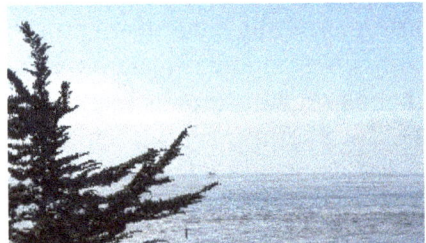

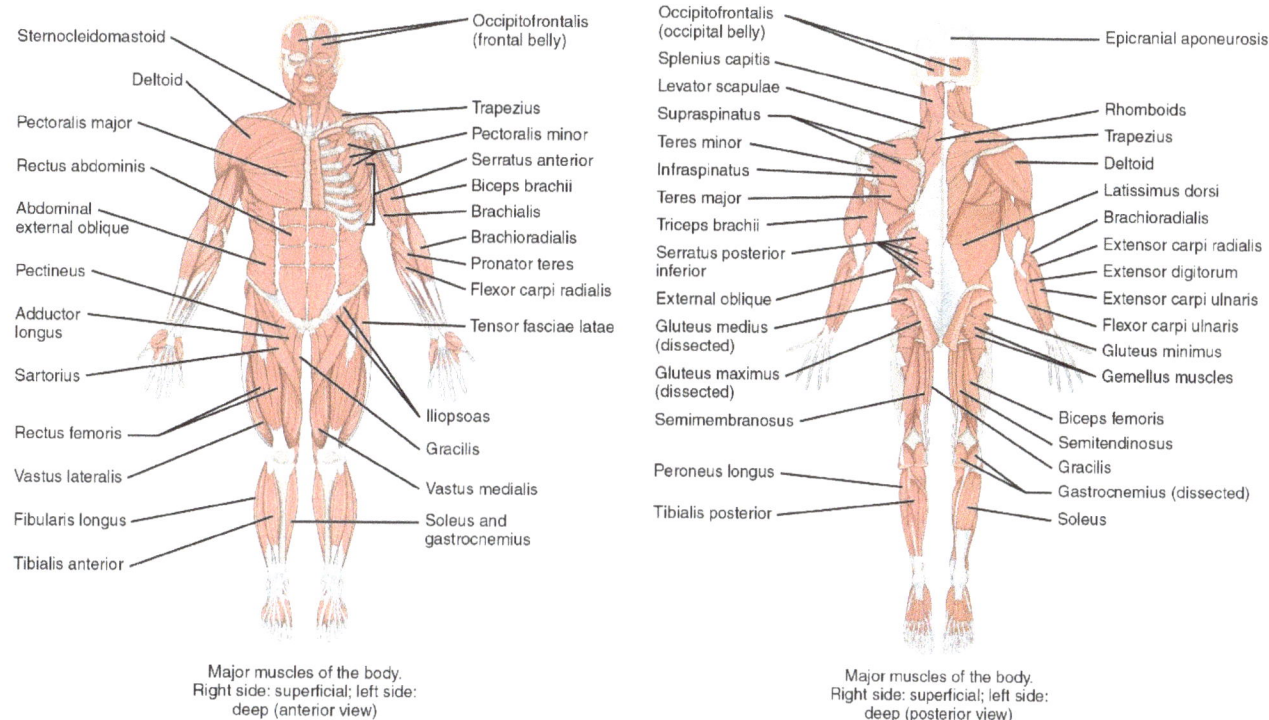

**Figure 1.21** Major muscles – anterior and posterior view. (Data source: OpenStax; https://commons.wikimedia.org/wiki/File:1105_Anterior_and_Posterior_Views_of_Muscles.jpg; Creative Commons Attribution 4.0)

## *Muscle Functions*

Muscle tissue specifically developed or evolved to support or facilitate movement, whether voluntary (by striated muscles) or involuntary (by smooth and cardiac muscles), in comparison to connective tissue, which specifically developed or evolved to provide stability across structures, protect organs and skin, and strengthen joints. Muscles evolved to stretch and contract, to have elasticity that returns them to anatomical position after contraction or stretching. Connective tissues, on the other hand, evolved to hold the body together and to give it shape; they are specifically designed for stability and have no to limited elasticity. This crucial difference between muscular and connective tissue can be well exemplified by contrasting muscle elasticity and resilience with features of ligaments. Ligaments, if (over)stretched are sprained and then less able to serve their stabilizing function for the joint they are supposed to protect. Due to poor blood supply, injuries to ligaments heal very slowly and often never completely, leaving the affected joint weaker (less protected) and more prone to injury.

It is true that muscles are most readily associated with movement, due to their capacity to contract and release to change the position of bones to generate locomotion or support posture. However, muscles are vastly more complex and multifunctional than their most obvious function suggests. Composed of highly specialized cells, muscle tissue possesses *excitability* (the ability to respond to neural stimulation), *contractility* (the ability to shorten and generate force), *distensibility* (the capacity to stretch), and *elasticity* (the ability to return to resting length after stretching or contracting). These intrinsic properties allow muscle to perform a wide range of essential, and sometimes surprising, physiological roles. Specifically, in addition to powering motion, muscles play a foundational role in maintaining internal homeostasis, regulating systemic functions, and supporting other tissues and organs. Muscle is increasingly recognized as a highly active endocrine organ, with emerging research continuously uncovering new muscular functions at the cellular and systemic level. Following is a look at the roles that muscles perform across the human body, looking beyond their capacity to affect movement.

### Maintaining Posture and Structural Integrity

Muscles are continually active, even at rest, to help us resist the gravitational pull of the earth. Postural control is largely unconscious and requires ongoing, low-level muscle activation across chains of muscles, particularly those organized along the superficial myofascial back line (described in the Anatomy Trains section below). This line includes structures such as the gastrocnemius, hamstrings, sacrotuberous ligament, erector spinae, and epicranial fascia, all of which contribute to upright posture. Postural muscles are tonic in nature; they are built for endurance and sustained contraction. Their health and responsiveness are central to balance, coordination, and injury prevention.

### Moving and Stabilizing Bones and Joints

Muscles generate movement by actively exerting force on bones across joints. This action, combined with precise neuromuscular control allows for fine motor skills as well as complex whole-body movements. However, movement is only one part of the story: muscles also help create stability across joints. For example, the rotator cuff muscles act less to produce large movements and more to hold the humeral head (the uppermost structure of the upper arm bone) centered in the glenoid fossa (or shoulder socket), providing dynamic joint stability during arm movements. Stabilization is particularly important in joints with wide ranges of motion (e.g., shoulder, hip) or joints under constant load (e.g., knees, ankles). The interplay of mobility and stability facilitated by muscles in collaboration with tendons and ligaments is a key consideration in functional movement and yoga *asana* practice. Too often yoga practice is about movement, mobility, and range of motion – rather than about stabilization and equilibrium. Skillful yoga professionals achieve a better balance between the body's capacity to move freely and to stabilize securely.

### Supporting and Protecting Internal Organs

Muscles are not simply responsible for moving the external body; they also support internal structures. Muscles of the abdominal wall and pelvic floor help hold abdominal and pelvic organs in place, preventing prolapse and contributing to intraabdominal pressure. These muscles participate in functional processes such as defecation, urination, childbirth, and coughing. Respiratory muscles, such as the diaphragm and intercostals, not only move air in and out of the lungs, but also help maintain the mechanical positioning of the thoracic organs.

Several organs rely directly on muscular activity to function. Smooth muscle tissue, found in the walls of blood vessels, gastrointestinal tract, bladder, and respiratory passages, is responsible for involuntary actions such as peristalsis, vasodilation, and bronchodilation. Cardiac muscle, found only in the heart, powers circulation of blood, whereas skeletal muscle contractions help support venous return (especially from the lower limbs; e.g., see the description of the soleus in Chapter 5) by compressing veins and pushing blood back toward the heart. This skeletal muscle action is at times referred to as a *muscle pump*.

*Thermoregulation: Producing and Conserving Heat*

Skeletal muscles play a central role in thermoregulation. As they contract, they generate heat as a byproduct of cellular metabolism. This heat helps maintain the body's core temperature, especially in cold environments. In fact, skeletal muscle accounts for approximately 85% of the body's heat production during vigorous activity. When additional heat is needed, the body can initiate shivering, a form of involuntary muscular contraction that helps elevate body temperature.

> Average normal body temperature is commonly cited as 98.6°F (37°C), but (hopefully not surprisingly by now) this is better viewed as a general guideline rather than a fixed number. Research suggests that normal resting body temperature for healthy adults is slightly lower and best reflected as a range (rather than an average) from **97.5°F to 98.9°F** (36.4°C to 37.2°C). Further, individual body temperature can vary significantly based on factors such as:
> - *Time of day* (lower in the morning, higher in the late afternoon)
> - *Age* (older adults tend to have slightly lower baseline temperatures)
> - *Sex and hormonal fluctuations* (during ovulation, body temperature may rise)
> - *Level of physical activity* (exercise generates heat)
> - *Body location where temperature is measured* (oral, axillary, tympanic, rectal)

*Secreting Health-Promoting Molecules: Muscles as Endocrine Organs*

Perhaps most surprising is the discovery that skeletal muscle functions as an endocrine organ, secreting a class of signaling molecules called myokines. These chemicals are released into the bloodstream during active muscular contraction and exert widespread effects on immune function, metabolism, inflammation, and even tumor suppression. Importantly, these protective effects only occur in response to contractile activity, not simply in the presence of muscle mass. In other words, it is muscle use, not muscle size, that promotes health. These amazing recent discoveries continue to redefine and refine the understanding of how muscles, physical movement, and vital engagement protect and enhance health at the cellular level. Two of the best-researched myokines include:
- *Oncostatin M*: This molecule, released through muscular exertion, has been shown to inhibit the growth of breast cancer cells, among other anti-cancer effects.
- *Interleukin-6* (IL-6): When produced by active skeletal muscle in motion (as opposed to in inflammatory states), IL-6 acts as a potent anti-inflammatory signal. It helps downregulate tumor necrosis factor-alpha (TNF-α; a pro-inflammatory cytokine), high levels of which are linked to heart disease (Dimitrov et al., 2017). It mobilizes natural killer cells (which attack and destroy cancer cells) if produced via active muscular exercise (McGonigal, 2019).

Clearly, muscles do far more than move the body. They are biomechanical stabilizers, thermal regulators, structural supports, organ function facilitators, and molecular communicators. Their contributions span the musculoskeletal, cardiovascular, respiratory, immune, and endocrine systems, making muscular health and activation central to holistic wellbeing. This understanding reinforces the idea that movement practices, especially those emphasizing conscious, whole-body engagement, such as yoga *asana* and flow practices, can influence not simply structure but systemic health and cellular function. No doubt, activation of muscle via yoga *asana* and other yoga-based movements can help explain the wide range of documented benefits of a regular yoga practice. This fact can be shared by yoga professionals with clients to support motivation to persevere in a committed daily yoga practice that is well-rounded, including activation and calming (i.e., honoring all limbs of yoga).

## *Muscle Types and Muscles as Neuromuscular Tissue*

Muscle has been discussed as highly complex in its profound linkages to other structural systems, such as fascia, tendons, ligaments, and bones. Muscular tissue is also complex in the sense that it is highly innervated and closely linked to the nervous system, as well as to human psychology and emotions. There is growing recognition that what we have traditionally called muscle tissue might be more accurately described as neuromuscular tissue, a term that better reflects the intimate and continuous relationship between muscle fibers and the nervous system. The idea that muscle is better viewed as neuromuscular tissue is supported by research that gains in muscular strength or power are attributable not only to muscle fibers contractility (Gross, 2025), but due to changes in the ease of signaling between muscles and the nervous system (Enoka, 2025). Even attentional focus and emotional arousal can affect physical performance, including strength and power (Wulf, 2013). Thus, the shift in language is not simply semantic; it speaks to a more integrated understanding of how movement arises and is regulated in the body. There are three primary types of muscles (smooth, cardiac, and skeletal), each type closely tied to its function as well as its relationship to the nervous system.

Although the term neuromuscular conventionally brings skeletal muscle to mind first, each type of muscle participates in a network of sensory-motor regulation that connects tissue-level activity with systemic functions and psychological experiences. All muscle types are in constant dialogue with the nervous system, each in its own way:
- *Smooth muscle* is neuromuscular through autonomic regulation of internal environments.
- *Cardiac muscle* is neuromuscular through intrinsic rhythm modulated by neural and emotional states.
- *Skeletal muscle* is neuromuscular through somatic voluntary and reflexive pathways.

These insights are not entirely new – they are reflected in the holistic integrated perspective on yoga (Brems, 2024b, 2025), as well as in polyvagal theory (Porges, 2009, 2022; Sullivan et al., 2018). It is a worthwhile interpretation of muscle activity for yoga professionals as it reminds us of the complex embeddedness of humans in all of their layers of experience (i.e., *koshas*) and their biopsychosociocultural context and interpersonal matrix. Let us look now at each type of muscle tissue holding this complex and holistic perspective in mind.

## Smooth or Involuntary Muscle

*Smooth or involuntary* muscle, found in the walls of hollow organs (e.g., intestines, blood vessels, and respiratory tracts), is under autonomic nervous system control because the functions it serves need to unfold automatically. Digestion needs to process ingested material constantly; arteries need to transport blood continuously and adaptively; intestinal motility needs to adaptively move contents along; and respiration needs to keep us alive. Smooth muscle is innervated by the autonomic nervous system (ANS), specifically the sympathetic and parasympathetic branches. Neural regulation is about modulating rate, tone, and rhythm of contraction in response to internal states (e.g., blood pressure, digestion, emotional stress) and external demands. Although we cannot consciously engage smooth muscle, our mind state and emotional reactivity (our polyvagal state or *guna*) directly influences it. For example, anxiety can cause bowel spasms, breath dysregulation, or rapid heartbeat. Stress can increase blood pressure and may disrupt digesting. Thus, smooth muscle is neuromuscular in a visceral and autonomically-regulated sense. It participates in the mind-body-spirit dialogue, particularly in the interface between the nervous system and internal organs (the enteric nervous system being a prime example of this integration).

## Cardiac Muscle

*Cardiac* muscle, a unique muscle tissue found in the heart only, supports the pumping of blood throughout the body. Cardiac muscle is highly unique, a hybrid between smooth and skeletal muscle. Like smooth muscle, it is involuntary and autonomically regulated. Cardiac muscle has its own intrinsic pace-making system: the sinoatrial (SA) node, a specialized group of cardiac cells that generate rhythmic impulses independently of the brain. However, the autonomic nervous system (via the vagus nerve and sympathetic cardiac nerves) modulates heart rate in response to physiological and emotional demands. Cardiac muscle tissue can be considered neuromuscular due to its responsiveness to neural input, whether from physical exertion, emotional arousal, or deep relaxation. For example, yoga practices that stimulate the parasympathetic nervous system (such as long exhalations or meditative focus) can decrease heart rate, increase heart rate variability, and enhance cardiac coherence. In this way, the heart is a neuromuscular organ whose function is closely linked to physiological states, emotional reactivity, arousal level, and affective tone.

## Skeletal or Voluntary Muscle

*Skeletal or voluntary* muscles are under voluntary control; however, and very fortunately, they also work as directed by the ANS (thank goodness we do not have to give conscious commands to walk, eat, talk, bicycle, wash dishes, or take a shower). Skeletal muscles are crucial to the human ability to take conscious charge of how we move our various body parts, stabilize our posture, or hold ourselves in yoga shapes, among others. Skeletal muscle is voluntarily controlled primarily through somatic motor neurons. However, even here, not all control is conscious; that is, reflex arcs, habituated motor patterns, and subconscious postural adjustments all blur the line between voluntary and involuntary control. Sensory structures like muscle spindles and Golgi tendon organs create a constant feedback loop between muscle tissue and the central nervous system. Because it responds to both conscious intention and reflexive neural feedback, skeletal muscle is a star example of neuromuscular function.

Skeletal muscle is densely innervated, meaning it is deeply permeated with sensory and motor nerve endings. These nerves do not just animate the muscle; they monitor and respond to its internal state in real time. Embedded within each muscle fiber are *muscle spindles* that serve as sensory receptors, detecting changes in muscle length and rate of stretch. When muscle spindles perceive a muscle as being stretched too far or too quickly, they send afferent (sensory) signals from the bottom up to the spinal cord. These signals are processed and responded to by the central nervous system, which then sends efferent (motor) impulses back to the muscle, creating a reflexive contraction to protect muscle from overstretching. Likewise, at the transition from muscle to tendon, *Golgi tendon organs* detect tensile load, that is, how much force is being exerted through the tendon. If tension on the tendon becomes excessive, the Golgi receptors send bottom-up sensory input to the spinal cord, initiating a motor response that down-regulates contraction in the muscle to prevent tendon injury. This sophisticated and instantaneous feedback loop of sensing, integrating, and responding is constantly active, modulating every muscular engagement and release.

Feedback mechanisms between muscle, tendon, and nervous system are the reason why it is not accurate to say that muscles (or humans) simply 'choose' to contract or relax. Muscle behavior emerges from a dynamic and ongoing conversation between the tissues themselves, the peripheral and central nervous systems, and the external environment. Moreover, as reviewed previously, muscle tissue is also richly embedded in myofascial networks. Feedback from the myofascia adds more information that is used by the nervous system to transform into action. Not surprisingly, the neuromuscular system does not operate in isolation from the psyche, from our mind with its preconceived ideas, strong beliefs, personal and cultural conditioning, emotional reactivity, and so on (a review of the relevant yoga psychology – namely the *vrittis* as affected by the *kleshas*, *vedana*, and *gunas* – can be reviewed in Volume 1 of this series, *Integrated Holistic Yoga Psychology*). Movement is never purely mechanical; it is psychophysiological. Our human nervous system is shaped by past experiences, beliefs, emotions, and states of mind as well as by expectations about our safety in each moment and about what is likely to occur next or may be a most auspicious choice for action.

Translating this notion into yoga *asana* practice, for example, a shape like Headstand is not simply physically challenging; it also calls up psychological, mental, and emotional responses, experiences, and expectations (i.e., *vrittis* and *samskaras*). One practitioner may receive a top-down inhibitory signal from the prefrontal cortex warning of risk and danger, causing hesitation or muscle guarding. Another student may receive an overconfident signal of invincibility that overrides caution. In both cases, tone and timing of muscular activation are influenced by psychological and emotional factors, not simply by biomechanics.

Similarly, for individuals living with chronic pain or movement inhibition, psychoneuromuscular dynamics may become especially apparent. Guarding patterns and protective tension are often less about the actual state of the tissue and more about learned associations and fear responses encoded in the nervous system (cf., polyvagal theory and *gunas*). These examples give added evidence to the appropriateness of the term *neuromuscular tissue*, a frame that deeply honors the complexity of movement as an expression of biological, neurological, and psychological integration. It reminds us that every gesture, every contraction, every moment of stillness or effort, arises from a deeply intelligent system that spans from tendon to cortex, from reflex to belief, from *annamaya kosha* to *anandamaya kosha*.

## Skeletal Muscle

Although skeletal muscle tends to be the primary focus of interest for yoga teachers and other yoga professionals, it is helpful to keep in mind the many functions and contributions of smooth and cardiac muscles and profound effect on these autonomically steered muscles of yoga practices such as *pranayama*, *pratyahara*, *dharana*, and *dhyana*. Breathing and interior practices of yoga have been well documented to support calming of the autonomic nervous system, shifting it toward a ventral vagal parasympathetic state that supports social engagement and connection (Brems, 2024b, 2025; Schwartz, 2024). They also have life-changing effects on mind states and emotional reactivity, which, in turn, can deeply affect the health of human digestive, immune, and other functions. Nevertheless, given the movement focus of this book, from here our attention will largely shift to working with skeletal muscle.

Voluntary or skeletal muscles are of greatest interest and importance to yoga professionals as they are responsible for postural alignment, movement, and action in *asana*. They most typically connect or attach to bones on either end of a muscle via a tendon. This placement, in combination with the contractile action of skeletal muscle, results in movement in the joints crossed by a particular muscle or set of muscles. The places where muscles (via tendons) meet bone have numerous labels, including insertion, attachment or origin.

Following are some clarifying definitions:
- The stationary (typically most proximal) end of a muscle is the *origin;* more accurate language might be *proximal attachment*.
- The moving or more distal end of the muscle is the *insertion*; more accurate language might the *distal attachment*.
- Many muscles have multiple insertions or multiple heads.

Muscles (primarily) move bones around the joints they cross. As some muscles cross more than one joint, they can affect movement in all joints across which they extend. For example:
- Rectus femoris crosses the knee and hip joint and hence can create movement in both joints, extending the knee and flexing the hip.
- The hamstrings cross the hip and knee as well; they contribute to knee flexion and hip extension.

Of course, due to their embeddedness in fascial and other connective tissue structures, muscles may have more effects than joint movement and may, in turn, be affected by the movement of other muscles and tissues. It is helpful to recall that all muscle fibers and each muscle overall are wrapped in fascia – another contributor to range of motion (as well as sensation of stretch and pain). Figures 1.22 and 1.23 illustrate fascia in the form of fascicles as well as in the form of muscle transforming into tendon.

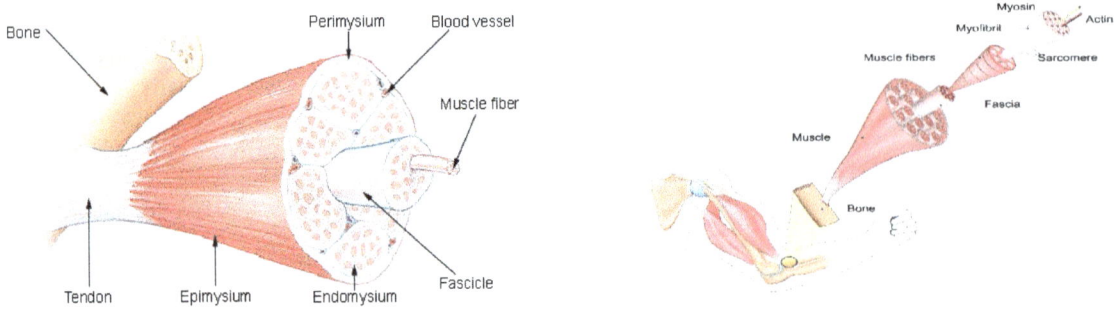

**Figure 1.22** Skeletal muscle structure. (Data source: https://commons.wikimedia.org/wiki/File:Illu_muscle_structure.jpg; public domain)

**Figure 1.23** Skeletal muscle structure. (Data source: Istock)

## Types of Movement in Joints Facilitated by Skeletal Muscle

Three types of skeletal muscle movement are important to differentiate and have crucial implications for how we work as yoga professionals guiding students or clients into yoga *asana*. This information is overlapping with active and passive movements across joints, covered above. The same cautions and implications apply for yoga *asana* cueing and assisting.

- *Active* movement refers to voluntary movement initiated by the individual engaging in the movement – engaging in the movement under their own muscle power, without external assistance.
- *Passive* movement refers to movement across a joint that is powered by an external force. This may be movement that is done to us by some<u>one</u> else (e.g., teacher moving a body part; massage therapist moving a specific muscle) or by some<u>thing</u> else (e.g., strap, block, other props). As noted in the context of joints above, but it bears repeating, passive movement has more risk of injury, especially if there is no active feedback loop between the individual being moved and the person or thing moving the individual. As yoga professionals, we ask students or clients to move with awareness if we ever engage them into passive movement via use of prop use (such as using a strap to find a new range of motion, or hands to increase the active range of a set of muscles and joints). Similarly, we ask for permission and feedback if we ever move an individual into passive movement through hands-on intervention. The latter needs to have a very specific purpose and it is key to review Section 2 of Volume 1 (p. 279 onward) as related to hands-on touch in teaching yoga *asana*.
- *Accessory or synergistic movement* refers to movement in structures that move because we move another body part; accessory movement has to happen for this movement to take place. For example, when we move our shoulder, the clavicle moves along with that movement automatically. In fact, the clavicle can only be moved via accessory movement. It cannot be moved actively or passively.

## Three Types of Contractions of Skeletal Muscle

Although explained separately below, the first two types of actions (active and passive) are both isotonic and always co-occur. As noted, the body is a biotensegrity and nothing ever moves in isolation. All actions require a multitude of muscles, agonists, antagonists, and stabilizers to work together to create strength, efficiency, and stability. Skeletal muscles are governed by the law of reciprocal innervation, which means that isotonic contractile force in the agonist (the activated muscle) is accompanied by a commensurate degree of diminishing contractile force in the antagonist; one contracts eccentrically, the other concentrically. Isotonic muscle movement always involves either lengthening or shortening of muscles; isometric muscle movement, on the other hand, is a movement through which muscle tension is held (via muscle contraction) in the absence of any outer movement. A bit more explanation is necessary for each type of contraction.

### Concentric Isotonic Contraction

Concentric contraction, also known as concentric shortening or a shortening contraction, occurs when a muscle generates force while actively shortening, bringing its origin and insertion points closer together under load. This is a dynamic form of contraction during which the muscle is actively working to produce movement. Concentric contractions are typically involved in movements that work against gravity, such as lifting a limb or rising out of a squatting position. For example, when lifting the leg into a standing Warrior 3, the quadriceps and hip flexors engage concentrically to raise the leg against gravity, shortening as they create the action of hip flexion and knee extension.

However, concentric contractions are not limited to anti-gravity movements. They also play a vital role in gravity-neutral or rotational actions, such as in twisting shapes like Revolved Triangle, during which the internal and external obliques concentrically contract to rotate the torso. In yoga practice, understanding where and how concentric contractions are occurring allows practitioners and teachers to identify active engagement and to exert conscious control. Shortening contraction is often used to initiate or maintain structural stability during transitions or while actively holding a shape. Notably, overuse or poor alignment during repetitive concentric effort can contribute to muscular imbalances or strain over time – not just in yoga shapes but any repetitive movement pattern. Therefore, it is helpful to balance concentric work with eccentric control and appropriate joint support for safe and effective practice and lifestyles.

### Eccentric Isotonic Contraction

Eccentric contraction, also called eccentric lengthening or lengthening contraction, occurs when a muscle generates force while lengthening under load. Rather than initiating movement, the muscle resists it, providing controlled deceleration or stabilization. In this type of contraction, origin and insertion of a muscle move farther apart even as the muscle remains active. Eccentric contractions are often gravity-assisted and typically occur when the body is moving in the direction of gravity, as in lowering or descending actions. A yoga example is the transition from Mountain to a Standing Forward Fold: as the hip joint flexes, spinal extensors remain engaged, but lengthen under load to prevent the trunk from moving forward too quickly. The same principle applies when slowly lowering through a yoga pushup; during this transition, the triceps eccentrically contract to control elbow flexion against gravity.

Unlike passive stretching, eccentric contraction provides an active and neurologically rich form of lengthening, sometimes described as resistance stretching. The muscle is working while elongating, which enhances tensile strength in the muscle and associated connective tissue, an action that is highly effective for joint stabilization and injury prevention. Notably, the body is stronger in eccentric (as opposed to concentric) contraction, being able to resist greater load in the lengthening than shortening phase. This type of engagement also demands higher cognitive input, requiring cortical motor control to coordinate the nuanced balance between effort and ease. In yoga *asana*, recognizing and intentionally cueing eccentric contraction supports safer transitions, more effective development of resilience, and long-term health in muscular and fascial systems.

### *Isometric Contraction*

Isometric contraction, also known as static contraction, involves muscular effort without visible change in muscle length. During isometric contraction, the muscle generates force to hold steady under load or resistance; there is no joint movement because the force produced by the agonist is equal to the opposing force of the antagonist. The term 'isometric' reflects this balance in that the 'iso' translates as *same*, and 'metric' refers to length. Unlike isotonic contractions, which involve movement through muscle shortening or lengthening under constant load, isometric contractions maintain tension without altering muscle length.

In yoga, isometric contraction is present when a posture is held in stillness with deliberate engagement. For instance, when holding Warrior 2, the quadriceps, glutes, and shoulder stabilizers engage isometrically to maintain the shape against gravity. This action creates a protective and neurologically safe environment because affected joints remain stable, and the nervous system is not challenged by movement, but by sustained effort. Isometric contraction can gradually increase range of motion by allowing the body to safely adapt to load or stretch, potentially improving joint flexibility (Mitchell, 2019). Additionally, it can provide an analgesic effect, offering consistent sensory input to the nervous system that can help override pain signals (Rio et al., 2017). This makes isometric holds particularly valuable not only for stability and strength but also for nervous system regulation and injury recovery.

> **Sample Application to Yoga: Types of contraction the triceps are engaged in while in**
> - High Plank → *isometric*
> - Moving into Low Plank (*chaturanga dandasana*) → *eccentric contraction*
> - Pushing back up from Low to High Plank → *concentric contraction*

### *Other Skeletal Muscle Contraction-Related Issues*

Muscles are less likely to be injured while contracted (as opposed to relaxed). All contractions are good for us, especially with high load as this builds resilience and strength. If there is no nerve impulse telling a muscle to contract, it will relax – though this is a relative term because muscles are always under some level of tension or contraction. Once 'relaxed', a muscle can stretch, either with time (active stretch) or with assistance from another external force (i.e., via passive stretch; see cautions above). Moving too quickly when a muscle is relaxed, can decrease its stretchability as pain or surprise cause the muscle fibers to contract; such pain or surprise inhibits lengthening and prevents relaxation of the muscle (Coulter, 2001).

Contraction can occur at different points along a muscle's available length, and this has meaningful implications for strength development, proprioception, and joint health in yoga *asana* and other movement practices (Coulter, 2001; Mitchell, 2019). The range at which a contraction occurs (short, mid, or long) refers to the position of the muscle relative to its neutral or anatomical resting length. Understanding and intentionally exploring these ranges in practice allows for more complete muscular conditioning and neuromuscular control.

*Short-range contraction* happens when a muscle is already in a shortened state relative to neutral, and then contracts further. This can be less mechanically efficient, as fewer cross-bridges are available between actin and myosin filaments, limiting force production. However, it is still highly functional in many movements. For example, in Bridge, the hamstrings and glutes may contract in a relatively shortened state to maintain pelvic lift, especially as the hips rise higher. Training short-range contractions supports control and strength in compact positions.

*Mid-range contraction* occurs when the muscle is contracting near its neutral anatomical length; this is typically where the muscle has the most mechanical advantage and can produce the greatest force. In yoga, this might correspond to a steady engagement of the biceps in Mountain with the arms held forward at shoulder height. Because this is the range and plane of movement in which where these muscles tend to be naturally strongest, it is often the starting point for building awareness of engagement.

*Long-range contraction* involves activation while the muscle is lengthened beyond its neutral position. This is particularly important for building strength in stretched positions and increasing joint stability at vulnerable end ranges. For example, in a wide-legged Forward Fold, engaging the adductors and hamstrings (while they are lengthened) supports pelvic control and protects the involved joints. Long-range contractions also enhance proprioceptive feedback and contribute to injury resilience by strengthening connective tissue and increasing tolerance to stretch under load. For yoga practitioners, training contraction across all ranges enriches joint stability, improves neuromuscular intelligence, and ensures that strength and control are available not only in familiar positions but also at the extremes of motion. It encourages a more responsive, adaptable, and resilient movement system.

### *Types of Contractile Fibers in Skeletal Muscle*

Three types of muscle fibers (i.e., *muscle cells* – in the same way that neurons are the cells that comprise nerves) reflect muscle specialization either for power or endurance. Skeletal and cardiac muscles are striated muscles, which contract to produce movement and generate force for activities like movement, posture, and pumping blood. Striated muscles have a striped appearance that results from the structure underlying their functionality. The striations reflect the structures within the muscle fibers that are the level of muscular tissue responsible for contraction or release of muscle overall.

As shown in Figure 1.24, striated muscles have sarcomeres that contain actin and myosin filaments that overlap (or cross-link via elastic and binding proteins) to greater or lesser degrees depending on the state of contraction or relaxation, respectively. If the filaments slide apart during relaxation, the muscle is essentially weaker as the sarcomeres are stronger the more the filaments overlap or are cross-linked (and "hook" into each other). Thus, as a muscle comes out of relaxation, it is best to support it briefly while the sarcomeres once again contract and the actin and myosin filaments again begin to overlap and cross-link. Once they have cross-linked again, the muscle's strength is regained. Engaging the muscles too quickly and without support when coming out of a state of relaxing that muscles can strain the sarcomeres.

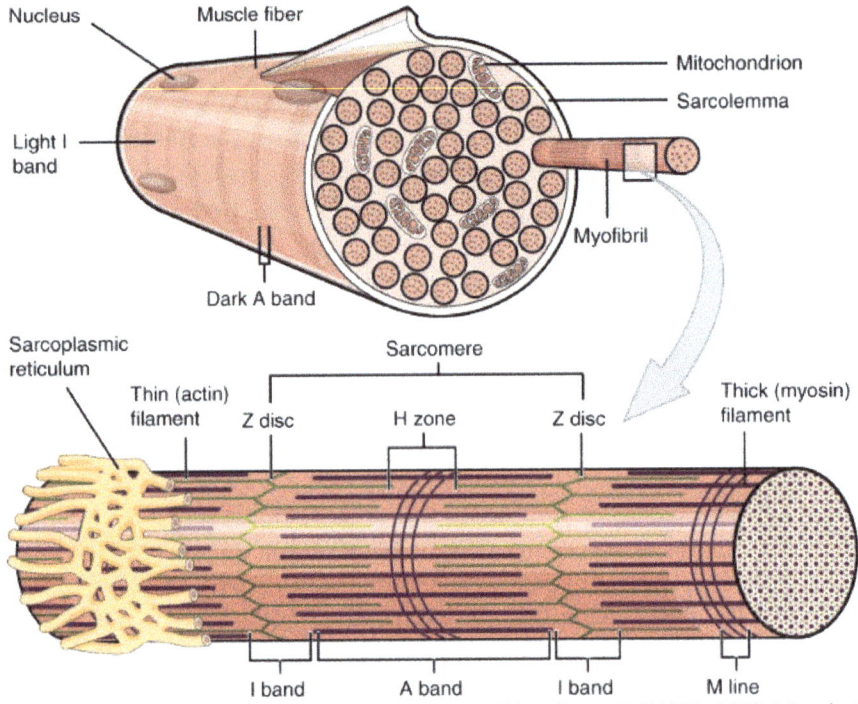

**Figure 1.24** Muscle fibers. (Data source: OpenStax; https://commons.wikimedia.org/wiki/File:1022_Muscle_Fibers_(small).jpg; Creative Commons Attribution 4.0)

The three types of fibers are *slow-twitch* (endurance), *fast twitch* (power), and *intermediate twitch*. The practical translation of this specialization is the fact that some muscles are evolved or specialized for speed and power, others for endurance, and others yet for a mixture of both Proportion of muscle fibers types in a given muscle contributes to the function (habitual and/or genetic) of that particular muscle. There is strong genetic predisposition for proportionality, which may explain why some humans excel at endurance activities (e.g., long distance runners) and others at power (e.g., high-jumpers; (Lieberman, 2021). Animal species other than humans also have distinct patterns of types of muscle fibers.

### *Slow-Twitch Muscle Fibers*

Slow twitch or red muscle fibers, also known as Type I fibers or 'red meat', are muscle cells specialized for endurance and sustained activity. These fibers are rich in capillaries and mitochondria, giving them their distinct red hue and enabling them to use oxygen efficiently through aerobic metabolism. Structurally, they are smaller in diameter and less defined in bulk compared to fast-twitch fibers, which is why muscles with a higher proportion of Type I fibers tend to appear leaner and less prominent, anatomically echoed in the long, sleek build of endurance athletes like marathon runners.

These fibers are not designed for speed or power; rather, they contract slowly and generate relatively low force. However, what they lack in intensity, they make up for in stamina and resistance to fatigue. Red muscle fibers are the backbone of postural stability and low-intensity, sustained activities such as standing, walking, or maintaining a yoga shape over time. In yoga practice, these fibers are especially engaged in static holds and subtle postural adjustments, such as in the deep stabilizing work in standing shapes like Mountain or Warrior 2, or the continuous, quiet support offered by the spinal extensors during seated meditation. Cultivating awareness and endurance in slow-twitch fibers allows for greater ease in maintaining alignment, breathing steadily, and sustaining internal focus during prolonged practice. They remind us that strength is not always about force; it is perhaps more often about quiet and enduring support. For a great visual of Type 1 fibers, see *Musculoskeletal System | Type I Muscle Fibers* by Ninja Nerds at https://youtu.be/EH_Eem-VBZg =

### *Fast-Twitch Muscle Fibers*

Fast-twitch muscle fibers, also known as white or light pink muscle cells, are Type IIX fibers specialized for power, speed, and short bursts of high-intensity effort. These fibers have a moderate diameter but are not well supplied with capillaries, which limits their oxygen use and gives them a pale color compared to the rich red of slow-twitch fibers. Instead of relying on oxygen, they burn glucose anaerobically to generate quick, explosive energy. This fact makes them ideal for short-duration, high-force actions such as sprinting, jumping, or lifting heavy loads. Athletes like powerlifters or sprinters typically have a high proportion of fast-twitch fibers, reflected in muscular and well-defined physiques.

However, power comes with trade-offs. Fast-twitch fibers fatigue quickly and lack endurance, as they cannot sustain effort for long periods. In yoga, these fibers are called upon in dynamic transitions, strong muscular engagements, or when holding demanding shapes that require sudden activation, such as lifting into Crow or jumping through in a *vinyasa* sequence. While yoga is not typically fast-paced or explosive, integrating short, intense actions (like engaging the glutes in a powerful Bridge lift or springing forward from Downward Facing Dog) can stimulate fast-twitch recruitment. Balancing the development of these fibers with slow-twitch endurance fosters a well-rounded, resilient, and adaptable body. From a teaching perspective, encouraging variety in tempo and load can help engage both fiber types, promoting adaptive responsiveness in the musculoskeletal system.

### *Intermediate-Twitch Muscle Fibers*

Intermediate-twitch muscle fibers, also known as pink fibers or Type IIA fibers, serve as a functional bridge between the endurance-focused red fibers and the high-power white fibers. Pink fibers are large in diameter, well-supplied with capillaries (giving them their characteristic pink coloration), and use oxygen efficiently to generate force aerobically. They are built for versatility, offering a balance of strength and stamina. Although not as fatigue-resistant as slow-twitch fibers or as powerful as fast-twitch fibers, intermediate fibers provide moderate power with moderate endurance, making them well-suited for sustained but demanding efforts such as a moderately intense yoga class, a hike, a long walk or swim, or a mid-distance run.

In a yoga context, pink fibers are actively recruited in dynamic sequences and sustained flowing movements, such as a strong standing series held with steady breath and muscular engagement. They support transitions between postures, especially when those transitions require strength and control but are not maintained for a long period of time. For example, stepping forward from Downward Facing Dog into a Lunge or moving through a series of Sun Salutations engages these fibers consistently. Training intermediate-twitch fibers through varied movement intensity and duration in yoga *asana* builds functional strength and enhances muscular adaptability and responsiveness. Encouraging a practice that mixes isometric holds, fluid movement, and moderate effort helps condition these fibers, supporting overall endurance and control without excessive fatigue. For a great video about Type 2 fibers, see https://youtu.be/bMV5BDoP8dY = Musculoskeletal System | Type II | Type IIa & IIx by Ninja Nerds.

## Skeletal Muscles by Types of Action

There are two ways to describe muscle actions. The first categorization uses the muscle's role and differentiates agonists, antagonists, and synergists. The second categorization defines type of action via their functions as flexors, extensors, or stabilizers.

### Categorization of Muscles by Role

In any given movement, muscles work together in coordinated roles to produce smooth and controlled action. The agonist, or prime mover, is the main muscle responsible for initiating a specific movement. It generates the majority of force and is typically supported by synergists that are located on the same side of the joint and assist through complementary, though weaker, actions. Synergists help refine movement by adding precision, stability, and subtle control, allowing the agonist to work more efficiently without overcompensating.

Opposing this movement is the antagonist, a muscle located on the opposite side of the joint. The antagonist does not simply relax; it co-contracts in coordination with the agonist but at a lower intensity. This co-contraction helps stabilize joints, monitor actions, and prevent overshooting or abrupt motion. For example, in a slow and controlled biceps curl, the biceps brachii acts as the agonist, the brachialis may assist as a synergist, and the triceps brachii functions as the antagonist. The balance between agonist, synergist, and antagonist activity is constantly at play in yoga *asana* practice that involves mindfully sustained engagement, nuanced motor control, and conscious joint protection. Whether lifting into a strong Backbend or softly lowering into a Forward Fold, the integrity of a yoga shape depends on the prime movers in collaboration with supportive and opposing muscle groups, all working together through a deeper intelligence, perhaps well understood as active involvement of *vijnanamaya kosha* in the physical practice. Figure 1.25 shows an example of agonists and antagonists.

**Application to Yoga: Sample Agonists and Antagonists** in Triangle:
- rectus femoris → hamstring (forward leg)
- psoas major → hamstrings (forward leg)
- gluteus maximus → biceps femoris (extended leg)
- triceps → biceps (arm)

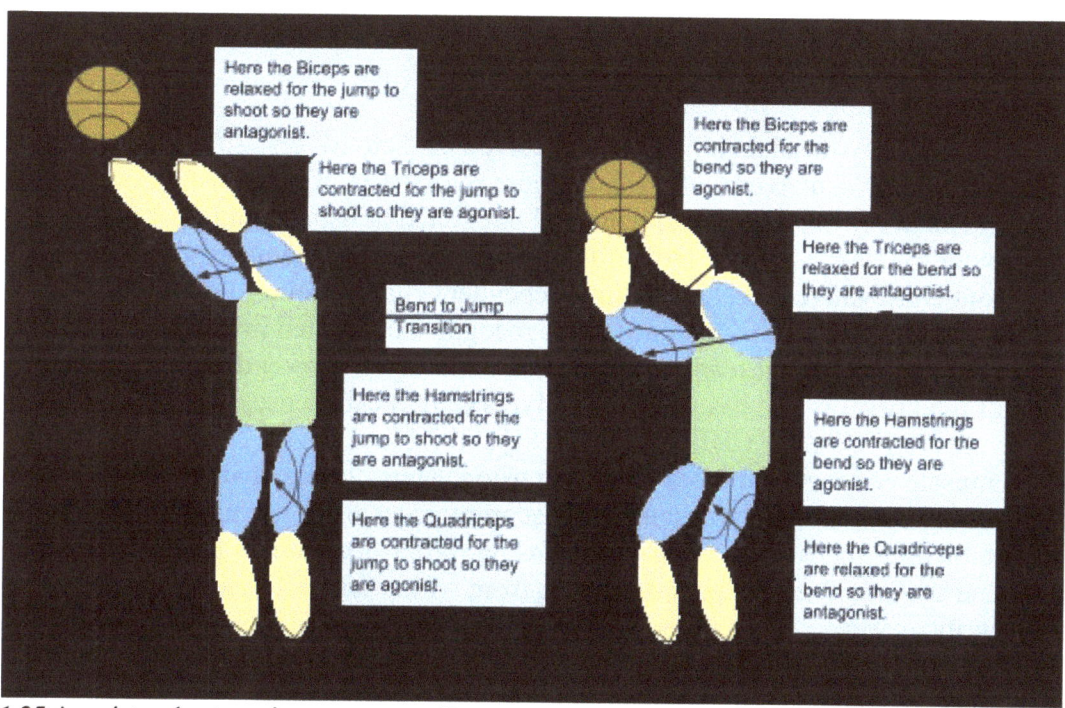

**Figure 1.25** Agonist and antagonist movements. (Data source: Thaer.Makdsi; https://commons.wikimedia.org/wiki/File:Final_Thaer_Ghassan_Makdsi_-_Wikipedia_Digital_Diagram.svg; Creative Commons Attribution 4.0

### *Categorization of Muscles by Function*

Flexors, extensors, and stabilizers each play distinct but interrelated roles in movement and postural integrity. Flexors are muscles that draw bones closer together around a joint, such as bending the spine forward or folding the limbs (e.g., elbow or hip flexion). These muscles shorten as they contract, decreasing the angle between body parts. In the upper body, flexors often work against gravity, for instance when holding the arms out in front or lifting a leg into a Forward Fold. Extensors, by contrast, move the limbs in the opposite direction, increasing the distance between bones at a joint, as in straightening the arm or leg, or arching the spine into extension. They are crucial for actions such as standing upright, backbending, and pushing movements; in the lower body, they typically resist gravity to maintain posture and upright movement (such as walking).

Working in the background of both flexion and extension are the stabilizers, the muscles whose primary role is not to create movement but to prevent unwanted movement in other parts of the body. Sometimes called neutralizers or fixators, stabilizers coordinate with agonists to secure the joints, ligaments, and supporting muscles around the moving parts, ensuring safe and efficient action. Rather than producing forceful contractions, they maintain steady, low-level engagement over time. This role makes them especially responsive to slow, mindful movement, balance challenges, and higher repetition activities. Yoga, with emphasis on sustained shapes, conscious transitions, and integrated breathing, is uniquely suited to train and tone stabilizer muscles. Whether holding a balancing shape such as Tree or moving slowly through a flow sequence, yoga helps develop the stabilizers' endurance and responsiveness, creating a foundation for safe, skillful movement across all physical activities.

## One More Note about Anatomy Trains

Anatomy trains (aka myofascial meridians), conceived by Tom Myers (2022), are the anatomical expression of the body's interconnection and a more recent way of conceiving how to teach movement and anatomy in general, and yoga and integrated holistic yoga in particular. It offers a helpful reminder to think less about individual muscles, tendons, ligaments, bones, and so on – and more about entire interconnected and interdependent chains of muscles, connective tissue, fascia, bones, organs, and so on. Anatomy trains recognize integrated myofascial pathways that transmit stability, strain (stretch), and response. Additionally, the body does not simply have this integration or integrity – it also has what Tom Myers (2022) calls tensegrity; others [e.g., Stephen Levine (1997), Bernie Clark (2016, 2018)] call it biotensegrity. This means that whenever a muscle contracts it creates force or tension. Thus, we are always in tension, which is life-giving and energetic. Fascia transmits and accommodates force throughout the body and is the basis of biotensegrity. In fact, much body sensing (proprioception) is fascial; many injuries are fascial; and a large portion of pain originates from within fascia. Organs may play a role in our biotensegrity as well. We can think of the internal organs as being aligned in an organ column (akin to our spinal column) that contributes to posture and alignment (Lasater, 2009, 2020; Moyer, 2015).

The body viewed from this perspective is a tension structure with biotensegrity. We are always under load, compressive and tensile. It is the tension that gives us our outer shape. Buckling or collapsing happens when the tension collapses and the structure collapses (gives in to gravity). Bracing or gripping happens when the tension becomes rigid and then the whole structure becomes rigid (fighting gravity). Yielding or stabilizing works adaptively with the structure's tensegrity (working with gravity).

Understanding the body through the lens of myofascial meridians and biotensegrity offers yoga teachers and therapists a powerful framework for cueing integrated holistic movement, refining alignment, and recognizing compensatory patterns. Myofascial lines trace the continuity of connective tissue across the body, revealing how distant structures influence one another through tension, load, and movement – through biotensegrity. A few sample anatomy trains may be illustrative of this integrative paradigm of understanding human anatomy. Each sample includes a functional description; basic anatomical pathway; notes on posture, movement, or imbalance; relevance to yoga; and two specific *asana* examples.

## Superficial Front Line

The Superficial Front Line consists of many fast twitch muscles as it is activated in reactive movements. It is essential to posture, especially in relation to providing a balance to the superficial back line. If it is shortened, it contributes to anterior head carriage. This anatomy train also defines the posture we have when we startle or have a fright and move into a self-protective stance. This line is often tight (and shortened) from sitting or habitual forward flexion. The Superficial Front Line flexes the body and its path is as follows:
From tops of toes → tibialis anterior → quads → rectus abdominis → sternal fascia → scalp

Yoga can support this line auspiciously by balancing it, improving postural ease and breath capacity. Yoga *asana* are healthful for resolving tension or shortening in this line are as follows:
- *Cobra*: Opens the front line from the tops of the feet to the chest
- *Camel*: Deep stretch and toning for the entire Superficial Front Line

## Superficial Back Line

The Superficial Back Line consists largely of postural, endurance-oriented muscles and connective tissue. It maintains extension and provides support during upright standing and walking. When shortened, this anatomy train can contribute to limited forward folding and compression in the posterior chain. It often holds tension related to over-effort, hypervigilance, or standing fatigue. A chronically loaded superficial back line may result in discomfort in the low back, hamstrings, or neck. The Superficial Back Line extends and supports the body's upright posture and plays a crucial role in resisting the pull of gravity. Its path is as follows:
From plantar fascia → Achilles tendon → gastrocnemius → hamstrings → sacrotuberous ligament → erector spinae → scalp fascia

Yoga can support this line by lengthening it gradually and rhythmically, particularly through slow forward bends and practices that encourage softening rather than pulling. Yoga *asana* examples that are healthful for this line include:
- *Standing Forward Fold:* Creates gradual length through the posterior chain from feet to head
- *Downward Facing Dog:* Gently stretches the entire line while allowing for spinal traction

## Deep Front Line

The Deep Front Line is composed of deep stabilizing muscles and fascial structures. It is essential for postural integrity, breath regulation, and smooth, balanced movement. It supports axial elongation, spinal stabilization, and diaphragmatic function. Because it spans the pelvic, abdominal, and thoracic cavities, dysfunction in the Deep Front Line can contribute to core instability, shallow breathing, or tension patterns that are harder to sense. This line stabilizes the core, supports breath, and links the body's central vertical axis. Its path is as follows:
From inner arch → tibialis posterior → adductors → pelvic floor → psoas → diaphragm → anterior spine and mediastinum → scalene muscles → deep throat and tongue

Yoga practice can enhance awareness and tonicity of this line through subtle engagement, gentle spinal undulation, and breath-centered movement. Healthful yoga *asana* examples include:

- *Mountain with diaphragmatic breathing*: Supports vertical integrity and access to the Deep Front Line's deep support and muscle tone
- *Constructive Rest* with mindful breath and pelvic floor awareness: Restores parasympathetic balance and integration of this line

## Lateral Line

The Lateral Line governs side-to-side movement and postural adjustments, especially when weight-bearing asymmetrically. It is crucial for maintaining equilibrium in walking, single-leg balance, and lateral reach. When tight or imbalanced, the Lateral Line may contribute to hip hiking, scoliosis patterns, or uneven spinal curves. Tension here may also impact breathing through asymmetrical rib basket mobility. This line stabilizes the body side-to-side and supports lateral flexion and balance. Its path is as follows:

From peroneals → iliotibial tract (IT band) → obliques → intercostals → lateral neck muscles (sternocleidomastoid and scalenes) → ear fascia

Yoga can tone and lengthen the Lateral Line through lateral bends, standing balances, and spiral movements that challenge stability. Healthful yoga *asana* examples are as follows:
- *Gate:* Opens and lengthens the side body along the entire line
- *Half Moon:* Engages the Lateral Line in support of balance and side-body lift

## Spiral Line

The Spiral Line wraps diagonally around the body in a helix-like fashion. It facilitates rotation and counter-rotation, helping the body stabilize during walking, spiraling, and dynamic transitions. This anatomy train works with other lines to prevent torque injuries and ensure integrity in cross-body movement. When imbalanced, this line may contribute to asymmetrical tension, SI joint strain, or over-rotation in the thoracic spine. The Spiral Line coordinates cross-body movement and integrates rotation and stabilization. Its path is as follows:

From occiput → rhomboids → obliques → tensor fasciae latae → outer leg → fibularis longus → arch → looping back up the opposite side

Yoga that includes twisting, oppositional reaching, and contralateral engagement helps balance this line and promote integrated movement patterns. Health yoga *asana* examples are:
- *Revolved Triangle*: Activates contralateral spirals across the torso and legs
- *Thread the Needle*: Opens and integrates spiral fascial connections through a supported twist

## What's Ahead

Having now explored the general concepts of human movement, anatomy, and physiology, a closer look is needed at the human body from a movement and yoga perspective. The next three chapters cover the axial, upper appendicular, and lower appendicular regions of the body. For each, bones, joints, muscles, and movement patterns are explored. Many tables and lists are offered to make the information more digestible and easier to peruse. Section Two of the volume then takes these concepts and applies them to yoga *asana* teaching and therapeutics in the context of the various types of yoga *asana*, from basic standing shapes to complex inversions.

# Chapter 4: Anatomy of the Axial Region of the Body

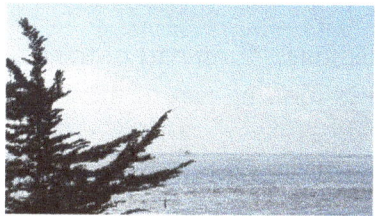

This chapter explores the anatomy of the axial region of the body, from the head to the vertebral column and thorax, with special emphasis on the spine. For each section in that body region, the chapter offers information about key structures – bones, joints, muscles, and movement patterns. It does so sequentially and assumes the reader's understanding (that was hopefully created in prior chapters) that these structures are, of course, completely interdependent, co-regulated, and connected. They never work in isolation of one another, nor of any other body regions and *koshas*. The sequential approach was chosen for ease of communication.

## Head

The head is the uppermost region of the body and houses key structures that support perception, communication, balance, and neural integration. In the context of yoga *asana* teaching and therapeutics, the head is significant as the site of major sensory organs, brain, and cranial nerves, all of which influence posture, breath, and autonomic function. Awareness of the head's orientation and support – particularly in relation to the cervical spine and jaw – can affect nervous system regulation, muscular tension, and proprioceptive feedback throughout the body.

## Bones and Joints of the Head

### *Bones of the Head*

(Note that the bones of the neck will be covered in the spine section.) Bones of the skull proper are fused. This is not terribly relevant to yoga but very relevant to other therapies, such as craniosacral work. The fused bones of the skull include the frontal bone (forehead), temporal bone, parietal bone, and occiput.

The bones in the face consist of a series of bony arches. These arches evolved from the hard parts of the gill arches of fish and obtain their arch shape from this origin. As an aside, the soft parts of the gills evolved into our lungs. The facial arches, from the eye on down, include the zygomatic arch, maxillary arch, mandibular arch, hyoid bone, and the laryngeal and tracheal cartilages – all arch-shaped. The face, also known as the facial skeleton or viscerocranium, consist of 14 bones (or bony structures) that primarily support facial structure, house sensory organs, and provide attachment points for facial muscles. These bones collectively shape the face; support essential functions like breathing, chewing, and speaking; and form the bony framework that interacts with soft tissues during yoga practices such as breath awareness, jaw release, and sensory focus. These bones (shown in Figure 1.26) include:

- *Nasal bones* (2) – form the bridge of the nose
- *Maxillae* (2) – form the upper jaw, support the upper teeth, and contribute to the orbit and nasal cavity
- *Zygomatic bones* (2) – the cheekbones; form part of the lateral wall and floor of the orbit
- *Lacrimal bones* (2) – small bones forming part of the medial wall of each orbit; house the lacrimal sac
- *Palatine bones* (2) – form the posterior part of the hard palate and part of the nasal cavity and orbit
- *Inferior nasal conchae* (2) – curved bones within the nasal cavity that help warm and humidify inhaled air
- *Vomer* (1) – forms the inferior portion of the nasal septum
- *Mandible* (1) – the lower jawbone; the only moveable bone of the facial skeleton and the strongest facial bone

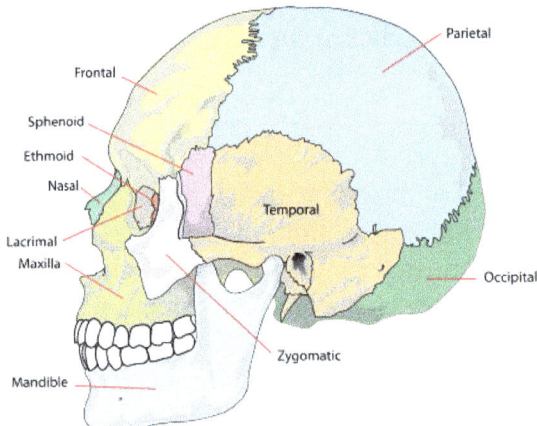

**Figure 1.26** Human skull bones. (Data source: LadyofHats; https://commons.wikimedia.org/wiki/File:Human_skull_side_simplified_(bones).svg; public domain)

## Joints of the Head

The two primary joints types in the head are the skull sutures (essentially non-movable fibrous joints) and the temporomandibular joint (TMJ). The latter is a hinge and gliding joint (gliding away from the ear forward). It functions as a hinge when we talk, but acts as a gliding joint when we eat and/or open the mouth wide. The gliding action of the head of the mandible at the ear can be felt when we open and close the mouth. Once we open wide enough, we can feel the gliding motion of the jaw with the heads of the mandible moving away from the ear. If the two sides of the TMJ move at the same time and speed, the jaws are *tracking*; if they do not, then the jaws are misaligned.

Discomfort can be experienced in the TMJ due to many factors, including bruxism (grinding teeth), trauma, stress, and tension. Symptoms include jaw pain, limited motion, and headaches. Lion's Breath works on the temporomandibular joint, by reducing stress and tension in the joints and surrounding tissue. Another method to address TMJ discomfort is to lie prone and fix the jaw on the floor; then open and close the mouth, letting head move via the opening of the jaw as opposed to moving the jaw when the head is fixed.

### Bony Landmarks on the Head

- *Zygomatic arch* – lower bony edge at the temple – the opening for the temporalis muscle (the muscle that produces the force to close the jaw)
- *Ramus* of the mandible – corner of the jaw
- *Coronoid* process of the mandible - knobby thing at the top of the mandible that serves as attachment site for the temporalis muscle
- *Base of skull* – essentially the sitz bones of the skull, where the skull meets the spine (at the atlas, the topmost vertebra)

## Muscles of the Head, Face, and Neck

There over 30 pairs of muscles in the head, face, and neck (see Figures 1.27 and 1.28). Covered here are only those most relevant to yoga practice (though, as yogis, perhaps we do not do enough face yoga, which can actually be quite helpful). The anterior and lateral neck muscles move the head and neck, contribute to swallowing actions, and help lift the rib basket during breathing. The posterior neck muscles act on the cervical spine and neck – the primary focus here. (Note: although the trapezius muscles extend all the way up the head, they are discussed under the back muscles and muscles of the shoulder girdle).

Several key superficial muscles of the face and jaw influence expression and functional movement, elements that can subtly affect yoga practice, especially in restorative and breath-focused work. The platysma, a thin, superficial muscle of the anterior neck, draws the lower lip and corners of the mouth downward and laterally; it originates from the fascia of the pectoralis major and deltoid and inserts into the mandible and surrounding facial muscles. The temporalis and masseter are primary muscles of mastication that move the jaw; they originate from the skull and zygomatic arch, respectively, and insert onto the mandible. Notably, the masseter often holds tension associated with stress or aggression. In yoga, mindful awareness of these muscles during breathwork, meditation, or relaxation practices can help release unconscious gripping or bracing in the jaw and throat, supporting a more easeful, open posture and breath. The fascial muscles also support a gentle smile – a beautiful way to find a joyful expression of any yoga *asana* shape.

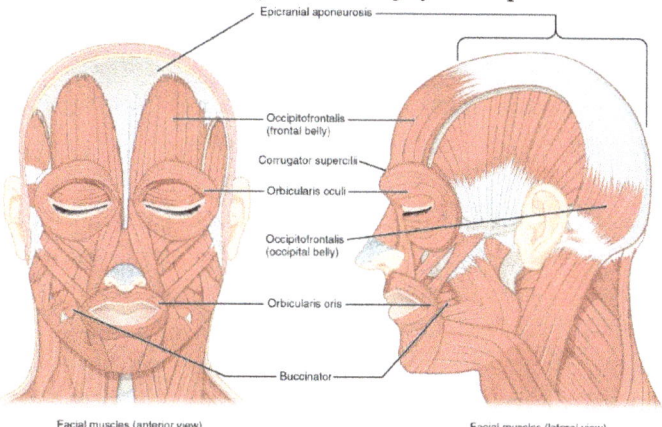

**Figure 1.27** Facial muscles. (Data source: OpenStax; https://commons.wikimedia.org/wiki/File:1106_Front_and_Side_Views_of_the_Muscles_of_Facial_Expressions.jpg; Creative Commons Attribution 4.0)

Next, the scalenes are important muscles located in the lateral neck that contribute to cervical movement and respiration. Comprised of three sections (anterior, middle, and posterior) these muscles originate from the transverse processes of the cervical vertebrae and insert on the first and second ribs. Their actions include neck flexion, contralateral rotation, and side bending. In addition, the scalenes can play a role in breath mechanics as they help elevate the first two ribs which may happen during stressed or effortful inhalation. In yoga *asana*, the scalenes support healthy neck alignment; in *pranayama*, their conscious relaxation supports easeful nasal and diaphragmatic breath that is subtle and smooth.

The sternocleidomastoid (SCM) muscles, with origins on sternum and clavicles and insertions on the mastoid process of the skull, are responsible for contralateral rotation and ipsilateral lateral flexion of the head. When both SCMs contract simultaneously, they contribute to forward head posture, a common pattern in states of stress or fear, but also in modern life where devises pull our heads forward. In this position, the lower cervical spine flexes and the upper cervical spine hyperextends. This dysfunctional pattern often correlates with a compensatory shift in the pelvis and ribcage, restricting breath and perpetuating tension. In yoga, opening and balancing the SCMs can help restore more neutral head alignment and improve breath capacity.

Longus colli and longus capitis are deep cervical flexor muscles that run alongside the posterior longitudinal ligament of the neck. They are key to maintaining cervical alignment and preventing hyperextension of the neck. When these muscles are weak (e.g., due to SCM overactivation), they permit forward head posture and instability. Strengthening the longus colli and capitis through controlled movements that strengthen the neck (e.g., vertebra-by-vertebra rolling down from Bridge) can help restore cervical stability.

Rectus capitis anterior and lateralis are small muscles that assist with flexion, rotation, and side bending of the head. They originate from the atlas and insert on the occiput. Though subtle in their actions, these muscles contribute to refined control of the head and neck, supporting balance and coordination during movement. Also in this body region, levator scapula plays a less obvious but important role in cervical stability. While traditionally known for its role in elevating the scapula, this muscle also acts to prevent excessive forward head posture. In yoga practice, its involvement becomes particularly relevant when addressing imbalances between the neck and shoulder girdle. More about this muscle below.

Collectively, these muscles profoundly influence posture, neck movement, and breathing, making them highly relevant in yoga *asana* and *pranayama* practice. Patterns of neck tension, forward head posture, and shallow chest or clavicular breathing often reflect underlying imbalances among these muscles, imbalances that can be addressed through intentional *asana*, breathwork, and inner awareness. Shapes and movements that emphasize spinal alignment, balanced head positioning, and core engagement can help restore functional relationships among these muscles. Integration of breath awareness and optimal functional breathing can down-regulate the stress responses, reducing habitual tension in the SCMs and scalenes, while deep flexor engagement supports an upright, easeful posture. For yoga practitioners and yoga professionals alike, understanding these muscular relationships enriches the precision and the therapeutic potential of several of the eight-limb practices as they support *asana*, *pranayama*, and posture during the inner practices.

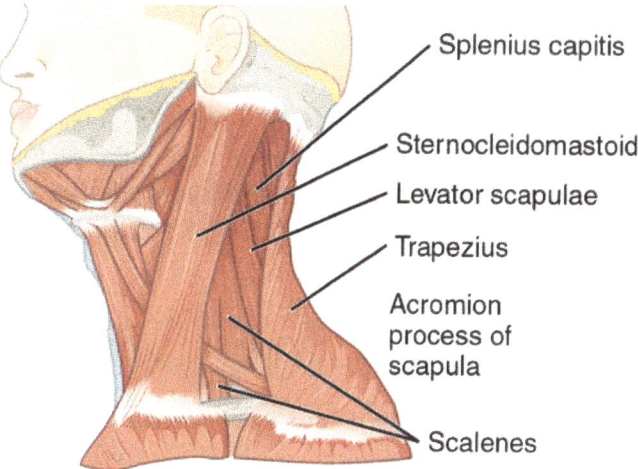

Figure 1.28 Neck muscles. (Data source: OpenStax; https://commons.wikimedia.org/wiki/File:1111_Posterior_and_Side_Views_of_the_Neck_Lateral_view.png; Creative Commons Attribution 3.0)

## Vertebral Column and Thorax

The vertebral column forms the central axis of the body, providing structural support and mobility while protecting the spinal cord. In yoga *asana* teaching and therapeutics, it is essential to understand the spine's role in transmitting force, coordinating movement, and supporting neural communication. Its curves, segmental motion, and relationships with surrounding musculature influence posture, breathing, balance, and systemic regulation. A functional spine supports adaptability and ease, while restrictions or misalignment can contribute to compensatory patterns across the entire body.

The thorax encompasses the rib basket, thoracic spine, and diaphragm, forming a protective enclosure for the heart and lungs. This region is integral to respiratory function, spinal mobility, and core stability. The dynamic relationship between breath and thoracic movement directly can affect autonomic nervous system state (or *guna*), circulation, and postural support. Understanding the thorax as both a container and a responsive structure allows for more accurate cueing guidance during breath-based and therapeutic movement practices.

## Bones of the Vertebral Column and Thorax

The spine's primary function is twofold: to provide structural support for the body and to protect the spinal cord. Structurally, it bears and transmits weight from the head and torso to the pelvis and lower limbs, maintaining upright posture and facilitating movement. Functionally, it houses the spinal cord within the vertebral canal, shielding this vital part of the central nervous system from mechanical injury. The spinal cord relays sensory information from the body to the brain and motor commands from the brain to the body, enabling coordinated movement and reflexes. The spine's design – combining strength, flexibility, and protection – makes it indispensable to both locomotion and neural integrity.

## Overview of the Vertebral Column, Thorax, and Vertebrae

There are on average 33 bones along the length of the spine, called vertebrae and divided up across five sections of the spinal column (shown in Figure 1.29): cervical, thoracic, lumbar, sacral, and coccygeal. Of these ~33 vertebrae, 24 are movable; the rest are fused. Vertebrae are numbered consecutively from the top down and lettered based on the section of the spine (e.g., C1 = first [most superior] vertebra of the cervical spine; L5 = fifth [most inferior] vertebra of the lumbar spine).

### Cervical Spine (aka Neck)

The cervical spine is the uppermost portion of the vertebral column, consisting of seven vertebrae that support the head, protect the spinal cord, and allow for a high degree of mobility in the neck. It plays a crucial role in posture, proprioception, and the integration of neural, vascular, and muscular functions between the head and the rest of the body. Its bony features include:
- Seven cervical vertebrae (C1-C7); C1 + C2 = upper cervicals; C3 – C7 = lower cervicals
- C1 connects to the base of the skull and supports the head
- Each cervical vertebrae has a transverse foramen that allows the cranial arteries to supply the brain with blood
- The atlas (aka C1) is the most superior cervical vertebra and holds the head; it has no body (just a strong bony ring) and no spinous process to allow the head to bend back)
- The axis (aka C2) sits below the atlas; it has an extension called the dens that connects it to the atlas in a special joint that allows the head to move side to side (in fact, this is the location where the bulk of neck rotation takes place)

### Thoracic Spine and Rib Basket

The thoracic spine and rib basket form the central portion of the axial skeleton, providing structural support, protection for vital organs, and a dynamic foundation for breathing. This region balances mobility with stability, integrating spinal movement with respiratory function and playing a key role in posture, core support, and nervous system regulation. Its bony features include:
- Twelve thoracic vertebrae (T1-T12), attached to 12 pairs of ribs
- Rib pairs 1 to 7 attach posteriorly to T1 to T7 and anteriorly directly to the sternum via a section of cartilage
- Rib pairs 8 to 10 attach posteriorly to T8 to T10 and anteriorly to cartilage that attaches to the sternum via an even longer section of cartilage
- Rib pairs 11 and 12 attach posteriorly to T11 to T12 and have no anterior attachment
- The discs between T2 to T9 are best hydrated via back breathing
- The anteriorly located sternum has three bones: manubrium, sternum proper, and xiphoid process; an important landmark is the sternal angle (a tiny bump about 3 cm below the manubrium that marks the second rib)
- *Landmarks*:
    o lower border of the rib basket is called the costal margin

- moving along the costal margin posteriorly helps locate the 10th rib above the anterior superior iliac spine (ASIS) (unless this rib is fused at the costal margin)
- the 11th rib is palpable above the iliac crest
- the 12th rib is above the posterior superior iliac spine (PSIS) (unless it is too deep because of poor posture [leaning back into the rib basket], which can actually press the 12th rib into the kidneys)

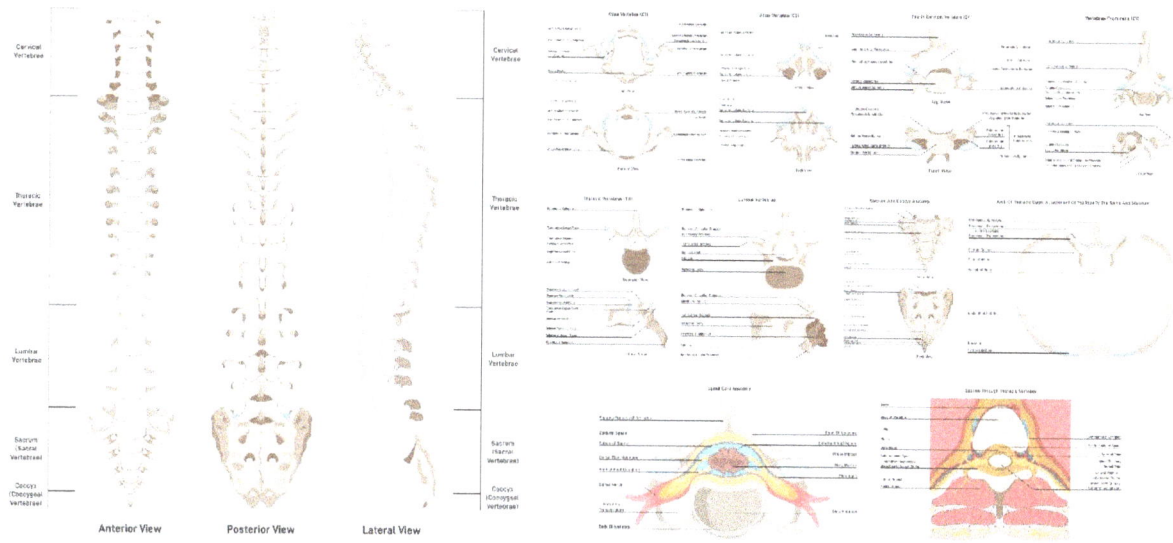

**Figure 1.29** Human spine anatomy. (Data source: Istock) -- see Pages 127 and 128 for an expanded version

## *Lumbar Spine, Sacrum, and Coccyx*

The lumbar spine, sacrum, and coccyx make up the lower portion of the vertebral column, providing a strong, stable base for weight-bearing, movement, and support of the upper body. Together, they absorb compressive forces, protect the lower spinal cord and cauda equina, and play a central role in load transfer between the spine and pelvis, making them crucial to postural integrity and functional movement in yoga practice. In typical anatomy convention, the lumbar spine plus sacrum are collectively referred to as the low back or lower back. Their bony features include the following:

- Lumbar Spine:
  - Five lumbar vertebrae (L1-L5)
  - L5 connects to the sacrum at a relatively vulnerable joint with S1; because of the anterior tilt of the pelvis, L5 could slide forward on S1 if it were not for very strong ligaments protecting this joint by lending enormous stability and support
- Sacrum:
  - Flat triangle in the low back below lumbar spine; part of the axial skeleton (lowest part of the spine)
  - Five sacral vertebrae (S1-S5) that are separate at birth and fully fused by age 6
  - Location where the axial skeleton (sacrum) meets the appendicular skeleton (ilia) at the sacroiliac joints (see below), stabilized by very strong ligaments (see below)
  - Tom Myers says that the fact that the sacrum is mobile during infancy and toddlerhood calls into question the shape of car seats which may put too much of a curve into the

sacrum – then as the sacrum fuses, that excessive curve may remain in the sacrum forever, further encouraged by slouched sitting at computers and on couches
- Coccyx
    - Also known as the tailbone, the coccyx is made up of three to five fused coccygeal vertebrae that cannot be differentiated (unlike in the sacrum, where the fusion points are easily discerned).
    - A broken tailbone at the joint with the sacrum can cause lots of problems, including back aches, neck aches, even headaches.

## *Anatomy of the Vertebrae*

The vertebrae together, via connections to each other by intervertebral discs and long ligaments, form the spinal column. Thanks to their shapes and functions, mobility increases as we move up the spine (i.e., more range of motion) and stability increases as we move down the spine (i.e., more load-bearing). Their parts and functions are nothing short of miraculous.

### *Parts, Functions, and Relationships of the Vertebrae*

Each vertebra has a vertebral body and bony ring, complex structures with key functions. Vertebral bodies are located at the anterior portion of the spine and are spongey, which is not ideal for load bearing. The bony rings at of the posterior region of the spine (called the spinous and transverse processes) therefore are key to sharing the load on the spine. The *vertebral bodies* come in different shapes and sizes depending on the location in the spine, adapted to the specific load bearing and functions needed in their respective spinal section. The shape of the vertebral bodies is mimicked by the intervertebral disc located between neighboring vertebrae.
- Cervical vertebral bodies (Figure 1.30) are oval to oblong and relatively small and thus less capable of load bearing. Notably, C1 (aka the atlas) has no vertebral body at all. The atlas makes a connection superiorly with the skull and inferiorly with C2 (aka the axis).
- Thoracic vertebral bodies (Figure 1.31) are heart-shaped and slightly larger and more load-bearing than those in the cervical region.
- Lumbar vertebral bodies (Figure 1.32) are round and large for maximum weight-bearing capacity in this stable and load-bearing part of this spine.
- Sacrum and coccyx have unique shapes by virtue of the fact that by adulthood, their vertebral bodies entirely fused (Figure 1.33). The sacrum is covered in more detail below.

A *bony ring* at the posterior and lateral portions of each vertebra has several distinct features, contributing to load bearing, stability, and movement in the spine (see Figure 1.30).
- The vertebral arch is essentially a bony ring posterior to the vertebral body with two anterior pedicles and two posterior laminae. This arch creates the opening for the spinal cord.
- Lateral transverse processes reach out to the side, emerging from between the arch's pedicles and laminae. The transverse processes are prime attachment sites for spinal muscles, ligaments, and fascia. They function like a handle bar: when the muscles on the right transverse process contract, the vertebra turns right; left contraction creates a left turn.
- The spinous processes are bony extensions to the posterior and can be easily palpated in the spine and seen during Forward Folds. They emerge from the laminae of the arch and serve as another important attachment point for muscles, fascia, and ligaments.

Finally, each meeting point between neighboring vertebrae also has a neural foramen (or opening; see Figure 1.30) that allows spinal nerves to exit from the spinal cord into the body.

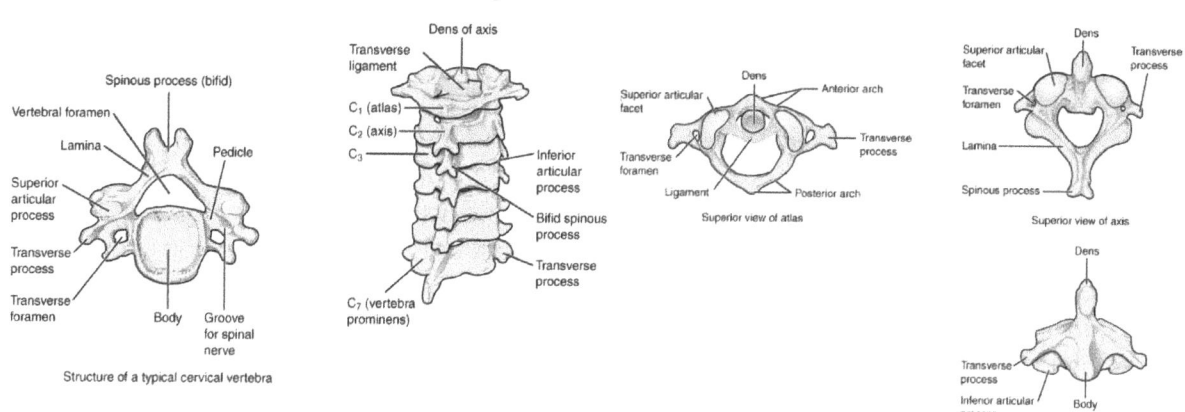

**Figure 1.30** Cervical vertebrae. (Data source: OpenStax; https://commons.wikimedia.org/wiki/File:723_Cervical_Vertebrae.jpg; Creative Commons Attribution 3.0)

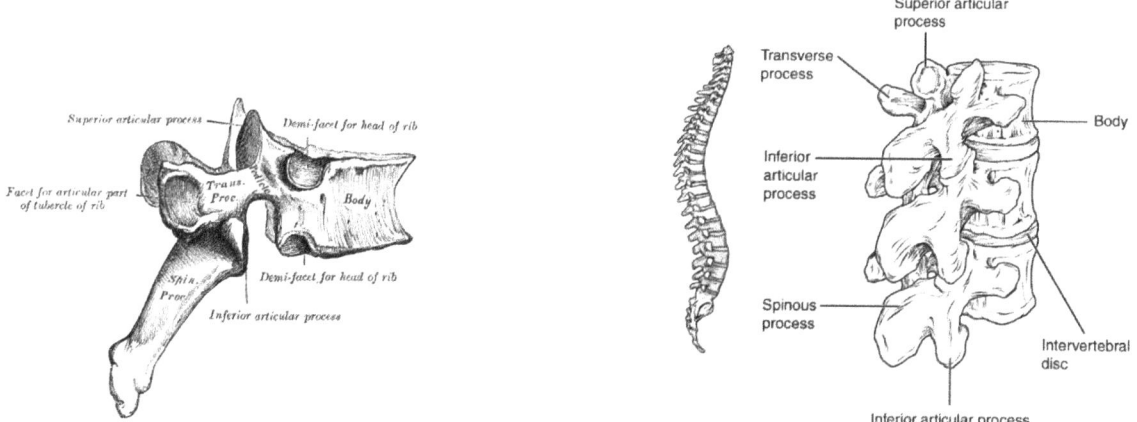

**Figure 1.31** Thoracic vertebrae. (Data source: Henry Vandyke Carter; https://commons.wikimedia.org/wiki/File:Brustwirbel_seite.png; public domain)

**Figure 1.32** Lumbar vertebrae. (Data source: OpenStax; https://commons.wikimedia.org/wiki/File:725_Lumbar_Vertebrae.jpg; Creative Commons Attribution 3.0)

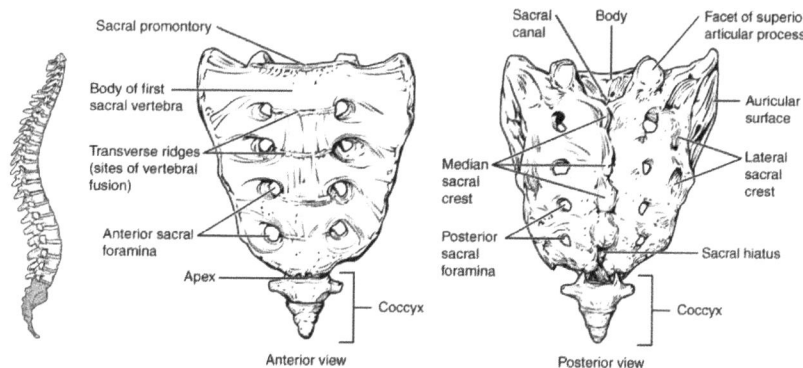

**Figure 1.33** Sacrum and coccyx. (Data source: OpenStax; https://commons.wikimedia.org/wiki/File:720_Sacrum_and_Coccyx.jpg; Creative Commons Attribution 3.0)

*Intervertebral Discs*

Intervertebral discs (Figure 1.34) are crucial components of the spine, serving as shock absorbers, spacers, and connectors between adjoining vertebrae. These discs, which constitute roughly 25% to 40% of the spine's length, are a type of cartilaginous joint and are part of the overall vertebral body joint (more about this below). They play a vital role in redirecting compressive forces, enhancing spinal stability, and contributing to the body's tensegrity. Structurally, each disc resembles the vertebral body it borders. Each disc has a soft, jelly-like center, known as nucleus pulposus, surrounded by a tough, fibrous outer ring called annulus fibrosus. Discs vary in thickness along the spine, being thinner in the cervical region and progressively thicker in the lumbar region. They have a slight wedge shape, oriented posteriorly in some spinal sections and anteriorly in others, which helps to create the spine's natural curves (kyphosis and lordosis). Disc hydration levels fluctuate throughout the day, being highest in the morning and lowest in the evening. Clark (2016) recommends delaying yoga practice for at least 30 minutes after waking, as spinal ligaments are most vulnerable when discs are most hydrated.

Prolonged sitting with lumbar flexion dehydrates the discs, making ligaments slacker and increasing vulnerability to injury; lumbar extension is recommended before lifting heavy objects in such cases. Although compression can contribute to disc hydration, disc issues generally arise not from sudden movements (except in high-force accidents) but from repetitive strain and habitual movement patterns, often leading to one-sided pain. In the lumbar spine, the annulus fibrosus is particularly susceptible to wear and tear from grinding. With age, the nucleus pulposus becomes more fibrous and less resilient, reducing spinal range of motion and increasing vulnerability to stress. Interestingly, the intervertebral discs in the cervical, lumbar, and lower thoracic spine are hydrated by movement. However, the upper thoracic spine (T2 to T9) relies primarily on back body breathing for disc hydration. Overall, intervertebral discs are adaptable structures with good capacity for healing.

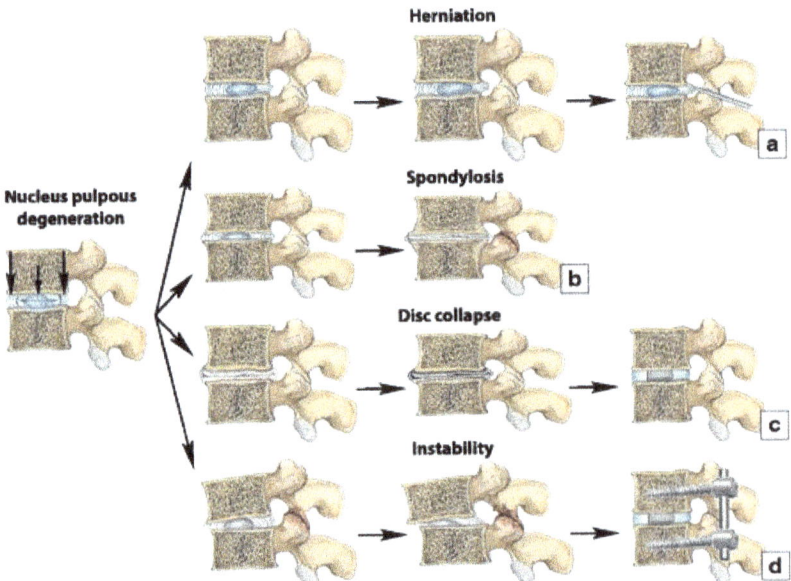

**Figure 1.34** Intervertebral disc degeneration. (Data source: Irina Nefedova; https://commons.wikimedia.org/wiki/File:Surgical_treatment_options_for_degenerative_changes.webp; Creative Commons Attribution 4.0)

## Joints and Ligaments of the Vertebral Column and Thorax

There are three types of joint categories in this region of the body: vertebral body joints, facet joints, and several specialized joints. It is helpful to have a clear understanding of each type of joints, its functions, and its vulnerability and strengths.

### *Vertebral Body Joints*

The vertebral body joints are the linkages between neighboring vertebrae and the intervening discs in one complex joint capsule (consisting of two vertebrae and one disc). They are the primary articulation points between vertebrae via the cartilaginous intervertebral disc between them. The following features and details are notable about vertebral body joints, all crucial to understand for the auspicious and safe teaching and application of therapeutic yoga *asana*:

- The whole vertebral body joint structure is encased in joint capsules, fascia, and ligaments; the joints can be thought of this as two separate joints, or symphyses – one between the lower vertebral body and the disc; and another between the upper vertebral body with the same disc
- These joints are at the anterior portion of the spine and function like a series of ball and socket joints; they can move in any direction but only a tiny bit at each joint; movement across all the vertebral body joints is additive to create complexity and range of motion of spinal movement overall
- Because the joints between the vertebrae and discs are cartilaginous (see Figure 1.35), they are less movable and more vulnerable to compression; hence the joints in the bony arch (covered below) provide the major weight-bearing and load transfer in the spine

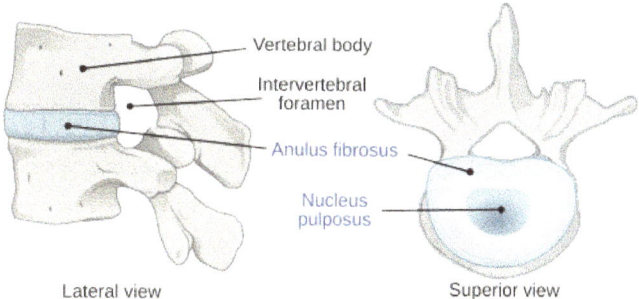

**Figure 1.35** Intervertebral disc. (Data source: Jmarchn, https://commons.wikimedia.org/wiki/File:716_Intervertebral_Disk.svg; Creative Commons Attribution 3.

### *Facet Joints*

Facing upward and downward from each vertebral arch are four facet joints: two facing up, one per side; two facing down, one per side (see Figure 1.36). They make up the secondary articulation points between vertebrae (with the primary articulation point being the vertebral body joint). Facet joints are gliding synovial joints with a small joint capsule filled with mechanoreceptors, proprioceptors, and nociceptors. These receptors provide feedback to the nervous system that affects activation of muscles and fascia, with effects on the degree of stability and load borne by the facet joints. The facets in each facet joints have particular angles that determine the type and depth of movement at that particular level of the spine (i.e., type of movement and range of motion are determined by the bony ring of the spine, not by the vertebral body).

- *Lumbar* facet joints face straight up and down in the sagittal plane and thus allow for ample flexion, extension, and lateral flexion, with limited rotation in anatomical position (only 5 degrees), a little more in a Forward Fold (because flexion creates more space between the facet joint), and even less in a Backbend (because even less space is available in extension). Rotations in backbends are not recommended for that reason; any rotation seen in this part of the torso comes from soft tissue rotating around the lumbar spine, especially from the internal and external obliques in the abdomen
- At the level of *thoracic* spine, alignment of the facet joints changes (starting at T1-T12) to lie in the frontal plane; this makes ample rotation and good lateral flexion possible, but limits flexion and extension
- At the level of the *cervical* spine, the facet joints are almost completely horizontal which allows for all movements – extension, flexion, lateral flexion, and rotation; however, the structure of the cervical spine does not allow for circumduction of the neck (in other words, although often encouraged in yoga, full range neck rolls can be harmful)
- The bony arch at the posterior region of the spine further contributes to what is and is not possible in terms of range of motion at each segment of the spine

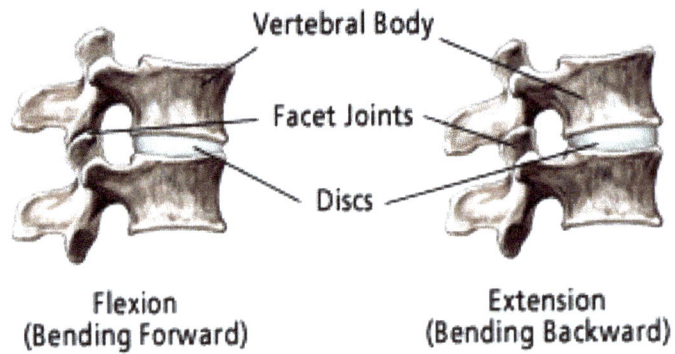

**Figure 1.36** Facet joints. (Data source: Dr.foksha; https://commons.wikimedia.org/wiki/File:Facet-joints.png; Creative Commons Attribution 4.0)

## *Specialized Joints Between the Vertebrae*

Several unique joints exist along the length of the spine. They are uniquely adapted to the specific functions and ranges of motion they facilitate. Importantly:

- *Atlanto-occipital joint*: C1 (aka atlas) meets the occiput of the skull without a disc between them – a completely horizontal joint; sometimes called the *yes* joint as neck flexion and extension (nodding the head as in saying yes) happen here because there are no spinous processes to limit that range of motion; also allows lateral flexion and rotation
- *Atlanto-axial joint*: C1 meets C2 (aka axis) – an almost horizontal joint; sometimes called the *no* joint as neck rotation happens here (as in shaking the head no)
- *C7 meets T1* as a transitional joint where cervical lordosis changes over to thoracic kyphosis – this joint is vulnerable because of this transition, especially if the individual tends to slouch or hunch (i.e., does not maintain good posture in this region of the spine)

- *L5 with S1* allows a little bit more rotation than most of the rest of the lumbar spine (only L4-L5 allows for more rotation); L5-S1 joint is a heavy weight bearing joint and also the junction in the spine where the load from the torso is transferred onto the pelvis

## Sternochondral Joints

A notable feature of the thorax is the presence of sternocostal joints, the articulations between the sternum and the cartilage extensions of the ribs. These sections of cartilage and the sternocostal joints allow the rib basket to expand and contract, facilitating respiration. This structural arrangement provides the rib basket with the capacity to absorb significant frontal impact, such as might be experienced during a car accident, without resulting in bone fractures.

## Ligaments Across the Joints of the Vertebral Column and Thorax

Successful functioning of the vertebral columns is supported by a wealth of ligaments that connect the spine along its length, as well as across the many articulations between adjoining vertebrae (Figure 1.37). The complexity of these ligaments supports the incredible range of motion and complexity of movements in the spine – supporting both stability and mobility. (Note: also see ligaments of the pelvic girdle for ligaments around the SI joints in Chapter 5.)

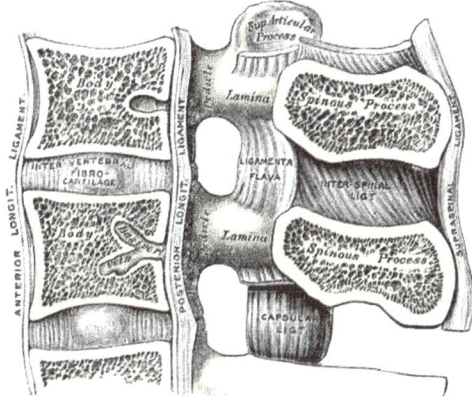

**Figure 1.37** Ligaments of the spine. (Data source: Henry Vandyke Carter; https://commons.wikimedia.org/wiki/File:Gray301.png; public domain)

Two ligaments run along the full length of the spine and are often implicated in strong sensations during yoga *asana* practices that flex or extend the spine. They are the anterior (forward on the vertebral bodies) and posterior (on the backside of the vertebral bodies) longitudinal ligaments.

The *anterior longitudinal ligament* (ALL) is a strong, fibrous band that runs along the anterior surface of the vertebral bodies, from the base of the skull to the sacrum. It plays a crucial role in spinal stability by limiting hyperextension and preventing excessive anterior displacement of the vertebrae. Notably, the ALL also serves as a point of attachment for fascial connections that suspend the abdominal organs, highlighting its integral role in the Deep Front Line of the body and its relationship to the organ column and its role in core stability. Unlike muscles, the ALL possesses limited elasticity, which can significantly restrict spinal extension (for good reasons). This characteristic is particularly relevant in yoga *asana* practice during backbends. Pain experienced in the low back, especially at the L5-S1 junction, during backbends can often be attributed to tension or restriction within the ALL or other Deep Front Line structures, rather than the posterior structures. This restriction can force the lumbar spine to hinge, leading to discomfort and the potential for repetitive stress injuries if engaged in regularly.

Yoga teachers and therapists best emphasize a gradual approach to Backbends, prioritizing spinal elongation and core engagement to distribute extension evenly along the spine (including whatever limited range of motion is available in the thoracic spine), rather than forcing the low back into excessive lordosis or hinging. It is important to respect the inherent limitations of the anterior longitudinal ligament's elasticity, focusing on fostering resilience and balanced support throughout the Deep Front Line rather than aiming for increased ligamentous length which, over time, will compromise spinal stability. To avoid pain and injury, patient and consistent work is needed, allowing months of practice to improve the resilience of the Deep Front Line and to correctly encourage safe backbending.

The *posterior longitudinal ligament* (PLL) is a vital structure for spinal stability that runs along the posterior aspect of the vertebral bodies, from the axis (C2) to the sacrum. Its primary function is to limit spinal flexion, effectively preventing excessive forward bending, and to restrict posterior displacement of the vertebrae. Additionally, the PLL plays a role in protecting the intervertebral discs by acting as a barrier against herniation, particularly in the lumbar region, where disc herniations are most common.

In yoga *asana* practice, this becomes highly relevant: forward folds, such as a Standing Forward Fold, stretch the PLL, potentially increasing its resilience but also demanding mindful engagement to avoid overstretching. Conversely, backbends, such as Camel or Cobra, create slack in the PLL, which is important to remember when working with students who have hypermobility or prior back injuries. Yoga teachers and therapists can help support the healthy engagement of the PLL by emphasizing controlled, gradual movements in forward folds and backbends, incorporating core engagement to support the spine and protect the PLL. Awareness of the PLL's role in spinal stability is essential for safe and effective yoga *asana* instruction, especially when addressing individuals with spinal concerns or injuries.

Several important stabilizing ligaments run between vertebrae at shorter distances, some between adjacent vertebrae, some crossing several. These shorter spinal ligaments include the supraspinous, interspinal, and transverse ligaments, as well as ligamentum flavum.

The *supraspinous ligament*, a highly elastic structure running along the tips of the spinous processes from the sacrum to the cervical spine (where it transitions into the nuchal ligament), facilitates spinal flexion by allowing for significant movement between the vertebrae. This elasticity, while beneficial for forward folding, necessitates careful consideration in yoga *asana* practice to prevent overstretching. Complementing the functions of the supraspinous ligaments, *interspinal ligaments* (connecting adjacent spinous processes) and *intertransverse ligaments* (linking adjacent transverse processes) provide additional stability and limit excessive lateral movement.

The *ligamentum flavum*, a unique and highly elastic ligament, connects the laminae of the vertebral arches from the second cervical vertebra (C2) to the sacrum, contributing significantly to spinal stability and assisting in returning the spine to a neutral position after flexion. In yoga *asana*, understanding these ligamentous roles is crucial for safe and effective practice. Teachers optimally emphasize controlled movements, especially in flexion, to respect the supraspinous ligaments' elasticity. Moreover, awareness of interspinal, intertransverse, and ligamentum flavum's functions informs the approach to lateral flexion or side-bending and backbending, ensuring stability and preventing injury. When working with clients, especially those with hypermobility or spinal concerns, it is vital to prioritize core engagement and mindful movement to protect these ligaments and promote healthy spinal alignment.

## Muscles along the Vertebral Column and Thorax

### Muscles of the Back

Spine health is not only about the ability to hold a particular position (i.e., stability) but also about the ability to move (i.e., mobility). Important to stability, *lumbodorsal connective tissue* shares the load with spinal muscles and has been described to have the tensile strength of steel (Mitchell, 2019). The spine is designed to move in all directions and some yogis say that we are only as old (biologically) as the spine is flexible. Three levels of spinal muscles are supported, of course, by all types of connective tissues that help facilitate stability and mobility along the spine: *superficial*, *intermediate*, and *deep*. The deepest layer of spinal muscles is most important to posture (or postural stability). The other layers are more involved in facilitating spinal movement as well as mobility in connected structures, such as the shoulder girdle and rib basket.

### Superficial Layer of Back Muscles Along the Spinal Column

All superficial back muscles support the movement of the shoulder. All have origins on the vertebral column and insertions on the bones of the shoulder girdle (i.e., on the clavicles, scapulae, and/or humeri). There are four key sets of superficial back muscles, the levator scapulae, latissimus dorsi, rhomboids, and trapezius muscles (see Figure 1.38). These muscles are referred to as the superficial back muscles and overlap with the muscles of the shoulder, as well as coordinating with the muscles of the chest.

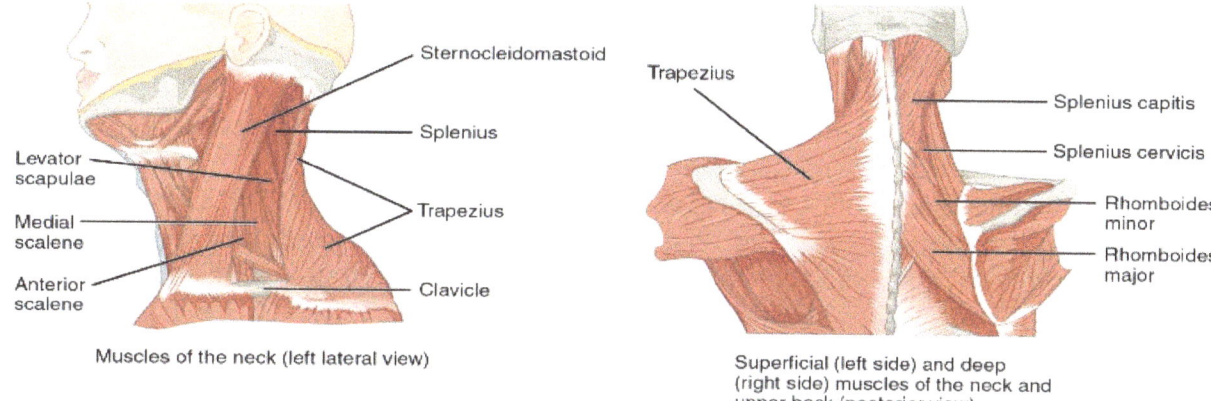

**Figure 1.38** Muscles of the neck and back. (Data source: OpenStax; https://commons.wikimedia.org/wiki/File:1117_Muscles_of_the_Neck_and_Back.jpg; Creative Commons Attribution 4.0)

The levator scapulae muscles, one on each side of the neck and upper back, originate from the transverse processes of the first four cervical vertebrae (C1–C4) and insert on the medial borders of the respective scapulas. Although traditionally known for their role in elevating the scapulae, these muscles more commonly function in daily life to stabilize and counter anterior head carriage (i.e., forward head or tech neck) by helping prevent excessive anterior translation of the cervical spine. They contribute to scapular depression and rotation, as well as lateral flexion and rotation of the neck, especially when the scapula is fixed. In yoga *asana*, the levator scapulae play an important role in neck positioning, scapular stability, and upper back tension, particularly in shapes that involve head-turning, weight-bearing through the arms, or postural correction. When overactive or shortened (often due to screen use or habitual slouching), they can restrict cervical mobility and contribute to upper back discomfort. Balanced activation and length in these muscles support functional neck alignment, efficient scapular movement, and more easeful breath and posture on and off the mat.

The latissimus dorsi muscles, one on each side of the back, are broad, powerful structures that span from the thoracic spine, thoracolumbar fascia, and iliac crest to insert on the anterior aspect of each upper arm bone. Acting bilaterally, they assist in spinal extension and postural support. When acting unilaterally, they generate arm extension, adduction, and medial rotation, and contribute to depression and retraction of the shoulder (though not of the scapula, as they do not attach to it). These muscles are heavily engaged during swimming, especially in strokes such as freestyle and butterfly, where they drive the arms through water in coordinated pulling motions that strengthen their connection between the spine, pelvis, and upper limbs. In yoga *asana*, the latissimus dorsi play a central role in backbends, weight-bearing arm postures, and overhead movements, where their tone and flexibility influence shoulder mobility, thoracic expansion, and postural alignment. Overuse or tightness can contribute to compensatory movement patterns and limit shoulder flexion, whereas balanced strength and length support spinal integration, breath capacity, and efficient arm mechanics, all key elements in dynamic and stabilizing postures.

Rhomboids major and minor, located on either side of the upper back, span from the spinous processes of C7 to T5 to the medial border of the scapulae, forming one half (along with the trapezius muscles) of an X-shaped support structure between the spine and shoulder blades. These muscles are responsible for retraction, stabilization, and rotation of the scapulae, working in tandem with serratus anterior to maintain healthy scapular positioning. In an ideal balance, the rhomboids and serratus muscles act like a functional sling, stabilizing the scapulae during weight-bearing arm shapes such as Plank, *Chaturanga*, and Downward Facing Dog. However, imbalances are common. For example, yoga practitioners may overly strengthen or concentrically load the rhomboids (along with the trapezius, as explored below), leading to restricted mobility and a chronically 'open chest,' whereas weightlifters may overdevelop serratus anterior, causing the rhomboids to become weak and overstretched. In yoga *asana*, balanced engagement of the rhomboids supports shoulder girdle stability, smooth scapular gliding, and integrated upper body strength, perhaps preventing compensatory tension patterns as well as maintaining spinal alignment and freedom of breath.

The trapezius muscles, which span the upper back from the occipital bone and cervical spine down to the lower thoracic vertebrae, are divided into upper, middle, and lower fibers, each contributing distinct actions that influence scapular movement and postural integration and stability. The upper trapezius elevates and assists in upward rotation of the scapula during arm abduction; the middle trapezius retracts the scapulae. The lower trapezius (which originates from T4 to T12 and inserts on the medial scapular border) depresses and rotates the scapula downward, forming the other half of an X-shaped sling across the upper back in coordination with the rhomboids. Functionally, the trapezius muscles need to be balanced with the pectoralis minor muscles of the chest, which draw the scapula forward and downward. When this balance is lost, especially if pectoralis minor muscles are short and tight, postural kyphosis and limited scapular mobility may result. In yoga *asana*, the trapezius plays a vital role in shoulder stabilization, spinal support, and overhead arm movements. Weakness, especially in the lower fibers, can undermine strength and alignment in shapes such as Cobra, Upward Facing Dog, and Plank. Awareness of the scapulothoracic sling formed by the trapezius and pectoral muscles is essential for cueing postural integrity, supporting spinal decompression, and maintaining functional shoulder mobility.

Overall, the superficial back muscles have many important functions that can inform skillful yoga *asana* teaching and therapeutics. A few insights are shared here, though they can, by no means, detail all functional aspects of these muscles in daily life and in yoga *asana*.

- *Role in breath and rib basket movement* – Although these muscles are not primary respiratory muscles, they indirectly influence breathing by affecting rib basket position and scapular mobility. For example:
  - tight upper trapezius or rhomboids may limit upward rotation of the scapula, which can restrict rib basket expansion in overhead shapes and breathwork
  - shortened latissimus dorsi can inhibit thoracic extension and posterior rib movement, both of which are essential for full diaphragmatic and posterior-lateral breath
- *Relationship to postural habits and modern lifestyles* – These muscles are affected by habitual posture, creating imbalances that can be addressed through lower trapezius strengthening and pectoralis minor releases; specifically, the challenging habits related to *samskaras* in these muscles include but are not limited to:
  - forward head posture
  - protracted shoulders from screen use or driving
  - sedentary behavior which contributes to weakness in the lower trapezius and over-reliance on the upper trapezius
- *Relationship to coordination and timing of movement* – In yoga *asana*, strength is often less important than timing and coordination of these muscles. For example:
  - serratus anterior and lower trapezius need to co-contract to support upward rotation of the scapula during overhead movements such as in Handstand (part of the glenohumeral rhythm covered in Chapter 6)
  - overemphasis on using these muscles for scapular retraction (common in 'heart-opening' cues) may overengage rhomboids and middle trapezius, reducing fluid scapular motion that is needed for sustainable shoulder mechanics and increasing the likelihood of bracing
- *Importance in eccentric control* – Many yoga *asana* transitions require eccentric control of these muscles, especially during lowering movements in prone positions with weight-bearing in the arms. For example, eccentric engagement supports:
  - Yoga Pushup (latissimus and trapezius support spinal and scapular stability)
  - transitioning from Plank to Cobra (eccentric lengthening of the trapezius and rhomboids)
  - controlled lowering of arms from overhead (lats and trapezius decelerate the motion)

*Intermediate Layer of Back Muscles along the Spinal Column*

The intermediate layer of (almost all) back muscles are breathing muscles. They elevate and brace the ribs and are covered again in detail in Volume 3 of the series, as well as in *Therapeutic Breathwork* (Brems, 2024b).

- *Internal and external intercostals* – These muscles facilitate the movement of the rib basket. According to some anatomists they may be accessory in breathing. Tom Myers describes them as more crucial to the <u>movement</u> necessary in the rib basket to allow for the coordination of walking and breathing. Their origins are on the vertebral column; insertions are on the rib basket (see Figure 1.39).
- *Scalenes* – These muscles in the neck region have their origins on the cervical vertebrae and insertions on the first two ribs. They support breathing by lifting up the rib basket. Their function related to the neck is detailed in the Head and Neck section. They also help hold the shape of the thorax.
- *Serratus posterior (superior and inferior)* – These muscles support breathing. They have origins on the neck and upper back (nuchal ligament and C7 to T2) and insertions on the second to fifth ribs.

Together, the intermediate layer of muscles along the spine play a key role in integrating breath with posture and movement. Although traditionally categorized as accessory respiratory muscles, they contribute meaningfully to both rib basket mobility and thoracic stability, especially during dynamic actions, such as walking, transitioning between yoga *asana* shapes, or coordinating breath with movement. Their strategic positioning, linking the spine to the rib basket, means they not only assist in respiration but also help maintain the structure and responsiveness of the thorax. In yoga *asana* and *pranayama*, this layer of back muscles becomes especially relevant when exploring breath-guided movement, thoracic expansion, and sustained spinal alignment, offering subtle but crucial support for practices that rely on breath-based engagement and postural integration.

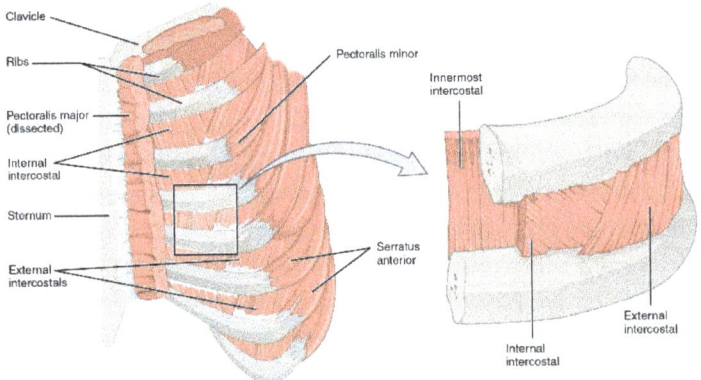

**Figure 1.39** Anatomy of the intercostal muscles. (Data source: OpenStax; https://commons.wikimedia.org/wiki/File:1114_Thorax.jpg; Creative Commons Attribution 4.0)

*Deep Layers of Back Muscles Along the Spinal Column*

The deep layer of intrinsic back muscles has three distinct layers of its own, the *deepest deep, intermediate deep,* and *cervical deep muscles*. These deep layers are essential to postural stability as well as to intricate movements of the spine in all directions. All deep back muscles have a preponderance of slow twitch fibers because they have to stay engaged all day, being responsible for movement of the spinal column and upright standing posture. These muscles are strong back extensors and lateral flexors. They engage in extension mostly to support lifting us from flexion. The deep layers of back muscles support all intricate movements of the spine at the level of the vertebrae. Not surprisingly, they extend from sacrum to the base of the skull, crossing one, a few, or several vertebrae per muscle (visible in Figure 1.40).

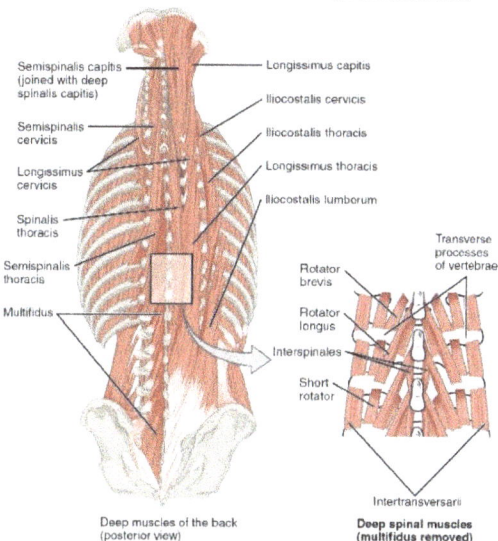

Figure 1.40 Deep muscles of the back. (Data source: OpenStax; https://commons.wikimedia.org/wiki/File:1117_Muscles_of_the_Neck_and_Back.jpg; Creative Commons Attribution 4.0)

### *Deepest Deep Back Muscles – or Transversospinalis Group*

The first of the three deep layers, the deepest deep layers of the intrinsic back muscles, is also collectively known as the transversospinalis group, and plays a crucial role in stabilizing and rotating the spine and head. The muscles in this group (namely, the semispinalis, multifidus, and rotatores) originate and insert along the transverse and spinous processes of the vertebrae, allowing for precise and controlled movements. The semispinalis muscles, extending across several vertebral segments, contribute to extension and rotation of the spine and head. The multifidi, a series of short, triangular muscles, provide segmental stability and play a significant role in proprioception, crucial for maintaining spinal awareness and control. The rotatores, the deepest of these muscles, are primarily responsible for rotational movements of the spine.

In yoga *asana* practice, engaging these deep muscles is essential for maintaining spinal integrity and preventing injuries, particularly during spinal rotations and extension. Cultivating awareness of these muscles through targeted and mindful movement can enhance spinal stability and improve postural stability and alignment. Yoga teachers ideally emphasize the importance of core engagement and controlled movements to activate the transversospinalis group, promoting healthy spinal alignment and preventing excessive strain. Furthermore, the multifidi's role in proprioception make them invaluable in therapeutic yoga interventions, especially for individuals with back pain or postural imbalances, as strengthening these muscles can improve spinal awareness and stability, leading to pain reduction and increased functional movement capacity (Johnson, 2002).

### *Intermediate Deep Back Muscles – or Erector Spinae Group*

The intermediate deep layers of the intrinsic back muscles, collectively known as the *erector spinae* group, are vital for stabilizing and moving the spine, particularly in flexion and extension. This muscle group, comprised of the spinalis, longissimus, and iliocostalis muscles, originates from various points including lumbar and thoracic vertebrae, sacrum, posterior iliac crest, and sacroiliac and supraspinous ligaments, providing a broad base of support for the spine. Spinalis muscles, located closest to the spine (i.e., deepest), primarily contribute to spinal extension. Longissimus muscles, situated laterally, also extend the spine and assist in lateral flexion. Iliocostalis muscles, the most lateral of the group, extend the spine and play a role in lateral flexion and stabilization.

Strengthening these intermediate deep muscles promotes healthy posture in daily life and yoga *asana* and provides support for the spine. In yoga *asana* practice, mindful engagement of the erector spinae is crucial for maintaining spinal alignment, especially in shapes or movements that involve backbending and forward folding. Yoga teachers ideally emphasize the importance of balanced muscle activation to prevent imbalances and potential injuries. In yoga therapy, understanding the erector spinae's role is essential for addressing back pain and postural misalignment. Targeted work can create strength and resilience in these muscles, support spinal stability, reduce discomfort, and enhance functional movement. Awareness of the erector spinae's origins and insertions allows for precise cueing and verbal adjustment, helping clients engage these muscles safely and effectively.

### *Cervical Deep Back Muscles – or Head Rotators Group*

The cervical deep muscles, primarily responsible for head rotation, are collectively known as the head rotators and include splenius capitis and splenius cervicis. These muscles play a vital role in the complex movements of head and neck, contributing to rotation and lateral flexion. Splenius capitis, originating from the spinous processes of the upper thoracic and lower cervical vertebrae, extends upward and laterally to insert on the mastoid processes and occipital bones, enabling rotation and extension of the head. Splenius cervicis, situated deeper, originates from spinous processes of the lower thoracic vertebrae and inserts on the transverse processes of the upper cervical vertebrae, primarily facilitating neck rotation and lateral flexion.

In yoga *asana*, mindful engagement of these muscles is key to maintaining cervical stability and preventing neck strain, particularly in shapes involving head movements and inversions. Yoga professionals can emphasize controlled, gradual movements and encourage students or clients to maintain a natural cervical spine to avoid overworking these muscles. Awareness of these muscles is especially important in yoga therapeutics, through which targeted exercises may help address neck pain, tension headaches, and postural imbalances. Strengthening and lengthening the head rotators can improve cervical stability, enhance head and neck mobility, and promote overall auspicious head alignment. Furthermore, understanding these muscles' actions allows for precise cueing and adjustments, helping students cultivate a healthy relationship with their cervical spine.

## *Muscles of the Core*

These muscles have to be understood in the context of the abdominal cavity. The abdominal cavity can change shape, but not volume (unlike the thoracic cavity, which can change both shape and volume). It is lined with a membrane called the parietal peritoneum. The peritoneum secrets moisture to ease the movement of the organs and holds the organs in place via folds called the mesentery. The core muscles are part of the abdominal wall, which creates a firm boundary and protection for the viscera, assists in forceful exhalation, contributes to stabilization of the torso, spine, and pelvis, and helps increase/maintain intraabdominal pressure [such as in child birth and during coughing, sneezing, vomiting, laughing, etc.]. The abdominal muscles (shown in Figure 1.41) are completely integrated with the skin, superficial fascia, and parietal peritoneum. They consist of flat muscles that have fibers in crossing directions and entwine at the midline as the linea alba, a strong, flat band of connective tissue at the front of the abdominal cavity, as well as vertical muscles.

While they also support spinal flexion, the abdominal muscles' primary function is stabilization of the trunk, spinal column, ribs, and pelvis. Stabilization means that these muscles act to hold a part of the body steady while another part moves, making the movement in the active part of the body easier and more efficient through the stabilization of the parts that need not or should not move (e.g., if we lift the neck while lying supine, we can clearly notice how the abs stabilize the ribs and pelvis). The abdominals fire any time we have to stabilize the trunk against gravity. The stabilization function of the abdominals is less effective or powerful when the low back is arched, stretching the abdominals. Following are a few helpful additional details about these important muscles:

- Stabilization of the torso happens developmentally and by age six months babies have enough strength in the toro from their core muscles to sit upright.
- Stabilizing the ribs and pelvis is one of the abdominals' major jobs in sitting, standing, walking, and all daily activities and yoga postures. They draw the ribs toward the pelvis and the pelvis toward the ribs to create a sense of core integration through their origins and insertions along the ribs and pelvis.
- The abdominal muscles also create rotation and side-bending in the torso (internal and external obliques).
- The abdominal muscles work with the psoas group to help flex the trunk, especially in a supine position (by helping draw the ribs and pelvis toward each other).
- They are also in relationship with the psoas and diaphragm creating a core stabilizing complex that is essential especially during walking.
- The abdominal muscles are stretched via Backbends. While stretched, they are less powerful. [Note that Backbends can overly stress the linea alba during pregnancy and need to be used with caution at that time.]
- The abdominals are strengthened via shapes focused on stabilization (e.g., Boat or *navasana*; Table Top with one arm lifted and slowly moving the weight of torso forward step-by-step).
- Although abdominal muscles can help with forceful exhalation, they do not need to be involved in quiet or natural breathing (contrary to common belief and cueing in yoga classes). In fact, they can interfere with breathing when strongly contracted. The notable movement in the abdomen during breathing is initiated by the movement of the diaphragm and its slight displacement of abdominal organs, not by the abdominal muscles.

The muscles in the abdomen are arranged to make a cross and an X (see Figure 1.41). The cross is comprised of the transverse abdominis, which runs horizontally, and the rectus abdominis, which runs vertically. The X consists of the external obliques, which create the two top portions of the X and the internal obliques which create the two bottom portions of the X. Lasater (2020) indicates that the "abdominal muscles create a 'basket weave' effect on the front of the body and wrap around the sides of the body, so that when we stand erect or lift things or bend in all directions or walk, we are able to maintain our upright postures. The abdominals 'hold us together' in a sense…" (p. 115).

As an aside, all abdominal muscles are centered on the navel, leading Tom Myers to state that *"all roads in the belly lead to the umbilicus"* (personal communication in a workshop). From this perspective, the navel is considered a mechanical and emotional crossroads. The navel, of course, is formed from the severing of the umbilical cord after birth. The umbilical cord is a part of the fetus, not the mother. Recent research has demonstrated that the umbilical cord should not be cut prematurely, with premature severing being related to more respiratory and other distress in the neonate (Makary, 2024). The umbilical cord is actually long enough for the baby to reach the breast and is meant to stay attached until the placenta is delivered and the cord has turned grey, significantly enhancing the wellbeing and respiration of the newborn child.

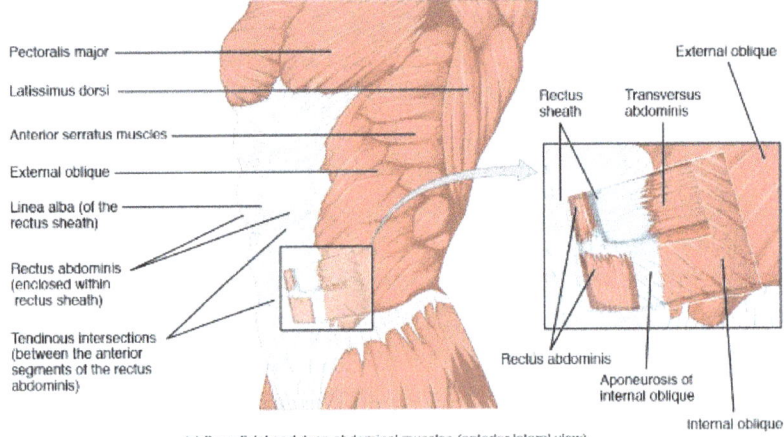

**Figure 1.41** Abdominal muscles. (Data source: OpenStax; https://commons.wikimedia.org/wiki/File:1112_Muscles_of_the_Abdomen.jpg; Creative Commons Attribution 4.0)

### *Rectus Abdominis*

The rectus abdominis is a vertically oriented muscle that runs straight up and down the front of the torso, from its origin at the pubis to its insertion at the 5th to 7th ribs and the xiphoid process of the sternum. The term *rectus* means 'straight,' and the muscle is marked by tendinous intersections that give rise to an appearance that has colloquially been referred as the 'six-pack' muscles. As the most superficial of the abdominal muscles, it is sometimes referred to as the superficial stomach muscle and forms the vertical axis of the abdominal cross mentioned above. Functionally, the rectus abdominis assists in compressing abdominal contents, flexing the lumbar spine against gravity, posteriorly tilting the pelvis when the rib basket is fixed, depressing the ribs when the pelvis is fixed, and stabilizing the pelvis and trunk during movement and load-bearing. It also supports forced exhalation and can contribute to intraabdominal pressure when needed.

### External Obliques (Abdominis)

The external obliques are the largest and second-most superficial of the abdominal muscles, forming the upper half of the diagonal X or basket-weave pattern of the abdomen (the internal obliques forming the lower half). These flat, broad muscles originate from the lower borders of the 5th to 12th ribs and insert on the iliac crest and iliac spine, with additional attachments to the xiphoid process, linea alba, and pubic bone. Functionally, the external obliques, upon contraction, rotate the torso to the contralateral side, assist in lateral flexion (side-bending) to the same side, and support the coordinated twisting action necessary for walking and gait stability. When both sides of the external obliques contract simultaneously, they contribute to spinal flexion and abdominal compression, playing a key role in core stabilization and trunk mobility.

### Internal Obliques (Abdominis)

The internal obliques lie deeper than the external obliques and form the lower half of the abdominal X or basket-weave pattern, working in coordinated opposition with the external obliques. These flat, layered muscles originate from the inguinal ligament, iliac crest, and thoracolumbar fascia, and insert into the linea alba, pubic crest, pectineal line, 10th to 12th ribs, and xiphoid process. Functionally, upon contraction, the internal obliques rotate the torso to the same side (in contrast to the external obliques, which rotate the torso to the opposite side) and assist in side-bending to the same side. They also support the twisting and stabilizing actions needed for walking, and when both sides contract together, contribute to spinal flexion and abdominal compression, enhancing core control and postural integration and stability.

### Transverse Abdominis

The transversus abdominis (TA) is the deepest of the abdominal muscles, wrapping horizontally around the torso like a natural girdle and making the other half of the muscular cross that was described above. The TA originates from the inguinal ligament, iliac crest, thoracolumbar fascia, and 7th to 12th ribs; it inserts into the xiphoid process, linea alba, and pubic symphysis. As the horizontal component of the abdominal cross, the TA plays a central role in compressing abdominal contents and stabilizing the trunk, especially during lifting or rising upward from seat or squat. When actively engaged, the TA can reduce pressure on intervertebral discs by up to 40%, particularly when working in coordination with the deep spinal stabilizers, such as the multifidi and erector spinae. Although the TA can assist with forced exhalation, its over-engagement in this regard can restrict abdominal breathing, making it important in yoga *asana* and *pranayama* practices to cultivate a balance between tone or effort and ease or release.

### Pyramidalis

The pyramidalis is a small, triangular muscle located just inferior to the rectus abdominis and is sometimes classified as an abdominal muscle. It originates from the pubis and inserts into the linea alba, where it functions to create tension and maintain tautness in the linea alba. Though not to be found in all individuals, when present, the pyramidalis may be considered functionally related to the pelvic girdle due to its location and attachment points. Its role is minor compared to the primary abdominal muscles but contributes to the integrity of the anterior abdominal wall.

As a whole, the core muscles (i.e., rectus abdominis, external and internal obliques, transversus abdominis, and pyramidalis) work as a highly coordinated team to support movement, posture, and internal regulation. Together, they generate intraabdominal pressure, stabilize the spine and pelvis, and facilitate functional movements such as walking, during which alternating patterns of rotation and side-bending are supported by the obliques and deep stabilizers. During breathing, particularly exhalation, the transversus abdominis and obliques can assist in drawing the rib basket downward and compressing the abdominal contents, maintaining sufficient tone to stabilize the spine and torso. These muscles work reflexively with spinal and pelvic musculature to maintain core stability under load or during transitions, protecting the spine and supporting efficient movement. In the context of yoga *asana*, understanding this muscular collaboration is essential for teaching practices that emphasize balanced core engagement without rigidity that might impede natural breathing. A well-integrated core supports spinal alignment, breath-guided movement, and easeful transitions between shapes and during flow practices. Yoga offers a unique opportunity to cultivate awareness of the strength and suppleness of the core muscles, essential for sustainable and functional movement on and off the mat. Essential movements that support awareness of core engagement and abdominal strengthening are offered in Section 2.

## Kinesiology of the Spine

Fundamentally, the spine is both a stabilizing axis and a mobile scaffold. Its intervertebral discs, vertebrae, facet joints, surrounding musculature, fascial connections, ligaments, tendons, and embeddedness in several crucial anatomy (or myofascial) trains, all work in careful collaboration and interdependence to provide nuanced control of movement or mobility, to create internal supports and pressure control (such as intraabdominal pressure and load bearing), and to be responsive to gravitational and ground reaction forces. The spine's kinesiology cannot be reduced to movement alone; it is a dynamic expression of the body's capacity to integrate support and fluidity in the context of upright living. Because it is an essential part of the human biotensegrity, it continually adapts and always moves in context with all other structures and outer environments. It is in constant communication with gravity, loads, compressive and tensive forces, movement-based variations in demand, and postural shifts. Without its profound connection to other structures, especially to fascial tissues, the bony structure of the spine would not be able to hold its shape, collapsing instead into its individual segments. Due to its profound connection to other structures, especially connective tissues, the bony structure of the spine continually moves, adjusts, and responds to inner and outer influences.

The kinesiology of the spine, in other words, is the very essence of an integrated holistic system and it is key to understand the spine (in fact the whole body) as such a living and adaptive system rather than looking at it from a mechanistic or reductionist perspective. Wholism is a key element in the biotensegrity that is the human body, with profound interconnection and interdependence across many structures, tissues, and organs. The spine's capacities for movement and stability are deeply connected to all *koshas* and biopsychosociocultural contexts – being influenced not only by genetics, biological structure, and other physical aspects of a human being, but also by personal experiences across the lifetime, cultural and socioeconomic influences, personal beliefs and attitudes, and behavioral patterns in relationship and in the environment in which the human being grows up and grows older.

The human spine is a structurally complex and functionally versatile structure, uniquely evolved to serve the dual demands of *stability* and *mobility* in an upright, bipedal body. It is made for complex movement and can easily handle situational distortions of the natural curves. In other words, while it is at its most stable in its natural curves, the spine can easily move through a wide range of motion that takes it out of its natural curves to meet situational demands. Distortion of the curves is only a challenge when it becomes habitual. The spine's architecture of carefully interconnected bones, fascia, muscles, tendons, and ligaments reflects an optimized balance between its load-bearing capacity and this dynamic adaptability. As described in detail above, comprised of 24 articulating vertebrae, along with the largely fused sacrum and coccyx, the spine is organized into distinct regions (i.e., cervical, thoracic, lumbar, sacral, and coccygeal), each contributing differently to overall spinal function and evolved to meet the demands that are unique to each specific region of the spine.

At birth, the human spine exhibits a single, continuous *kyphotic curve*, an adaptive outward convexity that spans from the base of the skull to the coccyx, molded to the fetal environment. This *primary curve* of the spine reflects fetal posture and provides a stable, flexed configuration suited to early life in a gravity-minimized environment. As neuromuscular development progresses the spine undergoes a significant restructuring as infants begin to lift the head, roll, crawl, and eventually stand. Through these movements geared toward an upright and bipedal life as a human being, a *secondary curve* in the spine begins to evolve that introduces anterior concavity, that is a *lordosis*, in the cervical and lumbar regions. These lordotic curves are not merely anatomical features but are functional adaptations necessary to support upright posture, load transmission through the spine, and head-to-pelvis alignment in bipedal locomotion (DeSilva, 2022).

As adaptive and essential as it is for bipedal life, spinal organization into primary (kyphotic) and secondary (lordotic) regions introduces inherent mechanical vulnerabilities (not to be confused with fragility). The lordotic segments, by virtue of their curvature and increased range of motion, are more susceptible to shear forces, disc compression, and muscular imbalances. Additionally, transitional zones (especially at the cervicothoracic, thoracolumbar, and lumbosacral junctions) bear increased structural demands as they mediate shifts between flexion- and extension-biased spinal regions. These areas experience concentrated mechanical stressors and hence are the more typical sites for spinal dysfunction, deviation, or injury. Understanding the developmental and structural origins of spinal curvature provides essential context for interpreting movement patterns, understanding the impact of postural tendencies, and creating healthful load-bearing strategies across the lifespan.

That said, the spine's natural curves (i.e., the sympathetic cervical and lumbar lordoses as well as the thoracic and sacral kyphoses) are essential and dynamic elements of the spine's dynamic efficiency and functional adaptability. Without them, bipedalism would not be possible. The alternating curves in the human spine help distribute axial loads, absorb shock, and maintain balance across this kinetic chain that is not in horizontal (as is true for most animals), but vertical alignment to gravity. The alternating kyphotic and lordotic curves have great value for posture, support a healthful walking rhythm, add shock absorption and transfer of load along the spine, optimize the placement of the organs (which are suspended from the anterior longitudinal ligament of the spine), and prevention of damage to the intervertebral discs (Bond, 2007; Brems, 2024b; Clark, 2018; Myers, 2022; Porter, 2013). The curves' alignment and responsiveness, so crucial to gait and postural control, are even essential to respiration.

In terms of specific directions of movement, the spine permits flexion, extension, lateral flexion, and axial rotation, and the capacity for these movements varies intelligently and adaptively by region. As explored in detail below, the cervical spine favors rotation and fine motor control, the thoracic spine is more limited due to its articulation with the rib basket, and the lumbar spine allows substantial flexion and extension with relatively less rotation. These region-specific capabilities contribute to the spine's ability to adapt to changing demands while preserving overall structural coherence. The spine, of course, moves in all planes of motion. For ease of understanding movement and stability in a yoga context, the spinal curves can be explored anatomically from the vantage point of two planes of movement: the sagittal plane that shows the lordotic and kyphotic curves of the spine; and the frontal plane that shows side-to-side deviation in the spine. The discussion here starts with the sagittal and then moves to the frontal plane.

## *Spinal Curves in the Sagittal Plane*

The first plane from which to explore the spinal curves is the sagittal plane (i.e., looking at the person from the side). The kyphotic and lordotic curves visible when assessing the human form from the side developed to support *"freedom of movement"* and *"the power of stability"*, unique to humans as bipedal creatures (Lasater, 2020). These spinal curves at center line of the sagittal plane come in two shapes – lordotic (concave into the back) and kyphotic (convex away from back). They, in essence, reflect the motions that happen in the sagittal plane – namely, flexion and extension.

In the neutral or anatomical position (in yoga called Mountain shape), the natural lordotic and kyphotic curves of the spine kick in and all vertebrae are stacked at all three joints (two facets of the transverse processes and one vertebral body), forming a tripod of weight transfer for maximum stability; all joints are optimally congruent and thus at their most stable position. The spine is a kinetic chain (i.e., a complex motor unit made up of several joints and segments that are arranged in a sequence); we can test for stability in Mountain (or anatomical position; see Chapter 8). The curves are supported by the wedge shape of the intervertebral discs, greater anterior thickness in lordotic parts of the spine and greater posterior thickness in kyphotic parts of the spine.

Given the unique construction along the spine, including the ingenious wedge shape of the discs, the spine is not and should not be straight; a straight spine is an anatomic impossibility and a very unhelpful yoga cue. It less helpful, and perhaps harmful, for yoga practice to be directed at straightening or flattening any part of the spine. For example, invitations to tuck the pelvis to remove lordosis from the low back can create havoc in any individual who has a perfectly healthy lordotic spine, but especially in people who are already hypolordotic (an increasingly common pattern); more about this below.

*Understanding Kyphosis and Lordosis*

Although the terms lordosis and kyphosis are often used as if they referred to unhealthful patterns in the spine, it is important to understand that there are natural and healthful curves in the spine, and exaggerated and unhealthful manifestations of these curves. That is, lordosis and kyphosis are natural to the spine; they are only a problem when they are exaggerated or missing.

*Types of Kyphosis*

As noted above, *natural kyphosis* is the primary convex curve with which we are born. At birth, it spans the full length of the spine. As we learn to walk and move in an upright posture, it remains expressed in the thoracic spine and sacrum. Excessive kyphosis is called *hyperkyphosis* and is manifested primarily in the thoracic spine (i.e., too much rounding of the thoracic spine). Hyperkyphosis in the thoracic region generally leads to excess lordosis in the lumbar and cervical regions, often in combination with forward head posture. A range of challenges can be associated with hyperkyphosis, including the following:
- Weight distributes poorly, which means more muscle efforts is necessary to maintain stability (leading to pain); this may lead to collapse in posture, compression, lack of integration in the core, and weak core muscles with overworking back muscles
- Spinal extension may be affected negatively and may also limit range of motion in the arms and shoulders; this may make it challenging to lift the arms overhead, either in shoulder flexion or abduction
- Tightness is increased in the hip flexors (though it is not clear which is cause and which is effect) and pectoralis and intercostal muscles; this can cause the ribs to be drawn inward and may restrict ease of breath and movement

The sacrum also needs to have a natural kyphosis and a proper 30° lumbosacral angle where the lumbar meets the sacrum. An overly tucked sacrum and tailbone can destabilize the spine and sacroiliac joints. Sacral over-tucking is becoming increasingly common due to too much sitting, using chairs with too much back support (causing the postural muscles to fail to engage), or sitting in chairs or seats that invite a slouch in the lumbar spine (e.g., car seats, couches).

*Types of Lordosis*

*Natural lordosis* is the developmental or secondary curve in the lumbar and cervical spines. These secondary or developmental curves are more vulnerable to injury and dysfunction (and thus pain). They move sympathetically with one another – when one flexes, so will the other (one can easily see and experience this link between the lumbar and cervical curve during movement in a Cat/Cow flow). Natural lumbar lordosis is essential to holding and supporting the weight of the organs (which otherwise drop their weight into the pelvis floor). *Lumbar hyperlordosis* (i.e., too much concavity in the low back) can cause compression of disks and nerves. It increases the lumbosacral angle and results in excessive forward tilting of the pelvis. Lack of natural lordosis, or *hypolordosis*, causes increasing amounts of pressure on the L4-L5 junction of the lumbar spine, drops the weight of the organs on the pelvic floor (which can cause incontinence), and decreases the lumbosacral angle. Modern postural habits and sedentary lifestyles have made lumbar hypolordosis more common than hyperlordosis. For yoga professionals, this may mean letting go of cueing that invites (further) tucking of the tailbone and encouraging students instead to embrace their natural lumbar curve. Natural cervical lordosis is essential to carrying the head's weight. Hypolordosis in the cervical curve can lead to neck compression, which may lead to compression of nerves, arteries, and veins (lots of which travel through the neck). It can also lead to headaches, backaches, and more.

### Unhelpful Patterns in the Spine Viewed from the Sagittal Plane

Unfortunately, as of recent, the evolution of human activities has increasingly shifted toward less movement, and more repetitive strain, habitual distortion, and forward curvature of the spine as a whole, especially in the thoracic spine and shoulders (see Figure 1.42). Although exercise-based and functional (or purposeful) rotation, flexion, extension, and lateral flexion of the spine are healthy and helpful, habitual distortion of the spine brings with it a plethora of challenges. Such habitual misalignment reverberates throughout the entire spinal column and its myofascial structures. It can cause structural changes (repatterning) that can create pain and improper weight distribution through the spinal column. For example, anterior head carriage has become an increasingly notable issue, especially among younger people. Unfortunately, for every inch that the head is forward of its center of gravity above the spine, the individual who has this pattern experiences 10 extra pounds of load.

Habitual distortion of the spine changes its whole environment – the whole biotensegrity, including discs, vertebrae, muscles, fascia, tendons, ligaments, nerves, even organs. Thus, it is important to notice spinal habits in yoga students or clients – either as seen in action during *asana* practice, as notable in habitual posture or movement, or as expressed in dysfunctional patterns and habits in their bodies. Misalignment in any portion of the spine reverberates through the entire column and all connective tissues; it affects the whole biotensegrity and all layers of human experience – yes, even thoughts, emotions, relationships, and psychology. Because of the deep connections of the spine with surrounding fascia and fascia's profound interrelationship across the organism due to their embeddedness in many anatomy trains, restrictions and changes anywhere along the spine create changes in all the curves above and below.

Yoga professionals need to understand these realities about the spine and need to be able to see a body and recognize the natural curves from the side. They need to be able to discern if the thoracic and sacral spinal regions give evidence to a natural kyphosis and if the lumbar and cervical spines are naturally lordotic. It is helpful to be able to look at a body from the side to discern whether the spinal curves are natural, overdeveloped, or underdeveloped. It is therefore important to explore these curves in a bit more detail, with implications for yoga teaching and therapeutics. The following table and figure provide guidance for observing spinal curves, looking at individuals from the side (i.e., exploring kyphosis and lordosis).

> *We can shake free of our knee-jerk behaviors and responses to life; we can let go of dissatisfying and unhealthy patterns. And, as we become more mindful, our innate wakefulness – our spiritual and inner wisdom – begins to blaze forth.*
> Lama Surya Das, 1999, Awakening to the Sacred, p. 191

> *Patient Self-Assessment and Clinician Observation of the Lordosis and Kyphosis*

1. Is the spine in its natural curves with a natural lordosis (curve) in the lumbar and cervical spine and a natural kyphosis in the thoracic spine and sacrum?
   - Is there:
     - hyper- (too much rounding forward) or hypokyphosis (standing at attention) in the thoracic spine?
     - hyper- (a hollow low back) or hypolordosis (slumping) in the lumbar spine?
     - distortion in the natural curve of the cervical spine, perhaps manifesting in forward head posture or hyperlordosis in the neck?
   - Is the pelvis overly tucked (flat) or tilted (with a hollow lumbar spine) or anchored in a natural and healthy balance that has a slight anterior tilt?
   - Is the low rib basket flared or too drawn in versus able to expand outward and upward with inhalation, and inward and downward with exhalation?
   - How do any distortions that are present in individual's typical spinal alignment seem to affect the breath?

2. How is the plumb line alignment? The line should pass:
   - Through the center of the ear
   - Through the center of the shoulder
   - Through the center of the waist
   - Through the center of the hip joint
   - Slightly anterior to the knee joint
   - Slightly anterior to the ankle and heel

3. Is there bowing in the spine and pelvic region forward or backward (beyond the natural curves)? Consider the following questions or dimensions:
   - Is any bowing distributed across the whole length of the body? Or are there opposing bows forward or backward in the upper versus lower portions of the body or in other portions?
   - Is the top of the ear slightly higher than the eyebrow (as opposed to chin jutting forward moving eyes higher than ears)?
   - Is the center of gravity of the head above the shoulders? Is the head forward of the body with the neck in too little extension at the upper cervical region?
   - Is the center of gravity of the shoulders above the hips?
   - Is the pelvis tilted anteriorly or tucked posteriorly?
   - Is the sacrum at its proper 30° angle (i.e., *not* vertical)?

4. Is there bowing elsewhere in the body forward or backward? Ponder the following questions or dimensions:
   - Are the hips above the knees?
   - Are the knees above the ankles?
   - Is there hyperextension in the knees?
   - Is there excessive plantar or dorsiflexion in the ankle?

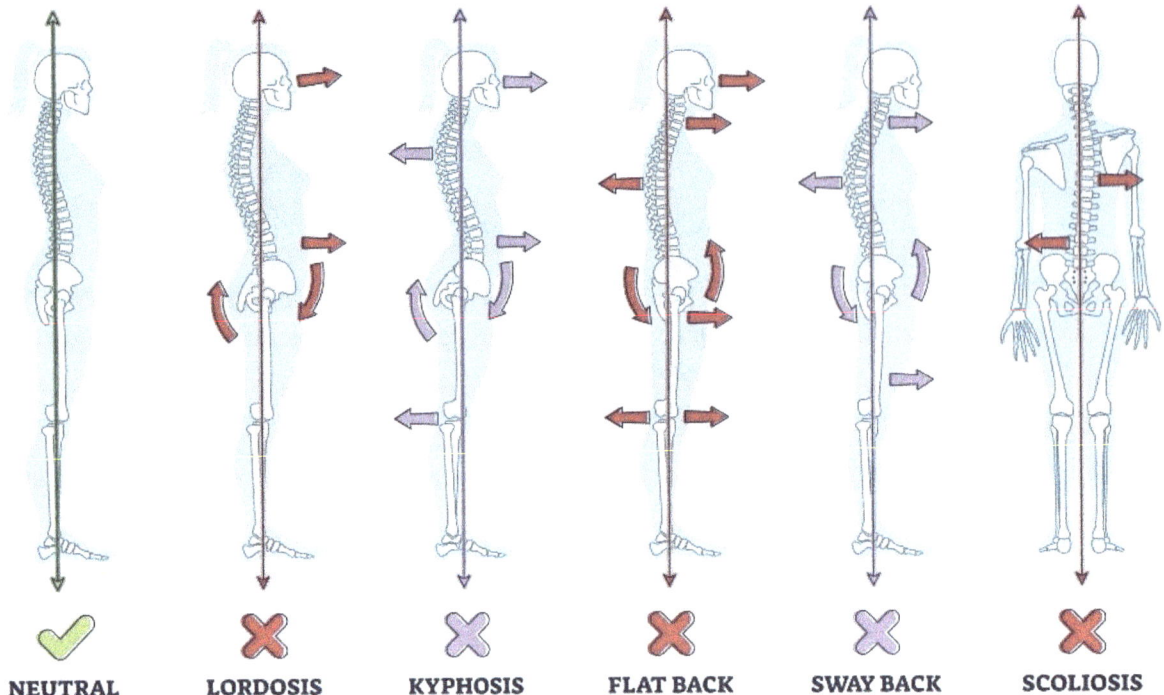

**Figure 1.42** Overview of spinal alignments – sagittal plane. (Data source: istock.com)

Particular spinal alignment dysfunctions have specific implications for muscular movements along the spine, assembly of organs in the abdominal cavity, range of motion of the diaphragm and other muscles along the spine, and movements of the rib basket. These postural changes create profound alterations in movement patterns and respiration. The implications for movement and breathing are varied, with tension, numbness, restricted ranges of motion, pain, labored breathing, shortness of breath, constricted or restricted breathing, gasping for air, and other possible effects. The following table provides an overview of spinal patterns in the sagittal plane and their effects on physical and respiratory patterns. These patterns also have effects on emotions and psychology – a reality that has much anecdotal and clinical evidence but less specific science.

| *Implications of Problematic Spinal Curve Patterns for Body And Breath* | | |
|---|---|---|
| *Type of Spinal Dysfunction* | *Physical Patterns* | *Impact on Breath* |
| *Hyperkyphosis* in thoracic spine = excessive forward curvature of the thorax with impact on the lumbar spine; likely posterior pelvic tilt (tuck) | • Shortened chest muscles (pectoralis minor, major, and fascia around them) and lax back muscles (rhomboids, mid traps)<br>• Tight external hip rotators, weak adductors, tight hamstrings<br>• May have back, sciatica, or disc herniations<br>• May experience numbness, tingling, or weakness in extremities | • Restricted breath<br>• Decreased rib basket resilience<br>• Restricted chest expansion<br>• Reducing lung capacity<br>• Shortness of breath<br>• Difficulty breathing |

| Implications of Problematic Spinal Curve Patterns for Body And Breath | | |
|---|---|---|
| *Type of Spinal Dysfunction* | *Physical Patterns* | *Impact on Breath* |
| *Anterior head carriage* = head is forward of shoulders; neck is likely hyperextended at C1 and C2 to keep gaze on horizon | • Tight chest muscles<br>• Restricted blood flow and nerve impingement in cervical spine<br>• Likely posterior tilt of pelvis<br>• Respiratory muscle weakness<br>• Decreased exercise tolerance | • Labored breath<br>• Decreased lung capacity<br>• Change in diaphragmatic function with over-recruitment of accessory muscles<br>• Shortness of breath |
| *Hyperlordosis* in lumbar spine = lumbar spine is too concave; thorax may be too flat; likely anterior tilt of pelvis | • Sway back posture has hips pushed forward and middle thoracic goes into kyphosis<br>• Tight hip flexors<br>• External rotation of hip joints and legs<br>• Respiratory muscle fatigue<br>• Overreliance on accessory muscles of breathing | • Restricted breath due to restricted rib basket mobility<br>• Diaphragm cannot contract effectively in inhalation<br>• Chest/thoracic breathing or reverse breathing<br>• Shortness of breath |
| *Overly tucked tailbone or sacrum* = sacrum is not at its proper 30° angle (excessively posterior), which results in destabilization of the spine and SI joints | • Creates excessive weight-bearing on vertebral body and discs; may compress discs<br>• Places the weight of the organs onto the pelvic floor, which weakens pelvic floor muscles, puts pressure on bladder, uterus, and prostate and may cause malfunction (e.g., incontinence) and/or prolapse<br>• May cause neck pain as entire spinal alignment is imbalanced | • Reduced diaphragmatic range of motion<br>• Shallow breathing with little abdominal movement<br>• Decreased lung ventilation and capacity<br>• Shallow breathing<br>• Labored breathing<br>• Excess recruitment of accessory breathing muscles |
| *Lack of natural curves in spine*, aka flat back = no natural lordosis in lumbar spine; no natural kyphosis in thorax and sacrum; cervical spine tends to be overly lordotic at the base and overly extended at the head | • Intervertebral joints compress and weight distributes poorly<br>• Likely shortening of hamstrings<br>• Pelvis tilt is off – either too posterior or anterior; more muscle power is needed to stay upright; can make sitting hard on discs<br>• Often accompanied by excessively externally rotated feet and knees and functional loss of height<br>• Can lead to chronic pain, tension in neck and cervical spine, pain in low back | • Reduced mobility in rib basket<br>• Reduced lung capacity and ventilation<br>• Diaphragm cannot contract effectively in inhalation<br>• Over-recruitment of accessory muscles leads to chest or clavicular breathing<br>• Shallow breathing<br>• Labored breathing |

*Considerations in Yoga Asana with Individuals With Spinal Deviations*

Clearly, deviations from the natural curves of the spine, such as excessive curvature as observed in hyperlordosis or hyperkyphosis; or reduction or flattening of these curves, such as in hypolordosis or hypokyphosis, can disrupt human biotensegrity with effects across the entire myofascial network, increasing risk of dysfunction or injury during yoga *asana* and other movement-based practices. A few contraindications, risks, and possible implications are offered below. These listings are meant as food for thought; they do not represent a complete analysis. Additionally, it is key not to overstep scope of practice and to work collaboratively with and prudently refer to other healthcare providers.

- Contraindications and risks related to therapeutic yoga:
  - loaded or end-range spinal movements (e.g., deep backbends or forward folds) may exacerbate stress on intervertebral discs, facet joints, and supporting ligaments when natural curvature is already compromised
  - compression risks are heightened in hyperlordosis, especially in the lumbar spine, potentially aggravating nerve impingement, spondylolisthesis, or facet joint irritation
  - flexion-dominant sequences may worsen thoracic hyperkyphosis or contribute to posterior disc bulges in those with diminished lumbar lordosis
  - weight-bearing shapes such as inversions or prolonged standing balances may challenge compensatory patterns, leading to over-recruitment of stabilizing musculature and fatigue-related breakdown of alignment
- Special considerations related to therapeutic yoga:
  - *observe and understand*: be attuned to students' spinal architecture through observation, functional movement screening, or collaboration with healthcare providers
  - *support natural curves*: cue neutral alignment over idealized "straight spine" positions. use props to sustain appropriate curvature in seated, supine, and standing postures
  - *offer gradual progression*: avoid abrupt introduction of shapes that intensify curvature extremes (e.g., Wheel, Camel) in individuals with known deviations or spinal sensitivity.
  - *support fascial adaptability*: integrate slow, myofascially-informed movement to support adaptive remodeling and tension redistribution across the spine's supporting structures
  - *avoid forced correction*: attempting to 'fix' spinal curvature through directive or forceful alignment cues are not appropriate as they may override helpful compensatory strategies and cause harm

### *Scoliosis or Spinal Curves in the Frontal Plane*

The second set of spinal curves can be observed in the frontal plane (i.e., looking at the person from the front or back). Exploration here is related to the identification of scoliosis, a side-to-side displacement of the spine, that is most easily noted when viewing students or clients from the back, especially in shapes such as Downward Facing Dog. Although most easily observed in the frontal plane, scoliosis is a three-dimensional deviation of the spine, primarily presenting as lateral curvature in the frontal plane, but often accompanied by rotational and sagittal plane changes. Although idiopathic scoliosis is the most common form, structural and functional variants each present unique challenges for movement-based practices. Sideways bows usually mean tightness and shortness on the concave (inwardly bowed) side and weakness and laxity along the convex (outwardly bowed) side. Other side-to-side difference can also be noted, such as asymmetries in the shoulders, chest, hips, knees, and feet. Scoliosis is often accompanied by changes in rib basket mobility, diaphragm function, and fascial tension.

*Understanding Scoliosis and Scope of Practice*

Awareness of asymmetrical loading patterns, altered proprioception, and compensatory tension is essential in a yoga context for supporting individuals with scoliosis safely and intelligently. Yoga professionals can understand scoliosis and become sensitive to how it translates for an individual client into movement and alignment patterns (a visual is provided in Figure 1.43). Yoga professionals also take care to be attuned to asymmetrical breathing patterns. In cases of severe curvature, pain, or known vertebral instability, collaboration with a physical therapist or scoliosis-informed clinician is essential. These healthcare professionals may even provide guidance to the yoga clinician about possible support to help students or clients lengthen the short concave side and strengthen the long convex side of their scoliosis. However, it is extremely important not to overstep scope of practice and to work collaboratively with the individual and in conjunction with relevant healthcare providers who may be involved in active treatment of the student or client.

Since the first step is awareness of what is present in students' anatomy, following are a few helpful hints about how to identify deviations in the spine as viewed from the frontal plane (i.e., from the back or front). That guidance is followed by a brief outline of major contraindications, risks, and cautions about engaging such individuals in yoga *asana*.

---

*Curves of the Spine from Frontal Plane*

Look at midline of the frontal plane (i.e., look at the person from the front and the back) to see if there is imbalance right to left. The view from the back is most helpful in a yoga position such as Downward Facing Dog. Ponder the following questions or dimensions:

1. From the front, notice all of the following:
   - Is there even openness in the front body?
   - Are the shoulders rolled forward (medial rotation of the scapula)?
   - Look at knees and feet – are the knees aligned or rotated internally or externally?
   - Is there excess inversion or eversion in the ankles?
   - Is the distance of one side flank shorter than the other? Which muscles seem to be involved in any notable one-sided shortening: quadratus lumborum, psoas, other?
   - Are the hips level to one another?
2. From the back, notice if there is any deviation side-to-side in the spine:
   - Is there a side-to-side curvature in the spine?
   - Where is the curve – thoracic, lumbar?
   - Where is/are the convex parts and concave of the curve? (Note: scoliosis is named for the convexity: e.g., right scoliosis has the convexity on the right side)
     - Can you notice that the muscles are shorter and tighter on the concave side?
     - Can you notice that the muscles are longer and weaker on the convex side (i.e., the side of the apex of the curve)?
   - Is the curve C-shaped (usually has some compensation in the other part of the spine, but less than in the S shape) or S shaped (more significant compensation for the primary curve)?

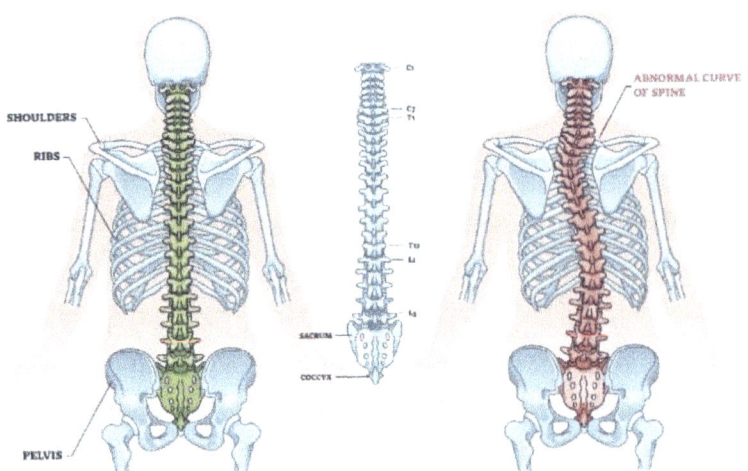

**Figure 1.43** Overview of spinal alignments – frontal plane. (Data source: istock.com)

*Considerations in Yoga Asana with Individuals With Scoliosis*

- Contraindications and risks in yoga *asana* practice
    - symmetrical shapes (e.g., Downward Facing Dog, Mountain, or Seated Forward Folds) may inadvertently reinforce asymmetrical muscle recruitment or feel uneven and unstable
    - deep spinal rotations can provoke discomfort or joint irritation when layered on top of existing vertebral rotation
    - long static holds, especially in sidebending or twisting, may strain already lengthened tissues on the convex side or compress shortened structures on the concave side
    - forceful cueing toward midline symmetry risks destabilizing compensatory strategies that may be protecting sensitive joints or neural structures
- Special considerations for yoga teachers and clinicians include the following, but need to be used with caution and only to the degree that the yoga professional has a clear understanding of what they are offering – staying within range of knowledge and scope of practice is key; additionally, power and agency is always with the client and not the yoga teacher
    - *understand structural vs. functional scoliosis*: functional curves are temporary and may be more responsive to movement and cueing; structural curves are more permanent and tend to require variation and modification, as well as stability-based approaches
    - *favor proprioceptive refinement over visual symmetry*: encourage clients to explore the four 'ceptions, breath patterns, and other mindfulness strategies (never enforcing external alignment ideals)
    - *include asymmetrical adaptations*: offering props, variations, or intentionally uneven loading can be useful to balance effort and ease across the spine; use them only with adequate knowledge and understanding of individuals' scoliosis; as always, students are in charge of alignment decisions and prop choices using the four 'ceptions to guide them
    - *prioritize spinal decompression and breath-based mobility*: supine practices, tractional orientations (e.g., hanging shapes, use of a wall), and directed breathwork can support elongation and reduce compressive strain – students need to have adequate interoceptive and proprioceptive skills for such practices
    - *avoid 'straightening' cues*; attempting to align a scoliotic spine to a textbook neutral can increase strain and ignore the body's adaptive intelligence; focus on function, stability, and spaciousness instead – inviting students to sense inward to create agency

## *Ranges and Directions of Motion across Spinal Sections*

We are always in motion, always readjusting to inner and outer factors that affect our posture, shapes, or movements. We are continuously rebalancing and readjusting to accommodate and meet all of the flowing influences and more:

- Environmental influences, such as soft or uneven surfaces, temperature, humidity
- Muscular involvement, including muscles that are relaxed versus engaged, active versus passive movement, bracing versus collapsing, habit versus novel movement, and more
- Joint alignment, both healthful alignment as well as extant injuries or pathologies
- Other connective tissue issues, including alignment that followed habitual function resulting in pattern locks in fascia, ligaments, and tendons, even bones
- Exteroceptive sensory inputs, such as visual distractions, nociception, noises, smells, inner ear balance, and more
- Inner sensory inputs, such as proprioceptive and interoceptive inputs, even neuroception
- Nervous system inputs, such as neuroception, polyvagal states or *gunas*, fears, and reactivity
- Affective, emotional and mental inputs such as *kleshas*, *vedana*, *vrittis*, and *samskaras*

It helps to notice these dynamic influences on and aspects of stability with wisdom, awareness, and compassion. This awareness-based approach leads to and, in fact, can define healthy postural alignment, much more so than an outer shape or an arbitrary alignment based on stereotypes and (social) media images of the various yoga *asana* shapes (Freeman et al., 2017; Razmjou et al., 2017; Vladagina et al., 2016).

As is hopefully clear by now, healthy directions of motion in the spine include flexion, extension, lateral flexion (side-bending), and rotation – all available along the length of the spine as well as to varying degrees in each specific section of the spine. Although we can elongate the spine overall, this axial extension is due to a flattening of the spinal curves, not due to muscular action separating the vertebrae from one another (muscles separating the vertebrae to create "length in the spine" do not exist). Specific movements and ranges of motion (ROM) vary greatly across the various sections of the spine. This is important to keep this in mind when cueing yoga *asana*, so as not to overemphasize or falsely cue motions in sections of the spine that do not allow for such directions or ranges of movement. A summary of spinal sections by type and range of motion is shown in the table below. Later sections in this chapter offer additional detail about ranges of motion specific to each individual section of the spine.

| **Summary of Range of Motion by Spinal Regions** | | | |
|---|---|---|---|
| *Type of Motion* | **Cervical Spine** | **Thoracic Spine** | **Lumbar Spine** |
| *Flexion* | 50-55° | 50° | 60-90° |
| *Extension* | 60° | Limited | 25-30° |
| *Lateral Flexion* | 45° | 45-50° | 20-45° |
| *Rotation* | 80-90° | 30-45° | 10-15° |

Based on: Krentzman (2016) and Lasater (2009)

Movements of the spine create various types of stresses, including tension, compression, torsion, and shear. As we move further away from the naturally curvy spinal alignment, load increases – all types of loads, especially shear. It is auspicious to reduce load in spinal flexion and extension via the use of props, (e.g., place blocks under the hands and arms in Camel to reduce load on the spine by co-carrying load in the arms; place blocks under the hands in a wide-legged Forward Fold, for the same reason). It is also auspicious to contract the muscles around the joints that are moving, even if this reduces range of motion. It also needs to be acknowledged that larger bodies have to bear a greater load when the spine departs from its natural curves. It is important to load properly and not to be tempted into excessive range of motion. Skinny people can have greater range of motion because their body weight gives them less load and their compression edges are wider (Clark, 2016, 2018). However, less body weight comes at a cost – heavier bodies are less likely to develop osteoporosis. Always practice in harmony with existing spinal structure.

> *Understanding the Stress/Stretch Spectrum* (Clark, 2018)
>
> **Stress**: *force applied to tissues*
> **Stretch**: *elongation of tissue under stress (also termed strain)*
> **Flexibility**: *range of motion of a joint*
> **Mobility**: *ease with which a joint can move through its range of motion*
> **Hypermobility**: *flexibility beyond the norm*
> **Dangerous hypermobility**: *flexibility beyond where the joint's tissues can provide stability*

To maximize healthy range of motion in the spine, muscles need to be at ease (note: this is *not* the same as not working or not contracting at all), not under load, especially not shear. Auspicious physical posture and embodiments of shapes are defined by ease (but not collapse); inauspicious postures or embodiments of shapes are defined by tension, pain, bracing, even fear. Interoceptive, proprioceptive, and neuroceptive awareness are key aspects to accessing auspicious alignment. To bear load, muscles need to contract around the joints that move which, in turn, limits range of motion in these areas of the body and creates a healthy trade off. In other words, it is important not to trade range of motion for risk of joint injury. As Clark (2018) stated, "*When under stress, stiffen; when enhancing movement, unload* (p. 9)."

Unfortunately, modern postural yoga is often perceived as being all about flexibility and large ranges of motion, instead of stability, auspicious healthful posture, and functional movement. Therapeutic and integrated holistic yoga *asana*, on the other hand, is about stability and strength *as well as* about healthful, conscious range of motion – both adapted to the reality of all factors of influence at hand in a given moment. A natural spine and posture is stable and at ease in the sense that there is the least amount of tension necessary given current circumstances as well as good bilateral balance in joints, fascia, other connective tissues, and muscles. This type of spinal stability is dynamic, not static (see following box); it is a constant adjustment to load factors such as compression, tension, torsion, and shear.

> ***Stability is marked by being dynamic, not static, and by the following traits:***
> - Endurance, steadiness, firmness, and sturdiness
> - Ability to reregulate after disturbance
> - Resilience and resistance to sudden force, load, or disturbance
> - Ability to adapt and regain postural equilibrium with mobility and ongoing micro-adjustments
> - Ability to support joints during movement
> - Defined by ease, not by tension

### *Cervical Spine Ranges and Directions of Movement*

The cervical spine is built for fast and free head movement and can move in all directions. This capacity to move freely and quickly is an important survival skill as neck and head need to move to orient all senses in relevant directions, that is, in the directions of possible danger or life threat. Following are a few specifics about ranges and directions of movement in the cervical spine:

- The "Yes" joint (which enables nodding the head up and down) is located between C1 and the skull and provides excellent capacity for flexion and extension.
- The "No" joint (which enables shaking the head left and right) at **C1–C2** allows flexion, extension, and rotation; in fact, 50% of total head rotation occurs at this joint. If a student is unable to rotate the head at all, the restriction is likely at C1–C2; if only partial rotation is present, the restriction typically lies in the lower cervical joints (below C2).
- In a natural cervical lordotic curve, the base of the skull and C7 should align in a vertical line.
- To tuck the chin and properly align the head with the spine (aligning the skull with C7), one should first flex the head by dropping the chin, and then move the chin back. Many yoga classes cue this movement in reverse, which can limit full range of motion and restrict healthy cervical function.
- The apex of neck extension occurs at C4, while the apex of neck flexion occurs at C5. Because the greatest range of motion in the cervical spine happens at these levels, it is not surprising that most cervical disc problems, especially herniation, occur at the **C4–C5** junction.
- During cervical flexion, the facet joints of the cervical spine move forward and upward; during cervical extension, they move downward and backward. These are the only two movement directions possible in the cervical facet joints.
- Since the cervical facets are not ball-and-socket joints, they are incapable of pure rotation. Instead, side-bending and rotation in the cervical spine are coordinated movements that rely on flexion and extension within the facet joints. As a result, side-bending and rotation happen on the same side: when the head rotates to the right, it also bends slightly to the right (causing the right side of the neck to shorten and the left side to lengthen), and the chin subtly drops. When the neck rotates right, the facet joints on the right move down and back, while those on the **left** move forward and up. This means that cervical movements such as dropping the ear toward the shoulder in yoga shapes naturally involve lowering the chin on the side toward which the head is bending or turning.

- Given that facet joints between the cervical vertebrae can only move forward and up and back and down, full neck rolls are not compatible with the nature of the cervical spine.
- Finally, C1 to C7 create a passageway through the transverse foramen on each side of the neck for the right and left vertebral arteries; simultaneous rotation and extension of the neck (i.e., tilting the head back while rotating the cervical spine) can result in occlusion of the vertebral arteries and thus restrict blood flow to the brain.

> *Neck Rolls Are Not a Good Idea*:
>
> Because the facets of the cervical vertebrae are oriented such that they only allow for flexion and extension (with rotation and lateral flexion being possible via carefully calibrated extension and flexion), there is no rotation during extension of the cervical spine. The facet joints do not allow for circling or rolling the head back (half-circles to the front tend to be okay for most individuals).
>
> Yoga professionals need to be aware of this cervical construction so they do not cue full neck circles or head rolls as they are:
> - Incompatible with the structure of the spine
> - Potentially risky to the nerves and arteries that pass through this section on the body

*Thoracic Spine Ranges and Directions of Movement*

The thoracic spine is built for protection of the heart and lungs. It has less mobility than the cervical spine due to the attachment of the rib basket and the orientation of its vertebral facets. Following are a few specifics about ranges and directions of movement in the thoracic spine:
- The C7-T1 junction is vulnerable and very much affected by poor posture, especially posture that involves anterior head carriage.
- Range of motion in the thoracic spine is limited by the rib basket, especially in flexion and extension. In fact, the thoracic spine cannot extend past straight up and down (i.e., there is no true backbending in this part of the spine); essential when in extension, it is flat – or straight.
- To protect the heart, the mid-thoracic vertebrae have spinous processes that are shaped such as to limit extension. The greatest amount of thoracic extension and flexion happens at the level of T11 and T12 (i.e., in the lower mid-back), which have facet joints that are more like the lumbar facets, and allow for slightly more movement here than further up in the thoracic.
- Flexion is also somewhat limited in the thoracic spine. This is less due to the shape of its vertebrae than due to the muscles and ligaments, especially the posterior longitudinal ligament, surrounding it. These structures add greatly to stability in this region.
- Side-bending and rotation are easy in the thoracic spine. They are relatively free and can range up to as much as 45°.
- In extension, side bending and rotation happen on opposite sides of each other in this portion of the spine. When we rotate the torso to the right, it bends to the left (i.e., right side lengthens and left side shortens). Notably, during side-bending, however, the rib basket rolls away from the side bend
- In flexion, side-bending and rotation occur on the same side

> *Feeling Thoracic Movement Quirks in the Body* -- Accessing Side Angle in two different ways:
> - First, come into the shape from the top down turning and bending before flexing
> - Second, enter the shape from the bottom up, starting in flexion and then turning the heart open
> - The first version will likely feel easier or more intuitive because it follows the natural combination of rotation, lateral flexion, and flexion

### Lumbar Spine Ranges and Directions of Movement

The lumbar spine is built for stability, with less mobility than the spinal sections above but more mobility than the sacrum below. It is most limited with regard to rotation. Following are a few specifics about ranges and directions of movement in the lumbar spine:

- The lumbar spine has very good flexion, being quite free as far as the vertebra are structured and the facet joints are oriented. Primary limitations to flexion in the lumbar are more typically associated with soft tissue limits rather than bony limits.
- As much as 50% of all flexion in the spine happens in the lumbar spine, with the majority happening in L5-S1 (*caution*: if overused, this range of motion and can put the disc into high-strain position). It is notable that the main muscles to flex the lumbar spine are the psoas and iliacus (i.e., the iliopsoas complex), as well as the abdominal muscles.
- The lumbar spine has very good extension, again being quite free based on vertebral shapes and facet joint orientation. Range of extension is limited largely by the anterior longitudinal ligament and internal organs.
- The anterior longitudinal ligament is quite strong in the lumbar region and limits extension (i.e., back-bending) to protect vertebrae from sliding forward (collaborating with several sacral ligaments as well).
- The posterior longitudinal ligament is weaker in the lumbar region, giving the lumbar discs less support in the back, which contributes to increased lumbar disc-related vulnerability during spinal flexion (or forward folding). This is an important caution for yoga *asana*.
- Limited rotation is possible in the lumbar spine (at most 10°), with most happening between L4-L5. the least amount of rotation is possible at L5-S1. Twisting in the lumbar spine must be approached with great caution and is covered in detail in the relevant sections below.
- Side bending is a moderate ~ 35°, limited by the low ribs and pelvis approaching each other. This can become a particular concern as individuals age and the discs between the spine become compressed.
- In extension, side bending and rotation happen on opposite side. This means that when the torso rotates to the right, it simultaneously bends to the left (i.e., right side lengthens and the left side shortens). When side bending, it can be noticed that the rib basket rolls away from the side bend.
- In flexion, side-bending and rotation occur on the same side.
- Rotation in the lumbar spine is easier when it is in its natural lordotic (slightly extended) state. Flexion in the lumbar limits rotation even further. The box that follows provides guidance about how to experience this nuance in the body.

> *Feeling Lumbar Rotation Quirks in the Body:*
>
> Access rotation in two ways:
> - First, sit in a slouch and twist to one side
> - Then sit naturally with a healthful lordosis in lumbar and try twisting to the side again
> → The second version will likely feel much easier as flexion (i.e., slouching) limits rotation in the lumbar spine

*Sacrum and Pelvic Girdle Ranges and Directions of Movement*

The sacrum cannot be discussed separately from the pelvic girdle; it is an integral part of the axial skeleton and yet also an integral aspect of the pelvis. It joints the pelvis via the sacroiliac (SI) joints. The SI joints form, quite literally, a keystone connection between the axial skeleton and the lower limbs, joining the sacrum to the two ilia of the pelvis. Unlike the highly mobile ball-and-socket hip joints in the anterior portion of the pelvic girdle, the SI joints are built primarily for stability. Their design allows only a very limited range of motion (generally less than two degrees), while supporting the substantial task of transmitting load from the spine into the lower body during walking, standing, and other functional movement.

A unique feature of the SI joints is their self-locking mechanism, particularly engaged in upright positions: when standing, seated, or transitioning through weight-bearing movement, the downward pressure of the torso compresses the sacrum between the ilia, reinforcing a close, interlocking fit. This *form closure* is enhanced by strong ligamentous supports (see Ligaments of the SI Joints in Chapter 5) and the tension created by surrounding musculature, particularly the abdominal and pelvic floor musculature. In seated positions, this interlock is slightly reduced due to decreased muscular engagement, resulting in a slight 'unlocking' effect that may increase vulnerability, especially when adding spinal rotations to seats.

> *Special Note for Yoga Professionals and All Humans*:
>
> The sacrum and pelvis need to be allowed to move in unison in rotations (i.e., twists) at the level of the lumbar and sacrum as there is virtually no rotation of the sacrum within the SI joints; yes, there is a tiny bit – so tiny, however, as to be negligible for all intents and purposes, especially in the context of yoga *asana* practice (Farhi & Stuart, 2017).
>
> In other words, it is not accurate or healthful to cue a planting of the sitz bones when moving into rotations as this may end up leading to torquing the sacrum inside the ilia at the level of the SI joints – not a good idea as this will destabilize this area over time, especially with repetition. This reality has functional implications.
>
> For example, when seated in a car's driver seat and twisting toward the backseat to help a child or retrieve a bag, the left sitz bone needs to lift and move into the turn with the entire pelvis.

Given the SI joints' architecture and purpose, introducing excessive or misdirected mobility (such as through excessive ranges of motion in the hip joints during yoga *asana*) can place strain on the supporting ligaments and threaten the joint's structural integrity. SI joint stability may be further compromised when hormonal fluctuations (as may occur during menstruation, pregnancy, and lactation) soften ligamentous tone, or when anatomical factors (such as wider pelvic breadth) alter load distribution across the joint. For these reasons, mindful attention to functional pelvic alignment and appropriate load-bearing is especially important in yoga *asana* practice. More detailed exploration of the SI joints, including their structural features and relevance to pelvic biomechanics, is offered in Chapter 5.

## What's Ahead

Having explored the axial region of the human body in some detail, it is now time to turn to this region's interaction with the appendicular regions. The discussion starts with the lower appendicular region, a logical approach given where the explorations in this chapter ended: namely, the relationship between the sacrum and the pelvis. The lower appendicular region of the body has profound importance in daily life and in yoga *asana* practice, especially since many yoga misconceptions and myths exist about this region.

**EXPANDED VERSION PART 1 OF Figure 1.29** Human spine anatomy. (Data source: Istock)

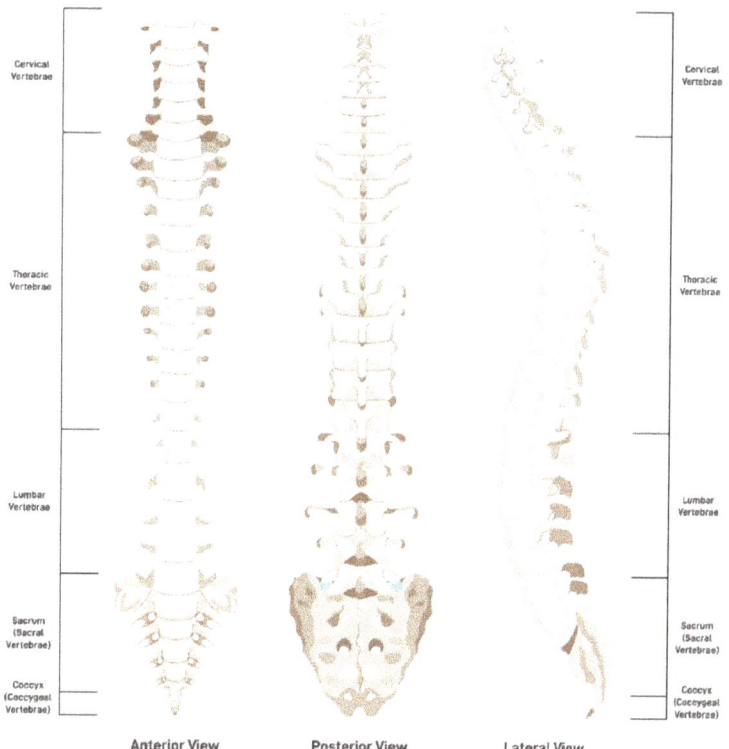

**EXPANDED VERSION PART 2 OF Figure 1.29** Human spine anatomy. (Data source: Istock)

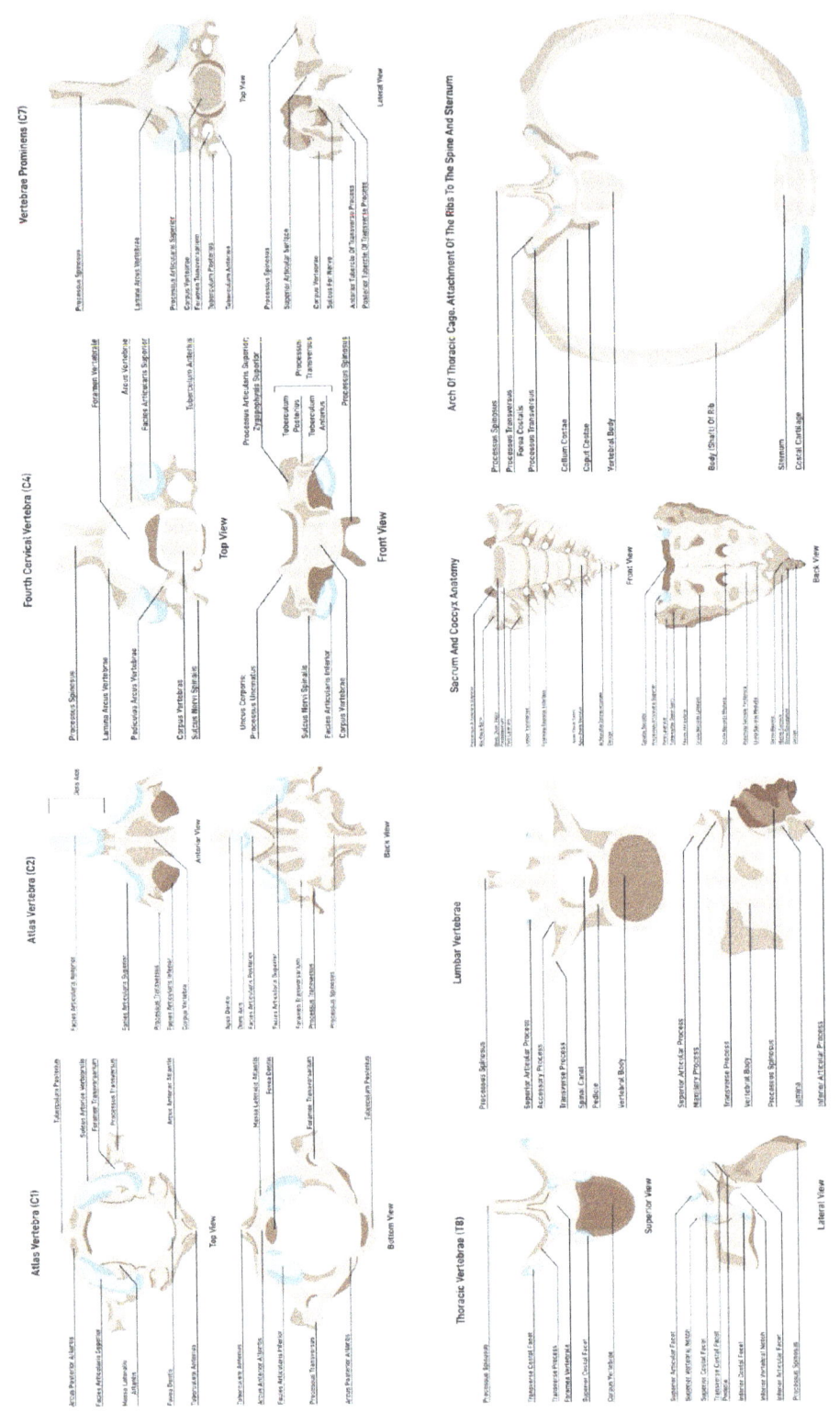

# Chapter 5: Anatomy of the Lower Appendicular Region

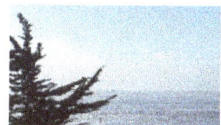

This chapter explores the anatomy of the lower appendicular region of the body, from the pelvic girdle and thighs to the lower legs, ankles, and feet. For each section in that body region, the chapter offers information about key structures – bones, joints, muscles, and movement patterns. It does so sequentially and assumes the reader's understanding (that was hopefully created in prior chapters) that these structures are, of course, completely interdependent, co-regulated, and connected. They never work in isolation of one another, nor of any other body regions and the *koshas*. The sequential approach is simply chosen (as always) for ease of communication.

## Pelvic Girdle and Thighs

The pelvic girdle forms the base of the spine and serves as a central hub for weight transfer between the upper body and lower limbs. It houses and protects pelvic organs, anchors key postural and locomotor muscles, and supports functions related to balance, stability, and internal pressure regulation. In yoga teaching and therapeutics, attention to pelvic alignment and mobility is crucial for spinal health, breath mechanics, and integration of core support with limb movement. The thighs connect the pelvis to the lower legs through the hip and knee joints, playing a primary role in locomotion, support, and force transmission. In yoga *asana* practice, the strength, mobility, and coordination of the thigh muscles influence not only standing and transitional postures but also the stability of the pelvis and spine. Therapeutic approaches often consider the thighs in relation to hip joint mechanics, gait patterns, and compensatory tension along the myofascial lines of the lower body.

## Bones of the Pelvic Girdle and Thighs

The pelvis is a bowl-shaped structure (shown in Figure 1.44) designed for exceptional strength as it receives and holds the weight of the entire upper body. The primary bony structures of the pelvic girdle and thighs are the ilia, ischium, and pubic of the pelvis; the sacrum; and the coccyx.

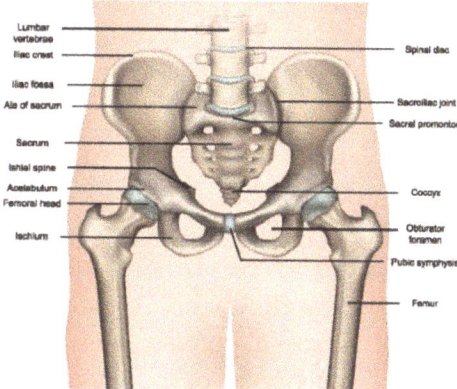

**Figure 1.44** Pelvic girdle and thighs. (Data source: istock.com)

The pelvic girdle forms a complex and vital junction between the axial and appendicular skeletons, supporting upright posture, load transfer, and coordinated movement through the lower limbs. In fact, the entire weight transfer from the torso and upper appendicular skeleton occurs at the level of the sacrum, most specifically at the sacroiliac joints where the sacrum of the spine meets the ilia of the pelvis. The pelvic girdle is composed of the sacrum and coccyx, both of which are of course essential parts of the spine and hence the axial skeleton (as discussed in Chapter 4), but not separable from the pelvic girdle; paired hip bones (ossa coxae) that are formed from three fused parts (namely, the ilium, ischium, and pubis each of which plays a distinct role while interacting to form a unified structure); and the femurs, which are technically part of the legs, but also an integral aspect of the pelvic girdle in terms of movements in the hip joints and reverberations into the pubis and sacroiliac joints. Understanding the structural integrity and integrated function of the bones in the pelvic region allows yoga professionals to develop anatomically meaningful *asana* sequences, auspicious and accurate weight-bearing cues, and therapeutic interventions tailored to the unique anatomy and needs of students and clients.

## Hip Bones

The hip bones, also known as *ossa coxae*, have three distinct, yet fused parts: two ilia, two ischia, and the pubis. The ilia form broad, curved plates that contribute to the figure eight shape of the pelvis when viewed from above. Prominent anatomical landmarks include the anterior and posterior superior iliac spines and the iliac crest. Posteriorly and inferiorly, the ischia contribute weight-bearing surfaces known as the ischial tuberosities, commonly referred to in yoga as the 'sitz bones.' The sciatic notches of the ischia mark the passageway for the sciatic nerve, a key structure to be considered in postures that load or stretch the posterior hip. Anteriorly, the pubic bones converge at the pubic symphysis, a fibrocartilaginous joint that adds anterior stability. Slight differences between male and female pelvises can be gleaned from Figure 1.45.

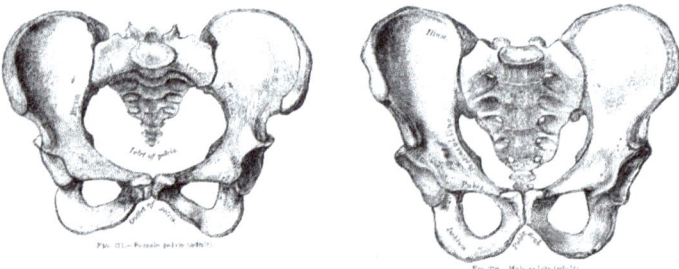

**Figure 1.45** Comparison of female and male pelvis. (Data source: Henry Vandyke Carter, https://commons.wikimedia.org/wiki/File:Comparison_human_male_and_female_pelvis.png; public domain)

## Sacrum and Coccyx

The sacrum is the flat triangle in the low back below lumbar spine. It is part of the axial skeleton and is one of the lowest parts of the spine (only the coccyx is lower). At the base of the spine, the sacrum completes the posterior wall of the pelvic girdle. It is formed from five vertebrae that are distinct at birth but typically fused by early childhood. As part of the axial skeleton, the sacrum articulates laterally with the ilia at the sacroiliac joints. These joints are strongly stabilized by major ligaments and serve as a crucial transfer point of load and movement between the spine and lower appendicular skeleton. Although fused in adulthood, the sacrum retains subtle capacity for movement, which plays a role in weight transfer and spinal shock absorption. According to Thomas Myers, premature and prolonged sitting in flexed postures, such as in infant car seats, may exaggerate sacral curvature during its formative fusion years, potentially influencing long-term spinal biomechanics.

Below the sacrum lies the coccyx, or tailbone, formed from two to five fused vertebrae. Though small, the coccyx anchors the pelvic floor musculature and contributes to spinal mechanics. Trauma at the level of coccyx may lead to dysfunctions extending as far as the neck and cranium, possibly making itself felt as back-, neck-, and headaches. Figure 1.46 shows both structures.

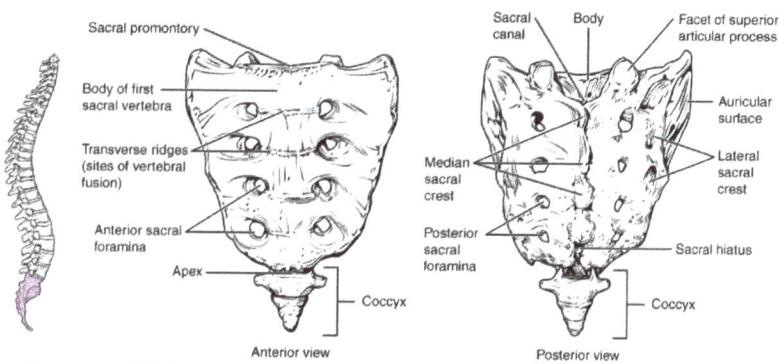

**Figure 1.46** Sacrum and coccyx. (Data source: OpenStax; https://commons.wikimedia.org/wiki/File:720_Sacrum_and_Coccyx.jpg; Creative Commons Attribution 3.0)

## *Femur*

The femur is the largest bone in the body, also known as the thigh bone. Although not part of the pelvis proper, the femur completes the functional articulation at the hip joint. The head of the femur fits into the acetabulum, the deep, cup-shaped socket formed where the ilium, ischium, and pubis meet, to create a strong yet mobile ball-and-socket joint (more about this below). The femur's greater trochanter is a palpable landmark laterally and serves as a key site for muscular attachment. Its lesser trochanter, head, and neck lie deep within the body and are not directly palpable. Medial and lateral condyles of the femur are situated near the knee and are discussed in more detail below.

## Joints and Ligaments of the Pelvic Girdle and Thighs

### *Pubic Symphysis*

The pubic symphysis is the cartilaginous joint that unites the left and right pubic bones at the anterior midline of the pelvis. Structurally, it is classified as a secondary cartilaginous joint, composed of a fibrocartilaginous disc between thin layers of hyaline cartilage. Although the pubic symphysis allows only minimal movement under normal conditions (typically a few millimeters of translation or slight rotation), it plays a crucial role in maintaining the integrity of the pelvic ring. It functions as a stabilizing connection between the two halves of the pelvis, distributing load during standing, walking, and transitions between positions. During pregnancy, the hormone relaxin increases mobility of the pubic symphysis, allowing the pelvis to widen for childbirth. For yoga professionals, awareness of this joint is particularly relevant when cueing asymmetrical standing postures, hip openers, or transitions that challenge pelvic alignment. Overstretching or uneven loading, especially in students or clients with underlying instability, hypermobility, or a history of pelvic trauma, can irritate or strain the pubic symphysis, leading to discomfort or dysfunction. Encouraging balanced muscle engagement through the inner thighs (adductors) and pelvic floor, as well as offering symmetrical variations, can help support the pubic symphysis and promote safe, integrated movement across the pelvis.

### Ligaments Around the Pubic Symphysis

The stability of the pubic symphysis is reinforced by a network of ligaments that limit excessive motion and help maintain alignment between the two pubic bones. The primary supporting structures include the superior pubic ligament, which spans horizontally across the joint and resists separation of the pubic bones; the inferior pubic ligament (also known as the arcuate ligament), which forms a strong arch beneath the joint and provides support against vertical shearing forces; and the anterior and posterior pubic ligaments, which reinforce the front and back of the joint capsule. Together, these ligaments provide passive stability, resist multidirectional forces, and complement the dynamic support from surrounding musculature. Their integrity is essential for transferring loads effectively across the pelvis, particularly during weight-bearing movements and transitional actions common in yoga *asana*.

### Acetabulofemoral Joint

As noted, the femurs are the longest and strongest bones in the body, forming the upper segments of the legs and playing a central role in locomotion, weight-bearing, and postural support. Each femoral head articulates with the acetabulum of the pelvis, a deep, hemispherical socket formed at the convergence of the ilium, ischium, and pubis. This articulation forms the acetabulofemoral joint, more commonly referred to as the hip joint, a synovial ball-and-socket joint that allows for a wide range of motion: flexion, extension, abduction, adduction, internal rotation, external rotation, and circumduction.

The joint's considerable mobility is balanced by a structural demand for stability, particularly during transitions, load-bearing, and unilateral stances. The safe grounding of the femoral head within the acetabulum is supported by the acetabular labrum, a fibrocartilaginous rim that deepens the socket and enhances joint containment. Stability is further reinforced by a strong fibrous capsule and three key ligaments: the iliofemoral, pubofemoral, and ischiofemoral ligaments. Dynamic stabilization is further enhanced and supported by surrounding fascia, other connective tissue, and musculature, including the deep lateral rotators, gluteal group, and iliopsoas (discussed below), all of which play essential roles in contributing to motion, stability, and alignment.

### Ligaments Around the Hip Joint

As noted above, the hip joint capsule is reinforced by three primary ligaments, the iliofemoral, pubofemoral, and ischiofemoral ligaments, which work together to stabilize the femoral head within the acetabulum while still allowing a broad range of motion. The iliofemoral ligament, often considered the strongest ligament in the body, spans from the anterior inferior iliac spine to the intertrochanteric line of the femur and resists excessive extension and external rotation. The pubofemoral ligament arises from the pubic portion of the acetabulum and blends with the joint capsule anteriorly, helping to limit excessive abduction and extension. The ischiofemoral ligament, located posteriorly, spirals from the ischium to the posterior femoral neck and limits internal rotation and adduction. These ligaments are taut in different positions and contribute to passive restraint, ensuring joint congruency during movement and load transfer. For yoga professionals, understanding the supportive role of these ligaments is essential when cueing end-range hip shapes or weight-bearing transitions, as overstretching or poor alignment can challenge joint integrity, especially in students with hypermobility or hip instability.

## *Sacroiliac Joints*

These are the spots where the sacrum meet the ilia of the pelvis (Figure 1.47). The sacroiliac (SI) joints are cartilaginous gliding joints. They have to move to permit walking, during which it makes something of a nodding motion. We do not want too much or too little motion in these joints (i.e., we want these joints to be neither hypermobile nor hypomobile). Contrary to common belief (especially among yoga teachers), SI pain is more often due to hypermobility. It is contraindicated to stretch the SI joints more; instead it is important to stabilize it via strengthening all structures around it.

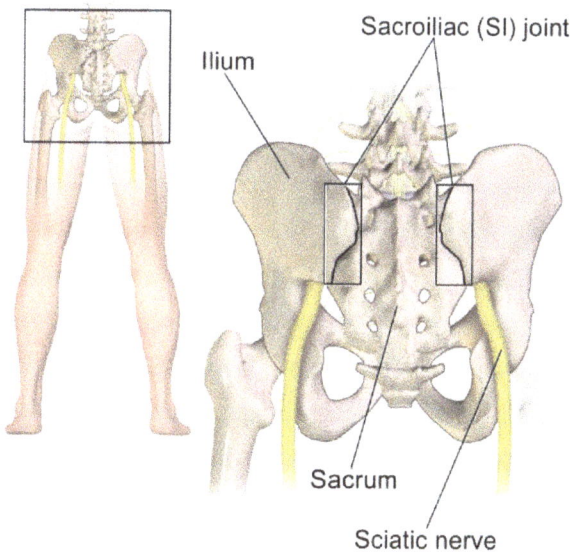

**Figure 1.47** Sacroiliac joint. (Data source: Medical gallery of Blausen Medical 2014, *WikiJournal of Medicine* 1 (2), DOI:10.15347/wjm/2014.010. ISSN 2002-4436; https://commons.wikimedia.org/wiki/File:Sacroiliac_Joint.png; Creative Commons Attribution 3.0)

## *Ligaments of the SI Joints*

The sacroiliac (SI) joints, where the sacrum meets the ilia on either side of the pelvis, are reinforced by a complex system of ligaments that provide crucial stability while allowing for limited motion. The anterior and posterior sacroiliac ligaments directly support the joint capsule, anteriorly spanning the front of the joint, and posteriorly forming the primary fibrous connection between the sacrum and ilia with thick, multidirectional fibers that fill the groove between the bones. These ligaments stabilize the sacrum, preventing it from shifting anteriorly or inferiorly under load and helping to distribute forces between the spine and legs.

Additional vertebropelvic ligaments further reinforce the SI joints. The sacrotuberous ligaments extend from the sacrum and posterior superior iliac spine to the ischial tuberosities, resisting anterior tipping of the sacrum (especially during forward folds) and connecting through the thoracolumbar fascia to the hamstrings, illustrating the strong anatomical link between the low back and posterior thigh. The sacrospinous ligaments are located deeper within the pelvis, stretch from the ischial spines to the sacrum and coccyx, and define the borders of the sciatic foramen. They work alongside the sacrotuberous ligaments to resist excessive pelvic torsion (or twisting), providing protection for the SI joints by helping control range of motion.

The iliolumbar ligaments, which run from the transverse processes of L4 and L5 to the iliac crest, prevent the upper sacrum from gapping and restrict L5 from moving forward over S1, playing a protective role against conditions like spondylolisthesis. These ligaments can be injured by forcing spinal rotation (twists) too low into the spine (ideally, twists occur only from L1 and up) and by rapid or forceful athletic movement. For yoga professionals, understanding the functional integrity of these ligaments is vital when cueing deep forward folds, twists, or jumping transitions, as excessive force or instability in the region can compromise the SI joints and affect the entire pelvic-lumbar relationship (see Figures 1.48 and 1.49).

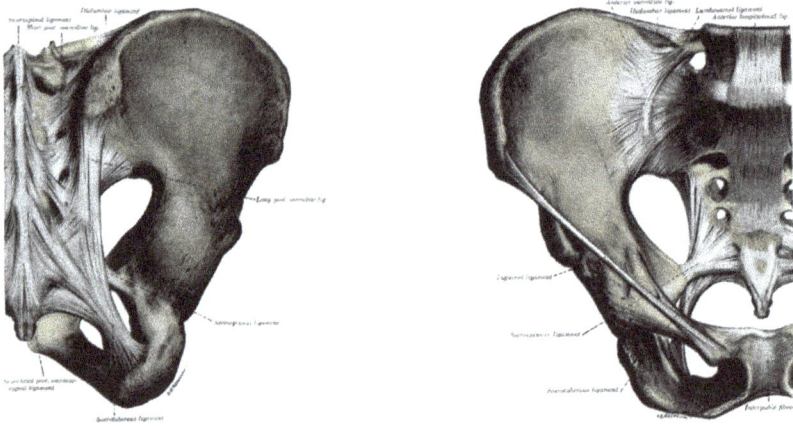

**Figure 1.48** Anterior view of sacroiliac joint. (Data source: Henry Vandyke Carter; https://commons.wikimedia.org/wiki/File:Gray320.png; public domain)

**Figure 1.49** Posterior view of sacroiliac joint. (Data source: Henry Vandyke Carter; https://commons.wikimedia.org/wiki/File:Gray319_with_Iliosacraljoint.png; public domain)

## Muscles of the Pelvic Girdle and Thighs

The muscles of the pelvic girdle form a dynamic and interconnected system that supports both movement and stability across the pelvis, hips, and lower spine. These muscles coordinate actions between the trunk and lower limbs, playing essential roles in postural integrity, load transfer, and functional movement. In yoga *asana* and other movement practices, a deeper understanding of these muscle groups can inform more effective cueing, reduce strain, and promote balanced engagement throughout the body. For clarity and functional relevance, the muscles of the pelvic girdle can be organized into the following groups, each explored in the sections that follow:

- Hip, spine, and lateral flexors, including muscles such as the iliopsoas and quadratus lumborum that influence both the spine and pelvis
- Deep gluteal muscles, such as piriformis and obturators, which stabilize and laterally rotate the hip
- Superficial gluteal muscles, including gluteus maximus, medius, and minimus
- Hamstrings, which span the hip and knee to extend the hip and flex the knee
- Quadriceps femoris group, responsible for extending the knee and assisting with hip flexion
- Adductors of the inner thigh, which draw the legs toward the midline and contribute to pelvic control
- Muscles of the pelvic floor, which provide foundational support for the organs and contribute to core stability

## *Hip Flexors, Spinal Flexors, and Lateral Flexors*

The hip flexors, spinal flexors, and lateral flexors work together to enable essential actions such as hip flexion, spinal flexion, and lateral bending of the trunk. These muscles also play important roles in maintaining core stability and coordinating walking and breathing rhythms. Central to this group is the psoas complex, comprised of the psoas major, psoas minor, and iliacus (Figure 1.50) and bridging the lumbar spine and femur. According to Tom Myers' Anatomy Trains model, the psoas complex is intimately linked to the diaphragm through both fascial and functional connections. Movement or tension in one can directly influence the function of the other. During walking, this relationship becomes dynamically active: as one leg swings forward, the corresponding psoas contracts and exerts a subtle pull on the diaphragm, alternating sides with each step. This rhythmic coordination contributes significantly to dynamic core stability, potentially even more than static engagement of the transverse abdominis.

The psoas major originates from the transverse processes and bodies of T12 to L5 and inserts into the lesser trochanter of the femur. It flexes the hip and assists in lateral flexion of the spine. The psoas minor, present in roughly half of the population, originates from T12 to L1 and inserts on the pelvic rim near the pubic bone, acting as a weak lumbar flexor. The iliacus, originating from the iliac fossa and inserting alongside the psoas major at the lesser trochanter, contributes strongly to hip flexion. These three muscles are often collectively referred to as the iliopsoas, though each has distinct anatomical features.

Also included in this group is the sartorius, the longest muscle in the body, which originates from the anterior superior iliac spine (ASIS) and inserts on the medial aspect of the proximal tibia. It crosses both the hip and knee joints, enabling hip flexion and external rotation, as well as knee flexion and slight internal rotation when the knee is flexed. Finally, the quadratus lumborum (QL), which arises from the iliac crest and inserts on the 12th rib and the transverse processes of L1–L4, plays a key role in stabilizing the lumbar spine and pelvis, especially during unilateral weight-bearing. It also contributes to lateral flexion of the spine. Together, these muscles form a foundational network that supports posture, breathing coordination, and integrated movement between the upper and lower body.

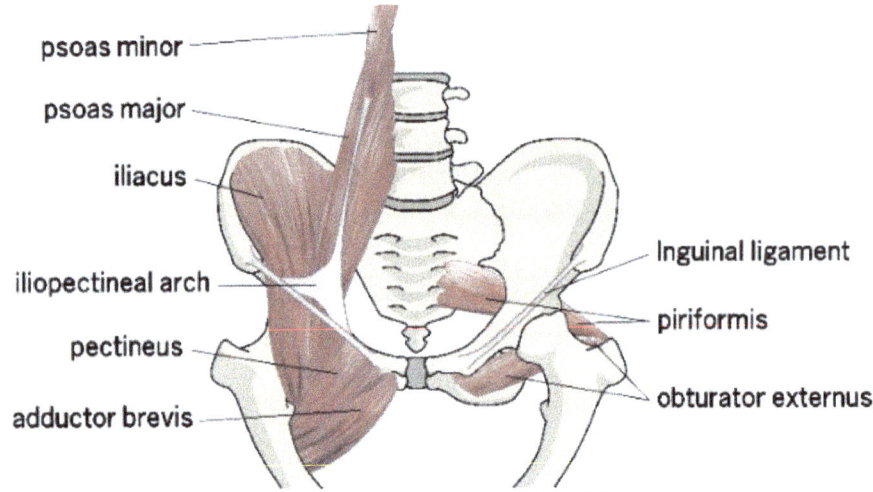

**Figure 1.50** Hip flexors and rotators – anterior view. (Data source: Istock)

## Deep Gluteal Muscles

The deep gluteal muscles, often referred to collectively as the *deep six* form a compact group of external (lateral) rotators that play a crucial role in controlling and stabilizing the hip joint. They include the following muscles, described in more detail below and shown in Figure 1.51, namely, piriformis, obturator internus and externus, superior and inferior gemelli, and quadratus femoris.

Positioned beneath the gluteus maximus, these muscles help rotate the femur outward when the hip is extended and abduct the femur when the hip is flexed. This shift in function, rotation versus abduction, depends on the orientation of the femur in the acetabulum, making their engagement highly relevant in movement practices such as yoga, particularly during transitions, standing balances, asymmetrical standing shapes (such as Warrior 2, Side Angle, and Triangle), and seated hip openers (e.g., Butterfly, Lotus). All of these muscles originate on the internal surfaces of the pelvis, spanning from the sacrum to the ischium, and insert on or around the greater trochanter of the femur, forming a stabilizing sheath of muscles around the back and sides of the joint.

The piriformis originates on the anterior surface of the sacrum (S2–S4), as well as the sacrotuberous ligament and the margins of the greater sciatic foramen, and inserts onto the greater trochanter. It externally rotates the hip in extension and contributes to abduction when the hip is flexed. The obturator internus and obturator externus both arise from the obturator foramen – internus from the internal surface of the pubis and ischium, externus from the external – and insert into the medial surface of the greater trochanter. These muscles share the functional shift from rotation to abduction based on hip angle and are key to stabilizing the femoral head during motion.

The superior and inferior gemelli, which flank the obturator internus tendon, originate from the ischial spine and ischial tuberosity respectively and insert alongside obturator internus into the greater trochanter. They reinforce the actions of their neighboring muscles and contribute to precise femoral tracking during hip rotation. The most inferior of the group, the quadratus femoris, spans from the lateral ischium to the intertrochanteric crest of the femur. It acts as a powerful lateral rotator and contributes to compressive stability at the back of the hip.

Though small and often overlooked, the deep gluteal muscles provide essential joint stability, particularly during asymmetrical or unilateral loading. For yoga practitioners and movement professionals, awareness of how hip angle affects their function can guide safer cueing in flexion, rotation, and balancing. Addressing imbalances or restrictions in this muscle group may also reduce compensatory strain in the low back or sacroiliac region.

### *Superficial Gluteal Muscles*

The superficial gluteal muscles, commonly known as the *glutes,* form a powerful and large muscular layer crucial for hip abduction, rotation, and extension. This group, working in concert with surrounding fascia and connective tissues, plays an indispensable role in stability and mobility of the hip joint, most notably in maintaining pelvic integrity in asymmetrical standing shapes and movements. They are profoundly important to the simple act of walking, as well as the more demanding action of completing an uphill section of a strenuous hike.

The collective strength of the glutes can influence range of motion in seemingly unrelated movements, such as forward folding in the context of yoga *asana* or daily life. Namely, strong engagement (contraction) of these powerful hip extensors and external rotators can create a natural resistance to deep hip flexion. Understanding this interplay is key to cueing that facilitates the most auspicious alignment and range of motion for affected yoga shapes. For example, cueing slight internal rotation of the femurs in Forward Folds can strategically off-load the external rotators within the gluteal group, allowing for greater ease in accessing the fold, particularly for individuals with less pronounced gluteal strength. However, this offered guidance requires careful tailoring. For hypermobile students or clients, actively maintaining external rotation and abduction through gluteal engagement is paramount for joint stabilization and preventing excessive movement.

The superficial gluteal group (also shown in Figure 1.51) includes four key players:
- *Gluteus maximus*, the most superficial and largest of the gluteal muscles, is a primary driver of hip extension (including movements such as rising up from a seat or climbing stairs) and contributes significantly to external rotation, especially during forceful movements such as running or climbing steep inclines. It also supports pelvic stabilization, trunk extensions, and in minor roles supports abduction and adduction. Hip position can affect the specific role of the gluteus maximus. For example, in a neutral hip position it functions as a primary extensor; however, in in flexion it assists abduction. Gluteus maximus originates broadly from the posterior aspect of the ilium, lower part of the sacrum, and coccyx, its fibers converging to insert onto the femur's gluteal tuberosity and blending into the iliotibial band. In *asana*, its engagement is palpable in powerful hip extension, such as the back leg in Warrior shapes.
- *Gluteus medius*, situated deep and slightly anterior to gluteus maximus, is a vital hip abductor that plays a nuanced role in medial and lateral rotation depending on degree of flexion in the hip joint. It acts as a dynamic stabilizer of the pelvis in single-leg shapes, preventing the contralateral hip from dropping, a key function observed in balances such as Tree or Eagle.

Its origin spans the lateral surface of the ilium, and its fibers converge to a strong insertion on the greater trochanter of the femur. Yoga teachers can indirectly cue engagement of gluteus medius by emphasizing maintaining a level pelvis in standing balances and asymmetrical (split leg) shapes.
- *Gluteus minimus*, the deepest of the three gluteal muscles, works synergistically with gluteus medius in hip abduction and contributes to medial rotation. It shares the crucial role of stabilizing the pelvis and preventing pelvic drop during single-leg weight-bearing. Originating from the lateral ilium, just below gluteus medius and along the margin of the sciatic notch, its fibers insert onto the anterior aspect of the greater trochanter of the femur. Awareness of gluteus minimus activation is essential in refining balance and stability in asymmetrical shapes.
- *Tensor fascia lata* (TFL), though often considered part of the lateral thigh compartment, works closely with the gluteals, particularly gluteus medius and minimus, to assist in hip flexion and internal rotation. Its unique origin is on the outer iliac crest and anterior superior iliac spine (ASIS); it inserts into the iliotibial band, a thick fascial structure that runs along the lateral thigh. Beyond its role in hip movement, TFL contributes to the stability of the knee during gait and assists in hip flexion, actions evident in stepping forward during Lunges or other standing transitions.

Understanding the distinct yet highly collaborative roles of the superficial gluteal muscles allows for cueing that is well-informed enough to translate yoga practice into functional movement patterns off the mat. Through yoga clinicians' precise guidance that encourages conscious engagement of these muscles, clients can learn to enhance stability, improve alignment, and address imbalances that may manifest in the low back or sacroiliac joint region. Recognizing how hip position influences their function allows for more nuanced and effective instruction in a wide range of yoga *asana* and movement practices.

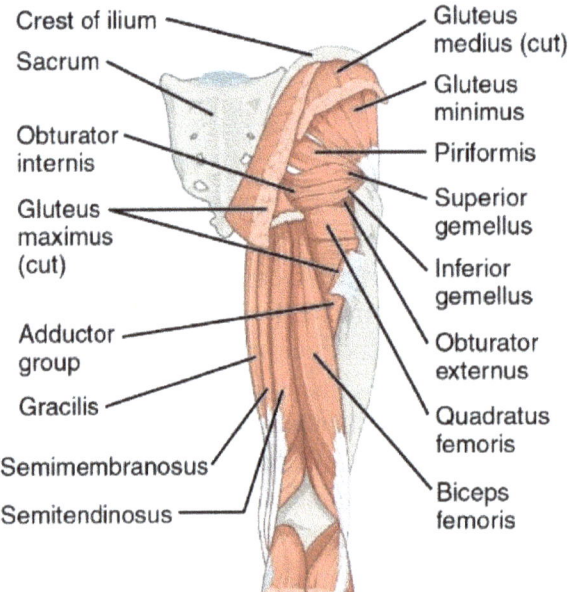

**Figure 1.51** Hip abductors, rotators, and extensors – posterior view. (Data source: OpenStax; https://commons.wikimedia.org/wiki/File:1122_Gluteal_Muscles_that_Move_the_Femur_c.png; Creative Commons Attribution 3.0)

## *Hamstrings*

The hamstrings are a group of four muscles located along the posterior thigh, functioning primarily as knee flexors and hip extensors. Though typically discussed as a unit, each muscle contributes in slightly different ways to coordinated movement and joint stability. The four muscles include the following and are detailed below and shown in Figure 1.52, namely, biceps femoris – long and short heads, semitendinosus, and semimembranosus.

The four hamstring muscles originate from the ischial tuberosity (except the short head of the biceps femoris, which originates from the femur) and insert on or near the bones of the lower leg. The biceps femoris inserts on the lateral head of the fibula, while the semitendinosus and semimembranosus attach medially on the tibia, with the semitendinosus also contributing to the pes anserinus tendon shared with sartorius and gracilis. The biceps femoris has a long head that crosses the hip and knee, and a short head that crosses only the knee. Together, the hamstrings contribute to hip extension, knee flexion, and external rotation of the tibia. The semitendinosus and semimembranosus support hip extension and knee flexion, while also contributing to internal tibial rotation when the knee is flexed.

To be very clear, these muscles span *two joints*: the hip and knee; this key feature helps define their function. From a movement perspective, understanding that the hamstrings have a narrow origin at the pelvis and a broad, complex insertion around the knee helps clarify why their influence is more pronounced at the lower (i.e., knee) joint. The hamstrings contribute to hip extension, particularly when the trunk is inclined forward or during the push phase of walking or running; however, their primary mechanical leverage is at the knee, where they control flexion and assist in rotating the tibia when the knee is bent. This tibial rotation plays a subtle but important role in stabilizing the knee during gait and pivoting actions. When the knee is extended, the hamstrings are less able to influence tibial position, and their focus returns to lengthening or contracting at the hip joint.

In yoga, awareness of hamstring function becomes particularly relevant during Forward Folds, when the hamstrings are often under tension, and in transitions that demand strength *and* length, such as in Lunges, Bridges, or standing balances. Overstretching or misaligning these muscles, especially without co-engagement from surrounding stabilizers (such as the glutes or adductors), can increase risk for strain either at the ischial origin or behind the knee. There are actions that can be taken in Forward Folds that decrease tension in the hamstrings and commensurate stress in the low back (which arises due to the origin of the hamstrings in the ischial tuberosities). As these muscles cross two joints, ease can be achieved either by decreasing hip flexion (e.g., rising to a prop or into a half lift from a Standing Forward Fold) or by decreasing knee extension (i.e., bending the knees). To address strength in these key muscles, balanced action in yoga and life addresses not simply flexibility, but also eccentric strength, joint coordination, and neuromuscular awareness across both joints influenced (i.e., crossed) by these muscles. This is addressed further in Section Two, in the context of yoga *asana*.

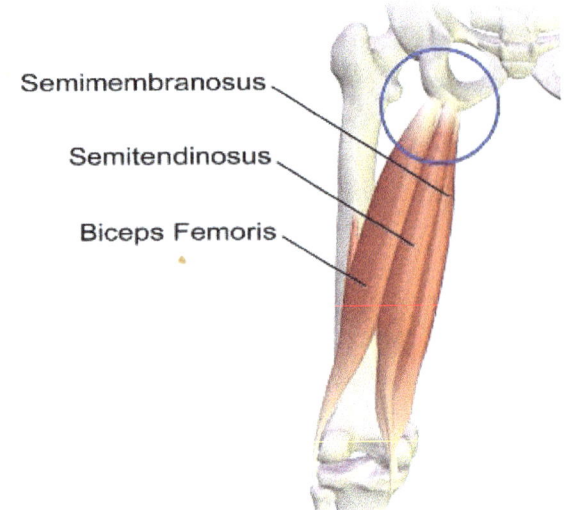

Figure 1.52 Hamstring muscles – posterior views. (Data source: Paul Hermns; https://upload.wikimedia.org/wikipedia/commons/2/2b/Opgespannen_hamstrings_%28cropped%29.jpg. Creative Commons Attribution 4.0)

## *Adductors*

The adductor group consists of five primary muscles detailed below and shown in Figure 1.53, located along the inner thigh, namely, adductor longus, adductor brevis, adductor magnus, pectineus, and gracilis.

Most of these muscles originate on the inferior pubic ramus, with the adductor magnus also arising from the ischial tuberosity, giving it a unique role that bridges adduction with hip extension. Their insertions vary along the medial femoral shaft, with the gracilis being the only one to cross the knee joint, inserting on the medial tibia as part of the pes anserinus ligament. This anatomical arrangement, a wide and fan-like origin on the pelvis converging toward narrower insertions on the femur and tibia, suggests that the greatest mechanical impact of these muscles is at the hip, not the knee.

Their primary collaborative functions are adduction and internal rotation of the hip joint, including drawing the femur inward toward the midline. During walking or other forms of forward locomotion, this effect on the femur prevents excessive hip abduction and lateral sway, making the adductors essential for maintaining efficient, straight-line forward motion. Their role in pelvic and femoral stability is often underestimated, but especially important during single-leg balances and lateral movements. Most adductors also assist with hip flexion, particularly in the first 45 degrees of this movement direction. Adductor magnus is unique for having both an adductor portion (which assists with flexion) and a posterior, hamstring-like portion that contributes to hip extension, especially when the hip is flexed. Gracilis also crosses the knee joint and thus plays a small role in knee flexion and medial tibial rotation; however, this is true only when the knee is flexed.

In a yoga *asana* context, the adductors often operate behind the scenes, contributing to pelvic alignment, stability in standing postures, and transitions involving lateral load shifts (such as

Warriors or wide-legged Forward Folds). Weakness or over-lengthening in this group can lead to instability in the pelvis or knees, while excessive gripping or asymmetrical loading may contribute to pubic symphysis irritation or medial knee strain. Supporting adductor function requires balanced flexibility and coordinated activation, especially in combination with the pelvic floor muscles, the gluteal muscles, and the deep core musculature, to promote safe, integrated lower body movement.

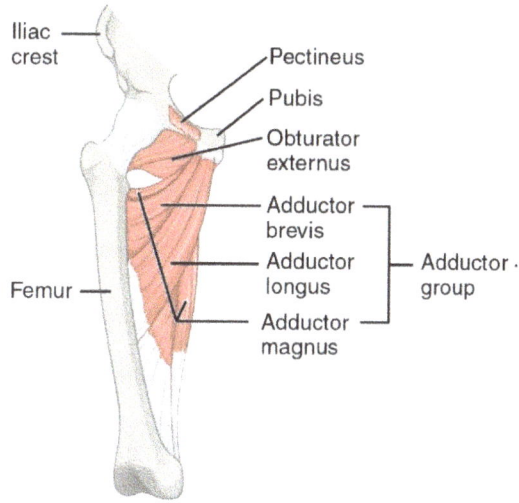

**Figure 1.53** Hip adductor muscle – anterior views. (Data source: OpenStax; https://commons.wikimedia.org/wiki/File:1122_Gluteal_Muscles_that_Move_the_Femur_b.png; Creative Commons Attribution 3.0)

## Quadriceps Femoris

The quadriceps femoris group consists of rectus femoris, vastus lateralis, vastus medialis, and vastus intermedius (Figure 1.54). Collectively, these muscles form the powerful musculature along the anterior thigh. Their primary function is knee extension, a foundational action for standing, walking, squatting, and most dynamic lower-body movements. All four muscles converge distally into the patellar tendon, which inserts onto the tibial tuberosity via the patella, which acts as a sesamoid bone that enhances the leverage and efficiency of knee extension. This shared insertion across the front of the knee provides a strong mechanical advantage, reinforcing the idea that the quadriceps' main action is on the knee.

Most of the quadriceps muscles originate high on the femoral shaft. However, rectus femoris is distinct in that it crosses two joints. It arises from the anterior inferior iliac spine (AIIS), making it not only a knee extensor but also a hip flexor. This muscles thus creates a functional link between the thigh and pelvis that is especially relevant in postures involving hip flexion under load (e.g., Lunges or Boat). Vastus lateralis and vastus medialis, located on the outer and inner thigh respectively, and the vastus intermedius, which lies deep to rectus femoris, contribute solely to knee extension. The vastus medialis, particularly its oblique fibers, is crucial to patellar stabilization, helping maintain proper knee tracking during movement.

Translating this to a yoga *asana* context, the quadriceps play a crucial role in stabilizing the knee joint, especially in weight-bearing positions such as Chair, Warrior, and standing balances. In addition to generating force, they provide eccentric control, resisting knee flexion during transitions such as descending into a squat or stepping back from a Lunge. Imbalances in quadriceps strength, or chronic overuse (especially of rectus femoris), may contribute to anterior knee pain, patellar tracking issues, or strain in the hip flexors. Balancing strengthening and stretching is crucial, particularly when sequencing movements that load the quads, involve long holds, or require active knee extension.

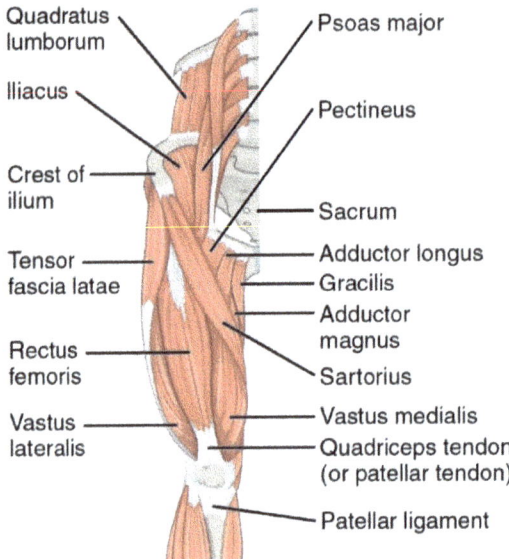

**Figure 1.54** Overview of the major muscles creating movement in the hip and knee joint – anterior view. (Data source: OpenStax; https://commons.wikimedia.org/wiki/File:1122_Gluteal_Muscles_that_Move_the_Femur_a.png; Creative Commons Attribution 3.0)

## *Muscles of the Pelvic Floor*

The pelvic floor muscles, collectively also known as the pelvic diaphragm, form the muscular base of the pelvic cavity and play a significant role in structural support. Shaped like a hammock, this muscular complex spans the region called the perineum, a diamond-shaped area bordered by the pubic symphysis (anteriorly), ischial tuberosities (laterally), and the coccyx (posteriorly). The pelvic floor contains two key muscular components, the levator ani (which includes the pubococcygeus, puborectalis, and iliococcygeus) and the coccygeus (or ischiococcygeus), integrated with associated fascia and connective tissues. Collectively, they create a dynamic support structure with urogenital and rectal hiatuses (i.e., openings) for the urethra, vagina (in biologically female bodies), and rectum.

Functionally, the pelvic floor is vital for supporting the abdominopelvic viscera, maintaining urinary and fecal continence and modulating intraabdominal pressure during actions such as coughing, sneezing, heavy lifting, and childbirth. The pelvic diaphragm also assists in postural and core stability, functioning in coordination with the diaphragm, transverse abdominis, and deep spinal muscles to create a central stabilizing system for the human bipedal, upright structure. In yoga and movement practices, the pelvic floor can be lifted to create subtle engagement that can be particularly helpful in shapes and movements that involve lifting, inverting, or increased demand for core engagement.

Notably, the piriformis and obturator internus, though categorized as deep gluteal muscles, are embedded in the posterior pelvic wall and help form the structural container that supports the pelvic floor. Optimal functioning of the pelvic diaphragm further depends on healthy fascial tone, including continuity with the perineal body, sacrospinous and sacrotuberous ligaments, and the endopelvic fascia. Dysfunction in the pelvic floor (whether from trauma, overuse, underuse, or poor neuromuscular coordination) can contribute to pelvic pain, incontinence, low back discomfort, and postural imbalances. For yoga professionals, understanding these muscles can inform nuanced cueing related to pelvic awareness, breathwork, and mindful engagement in shapes that load or decompress the pelvic bowl.

## Kinesiology of the Pelvic Girdle and Thighs

As discussed in greater detail for each *asana* in Section Two, one of the most effective and sustainable focal points for cueing yoga *asana* and functional movement is to begin with an emphasis on natural pelvic orientation, which, in most individuals, means a slight anterior tilt. This position reflects the pelvis's anatomical alignment when the spine's physiological curves are at their most natural: lumbar lordosis is maintained, the sacrum is neutrally angled into the ilia, and the hip joints are neither compressed nor overly slack. This foundational alignment is especially relevant in standing and seated shapes, but also underpins transitions and load-bearing shapes across all categories of *asana*. The position of the pelvis affects alignment upward and downward the kinetic chain: the spine and head, as well as the knees and feet.

Patterns of pelvic positioning vary greatly – they are highly bioindividual, partly shaped by genetics and partly by postural habits. Some individuals exhibit chronic (excessive) anterior tilt that causes the top of the pelvis to tip forward and the lumbar spine to become excessively lordotic. Other individuals tend toward a posterior pelvic tilt, often characterized by habitual tucking of the tailbone and flattening of the lumbar curve. Both extremes can contribute to musculoskeletal compensation and dysfunction. Helping students find their 'natural' pelvic position (i.e., the middle way between over-arching and over-tucking) is supportive of sacroiliac joint integrity, lumbar decompression, and efficient load transfer through the axial and into the lower appendicular skeleton. Healthful position of the pelvis can be transformative as the pelvic girdle is the base of locomotion – walking, running, skipping, jumping, and doing yoga *asana*.

During yoga *asana*, cueing from a naturally aligned pelvis upward encourages the spine to elongate from a stable base, preserving its natural curves and promoting postural integration. A natural pelvic base facilitates balanced diaphragmatic breathing, optimizes alignment of internal organs, and allows for more sustainable muscular engagement across the spine, core, and lower limbs. Importantly, natural pelvic alignment is not a fixed *external* shape, but a dynamic and interoceptively guided orientation. Students benefit most from invitations to explore their own proprioceptive feedback, using breath, micro-adjustments, and somatic awareness to feel their way into an individualized alignment that feels balanced, grounded, and responsive. In other words, rather than prescribing a singular location or angle for the pelvis, effective guidance centers on interoceptively-based inquiry and exploration, allowing for individual expressions of body structure, mobility, and alignment. Over time, students may come to recognize how pelvic orientation subtly informs their entire posture, breath, and felt sense of integration in practice.

> *Cueing Guidance*:
>
> To help individuals access a naturally slightly anterior pelvis, it serves to explore extremes of positioning, such as an excessive lumbar curve with excessive anterior rotation of the pelvis versus a flat lumbar spine with the rib basket leaning toward the back, and excessive posterior rotation (or tucking) of the pelvis. Yoga professionals can offer practices that help students feel the extremes to facilitate accessing natural alignment in the middle. This can happen in tabletop, seats, standing, and supine positions. For some, this can even be accessed in inversions.

## *Understanding Movement in the Acetabulum*

Clear and nuanced understanding of femoral articulation empowers yoga professionals to offer safe and skillful variations of traditional postures that tend to stress this joint, to cue alignment that honors each student's unique bony architecture, and to preserve both in-the-moment comfort and long-term health of the hip joint.

In yoga practice, understanding the structure and function of the hip joints is essential, as positioning and movement of the femurs within the acetabula directly influence joint loading and alignment patterns throughout the pelvis, including reverberations into the sacroiliac joints. For example, femoral movements involving flexion, adduction, and external rotation (especially passive movements created by using hands, body weight, or props to increase active or even natural range of motion), as commonly seen in yoga shapes such as Pigeon or Lotus, can increase stress on the anterior joint capsule, particularly in practitioners with hypermobility, reduced labral integrity, or unbalanced muscular engagement. Femoral torquing or forcing (i.e., passive movement) can disrupt the sacroiliac joints as the power of the femur is used to create movement that exceeds the healthful range of motion in the hip joint proper (Farhi & Stuart, 2017) and creates movement of between the ilia and sacrum that exceeds it natural range of motion. Over time, this pattern can lead to hypermobility in a joint specifically designed for stability (Clark, 2016).

Understanding natural movement of the femoral heads in the acetabulum is helpful to find more ease in forward folding. It can facilitate auspicious cueing that is accurately tailored to what may be happening in the hip joint during various shapes and movements. The table below provides *asana*-specific information and guidance to counter the commonly less-than-auspicious cueing related to this topic for specific types of *asana*. Additionally, following are pointers about anatomical understandings of femoral movement in the acetabulum and its implications:
- Positioning of the femoral head in the acetabulum can support or detract from stability in this joint. Specifically, according to Lasater (2009, 2020), the joint is in its:
  - *least stable position* when in flexion + adduction + external rotation = head of femur out of the socket with ligaments slack around the joint
  - *most stable position* when in extension + internal rotation + abduction = head of femur in closed packed position with ligaments strong and tight around the joint
- Internal rotation of the femur is auspicious as it helps plant the femoral head in a more natural, stable, yet easeful position in the acetabulum. Specifically:

- o femurs internally rotate on hip flexion (e.g., in Downward Facing Dog, the femurs rotate internally, which also helps stabilize the knees; more about the knees below)
- o internal rotation of the femur stretches and releases the external hip rotators (including the glutes), which allows the pelvis to move more freely – more about this later
- The gluteal muscles are strengthened by hiking and walking, with impact on yoga *asana*:
  - o very strong glutes can limit forward folding; in other words, limitations in forward folding may not always be a hamstring or superficial backline issue
  - o internal rotation in the thighs during forward folding can take the glutes off line a bit, essentially taking limitations based on external rotators tightness out of the equation
  - o cueing internal rotation in forward folding is helpful for many yoga practitioners – unless they are hypermobile; for such students, internal rotation is not cued; instead gluteal engagement may create needed joint stability (see Chapter 12)
- Femurs externally rotate on hip extension (e.g., Camel) making the joint naturally more vulnerable and necessitating care in cueing and alignment. Thus:
  - o to enhance joint integrity during hip extension, engagement of the adductors can support stability (e.g., squeezing a block between the legs); this adduction of the legs is key especially in shapes where the legs are abducted (yes, this sounds contradictory; however, remember that adduction is a *direction* of movement [not a position]; it can be cultivated even while the legs are wide apart)
  - o to create more interoception and thus joint integrity, it can help to cue active engagement of the external hip rotators
  - o to support integrity in the lumbar spine (and upward), it can be auspicious to invite a lifting upward and backward of the anterior superior iliac spine (yet without flaring the low ribs)

| *Sample Shapes* | *Anatomical Considerations* | *Cueing Suggestions* |
|---|---|---|
| **Hip Flexion + External Rotation** | | |
| *Pigeon, Lotus, Seated Twist* | Places anterior capsule and labrum under tension; vulnerable in hypermobile or shallow-hipped practitioners; stresses the SI joints; can stress the knees | - Support front knee or hip with props<br>- Encourage active hip flexion, not passive 'sinking' or bouncing<br>- Let the shin angle naturally in seats; do not force it parallel |
| **Hip Flexion + Internal Rotation** | | |
| *Cow Face, Eagle* | Less range available in most bodies; challenges deep rotators and posterior joint capsule | - Avoid torquing the knees into position<br>- Elevate hips if knees lift<br>- Ground sitz bones to support pelvic neutrality |
| **Hip Extension** | | |
| *Warrior 1, Bridge, Bow, Upward Dog* | Femur moves posteriorly in the acetabulum; anterior structures are lengthened | - Engage glutes without over-squeezing<br>- Cue a lift through the front of the hip to prevent lumbar compression<br>- Ground through the big toe mound to activate adductors |

| Hip Abduction + External Rotation | | |
|---|---|---|
| *Tree, Triangle, Half Moon, Warrior 2* | Femur shifts laterally in socket; stability depends on balanced muscle engagement; can stress the SI joints and knees | - Root through center of the heel<br>- Engage gluteus medius<br>- Avoid passive turnout of the lifted leg |
| **Deep Flexion under Load** | | |
| *Chair, Crow* | Increases joint compression, especially anteriorly and superiorly in the acetabulum | - Lengthen spine to reduce joint compression<br>- Engage hip flexors and pelvic floor<br>- Support heels or hips to avoid excessive pelvic tilt |
| **Transitions / Asymmetrical Loads** | | |
| *Lunge, Balancing Transitions* | Demands dynamic control of femoral head in socket; risk of uneven pelvic and sacroiliac loading | - Cue slow, mindful transitions.<br>- Ground all four corners of the foot<br>- Avoid flinging the leg; move with core strength support |

### *Understanding Movement in the Sacroiliac Region*

The sacroiliac (SI) joints represent the most crucial connection between the axial and appendicular skeletons. They are the meeting point of the sacrum at the base of the spine with the ilia of the pelvis. Structurally, the SI joints are a keystone articulation (quite literally akin to a keystone structure in an architectural arch; Figures 1.55 and 1.56), thus clearly built for stability much more so than mobility. With less than 2 degrees of total movement available in healthy SI joints, they function primarily to receive and transfer load between the spine and pelvis. The SI joints are reinforced by a thick web of ligaments and supported by a bony interlocking mechanism that becomes particularly stable when the human body is in its fully upright bipedal position, in which the weight of the trunk wedges the sacrum securely between the ilia. This is referred to as the joint's self-locking or *form closure* system.

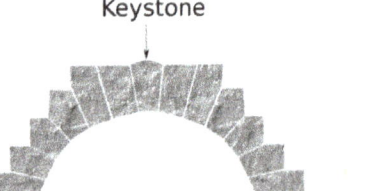
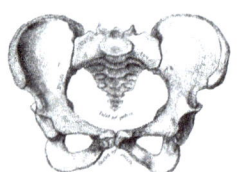

**Figure 1.55** Keystone arch in architecture. (Data source: Jhbdel; https://commons.wikimedia.org/wiki/File:Arch_voussoirs.svg#:~:text=https%3A//upload.wikimedia.org/wikipedia/commons/2/24/Arch_voussoirs.svg; creativecommons.org 3.0)

**Figure 1.56** Pelvis with sacrum as keystone. (Data source: Henry Vandyke Carter, https://commons.wikimedia.org/wiki/File:Comparison_human_male_and_female_pelvis.png; public domain)

Since the SI joints inhabit the same pelvis as the hip joints, they can be deeply affected by movements that occur in the hip joints. Healthful biomechanics in this entire region rely on clear differentiation between femoral movement in the acetabulum, pelvic or sacral movement around the SI joints, and spinal movement in the lumbar spine and lumbosacral junction. It all starts with the hip joint: the wide variability in hip socket orientation and femoral neck angles across individuals translates into highly diverse ranges of motion in this joint, meaning that alignment is not based on outer shape but relies on inner experience of natural bony limits. Exceeding the bony limits within the hip joint through force is a significant risk for SI irritation, even in the presence of great flexibility of soft tissues around the joint. Healthful movement thus means that hip joint range of motion is respected for its structural limits and the femur moves inside the acetabula in a natural range of motion (i.e., without force, especially force created by passive movement). When this is the case and motion is isolated appropriately in the hip joint, the pelvis is truly a stable and integrated whole, a reliable base. However, when teachers invite and students to seek more range than the bony architecture of the hip joint allows, resulting strain often transfers to the SI joints (as well as the lumbosacral joint).

Due to its relationships within other structures in the pelvis and lumbar spine, SI joints are vulnerable to *excessive* stress and *forced* misalignment, particularly during yoga *asana* practices or other movements that create shear at the level of the spine or torque between the sacrum and ilia. Shear forces, torquing, and asymmetrical loading can compromise the region's ligamentous integrity, especially among individuals with naturally looser connective tissue (e.g., hypermobility) or experiencing hormonal fluctuations (e.g., during menstruation, pregnancy, or postpartum). Biologically female bodies, whose pelvic architecture tends to have a wider interacetabular distance, may be particularly prone to SI joint instability. Yoga cueing and practice needs to prioritize biomechanical integrity of the SI joints by avoiding, rather than introducing (inadvertently and unknowingly) introducing, destabilizing forces. Three primary mechanisms can create stress on the SI joints (and the lumbar spine) and warrant close attention in terms of common yoga cueing and practice: *corkscrewing*, *spinal leveraging* and *femoral leveraging* (Farhi & Stuart, 2017). While described separately, they often overlap and co-occur in the same shapes or movements.

### *Femoral Leveraging*

Femoral leveraging describes a situation in which the femur and pelvis are forced to move as a single unit (rather than the femur rotating independently within the acetabulum). Such movement is typically forced – it does not happen naturally; it requires overpowering natural wisdom with the willpower or desire to please a teacher or find a particular outer shape. Femoral leveraging occurs when movement of the femur in the acetabulum exceeds its natural range of motion and essentially forces a bypassing of the hip joint – movement is continued, instead of ending at maximum healthful range, and pries excessive movement into the SI joints. This stress on the SI joints occurs most commonly when a practitioner pushes beyond the available range of hip *abduction* or *external rotation*. Shapes such as Side Angle and Warrior 2 are common culprits, especially in the presence of cueing that is focused more on outer shapes than inner experience and that does not carefully prepare the individual through generating core strength and keen attention. This may also occur in Butterfly or Wide-Legged Forward Folds, whether seated or standing. Rather than simply moving in its natural ranges of motion within the acetabulum, forced movement in the femur moves one entire side of the pelvis, creating stress in the SI joints.

### *Sacral or Lumbar Corkscrewing*

Sacral corkscrewing refers to spinal movements and alignments (intentional or inadvertent) that create shearing or rotational forces into the lumbar spine and/or the connection between sacrum and ilia (essentially torquing the sacrum inside the ilia). In yoga *asana*, such a situation occurs most commonly in shapes that bring rotational movement into this region of the spine. *Sacral torquing* can arise alongside femoral leveraging, exemplified by (less than natural) movement patterns in Warrior shapes. In Warrior 2, this type of stress occurs if alignment cueing forces outer shapes such as a pelvis aligned (arbitrarily) with the long edge of the mat. Similarly, in Warrior 1, sacral torquing can occur if the sole of the back foot is forced to meet the ground aligned parallel to the short edge of the mat. Sacral corkscrewing arises from twisting shapes (especially seated) in which the pelvis is not allowed to move freely into the twist. Such outer-alignment based cueing does not serve as it invites students to engage in unnatural movements and forced alignments that result in the sacrum turning inside of the ilia, a shearing force that over time can be extremely destructive in this joint. It can also force rotation into the lumbar spine, which naturally has very little rotation. Any such rotation in the lumbar region that cannot be absorbed will be transferred as torquing stress into the SI joints.

## Spinal Leveraging

In spinal leveraging, the spine is jutting out (or cantilevering) to the side, hanging off the pelvis without core support from within or prop support (i.e., a stack of yoga blocks) on the floor, a common occurrence in Triangle. A great amount of shear and possibly rotational stress is created in the lumbosacral junction (i.e., between L5 and S1) and both SI joints. Additional stress on the whole kinetic chain that is the spine may be introduced with poor alignment elsewhere in the body. For example, the head hanging unsupported downward toward the floor and away from the midline tremendously increases load on the spine. Similarly, if the lower ribs are flaring forward with a commensurate loss of core integration, there is increased sacral and lumbosacral shear (as well as possible excessive torquing in the lumbar spine). Over time, repetitive engagement of such misalignment, without structural awareness of the stresses it creates, can destabilize the involved joints, essentially creating repetitive stress injuries in the SI and lumbosacral joints.

## Understanding the Lumbar-Sacral Rhythm

Another oft-mentioned concept in understanding healthy spinal and pelvic movement is the natural coordination between the lumbar spine and pelvis, known as the lumbosacral or spinopelvic rhythm. This rhythm describes how the lumbar spine and pelvis move in concert during flexion and extension, allowing for efficient load distribution and minimizing strain across the sacroiliac (SI) joints. In lumbar extension, such as in backbending, the pelvis naturally rotates anteriorly, the iliopsoas complex contracts to facilitate hip flexion, and the erector spinae activate to draw the pelvis forward. This anterior tilt is maintained through the full range of the backbend. Conversely, during spinal flexion (i.e., forward folding), the pelvis starts out in an anterior tilt and begins to rotate posteriorly as flexion deepens; the gluteal group and hamstrings engage to draw the ischial tuberosities downward, while the rectus abdominis and external obliques help draw the ilia upward.

A related and often misunderstood set of movements, called nutation and counternutation, describes the subtle rocking of the sacrum within the ilia. In lumbar extension, the sacrum nutates, meaning the sacral promontory (around S1) tips forward relative to the ilia. In lumbar flexion, it counternutates, tipping backward. These are small, natural motions, limited by robust ligamentous support. Excessive nutation, often caused by miscueing (e.g., urging a tucked tailbone in backbends), may destabilize the SI joints and contribute to dysfunction. Respecting the innate lumbosacral rhythm and the mechanics of nutation and counternutation supports spinal integrity, promotes balanced muscle activation, and protects the SI joints from undue stress.

Yoga teachers can serve their students best by encouraging awareness of the pelvis's natural anterior tilt and lifting through the front body to maintain length and space during backbends. In forward folds, movement is invited to initiate from the hip joints with a sense of the femoral heads being grounded securely in the hip sockets and the pelvis tilting anteriorly without spinal flexion. Once the fold deepens, a soft rounding of the spine and a gentle posterior tilt will occur naturally. Individual hip structures are honored by not cueing outer shapes but instead highlighting that not all students have the same degree of available hip flexion.

> *Yoga Guidance*:
>
> The best action for yoga professionals who are unsure about cueing related to these rhythms (especially nutation and counternutation) is *no* action. Most cueing related to these rhythms, if it does not come from a deep understanding, is counterproductive and can get in the way of students' natural wisdom and movement of the body.

## Lower Legs, Ankles, and Feet

The lower legs, ankles, and feet form the body's foundation and anatomical position, bearing weight, absorbing shock, and facilitating movement and balance. This region plays a crucial role in proprioception, postural alignment, and force transmission throughout the bipedal human kinetic chain. In yoga teaching and therapeutics, attention to foot placement, ankle mobility, and lower leg engagement can reveal and resolve imbalances that affect the entire body.

Human bodies have what is called a '1, 2, 3, 4, 5' bony construction in the upper and lower appendicular skeletons (i.e., the areas around the legs/feet and arms/hands). This construction allows for greater stability more proximal to the torso (i.e., near the shoulder girdle for the arms; near the pelvic girdle for the legs) and increasing mobility further along the limbs. Hands and feet have maximum mobility with many very small bones and many tiny joints. This structural complexity allows for the fine motor ability we need in our hands, and the mobility to navigate uneven terrain with the feet. The five levels of this complex structure in the limbs are as follows:

- There is *one large bone* in each limb *most proximally* to the torso (i.e., the humerus in the arms; the femur in the legs).
- There are *two bones further out along the limbs* (i.e., ulna and radius in the forearms; tibia and fibula in the lower legs).
- There are *three bones in the transition between the limbs and the appendage* (i.e., the hindfoot in the ankle; one set of carpals in the wrists)
- The 3-bone segment is then followed directly by a row of *four distinct small bones* (the midfoot in the foot; and the second set of carpals in the wrists)
- Finally, there are several sets of *five small bones* in the far extremity of the limbs:
  o one row of five metatarsals in the toes and metacarpals in the fingers
  o two rows of five and one row of four phalanges in the fingers and toes

# Bones of the Legs, Ankles, and Feet

## *Bones of the Legs*

The legs are comprised of a structured arrangement of long bones that progress from the thigh to the ankle, transitioning from maximum strength and stability in the upper segments to greater mobility distally. The femur, or thigh bone, is the longest and strongest bone in the human body. It articulates proximally with the acetabulum of the pelvis and distally with the tibia at the knee joint. Notable landmarks of the femur include the head and neck (both deep and not externally palpable), greater trochanter (palpable on the lateral hip), lesser trochanter, and medial and lateral condyles, which contribute to the knee joint surfaces.

The patella that caps off the knee is a sesamoid bone embedded within the quadriceps tendon. It sits anterior to the femur and is not directly part of the femur or tibia. Although it does not articulate in the conventional sense, it tracks within the trochlear groove of the femur and serves to increase the mechanical efficiency of knee extension. As will be explored below, it is surrounded and stabilized by several ligaments and fascial layers. The patella protects the knee joint from the front – making kneeling tolerable. Additionally, it functions as a lever, augmenting the power of quadriceps muscle to support knee extension, especially when extra force is needed (e.g., when kicking something).

Below the knee, the leg contains *two bones*: the tibia and the fibula (see Figure 1.57). The tibia is the larger and more medial of the two and is the primary weight-bearing bone of the leg. It articulates with the femur at the knee and with the talus at the ankle. Prominent landmarks include the tibial tuberosity, medial and lateral tibial condyles, and the medial malleolus at the ankle. The fibula lies lateral to the tibia and is slender and non-weight-bearing. Its anatomical roles include muscle attachment and contribution to ankle stability. Key landmarks include the fibular head (below the lateral knee) and the lateral malleolus, which forms the prominent outer portion of the ankle.

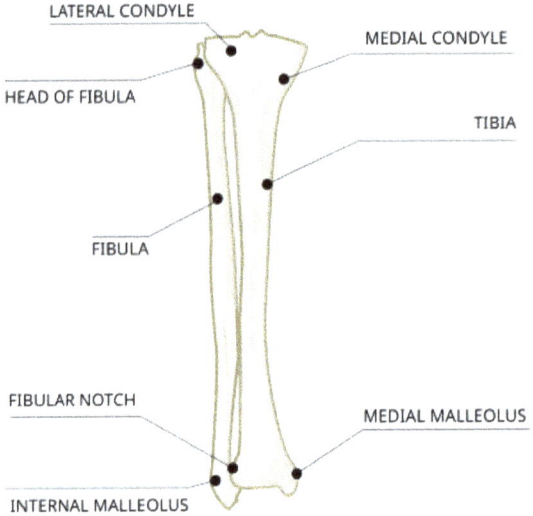

**Figure 1.57** Tibia and fibula. (Data source: OpenStax; https://commons.wikimedia.org/wiki/File:Tibia_fibula_svg_hariadhi.svg; Creative Commons Attribution 4.0)

## *Bones of the Ankles and Feet*

Each foot contains up to 26 bones (shown in Figure 1.58), organized into three primary regions: the hindfoot, midfoot, and forefoot. This complex bony architecture allows the foot to serve as both a strong base of support and a highly adaptable structure capable of nuanced movement.

The *hindfoot* consists of three bones and represents the transition from lower leg stability to foot mobility. The talus is a dome-shaped bone that articulates with the tibia and fibula above to form the ankle joint and with the calcaneus and navicular below. Uniquely, no muscles attach directly to the talus; it is stabilized by a robust capsule of ligaments and a surrounding cage of tendons. Inferior to the talus is the calcaneus, the largest bone in the foot, commonly referred to as the heel bone. Although it provides a base for the heel, it does not make direct contact with the ground due to a resilient fat pad and enclosing connective tissues. The navicular bone, located anterior to the talus, serves as a keystone between the hindfoot and midfoot. Its name reflects its boat-like shape.

The *midfoot* includes four bones: the cuboid laterally and the three cuneiforms medially, named medial (first), intermediate (second), and lateral (third) cuneiforms. These bones form the arching structure that connects the hindfoot to the forefoot and provide increasing mobility and flexibility, particularly in dynamic activities such as walking and balancing.

The *forefoot* contains several sets of five bones. The five metatarsals, numbered from medial to lateral (big toe to little toe), form the bridge between the tarsals and the toes. The second metatarsal is typically the longest and is aligned with the tibia, providing structural continuity sometimes referred to as the tibial array. The first and fifth metatarsals are commonly used as surface landmarks, and the navicular can be palpated approximately one inch in front of and below the medial ankle. A division exists between the third and fourth metatarsals, with the medial three contributing to the medial longitudinal arch and the lateral two to the lateral arch. Finally, the phalanges form the toes. There are 14 phalangeal bones in total: each toe contains three phalanges – proximal, middle, and distal – except for the hallux (big toe), which has only two. In some individuals, the fifth digit (little toe) may also lack a middle phalanx, a variation typically identified only through imaging. Together, these segments of the foot create an adaptable and layered support structure for the entire body.

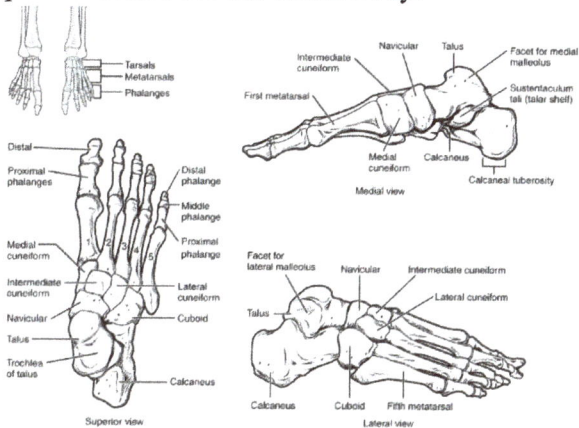

**Figure 1.58** Bones of the feet. (Data source: OpenStax; https://commons.wikimedia.org/wiki/File:812_Bones_of_the_Foot.jpg; Creative Commons Attribution 3.0)

# Joints and Ligaments of the Legs, Ankles, and Feet

## Knees

The knee joint (shown in Figure 1.59) is a complex synovial hinge joint that unites the distal femur with the proximal tibia. Although the fibula is part of the lower leg, it does not articulate at the knee and therefore is not considered part of this joint. Similarly, the patella does not articulate with the tibia and is not structurally part of the tibiofemoral joint, although it plays an essential role in the surrounding mechanism. The knee contains more cartilage than any other joint in the body, including two crescent-shaped menisci (medial and lateral) that deepen the joint surface, improve weight distribution, and contribute to joint stability. This cartilage is nourished primarily by synovial fluid, which is circulated through the joint capsule during movement, especially walking. The knee contains synovial recesses, or bursae, that receive this fluid during walking, which makes this basic activity essential for joint health. In contrast, running is typically too rapid and high-impact to effectively circulate synovial fluid, while passive techniques like leg-swinging with ankle weights can encourage fluid flow by temporarily distracting the joint surfaces.

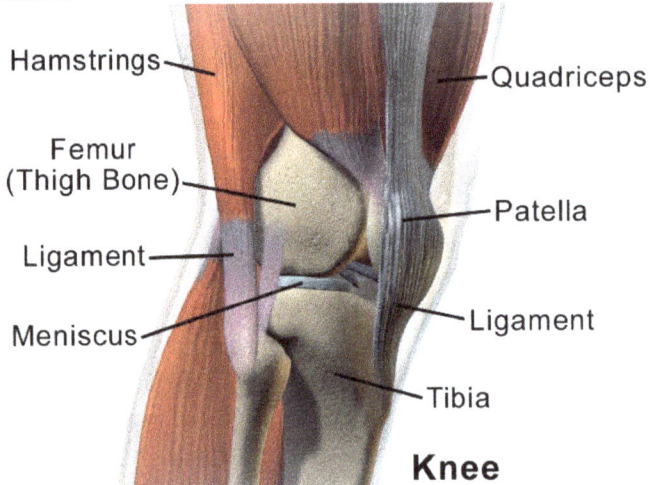

**Figure 1.59** Anatomy of the knee. (Data source: Medical gallery of Blausen Medical 2014, *WikiJournal of Medicine* 1 (2). DOI:10.15347/wjm/2014.010. ISSN 2002-4436; https://commons.wikimedia.org/wiki/File:Blausen_0597_KneeAnatomy_Side.png; Creative Commons Attribution 3.0)

### Ligaments of the Knee

The stability and function of the knee joint are reinforced by a network of ligaments and tendinous structures. The anterior cruciate ligament (ACL) and posterior cruciate ligament (PCL) cross inside the joint capsule, controlling anterior-posterior glide of the tibia relative to the femur and resisting rotational forces. The ACL prevents hyperextension in the knee joint; the PCL prevents anterior or posterior movement of the tibia or the femur at their articulation. On the outer surfaces, the medial collateral ligament (MCL) and lateral collateral ligament (LCL) stabilize the inner and outer aspects of the joint, protecting against valgus and varus forces respectively. The fibrocartilaginous menisci function as stabilizers, aiding in shock absorption and improving the congruence between femur and tibia. They are akin to the intervertebral discs in the spine in that they are like spacers, creating padding between the femur and tibia. The patellar tendon, technically a ligament, extends from the quadriceps tendon across the patella and attaches to the tibial tuberosity, acting as a key conduit for force transmission during knee extension. The patella itself, embedded within this tendinous structure, functions as a sesamoid bone, improving mechanical leverage for the quadriceps and ensuring smooth tracking over the femoral trochlear groove. It is noteworthy that knee injuries are more likely to result from repetitive stress (e.g., micro-misalignments during yoga), rather than from sudden movements (Lasater, 2020). Thus, any pain or discomfort in the knee joint during yoga *asana* deserves care and attention; pushing through knee pain is inauspicious. Given its great importance, a summary of the knee, adjoining bones, and supporting ligaments is offered in the table that follows.

| *Anatomy of the Knee Joint: Key Structures* | | |
|---|---|---|
| *Structure* | *Type* | *Function* |
| *Femur (distal end)* | • Long bone | • Articulates with tibia to form the knee joint |
| *Tibia (proximal end)* | • Long bone | • Main weight-bearing bone of the leg<br>• Articulates with femur at the knee joint |
| *Fibula* | • Long bone (not articular with knee) | • Does not participate in the knee joint<br>• Serves as attachment site for muscle and ligament |
| *Patella* | • Sesamoid bone | • Increases leverage of the quadriceps tendon to support knee extension<br>• Tracks within the femoral groove |
| *Medial and Lateral Menisci* | • Fibrocartilage | • Shock absorption and load distribution<br>• Joint congruency, and mobility support |
| *Anterior Cruciate Ligament* | • Intra-articular ligament | • Prevents anterior translation of the tibia<br>• Resists excessive rotation |
| *Posterior Cruciate Ligament* | • Intra-articular ligament | • Prevents posterior translation of the tibia |
| *Medial Collateral Ligament* | • Extra-articular ligament | • Stabilizes inner (medial) knee<br>• Resists valgus (inward) forces |
| *Lateral Collateral Ligament* | • Extra-articular ligament | • Stabilizes outer (lateral) knee<br>• Resists varus (outward) forces |
| *Patellar Tendon* | • Tendon (technically a ligament) | • Connects quadriceps tendon to tibia<br>• Enables knee extension |
| *Synovial Fluid and Recesses* | • Synovial structure | • Nourishes cartilage; fluid is circulated during walking and passive motion |

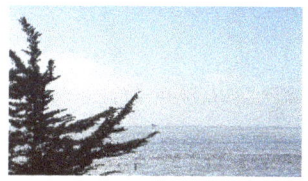

> *Knee Alignment Assessment*
>
> To assess the alignment in the knee, we can look for an isosceles triangle between lateral and medial superior edge of the patella to the tibial tuberosity
> - If there is no isosceles triangle (i.e., if one side of the triangle is longer than the other), the knee is rotated
> - If this is the case, do not parallel the feet or you will harm the knee:
> - That means for students with a rotated knee, the instruction is to face the knee caps straight forward (rather than cueing parallel feet), aligned with the hip joint
> - Make sure the knee hinge is aligned and not torqued (more about this in the kinesiology section below)

## *Ankles*

Although commonly referred to as a single structure, the ankle is composed of two distinct yet profoundly interrelated joints (Figure 1.60), each contributing to the complexity and mobility of the lower limb. The *tibiotalar joint* (also known as the upper ankle joint or *supratalar joint*) is formed by the distal ends of the tibia and fibula, which wrap around the dome of the talus. This joint primarily allows for dorsiflexion and plantarflexion and functions biomechanically like a hinge joint. Just beneath it lies the *subtalar joint* (or lower ankle joint), a more complex articulation involving the talus, calcaneus, and navicular bones. This joint allows for inversion (supination) and eversion (pronation) of the foot, enabling the foot to adapt to uneven surfaces and variable loads. Subtalar movement travels diagonally across the foot rather than straight through the second metatarsal line, and can be initiated either by movement of the leg over the foot or vice versa.

Although the tibiotalar and subtalar joints operate independently, they are contained within a shared ligamentous capsule, meaning that complex movements like ankle circling involve coordination of both joints. This shared capsule also explains why ankle sprains typically compromise multiple planes of motion, affecting both the hinge-like flexion and the side-to-side adaptability of the foot.

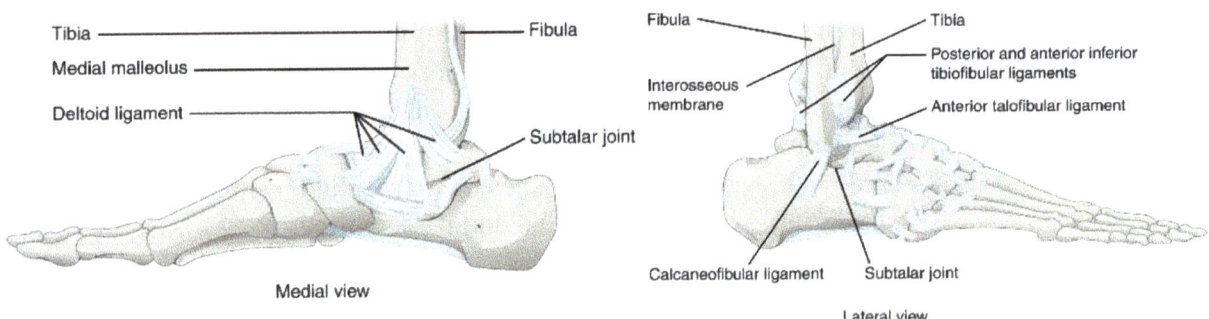

**Figure 1.60** Ankle and foot joints. (Data source: OpenStax; https://commons.wikimedia.org/wiki/File:919_Ankle_Feet_Joints.jpg; Creative Commons Attribution 3.0)

*Ligaments of the Ankles*

The ankle joints are stabilized by a dense and well-organized network of ligaments that balance mobility and injury prevention (Figure 1.61). On the medial (inner) side, the deltoid ligament, a strong fan-shaped structure, connects the tibia to the talus, navicular, and calcaneus, resisting excessive eversion. On the lateral side, a trio of ligaments, namely, the anterior talofibular ligament (ATFL), posterior talofibular ligament (PTFL), and calcaneofibular ligament (CFL), anchor the fibula to adjacent tarsal bones and primarily resist inversion. Notably, lateral ankle sprains are more common than medial ones. The interosseous membrane between the tibia and fibula, as well as the anterior and posterior tibiofibular ligaments, provide stability, especially during weight-bearing and dynamic movement. Together, these ligamentous structures protect against excessive translation and torsion across the ankle complex while permitting the flexibility necessary for grounded standing shapes and dynamic transitions in yoga *asana*. Given the complexity of the ankle region, a structural summary is provided in the table that follows.

| *Joints and Ligaments of the Ankle* | | | |
|---|---|---|---|
| *Structure* | *Anatomical Description* | *Function* | *Notes* |
| *Tibiotalar Joint* | Articulation of tibia and fibula (from above) with the talus | Allows dorsiflexion and plantarflexion (hinge-like motion) | Also called "supratalar joint" or "upper ankle joint" |
| *Subtalar Joint* | Articulation of talus with calcaneus and navicular | Allows inversion (supination) and eversion (pronation) | Motion runs diagonally through the foot; also called lower ankle joint |
| *Deltoid Ligament* | Medial side; tibia to talus, navicular, and calcaneus | Resists eversion | Very strong and broad; rarely injured |
| *Anterior Talofibular Ligament* | Lateral side; fibula to anterior talus | Resists anterior translation and inversion | Most commonly injured ligament in ankle sprains |
| *Posterior Talofibular Ligament* | Lateral side; fibula to posterior talus | Provides posterior ankle stability | Injured in more severe ankle sprains |
| *Calcaneofibular Ligament* | Lateral side; fibula to calcaneus | Resists inversion in a neutral or dorsiflexed position | Often injured along with the ATFL |
| *Anterior & Posterior Tibiofibular Ligaments* | Between distal tibia and fibula | Provide syndesmotic stability | Support the ankle mortise and are involved in high ankle sprains |

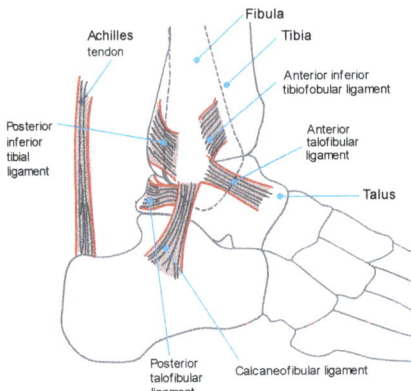

**Figure 1.61** Ligaments of ankle. (Data source: Jak; https://commons.wikimedia.org/wiki/File:Ankle_en.svg; public domain)

## Feet (Including Arches)

Each foot contains up to 33 joints, allowing for a remarkable combination of mobility, adaptability, and stability. The 14 interphalangeal joints, located between the phalanges of the toes, function primarily as hinge joints, designed for flexion and extension. These joints are considered prehensile, meaning they can grasp or grip objects to a degree, which is especially noticeable when walking barefoot or balancing on uneven surfaces. However, these joints do not allow for sideways movement.

At the junction of the toes and long bones of the foot lie five *metatarsophalangeal* (MTP) joints, commonly known as the balls of the feet. As a group, these joints function like a hinge, facilitating rolling through the foot during gait or transitions in yoga shapes. Uniquely, each individual MTP joint also allows for a small degree of axial rotation, enabling subtle torsional movements of the metatarsals around the phalanges. This makes the MTP joints especially relevant in standing balancing shapes, directional changes, and dynamic pivots on the foot. Unlike the gripping function of the toes, the MTP joints emphasize rotational control and weight transfer, enhancing balance and proprioception during yoga *asana*.

### Ligaments of the Feet

The structural integrity and functional precision of the foot are supported by a dense network of ligaments. These include the plantar ligaments, such as the long plantar ligament, short plantar ligament, and the plantar calcaneonavicular (or spring) ligament, which collectively stabilize the arches of the foot and provide passive tension to support load-bearing. Around the MTP and interphalangeal joints, collateral ligaments prevent side-to-side movement and reinforce joint alignment during motion. The deep transverse metatarsal ligament connects the heads of the metatarsals, stabilizing the forefoot and maintaining spacing between the toes. These ligamentous structures, along with a web of supportive fascia, ensure the coordinated interplay between rigidity and flexibility that defines healthy foot mechanics – an essential foundation for balance, strength, and mobility in daily life and yoga *asana*. The following table summarizes the joints and ligaments of the feet.

| Joints and Ligaments of the Foot | | |
|---|---|---|
| Structure | Type / Location | Function / Relevance |
| Interphalangeal Joints | Between phalanges (two per toe, except big toe with one) | Prehensile hinge joints; allow flexion/extension (gripping) but no side-to-side motion |
| Metatarsophalangeal (MTP) Joints | Between distal metatarsals and proximal phalanges (five per foot) | Function as a collective hinge; individual joints also allow axial rotation; critical for weight transfer and pivoting |
| Tarsometatarsal Joints | Between distal tarsals and bases of metatarsals | Support transverse arch; provide stability during gait and weight-bearing |
| Intertarsal Joints | Between tarsal bones (navicular, cuboid, cuneiforms, etc.) | Allow slight gliding motions; facilitate midfoot adaptability and shock absorption |
| Long Plantar Ligament | From calcaneus to cuboid and metatarsals | Supports the longitudinal arch; stabilizes lateral foot |
| Short Plantar Ligament | Deep to long plantar ligament (calcaneus to cuboid) | Stabilizes the calcaneocuboid joint and lateral arch |
| Spring or Plantar Calcaneonavicular Ligament | From sustentaculum tali of calcaneus to navicular | Supports head of talus; crucial to medial longitudinal arch; contributes to foot recoil |
| Collateral Ligaments | Flank MTP and interphalangeal joints | Prevent excessive side-to-side motion; stabilize toe alignment |
| Deep Transverse Metatarsal Ligament | Connects heads of all five metatarsals | Maintains metatarsal spacing and forefoot integrity |

*Arches of the Foot*

The arches of the feet form an intricate system of load-bearing and shock-absorbing structures that support locomotion, balance, and adaptation to uneven terrain. These arches are not static architectural features but living, dynamic systems sustained by muscles, tendons, ligaments, and the shape of the bones themselves.

Muscles of the lower leg (particularly the calf muscles) connect via tendons into the feet, where they integrate with intrinsic foot musculature and connective tissue to help maintain the shape and responsiveness of the arches. Strength and adaptability of the arches are closely tied to the health of the calves, which can be improved through practices that lengthen, load, and strengthen the posterior chain (e.g., hiking uphill, calf raises through full range of motion). Arch integrity also depends on stimulation through weight-bearing and barefoot movement. Overly supportive footwear, while sometimes medically necessary, can diminish intrinsic muscular engagement and lead to weakened or collapsed arches over time.

Each foot has four distinct arches, each contributing to a multidirectional support system:
- *Lateral Longitudinal Arch*: This arch acts as a lateral stabilizer, like the outrigger on a canoe. Formed by the calcaneus, cuboid, and 4th and 5th metatarsals, this arch is strong and rarely collapses. It receives influence from the fibula and is sometimes called the *heel foot* among movement therapists.
- *Medial Longitudinal Arch*: This arch functions as the primary shock absorber and propulsive structure in the foot. It includes the talus, navicular, cuneiform bones, and the 1st to 3rd metatarsals, and aligns with the tibia. This arch is more flexible and prone to collapse, a functional adaptation that allows the arch to absorb weight and then rebound during the gait cycle. When the lateral and medial arches are placed together side-by-side, they form a full dome.
- *Proximal Transverse Arch*: This arch spans the instep across the cuboid and cuneiform bones at the midfoot. It bears considerable weight and gains structural strength from the wedge-shaped bones that are narrower underneath and wider on top to create an exquisitely sculpted, nearly indestructible arch that contains small gliding joints that enhance mobility.
- *Distal Transverse Arch*: Also called the metatarsal arch, this arch spans the heads of the metatarsals at the balls of the feet. Ideally, only the 1st and 5th metatarsal heads contact the ground, allowing the central three to float in an arch formation. However, in many people this arch is underdeveloped, often due to weakness in the adductor hallucis muscle. Exercises such as marble pickups and towel-scrunching can strengthen the intrinsic muscles that support this arch.

### ASSESSMENT 1 – *Medial Arch Resonance*

Feel for resonance in the medial arch; tester places hands under testee's arches; testee crosses the arms and then rotates the spine side to side to simulate walking motion; tester should feel the collapse of the arch and then the rebound with each "step"; it does not matter if these arches are high or low; what matters is whether they are responsive or not (i.e., collapse and come back).

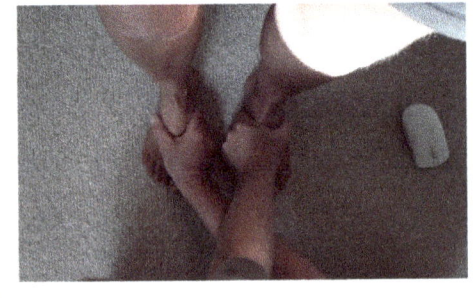

### ASSESSMENT 2 – *Distal Transverse Arch*

You can tell whether you have this arch by whether you have calluses under all balls of the toes or only where you should have them, under the 1st and 5th balls of the toes (i.e., under the *metatarsophalangeal joints*).

*Maintaining Health in the Feet And Arches*

The four arches of each foot work in concert to create spring, distribute load, and adapt dynamically with every single step. Their health is key to foot integrity, efficient movement, and overall kinetic chain function. To maintain their health, the following information may prove helpful. There are approximately 7,000 nerve endings in each foot – more nerve endings per square inch than in any other body part. This plethora of innervation is because feet need to translate the characteristics of the ground we walk into sensory signals to our nervous system which, in turn, sends motor signals that help with adapting foot movements to the surface on which we stand, walk, or run. It is important not to disrupt this feedback loop via thick-soled shoes. Myers (in workshop environments) called shoes sensory deprivation chambers or coffins for the feet. They deprive the feet of having to adapt to a variety of surfaces and to take on a variety of shapes. High arch support in shoes can interfere with proper pronation while walking: the medial arch cannot collapse and rebound which slowly extinguishes the responsiveness of the medial arch. Arch support is useful only when we have to stand for a long time (e.g., jobs like cashiers). Shoes with high arches may make little sense for running or walking.

To improve proprioception, stimulate nerve endings, and enhance reflexes (and improve low back pain, which is often linked to foot problems):
- Walk barefoot as often as possible and/or wear (transition to) barefoot shoes
- Engage in ball rolling of the plantar facia or marble clasping with the toes to make up for deprivation and bring health back into the feet

More fancy footwork options are offered in Section 2.

## Muscles of the Lower Legs, Ankles, and Feet

Several groups of muscles can be found in the lower legs, acting on the knee joints, ankles, and feet. Some muscles act on both joints; others act on a single joint.

### Muscles Acting on the Knee and Ankle

Several muscles in the posterior lower leg cross both the knee and ankle joints, enabling them to support locomotion by coordinating flexion of the knee and plantarflexion of the ankle. These muscles (see Figure 1.62 and 1.63) play important roles in walking, jumping, and posture, contributing to both movement and stabilization.

- *Gastrocnemius (medial and lateral heads)*: The gastrocnemius is the most superficial calf muscle and spans two joints. Its medial head originates from the medial condyle of the femur, while the lateral head originates from the lateral condyle of the femur. Both insert via the Achilles tendon into the posterior surface of the calcaneus. The gastrocnemius flexes the knee, plantarflexes the ankle, and contributes to supination of the foot. It plays a crucial role in raising the heel during walking and is one of the few muscles that act on both the knee and ankle joints.
- *Plantaris*: A small, vestigial muscle, the plantaris originates on the posterior femur above the lateral condyle and inserts on the calcaneus alongside the Achilles tendon. Though weak, it assists in knee flexion and ankle plantarflexion. Present in only 90% of people, it is considered a remnant of a more powerful ancestral muscle involved in plantarflexion.
- *Popliteus*: This deep posterior knee muscle originates on the lateral femoral condyle and inserts on the posterior surface of the proximal tibia. It does not act on the ankle. The popliteus weakly flexes the knee and medially rotates the tibia, especially to unlock the extended knee at the beginning of flexion. It also resists hyperextension of the knee and contributes to postural stability during standing.

## Muscles Acting Primarily on the Ankle

These muscles do not act on the knee but are essential for ankle motion and foot stability. Their coordinated actions support upright posture, balance on uneven surfaces, and dynamic propulsion.

- *Soleus*: Located deep to the gastrocnemius, the soleus originates from the posterior surfaces of the tibia and fibula and inserts into the calcaneus via the Achilles tendon. It does not cross the knee joint and therefore has no action at the knee. It plantarflexes the ankle and plays a major role in maintaining posture and returning venous blood to the heart, earning it the nickname second heart. Its tendon merges with that of the gastrocnemius and contributes to the structural support of the underside of the foot.
- *Peroneus Longus and Peroneus Brevis*: The peroneals form the lateral compartment of the lower leg. The peroneus longus originates from the head and proximal fibula, while the peroneus brevis originates from the distal fibula. Both muscles pass behind the lateral malleolus and insert onto the foot—longus on the base of the first metatarsal and medial cuneiform, brevis on the base of the fifth metatarsal. Together, they assist in plantarflexion and eversion of the foot. The peroneals stabilize the ankle on uneven terrain and contribute to the lateral arch. Working with the tibialis anterior, the peroneus longus forms part of a deep tendon sling (Steigbuegel) under the foot, helping to support all three major foot arches.

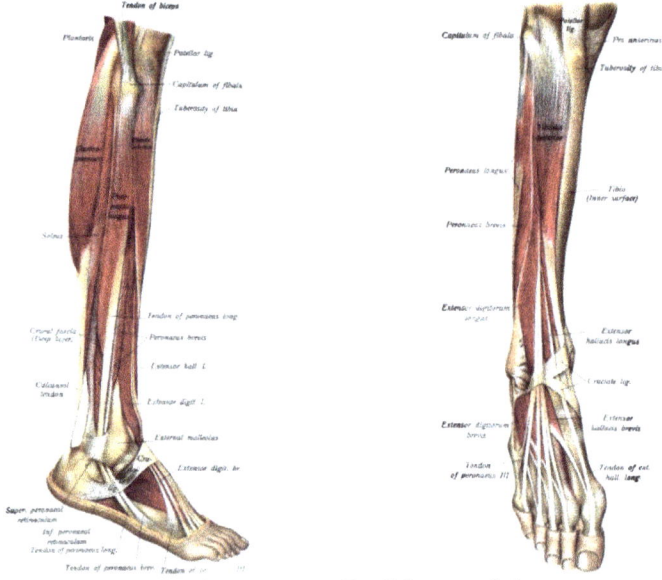

**Figure 1.62** Lateral view of the calf muscles (Data source: Dr. Johannes Sobotta; https://commons.wikimedia.org/wiki/File:Sobo_1909_307.png; public domain)

**Figure 1.63** Anterior view of the lower leg muscles (Data source: Dr. Johannes Sobotta; https://commons.wikimedia.org/wiki/File:Sobo_1909_306.png; public domain)

## Muscles Acting on the Ankle and Feet

The ankles and feet are controlled by both anterior and posterior muscle groups that enable dorsiflexion, plantarflexion, inversion, eversion, and toe movement. These muscles play key roles in both dynamic propulsion (e.g., walking and running) and maintaining postural stability, especially through the arches of the feet.

*Anterior Compartment: Dorsiflexors and Extensors*

Three muscles lie in the anterior compartment of the lower leg and are primarily responsible for dorsiflexion of the ankle. They are tibialis anterior, extensor hallucis longus, and extensor digitorum longus. Their tendons are held close to the ankle by a fascial strap called the extensor retinaculum, which acts like a pulley to prevent bowstringing during motion.

- *Tibialis anterior* originates on the lateral surface of the tibia and inserts on the medial cuneiform and base of the first metatarsal. It dorsiflexes the ankle and inverts the foot, helping lift the medial arch during gait.
- *Extensor hallucis longus* extends the big toe and assists in dorsiflexion and foot inversion.
- *Extensor digitorum longus* extends toes 2 through 5 and supports dorsiflexion.

*Posterior Compartment: Flexors and Propulsive Muscles*

These deep muscles lie in the posterior compartment of the leg and are involved in plantarflexion, inversion (supination), and toe flexion. They include tibialis posterior, flexor hallucis longus, and flexor digitorum longus. These muscles also contribute to the backline tension of the body and can restrict ankle mobility when overly tight. They are often overlooked in assessments of posterior chain flexibility and lower limb range of motion.

- *Tibialis posterior* originates on the posterior tibia and fibula and inserts broadly across the tarsal and metatarsal bones. It supports the medial arch and helps invert the foot.
- *Flexor hallucis longus* flexes the big toe and contributes significantly to propulsion during walking.
- *Flexor digitorum longus* flexes toes 2 through 5 and works with the tibialis posterior to maintain the medial longitudinal arch during push-off in gait.

## Intrinsic Muscles of the Foot

In addition to the extrinsic muscles acting on the ankle and toes, the intrinsic muscles of the foot originate and insert entirely within the foot. These intrinsic muscles originate and insert within the foot itself (unlike the extrinsic muscles which originate in the leg). They play essential roles in fine motor control, arch support, balance, and adaptability of the foot. Though small, these muscles are essential for refined balance, posture, and maintaining dynamic arch support. Many of them act in concert with the extrinsic muscles to create a responsive and adaptable base for locomotion and standing. Some intrinsic muscles lie on the dorsal (top) surface of the foot and assist in toe extension, while others are located on the plantar (bottom) surface and assist in toe flexion, abduction, and arch stabilization. Although many are rarely activated in modern shoe-dependent life, they can be reawakened through barefoot movement, yoga *asana*, and exercises like towel-scrunching and marble-picking.

Since there are many of these small muscles, a summary table is offered instead of narrative descriptions (also see Figure 1.64 below the table). For a great video about feet, check out the following YouTube video with Jim Dooner: https://youtu.be/wvIKHDiO-H0?si=4iTSLkfsGiakYjXK

| Selected Intrinsic Foot Muscles | | | |
|---|---|---|---|
| *Muscle* | *Location* | *Primary Action* | *Additional Notes* |
| *Extensor digitorum brevis* | Dorsal foot | Extends toes 2–4 | Assists with toe lift during gait |
| *Flexor digitorum brevis* | Plantar foot | Flexes toes 2–5 | Supports medial longitudinal arch |
| *Abductor hallucis* | Medial sole | Abducts and flexes big toe | Supports medial arch; commonly underused |
| *Abductor digiti minimi* | Lateral sole | Abducts and flexes 5th toe | Stabilizes lateral edge of foot |
| *Adductor hallucis* | Deep plantar foot | Adducts big toe toward midline | Crucial for distal transverse arch support |
| *Quadratus plantae* | Deep plantar foot | Adjusts pull of flexor digitorum longus | Helps direct toe flexion in line |
| *Lumbricals and interossei* | Between/toes | Fine toe control and arch support | Important for balance and proprioception |

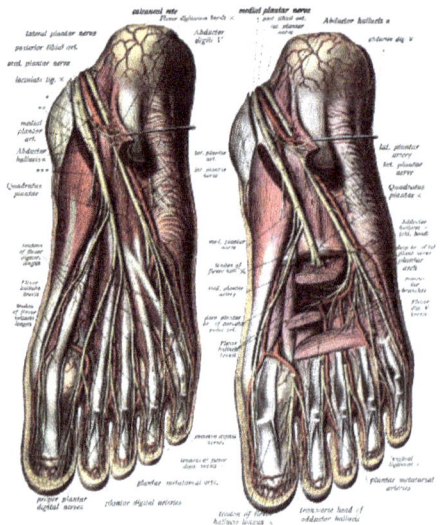

Figure 1.64 Foot muscles. (Data source https://commons.wikimedia.org/wiki/File:Sobo_1909_585-586.png; public domain)

## Kinesiology of the Knee, Ankle, and Feet

### Understanding Movement in the Knee

#### Anatomical Function and Joint Mechanics

The knee is a modified hinge joint located where the femur meets the tibia. As a hinge joint in the sagittal plane, it functions primarily in flexion and extension. Knee flexion is supported by the hamstrings, gastrocnemius, and other posterior muscles; extension is powered primarily by the quadriceps. Examples of these knee movements in yoga *asana* are transitions such as moving from Downward Facing Dog (both knees extended) to Low Lunge (forward knee moving into flexion), Child (which requires full knee flexion), or Triangle (which requires knee extension).

The knee is a joint between two joints: specifically, it transfers load and movement between the hip above and the ankle below. This intermediary role makes it particularly vulnerable to stress or strain when either of the adjacent joints lacks mobility or stability or presents with pathology. For example, when range of motion in the hip joint is restricted (e.g., limited external rotation or abduction), the knee may be forced to rotate or torque to compensate, even though it has limited rotational capacity. The knee also functions as a responsive stabilizer during movements and in various postural alignments. The menisci and ligaments contribute both mobility and stability, facilitating movement while protecting against excessive shearing or rotation. This role becomes especially important in yoga *asana*, particularly during standing shapes (e.g., Warriors) and sequences requiring knee flexion under load.

Notably, the knee joint also can move into a small degree of axial (internal and external) rotation of the tibia relative to the femur, a very limited range of about 10-15 degrees. The direction of the rotation depends on whether the knee is moved while the foot is fixed on the ground (creating a closed chain) or floating in the air (i.e., in an open chain such as while lying on the back with the leg in the air). In a closed chain (e.g., during walking or in yoga during a Warrior), flexion (i.e., the front leg in Warrior) creates external rotation and extension creates internal rotation (i.e., the back leg in Warrior). The combination of flexion and rotation is essential to facilitating movements such as walking, squatting, and rising. However, its healthy range is easily exceeded if torque is created because of limitations in range of motion in the ankle or hip joints. This reality introduces potential vulnerability to injury if the minimal rotational range of motion in the knee is abused and the knee is subjected to torquing forces that it is not built to withstand. For example, if the hip joint is restricted or the foot is fixed, the rotational capacity may be exceeded, straining the cruciate ligaments or compressing the menisci. Stabilization of the knee in healthful alignment is essential to yoga shapes that involve flexion with weight-bearing, a common occurrence. In that position, the congruence between the tibia and femur is lessened, making the knee more vulnerable – hence the great care we need to take as yoga professionals to understand how to align the knee in standing shapes involving a flexed knee, a reality that is explored in detail in Chapter 8 on Standing Shapes.

*Functional Role and Yoga Asana Relevance*

*Torque and Compensation in the Knee Joint*

The knee's position between the ankle and hip makes it susceptible to torque when those joints are limited in range or control. It is important not to cue in a manner that overrides healthy knee mechanics because of a desired outer shape or alignment. Instead, it is important to invite students to remain mindful of allowing the knee to track over the center of the ankle, allowing the kneecap to follow its natural path, which may be slightly medial for many bodies. Such careful tracking of the knee protects the collateral ligaments and encourages proper patellar tracking. It is important to avoid universal cues such as *'line up the foot with the side of the mat'* as this may misalign the knee depending on the individual's unique hip anatomy and femoral rotation.

For example, in Warrior 1, the unfortunate cueing of foot placement as parallel to the back of the mat (or even slightly angled forward but with the full foot planted) will likely exceed the natural range of motion in the back hip for most human beings. Most students who force this foot alignment unknowingly twist the front knee as they square the pelvis toward the front of the mat. This rotational compensation in the knee for unnatural and impossible range of motion in the hip joint stresses the ligaments of the knee. Similarly, attempting to square the hips to the side of the mat in Warrior 2 exceeds natural hip range for the majority of human beings (unless they are hypermobile) and results in inward buckling or torque at the front knee. Thus, in yoga *asana* it is helpful to invite students to allow the kneecap to point in its natural direction rather than attempting to force an outer alignment, shape, or placement of body parts on the mat. For almost all students, Warrior 2 requires a diagonal placement of the pelvis to prevent torque in the knees or excessive femoral leverage at the sacroiliac joints (Farhi & Stuart, 2017). In seated shapes, especially shapes such as Lotus or Half Lotus, it is essential to avoid sickling of the ankle as this greatly stresses the ligaments in the knee, especially putting excess pressure on the medial knee (Lasater, 2020). In seated Hero, the knee may be torqued as the vector of the lower leg is outward to the lateral sides of the pelvis. In this case, creating movement in the hip joint that rotates the head of the femur internally can prevent excessive strain on the knee (Clark, 2016). Alignment always need to prioritize functional joint health over arbitrary visual lines on the mat.

### *Valgus and Varus Stress in the Knee*

Valgus refers to inward collapse of the knees (colloquially called being knock-kneed), often seen when the knees buckle toward each other in weight-bearing shapes. This is a common pattern in Warrior 2, Chair, or squats. Valgus strain can overstretch the medial collateral ligaments (MCL) and compress the lateral joint space. Using a looped strap around the thighs, just above the knees, and asking students to press gently into it can activate the external hip rotators and strengthen the stabilizers of the knee. Varus, or outward drifting of the knees (colloquially called being bow-legged) is less common but can emerge in yoga contexts. When the knees drift outward excessively (e.g., in Mountain, Chair, or Lunge), placing a block between the knees and cueing a gentle squeeze will engages the adductors and bring better balance to the knee joint.

### *Supportive Use of Props for Knee Health*

The anterior portion of the knee contains minimal soft tissue and pressure during kneeling on the floor can irritate the bursa or press directly against bone. Thus, not surprisingly, kneeling may be painful for individuals with patellar tracking issues, bursitis, or a history of meniscal injury. Using a blanket, doubled-up mat, or cushion under the knee helps reduce compressive load and supports better alignment. In deep knee flexion (e.g., Hero or Child), a block or bolster under the hips can reduce strain on the knee joint and lessen the required internal rotation at the hip. In Easy Seat, it may be necessary to prop both an elevation of the pelvis and to provide a lift under the thighs if they are floating.

Yoga teaching embraces biomechanical individuality. Each student's alignment needs to reflect their skeletal structure and range of motion, especially at complex hinge joints like the knee. Healthy knees are not guaranteed by visual symmetry but by joint-friendly, patient-tailored biomechanics.

## Understanding Movement in the Ankle

### Anatomical Function and Joint Mechanics

The ankle complex is composed of two distinct but interconnected joints: the tibiotalar (or talocrural) joint and the subtalar joint. The tibiotalar joint, formed by the tibia and fibula gripping the talus from above, functions primarily as a hinge joint that allows dorsiflexion (toes moving toward the shin) and plantarflexion (pointing the foot downward). This movement is crucial in yoga transitions such as stepping forward from Downward Facing Dog (dorsiflexion of the front ankle) or rising to tiptoes in Chair (plantarflexion). Below this joint lies the subtalar joint, connecting the talus with the calcaneus and navicular bones. The subtalar enables inversion (turning the sole inward) and eversion (turning the sole outward), movements that are essential for balance on uneven terrain and controlled transitions on and off the mat. This joint's axis runs obliquely through the foot, which means that inversion and eversion do not occur in a straight line but rather in a diagonal pathway through the foot and lower leg.

Although often thought of as a single joint, the ankle's full range of motion, such as circling or rolling the ankle, is a result of combined movement from both the tibiotalar and subtalar joints. Because these two joints share a common ligamentous capsule, ankle injuries (such as sprains) frequently affect both hinge-like and side-to-side movement patterns.

### Functional Role and Yoga Asana Relevance

Just like the knee, the ankle sits between two influential joints: the foot and the knee. Limited dorsiflexion (whether due to tight calves, stiff talocrural joint, or habitual shoe use) can create compensatory patterns further up the chain. For instance, when the ankle cannot dorsiflex sufficiently in squats or Lunges, the heel may lift or the knee may collapse inward (valgus), stressing the medial knee and arch of the foot. In standing balancing shapes, weak or uncoordinated ankle musculature can cause wobbling or arch collapse.

The ankle functions as both a mobile lever and a stabilizer in yoga *asana*. In weight-bearing shapes such as Warrior or Chair, the ankle must support and adjust to subtle shifts in balance. In transitions like stepping from Down Dog to Lunge, the ankle helps absorb force and initiate forward propulsion. These tasks demand strength and mobility, particularly in the calves, peroneals, and anterior compartment muscles (like tibialis anterior).

### Support and Cueing Considerations

When cueing ankle position in yoga *asana*, it is prudent to avoid demanding *extreme* dorsiflexion (such as passively *forcing* the front knee far past the ankle in Lunges) or plantarflexion (such as extreme pointing in seated or prone shapes) without adequate muscular support. Invite students to work within their natural and active range of motion and with interoceptive and proprioceptive awareness, especially when transitioning between weight-bearing shapes. For students with a history of ankle instability, cueing to press down through the base of the big toe and the outer heel can help activate intrinsic foot and lower leg muscles that stabilize the ankle. Props such as wedges under the heel in squats and Downward Facing Dog can support students with limited dorsiflexion and reduce compensatory strain in the knees or spine. Similarly, strengthening barefoot practices and targeted balance work can restore proprioception and neuromuscular control around the complex ankle joint.

## Understanding Movement in the Foot

### Anatomical Function and Joint Mechanics

The feet serve as the primary interface between the body and the ground, adapting to both static and dynamic conditions. Structurally, feet are organized into three main regions: the hindfoot (talus and calcaneus), the midfoot (navicular, cuboid, and cuneiforms), and the forefoot (metatarsals and phalanges). The foot's stability and shock-absorbing capacity are supported by four primary arches (not three as commonly taught):
- *Medial longitudinal arch* – from the heel to the head of the first metatarsal
- *Lateral longitudinal arch* – from the heel to the head of the fifth metatarsal
- *Transverse arch* – across the forefoot at the level of the metatarsal heads
- *Proximal transverse arch* (also called the tarsal arch) – deep in the midfoot, near the cuneiforms and cuboid

These arches distribute load, store and release elastic energy, and enable foot adaptability across various surfaces. They are maintained by passive structures (such as ligaments and fascia) and active muscular support, particularly from the intrinsic foot muscles and deep lower leg muscles like the tibialis posterior and peroneals. The foot's joint mechanics are multidirectional, allowing for subtle adaptability that is critical in balance and weight distribution. The subtalar joint enables inversion and eversion, while the metatarsophalangeal (MTP) joints allow for toe extension and flexion, key movements in walking and in yoga shapes such as Tree or Warrior 3.

### Functional Role and Yoga Asana Relevance

The feet act as a foundation *and* a sensory platform. Their function deeply influences the biomechanics of the knees, hips, and spine. In yoga practice, particularly in weight-bearing standing shapes, alignment and engagement of the feet can either support integrated kinetic chain functioning or contribute to collapse and strain elsewhere in the body. For example, if arches collapse, especially the medial longitudinal arch, this can lead to internal tibial rotation, contributing to valgus collapse at the knee and medial ankle strain. Conversely, excessive supination or rigid arch lifting can limit shock absorption and challenge balance. Both underuse and overuse of the arches can lead to joint misalignments upstream.

Cueing the corners of feet is an accessible way to invite active arch support. Notably, some students experience four corners of the feet (distribution of weight through the base of the big toe and the base of the little toes and the inner and outer heel), whereas others sense three (even weight through the base of the big toe, the base of the little toe, and the center of the heel). Additionally, awareness of the corners of the feet can be integrated with awareness of the deeper structure of the four arches of the feet. For instance, lifting through the inner ankle can support the medial arch, while gently drawing the heads of the metatarsals toward one another can support the transverse and proximal transverse arches.

## Working with the Arches of the Feet

Effective support of the arches requires activation of intrinsic foot muscles, that is the muscles that originate and insert entirely within the foot, including flexor hallucis brevis, abductor hallucis, flexor digitorum brevis, and lumbricals and interossei. These muscles contribute to fine motor control, arch stability, and proprioception. Chronic shoe use, especially in stiff or (excessively) supportive footwear with high arch supports, can lead to deactivation of these muscles and increased dependence on extrinsic stabilizers (from the calf and shin).

To help reawaken and retrain the foot in yoga practice, yoga teachers or clinicians can cue intrinsic muscular control with suggestions such as the following:
- *Spread the toes wide, then press down gently through the balls of the toes to lift the arch.*
- *Draw the ball of the big toe and ball of the little toe toward one another to activate the transverse arch.*
- *Lift the inner ankle, but keep the big toe rooted, feel the inside of your foot 'hug' inward.*
- *In balance shapes, imagine suctioning the center of your foot up and in, like lifting a jellybean with the arch.*

Simple barefoot movements like rolling onto the balls of the feet, dome lifts, or holding standing shapes on a folded mat or balance pad can help restore intrinsic muscle strength and arch awareness. Using the toes to grip a strap other resistance band can bring strength and mobility. Squats and Toe Pose can help release plantar fascia; toe mobility can be trained and, while doing so, a folded blanket under the ankles or wedges under the toes may be helpful if there is severe stiffness or foot pain.

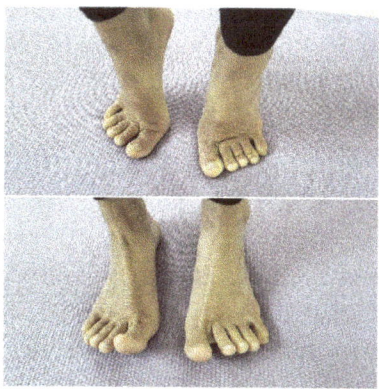
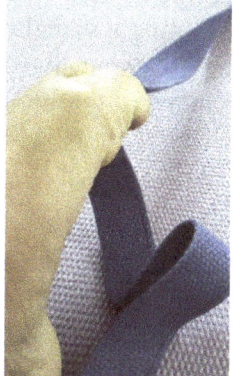

## Props and Adaptations for Foot Comfort

For students with foot discomfort, it is important to remember that certain structures (e.g., plantar fascia, sesamoid bones, or metatarsal heads) may be irritated by direct pressure. Props can be helpful in these cases. For example:
- A rolled blanket or a mat under the arches can enhance awareness and provide helpful tactile feedback.
- Blocks under the hands in forward folds can help offload sensitive feet – if just for a moment.
- A blanket or wedge under the heels during squatting can help individuals with limited ankle dorsiflexion or stiff plantar fascia feel more secure and supported – with less pain and strain.

- Toe separators or massage balls can be used to enhance proprioception and mobility over time.
- Massaging the bottoms of feet before and after standing shapes can be soothing and therapeutic.

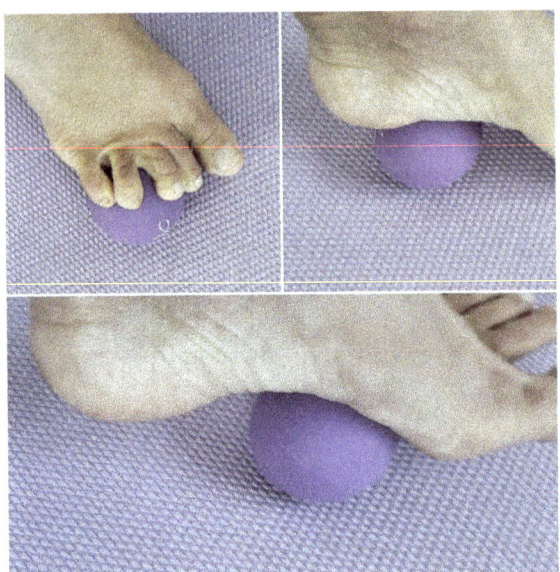
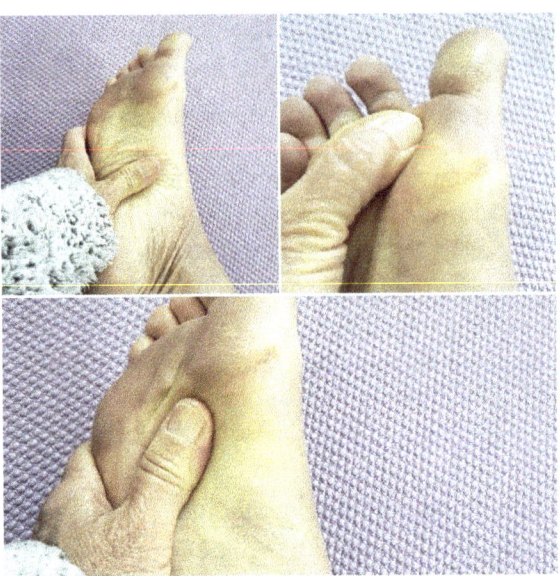

There is wide variability in foot structure due to skeletal shape, connective tissue tone, and training history. Not all humans can achieve high arches or even toe spreading. The goal is not uniformity, but responsiveness and stability. Yoga *asana* encourages students to explore what grounding and lift feel like in their own feet, and to use the feet as sensory organs for alignment feedback rather than meeting a visual or external standards. When feet are strong, sensitively engaged, and dynamically responsive, yoga *asana* practice and life off the mat become more integrated and sustainable, one grounded step at a time.

## What's Ahead

Having explored the lower appendicular region of the human body in some detail, it is now time to turn to the upper appendicular region. The discussion starts with the structures of the shoulder girdles and arms. It concludes with a detailed exploration of the kinesiology of this region of the body, focusing on understanding movement primarily in the shoulder girdle, but also in the wrists and hands. Applications to yoga are elucidated and then further addressed in the context of individual yoga *asana* practices in Section 2.

# Chapter 6: Anatomy of Upper Appendicular Region

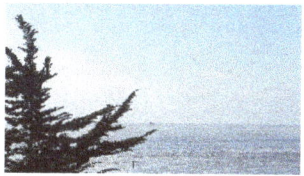

This chapter explores the anatomy of the upper appendicular region of the body, from the pectoral girdle and upper arms to the lower arms, wrists, and hands. For each section in that body region, the chapter offers information about key structures, including bones, joints, muscles, and movement patterns. It does so sequentially and assumes the reader's understanding (that was hopefully created in prior chapters) that these structures are, of course, completely interdependent, co-regulated, and connected. They never work in isolation of one another, nor of any other body region and *koshas*. The sequential approach is chosen for ease of communication.

## Pectoral Girdle and Upper Arms

The pectoral girdle, composed of the scapulae, clavicles, and arms, connects the upper limbs to the axial skeleton and provides a dynamic base for shoulder movement. In yoga *asana*, its mobility and stability are essential for effective weight-bearing, breath support, and upper body integration. The position and function of the scapulae influence spinal posture, cervical tension, and access to the full range of motion in the arms, making this region central to strength-based and restorative practices. The upper arms link the shoulders to the elbow and play a key role in positioning and mobilizing the hands. In yoga teaching and therapeutics, their function is closely tied to scapular stability, core support, and coordinated engagement of the entire shoulder complex. Balanced tone in the upper arms supports sustainable weight-bearing in postures such as Downward Facing Dog or Plank, while excessive tension or instability may signal compensatory patterns that benefit from refined alignment and muscular re-education.

## Bones of the Pectoral Girdle and Upper Arms

The pectoral gridle (commonly known as the shoulder girdle; Figure 1.65) consists of the two scapulae on the back body, two upper arms, and two clavicles at the apex of the chest. Unlike the pelvic girdle, the pectoral girdle is built for mobility, much more so than stability. The arms can move completely independently of one another. This is very unlike the legs, which are so connected as to affect each other noticeably when one leg moves. It is easy to try this in one's own body. If we move one leg and then pay attention to what happens in the pelvic girdle, we will note significant movement in the other leg. On the other hand, if we move one arm and pay attention to what happens in the shoulder girdle and the other arm, we may note that the other arm does not have to move at all. The connection between the two sides of the shoulder girdle is highly mobile and not constricted by a highly stable structure. In the pelvic girdle, on the other hand, the strong and integrated structure of the pelvis relays movement from one side of the lower body to the other, reverberating any movement throughout the entire structure.

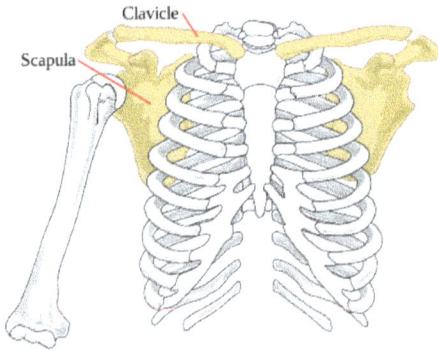

**Figure 1.65** Pectoral girdle. (Data source: LadyofHats; https://commons.wikimedia.org/wiki/File:Pectoral_girdle_front_diagram.svg; public domain)

## *Scapulae*

The scapulae, or shoulder blades, play a central role in stabilizing and coordinating movement in the shoulder complex. Although located on the posterior thorax, each scapula curves around the body to connect functionally to the upper arm. Its lateral edge forms the glenoid fossa, a shallow, anteverted socket that receives the head of the humerus. This glenohumeral joint allows great freedom of movement but depends heavily on muscular support for stability, as the bony congruence between the humeral head and glenoid is minimal – more like a plate than a cup. Several key landmarks on the scapula support the intricate muscular architecture of the shoulder girdle. The vertebral (or medial) border of the scapula should ideally lie parallel to the spine, approximately two inches away, but often it does not. Many individuals display a laterally displaced inferior angle compared to the superior angle, often due to imbalanced tone in the surrounding musculature. These inner angles frame the vertebral border and are useful landmarks for palpation. Just above the superior angle lies the levator scapulae, a muscle that often becomes tender or tight, especially in individuals with forward head posture or elevated shoulders.

One of the most prominent and palpable features of the scapula is the spine of the scapula (Figure 1.66), a thick, horizontal ridge that runs across its upper posterior surface. It divides the posterior scapula into the supraspinous and infraspinous fossae and serves as a major attachment point for the trapezius and deltoid muscles. At its lateral end, the spine broadens into the acromion process, the tip of the shoulder and a key point of articulation with the clavicle. The acromion provides the attachment site for the middle fibers of the deltoid, supporting both abduction and stabilization of the upper arm.

On the anterior aspect of the scapula, just beneath the clavicle and above the axilla, is the coracoid process, a small, hook-shaped projection often described as resembling a crow's beak (from the German *Rabenschnabel*). This bony point is a major muscular anchor, particularly for the coracobrachialis, short head of the biceps brachii, and pectoralis minor, all of which contribute to stability and control in movements of the arm and shoulder. Next, the inferior angle is also of great interest functionally. It serves as the attachment site for teres major, a muscle that assists in adduction and internal rotation of the humerus and also helps stabilize the scapula against the thoracic wall. Taken together, the vertebral border, spine, acromion, coracoid process, and inferior angle form an architectural scaffold for the muscles that stabilize and articulate the entire shoulder complex.

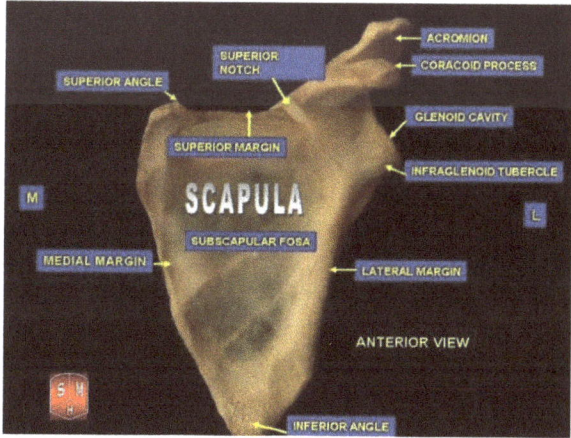

**Figure 1.66** Scapula. (Data source: Anatomist90,; https://commons.wikimedia.org/wiki/File:Anterior_surface_of_scapula.jpg; Creative Commons Attribution 3.0)

From a yoga perspective, healthy scapular motion – particularly upward and downward rotation, protraction, and retraction – is essential for functional arm movement and load-bearing shapes such as Downward Facing Dog, Plank, or *Chaturanga* (Yoga Pushup). Impaired scapular positioning can affect humeral alignment, limit shoulder range of motion, or contribute to strain in the neck, shoulders, or wrists. Teachers best cue not only shoulder blade movement but also emphasize the muscular engagement necessary to support the scapulae dynamically, especially when the arms are weight-bearing or overhead.

## *Clavicles*

The clavicles are slender, S-shaped bones that serve as vital connectors between the sternum and the scapulae (Figure 1.67). Each clavicle curves outward medially, then bends inward laterally, resembling an old-fashioned key – an image reflected in its German name, *Schlüsselbein*, or key bone. Functionally, the clavicles act as struts, holding the shoulder girdle out from the rib basket and preserving the width and shape of the upper thorax. Without this bony support, the shoulders would collapse inward, significantly compromising stability and range of motion.

A remarkable fact about the clavicle is that it forms the only true bony articulation between the upper appendicular skeleton (limbs and shoulder girdle) and the axial skeleton (spine and rib basket). This articulation is the sternoclavicular (SC) joint, located where the medial end of the clavicle meets the manubrium of the sternum. Despite its small size and subtle movement, the SC joint plays a crucial role in transferring force and coordinating motion between the trunk and arms. Through this joint, every movement of the shoulder and upper limb reverberates back into the axial skeleton.

Laterally, the clavicle articulates with the acromion process of the scapula at the acromioclavicular (AC) joint. If we palpate along the clavicle from the center of the chest outward, we can feel a slight dip near the shoulder where the bone ends – this is the location of the AC joint. Notably, the clavicle does not extend all the way to the edge of the shoulder; instead, it terminates just before it, leaving the outermost segment of the shoulder defined by the acromion.

Functionally, both the SC and AC joints contribute to the full range of motion available at the glenohumeral (shoulder) joint. When the arm is lifted or rotated, the clavicle moves in sympathy with the scapula, elevating, rotating, and tilting to increase the freedom of the arm. Although this movement is subtle and often overlooked, it is essential for the smooth and pain-free functioning of the shoulder complex.

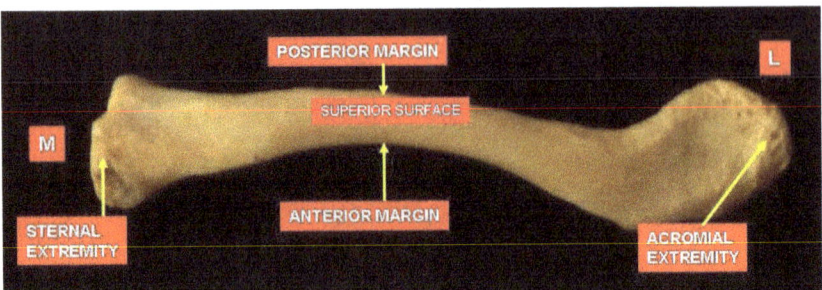

Figure 1.67 Clavicle. (Data source: Anatomist90; https://commons.wikimedia.org/wiki/File:Clavicle_4.jpg; Creative Commons Attribution 3.0)

From a yoga *asana* perspective, awareness of the clavicle's role can support healthier shoulder mechanics. For instance, in weight-bearing shapes like Side Plank or arm balances, cueing students to broaden across the collarbones can activate postural muscles that support scapular positioning and maintain space through the upper chest. In overhead shapes such as Warrior 1 or Extended Mountain, freedom in the clavicles contributes to the overall ease and range of shoulder elevation. Any rigidity or dysfunction at the SC or AC joint may restrict arm movement or place excess stress on the glenohumeral joint. In teaching and practice, it is helpful to consider the clavicle not simply as a passive bone, but as an integral part of the dynamic shoulder girdle that transmits force, enables motion, and sustains the open architecture of the upper body.

## *Humerus of the Upper Arm*

The humerus is the sole bone of the upper arm and the largest bone of the arm as a whole. Structurally robust and designed for leverage and load-bearing, the humerus forms the central strut between the shoulder and the elbow. Its design reflects the overall logic of the limbs: one large bone provides stability in the proximal segment (humerus in the arm; femur in the leg), followed by two bones in the next segment (radius and ulna in the forearm; tibia and fibula in the lower leg), and then increasingly complex bone arrangements through the wrist and hand, or ankle and foot, to maximize fine motor capacity and mobility.

At the proximal end, the humeral head articulates with the glenoid fossa of the scapula to form the glenohumeral joint (shoulder joint). The head of the humerus is rounded and fits into the shallow, slightly angled glenoid like a golf ball on a tee. This configuration prioritizes mobility over stability, making the shoulder the most mobile and one of the most vulnerable joints in the body. Distally, the humerus broadens and flattens to articulate with the bones of the forearm (the ulna and radius) at the elbow joint. The trochlea, a pulley-shaped structure on the medial side of the distal humerus, interfaces with the ulna, enabling the hinge-like flexion and extension of the elbow. Lateral to the trochlea is the capitulum, which receives the head of the radius. These articulating surfaces are accompanied by fossae (shallow depressions) that accommodate movement of the ulna during flexion and extension.

Several bony landmarks on the humerus serve as essential attachment sites for major muscles of the shoulder and upper arm:
- *Greater and lesser tubercles* near the proximal head anchor the rotator cuff muscles (supraspinatus, infraspinatus, teres minor, and subscapularis), which dynamically stabilize the shoulder joint.
- *Deltoid tuberosity*, halfway down the lateral shaft, serves as the insertion point for the deltoid muscle, one of the primary movers of the arm in abduction.
- *Medial and lateral epicondyles* at the distal end are prominent bony ridges that provide attachment for forearm flexors and extensors, respectively.

Functionally, the humerus is not only a structural bridge but a lever for upper limb movement. Muscles that move the shoulder, elbow, wrist, and even fingers either originate from or insert onto it. This makes the humerus a biomechanical conduit for force transmission throughout the upper limb. In yoga *asana* practice, the position and orientation of the humerus often dictate shoulder integrity and comfort. For example, in weight-bearing shapes like Downward Facing Dog, Plank, or Yoga Pushup, proper rotation of the humerus stabilizes the shoulder and prevents impingement. In overhead positions such as Extended Mountain or Warrior 1, awareness of humeral alignment can support freedom in the glenohumeral joint while minimizing compensatory patterns in the ribs or neck. Clearly, the humerus is a central pillar of the upper limb, linking mobility at the shoulder to stability at the elbow and serving as a structural and muscular hub for movement throughout the arm.

## Joints of the Shoulder Girdle

The shoulder girdle relies on the coordinated function of four primary joints; three of these contribute to stability and one prioritizes mobility. These structures link the upper appendicular skeleton to the axial skeleton and are essential to the complex mechanics of the upper body. Yoga professionals benefit from a detailed understanding of these joints to support shoulder health, prevent injury, and guide optimal alignment in postures. This section first outlines the scapulothoracic, acromioclavicular, sternoclavicular, and glenohumeral joints (see Figure 1.68). Then it shows how together, they form the stable base that supports movement at the glenohumeral joint.

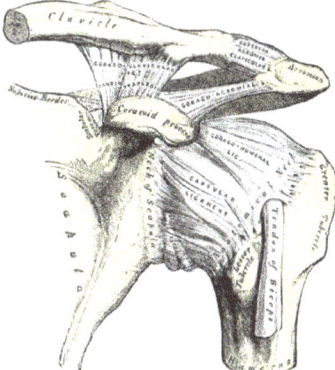

**Figure 1.68** Shoulder anatomy. (Data source: Henry Vandyke Carter; https://commons.wikimedia.org/wiki/File:Gray326.png; public domain)

## Scapulothoracic Junction

The scapulothoracic junction is not a true anatomical joint, as it lacks a synovial capsule and direct bony articulation. Instead, it is a functional interface between the anterior surface of the scapula and the posterior surface of the rib basket. This curved articulation bridged entirely by connective tissue allows the scapula to glide across the ribs with the aid of two primary muscular layers: the subscapularis on the underside of the scapula and the serratus anterior overlaying the ribs.

Although not technically a joint, the scapulothoracic junction plays a crucial role in shoulder stabilization and movement. It facilitates motions such as elevation and depression, protraction and retraction, and upward and downward rotation of the scapulae. These movements allow the shoulder girdle to adjust dynamically to arm motion, particularly in overhead postures. In yoga *asana* practice, optimal scapulothoracic mobility and neuromuscular control are essential for weight-bearing shapes such as Plank, *Chaturanga*, Handstand, and Downward Facing Dog, where scapular positioning contributes to force distribution and joint protection.

## Acromioclavicular Joint

The acromioclavicular (AC) joint is a small plane-type synovial joint located where the lateral end of the clavicle meets the acromion process of the scapula. It allows for subtle but vital gliding movements that accommodate larger motions of the scapula across the thoracic wall. This joint serves as a functional pivot point for scapular upward rotation during arm elevation and abduction. Though small, the AC joint plays a significant role in preserving overall mobility and mechanical integrity of the shoulder girdle. It transmits forces between the upper limb and axial skeleton and helps the scapula adjust to a wide range of upper limb positions. Dysfunction at this joint (e.g., through strain, instability, or degeneration) can limit shoulder mobility and alter the scapulohumeral rhythm, which may manifest as discomfort in shapes like Handstand, Reverse Warrior, or any other shape requiring full overhead reach.

## Sternoclavicular Joint

Amazingly, the tiny sternoclavicular joint is the only bony articulation between the upper appendicular skeleton and the axial skeleton. This joint forms where the medial clavicle meets the manubrium of the sternum and the first costal cartilage. Despite its small size, it is crucial to the transmission of load and motion between the trunk and upper limb. Functionally, the sternoclavicular joint allows elevation, depression, protraction, retraction, and limited axial rotation of the clavicle, key movements that support full range of motion in the shoulder.

Interestingly, in everyday biomechanics, the sternoclavicular joint also acts as a kind of mechanical safeguard. When a person falls and instinctively reaches out to catch themselves with an outstretched hand, the force travels up the limb and often dissipates through the sternoclavicular joint. This is the most common site of fracture or strain in such cases, not due to weakness, but rather because the joint acts as a sacrificial buffer, helping protect more vital soft tissues and preventing potentially more serious injuries to the thorax, spine, or internal organs. Although this design is protective, it also means yoga teachers need to be mindful of the sternoclavicular joint's potential vulnerability during transitions or falls in balances and inversions.

Because of its strategic location, the SC joint is highly relevant in yoga shapes involving arm elevation, suspension, or load-bearing. In inversions such as Headstand or Handstand, or in arm-supported shapes such as Crow and Side Plank, the sternoclavicular joint becomes a crucial conduit for load transfer from the thorax into the arms, shared with connective and muscular tissue through the arms, shoulders, and thorax (more about this below). Although well-stabilized by strong ligaments, this joint can be strained by excessive pulling or shearing, particularly in individuals with hypermobility or weakness in surrounding musculature.

> *Overall shoulder range of motion is the range of motion of three joints put together.*
>
> We can experience this complexity of shoulder movement by holding the acromioclavicular and sternoclavicular joints stable with our opposite hand notice how much less range of motion is now available in the shoulder:

### Glenohumeral (Shoulder) Joint

The glenohumeral joint is a *very shallow* synovial ball-and-socket joint formed between the glenoid fossa of the scapula and head of the humerus. In fact, the socket is more like a plate than a cup (unlike the acetabulum). Appropriately descriptively, *gleno-* refers to the shallow nature of the socket, which, unlike the deep socket of the hip joint, allows for tremendous freedom of movement. This joint is the most mobile joint in the human body, but this mobility comes at the cost of inherent instability, making the glenohumeral joint particularly susceptible to dislocation and strain, especially during load-bearing or extreme ranges of motion.

The glenoid fossa is anteverted, which means that it faces slightly forward rather than directly laterally. This anatomical feature has important implications for shoulder alignment and cueing in yoga *asana*. If the humeral head is pointed directly to the side, it is already externally rotated relative to the glenoid fossa. This has led some anatomists and physical therapists to question the overly rigid avoidance of *shoulders rolling forward*, pointing out that a slight anterior glide or protraction may, in fact, reflect the body's natural architecture rather than poor posture (Bond, 2007; Lasater, 2009, 2020; Porter, 2013).

The glenohumeral joint is least stable when the humerus is flexed, abducted, and externally rotated, and most stable in extension, adduction, and internal rotation (Lasater, 2009). As explored in the kinesiology section below, this reality has direct implications for yoga practice, particularly in arm-supported shapes. Another important fact about the glenohumeral joint is that it does not act alone. It works in concert with the other joints, as well as with several muscles and other shoulder structures to produce full range of shoulder motion. This coordinated movement is referred to as the glenohumeral rhythm or scapulohumeral rhythm and is addressed in detail in the kinesiology section below.

## Muscles of the Arms and Shoulder Girdle

Several sets of muscles collaborate to stabilize or mobilize the shoulder girdle, scapulae, and glenohumeral joint (Figure 1.69). Many have already been alluded to above; a detailed description with relevance to arm and shoulder movement follows.

### *Muscles that Stabilize the Scapulae on the Back Body*

Stability of the scapulae, so crucial for shoulder health and upper limb movement, relies on the complex interaction of muscles that connect the scapulae to the thoracic and cervical regions of the vertebral column and the rib basket. In yoga *asana*, especially in inversions and weight-bearing shapes such as Downward Facing Dog, Crow, and Handstand, these muscles are engaged in precise and coordinated balance to stabilize the shoulder girdle and protect the cervical and thoracic spine. Although often classified as back muscles, many of these scapular stabilizers also belong to myofascial lines that support upper limb function, such as the deep back line and deep front arm line.

#### *The "X" System of Scapular Stabilization*

The dynamic balance of scapular stabilization is often described as an X-shaped system on the upper back (e.g., Tom Myers in a workshop environment). On one diagonal, the rhomboids and serratus anterior work in coordinated opposition: the rhomboids retract the scapulae toward the spine, while the serratus anterior anchors them against the rib basket and pulls them forward into protraction. Some consider the rhomboids and serratus anterior a sling around the scapula, a sling that is a single myofascial structure. On the opposite diagonal, the lower trapezius and pectoralis minor also act in opposition. The lower trapezius sections on the back body draw the scapulae downward and inward toward the spine, whereas the pectoralis minor muscles in the chest pull them forward and upward. Each of these diagonal pairings function optimally when balanced in strength and length to maintain healthful scapular mechanics.

#### *Rhomboids and Serratus Anterior*

The rhomboid major and minor muscles have central responsibility in scapular stabilization, creating retraction and rotation. They form the upper portion of the posterior diagonal X and connect the vertebral column to the medial border of the scapula. Their action can be envisioned through understanding that rhomboid minor originates on the spinous processes of C7–T1 and inserts along the medial border of the scapula; and that rhomboid major originates from T2–T5 and inserts similarly on the medial border.

In yoga practitioners, imbalance between the rhomboids and the serratus anterior is common. For instance, rhomboids are often over-contracted or locked short in individuals who habitually open the heart by excessively retracting the shoulder blades (even when not necessary), leading to a weakening of the opposing serratus. Conversely, in athletes or weightlifters who overly strengthen the serratus, the rhomboids may become eccentrically loaded or locked long. For stable scapulae in inversions, rhomboids *and* serratus anterior ideally function in a balanced manner, being equally strong and evenly recruited.

### Trapezius and Pectoralis Minor

The trapezius muscles, spanning the back of the neck and upper thorax, play a crucial role in elevating, retracting, and rotating the scapula. They are composed of three distinct sections, each with specific roles:

- Lower trapezius muscles originate on T4–T12 and insert on the medial border of the scapulae. They are the only muscles that medially depresses the scapulae, pulling them down and inward. They partner with the pectoralis minor muscles of the chest to create the second diagonal of the X-shaped stabilization system. If the lower traps are weak or underactive, kyphosis may develop due to overpowering action from the front chest muscles. This pattern has been linked to modern posture when using various devices (such as phones and laptops).
- Middle trapezius muscles originate from C7–T3 and are primarily responsible for retracting the scapula, aiding in midline stabilization.
- Upper trapezius muscles originate from the occipital bone and nuchal ligament and elevate and upwardly rotate the scapulae, especially during arm abduction. Overdominance here can contribute to neck tension or the *shrugging of the shoulders* that is notable among many students in certain yoga shapes (e.g., Downward Facing Dog).

### Levator Scapulae

The levator scapulae muscles, extending from the transverse processes of C1–C4 to the medial scapular border, assist with scapular elevation and downward rotation. However, they also play an important role in cervical spine stability and lateral flexion, helping to resist forward head posture. Despite the name, these muscles may function more to stabilize head position than to elevate the scapula during dynamic movement.

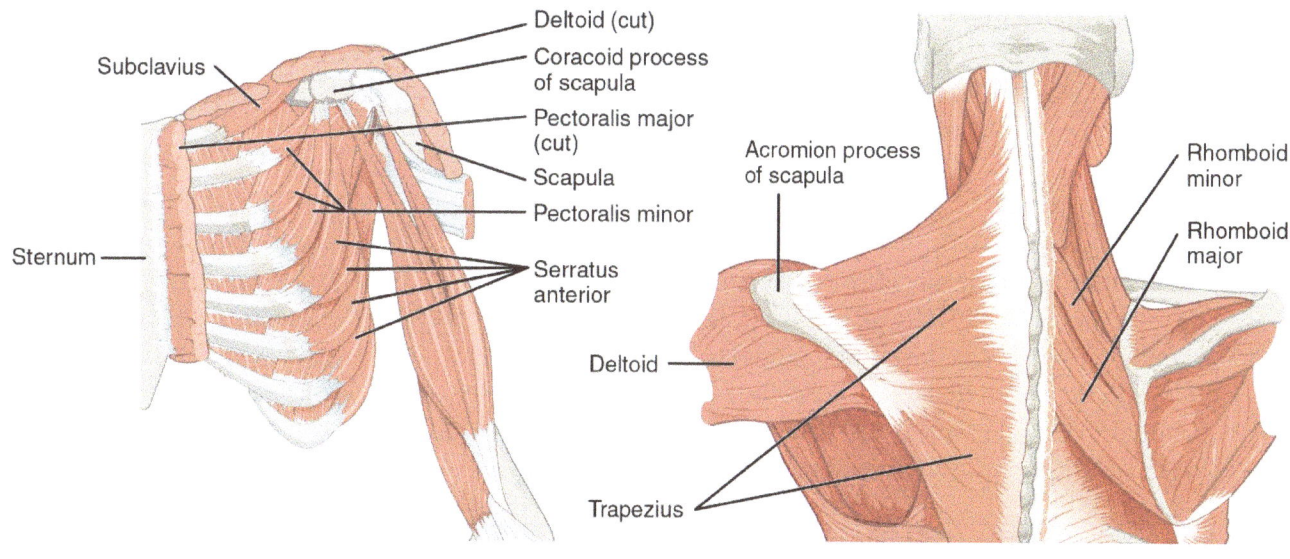

**Figure 1.69** Pectoral girdle muscles. (Data source: OpenStax; https://commons.wikimedia.org/wiki/File:1118_Muscles_that_Position_the_Pectoral_Girdle.jpg; Creative Commons Attribution 3.0)

## Muscles that Stabilize the Arms and Scapulae on the Front Body

While the muscles along the back body (Figure 1.70) play a dominant role in scapular stabilization, the anterior shoulder and chest muscles provide crucial counterbalance and control, especially in yoga shapes that involve arm support or shoulder loading. These muscles link the scapulae and arms to the rib basket and trunk from the front body, and their integrity and length directly influence shoulder mechanics, spinal posture, and scapular placement. In particular, serratus anterior, pectoralis minor, and latissimus dorsi serve essential and complementary functions in the stability and mobility of the shoulder girdle.

### Serratus Anterior

The serratus anterior muscles are broad, multi-bellied muscles with a serrated edge, described by Tom Myers as a "bunch of bananas" for their rib-wrapping visual appearance. They originate from the outer surfaces of ribs 1 through 9 and insert on the anterior surface of the medial border of the scapulae, effectively wrapping underneath the scapula and adhering it to the rib basket. Functionally, they are the primary scapular protractors and some of the most important scapular stabilizers in weight-bearing arm shapes such as Plank, *Chaturanga*, and Downward Facing Dog.

As noted previously, the serratus anterior muscles work in opposition to the rhomboids, forming one diagonal of the X-system described in above. For optimal shoulder mechanics, these two muscle groups are balanced in tone and strength. Weakness in the serratus anterior muscles contributes to scapular winging (during which the medial border of the scapula lifts off the thorax), destabilizing the shoulders and increasing shoulder vulnerability in shapes such as Headstand and Handstand. Yoga practitioners can activate the serratus anterior with cues that draw attention to the lateral ribs, such as gently drawing the lower ribs toward one another or spreading the shoulder blades wide across the back. Additionally, a cue to broaden the collar bones engages the rhomboids, creating balance from the back body. Consistent and mindful practice of weight-bearing shapes on the arms can strengthen this essential muscle group and helps retrain protraction mechanics without collapsing into the chest.

### Pectoralis Minor

The pectoralis minor muscles in the chest, though small in size, exert significant influence on scapular positioning. They originate from ribs 3 to 5 and insert onto the coracoid process of the scapulae, functioning to pull the scapulae forward and downward. They directly oppose the action of the lower trapezius muscles, which draw the scapula back and down, forming the other diagonal in the scapular X-system. Ideally, these two muscle groups work together to keep the shoulder blades securely positioned on the back.

However, shortness or tightness in the pectoralis minor, which is deeply embedded within the clavipectoral fascia, can lead to a forward-drawn shoulder posture, contributing to thoracic kyphosis and limiting range of motion in shoulder extension and retraction. In yoga *asana*, this restricted posture is especially evident in backbends such as Upward Facing Dog, where open shoulders and a lifted sternum are necessary. When pectoralis minor dominates, it becomes difficult to anchor the scapulae onto the back, compromising shoulder integrity in backbends and overhead inversions. To release and lengthen this area, mobility work (such as placing the armpit against a wall and sliding the arms in a slow upward motion) can be helpful. This technique targets pectoralis minor and its fascial continuity with deeper anterior tissues, such as the clavipectoral fascia.

### *Latissimus Dorsi*

Though technically superficial back muscles, the latissimus dorsi muscles also play a stabilizing role on the front body by acting on the arm and shoulder joint, not directly on the scapula. They originate along the thoracolumbar fascia (T7–T12), sacrum, and iliac crest, and insert on the intertubercular groove of the humeri. Functionally, latissimus dorsi supports arm extension, adduction, and internal rotation, and contributes to depression and retraction of the shoulder joint. Although it does not attach directly to the scapula, its influence is felt in weight-bearing shapes that involve pulling or extension actions (such as Downward Facing Dog, Locust, or arm balances). A shortened or dominant latissimus dorsi can limit overhead arm mobility and restrict scapular upward rotation. In yoga *asana*, thoughtful cueing of side body length, spinal extension, and softening of the front ribs can help modulate overuse of the latissimus while encouraging harmonious co-activation with other stabilizers.

### *Rotator Cuff Muscles*

The rotator cuff (Figure 1.71) is a deep, stabilizing muscular structure that encircles the head of the humerus and holds it securely within the glenoid fossa of the scapula. This group of four muscles, namely, supraspinatus, infraspinatus, teres minor, and subscapularis, commonly identified by the acronym SITS, originates on the scapula and inserts onto various aspects of the proximal humerus, forming what is often described as a muscular cuff that protects, centers, and orients the humeral head during all movements of the arm (akin to the small muscles surrounding the eyeball that direct the eyes in the direction of movement). As noted above, although the shoulder is a ball-and-socket joint, the glenoid cavity is relatively shallow compared to the head of the humerus. The rotator cuff provides the dynamic stabilization necessary to keep the humeral head seated in this shallow, plate-like socket, particularly during elevating, rotating, and load-bearing actions. Here are some details about each of these important and collaborative muscles that wrap the glenohumeral joint:

- *Supraspinatus:* The supraspinatus sits above the spine of the scapula, originating from the supraspinous fossa and inserting on the upper facet of the greater tubercle of the humerus. It initiates the first 15 degrees of arm abduction and contributes to superior joint stability by helping to center the humeral head within the glenoid fossa during elevation. This muscle is frequently engaged in yoga shapes that require arm abduction or elevation, such as Warrior 2, Triangle, or extended arm variations in standing postures. Due to its position and function, supraspinatus is vulnerable to impingement, particularly if the humerus is not allowed to externally rotate during arm elevation or if scapular upward rotation is restricted.
- *Infraspinatus:* Located on the posterior surface of the scapula below the scapular spine, the infraspinatus originates from the infraspinous fossa and inserts on the middle facet of the greater tubercle of the humerus. It is a primary external rotator of the shoulder and, along with its smaller counterpart, the teres minor, stabilizes the joint posteriorly. Infraspinatus is

essential in maintaining balance across the shoulder girdle, particularly in practitioners who favor internally rotated arm positions or with over-recruitment of the pectoral group. It becomes especially important in transitions such as lowering from Plank to Chaturanga or when bearing weight in shapes like Side Plank, where subtle external rotation may help secure the humerus.

- *Teres Minor:* Teres minor is the smallest of the rotator cuff muscles and shares a synergistic role with infraspinatus. It arises from the lateral border of the scapula and inserts on the lower facet of the greater tubercle of the humerus. Its main function is external rotation of the humerus, and it provides posterior-lateral stability to the shoulder joint. Despite its small size, teres minor is often a source of tenderness or trigger point activity, particularly in practitioners who load the shoulder without full awareness of rotator cuff engagement. It plays a quiet but crucial role in overhead motions of the arm in the glenohumeral joint.
- *Subscapularis*: The only anterior muscle of the group, the subscapularis lies deep to the scapula on its costal (or anterior) surface. It originates from the subscapular fossa and inserts onto the lesser tubercle of the humerus. Its primary action is internal rotation of the humerus; it also contributes to adduction and anterior stabilization of the shoulder joint. In yoga *asana*, subscapularis plays an active role in shapes that require the arms to rotate inward or draw across the front of the body, such as Eagle. It also resists external rotation in transitions like those into Cow Face or during externally rotated arm balances, functioning as a deep stabilizer when challenged eccentrically.

Without the constant, subtle adjustments of the rotator cuff muscles, the static ligaments of the joint would be insufficient to prevent instability or dislocation, especially in overhead or weight-bearing shapes. Rotator cuff function is addressed further in the kinesiology section in the context of its essential role in the glenohumeral rhythm. Yoga practitioners frequently place significant and repetitive demands on the shoulders through shapes such as Downward Facing Dog, *Chaturanga*, and inversions. In these positions, a well-conditioned rotator cuff is essential to maintain joint integrity. Imbalance, overuse, or underdevelopment of any one of these four muscles can compromise the entire shoulder complex.

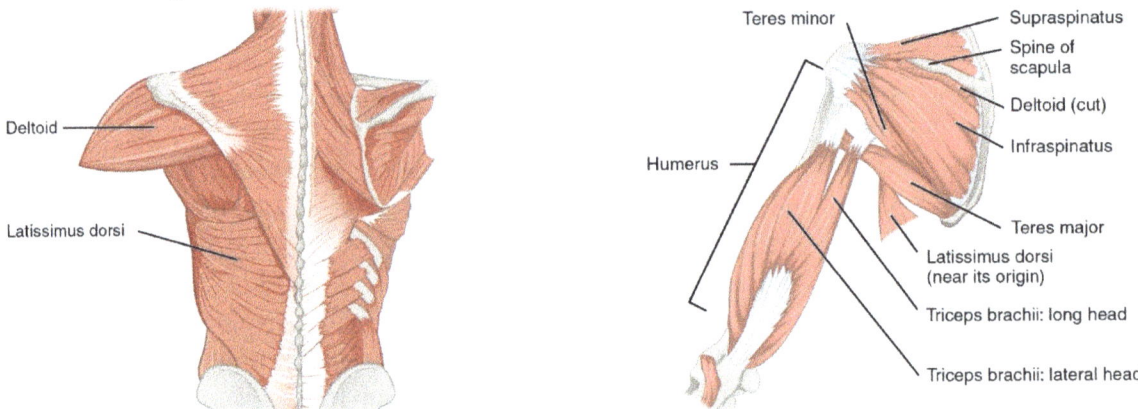

**Figure 1.71** Muscles creating movement in the humerus. (Data source: OpenStax; https://commons.wikimedia.org/wiki/File:1119_Muscles_that_Move_the_Humerus_b.png; Creative Commons Attribution 3.0)

**Figure 1.70** Muscles of the glenohumeral joint (and more). (Data source: OpenStax; https://commons.wikimedia.org/wiki/File:1119_Muscles_that_Move_the_Humerus_d.png; Commons Attribution 3.0)

## Muscles Connecting the Arms and Shoulder Joints

A few additional muscles generate powerful movements of the arm at the shoulder joint and deserve mentioning. These muscles do not always originate or insert on the scapula but nevertheless contribute to shoulder function and range of motion. They include pectoralis major, deltoid, teres major, and coracobrachialis, each influencing the positioning and movement of the humerus through different vectors of force (see Figure 1.72).

### Pectoralis Major

Spanning the upper chest from the sternum, clavicle, and upper ribs to its insertion on the lateral humerus, pectoralis major is a broad, superficial muscle responsible for adduction, internal rotation, and flexion of the humerus. It plays a dominant role in many arm-centric activities and is often over-recruited in modern postural patterns associated with forward rounding of the shoulders. In yoga *asana*, tightness in the pectoralis major can be a limiting factor in backbends and overhead arm positions. When this muscle, along with its fascial continuum in the clavipectoral fascia, becomes short or overactive, it can draw the humerus into internal rotation and anterior positioning, impeding scapular retraction and contributing to a collapsed chest. Creating resilience in this area and balancing its strength with posterior shoulder stabilizers is helpful for opening the heart region and cultivating healthy shoulder mechanics.

### Deltoid, Teres Major, and Coracobrachialis: Coordinated Movers

Although anatomically distinct, deltoid, teres major, and coracobrachialis muscles collaborate to mobilize the humeri through flexion, extension, rotation, and abduction. All three insert on the humerus and, collectively, bridge the scapulae or upper thorax to the arm. The deltoid wraps over the top of the shoulder, originating from three distinct points: the anterior clavicle, the lateral acromion, and the posterior spine of the scapula. These three segments allow the deltoid to produce a wide range of motion:
- Anterior deltoid contributes to shoulder flexion, internal rotation, and horizontal adduction.
- Middle deltoid is the primary abductor of the shoulder, especially from 15 to 90 degrees.
- Posterior deltoid assists in shoulder extension, external rotation, and horizontal abduction.

Teres major, sometimes called the 'little lat', originates from the inferior angle of the scapula and inserts on the medial lip of the intertubercular groove of the humerus. It assists in internal rotation, adduction, and extension of the shoulder – actions that mirror those of the latissimus dorsi, with which it often works synergistically. Coracobrachialis, though smaller, plays a supportive role in flexion and adduction of the shoulder. It arises from the coracoid process and inserts on the medial humerus. It contributes to arm control during transitions that require shoulder flexion with scapular stabilization.

Together, these muscles provide the power and control needed for large-range movements of the arm. Their function is most effective when integrated with the deeper stabilizing muscles in the region, particularly the rotator cuff and scapular muscles, to create a balanced shoulder complex that supports fluid, stable, and sustainable practice.

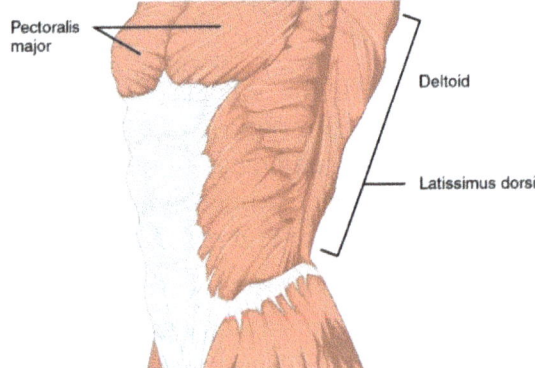

**Figure 1.72** Muscles affecting movement of the arm. (Data source: OpenStax; https://commons.wikimedia.org/wiki/File:1119_Muscles_that_Move_the_Humerus_a.png; Creative Commons Attribution 3.0)

## Kinesiology of the Pectoral Girdle

To recap, the pectoral girdle, the anatomical complex that links the upper limbs to the axial skeleton, includes the scapulae, clavicles, humeri and associated musculature. Its function depends not only on individual muscle and joint actions, but on the dynamic interplay between and collaboration of the glenohumeral joint, scapulothoracic articulation, and supporting structures of the thoracic spine (among others). For yoga practitioners and teachers, understanding the pectoral girdle as a network of interdependent parts is essential for supporting joint integrity, preventing injury, and enhancing functional movement on and off the mat.

### *Scapular Stabilization Through Anterior-Posterior Balance*

A central tenet of pectoral girdle function is the stabilization of the scapulae. Scapular positioning provides a foundation for humeral movement, particularly in overhead postures and transitions. This stability is not static; rather, it is the product of balanced tension between anterior stabilizers – namely, the serratus anterior and pectoralis minor – and posterior stabilizers such as the rhomboids and trapezius muscles. In a healthy shoulder girdle, these opposing muscle groups work in synergy to maintain a neutral, mobile scapular platform. Dysfunction arises when the anterior musculature becomes short and tight, often due to habitual posture or repetitive anterior-dominant movement patterns. The resulting forward-drawn scapulae disrupt healthy glenohumeral mechanics and may contribute to impingement, instability, or thoracic rigidity. Conversely, excessive tension in the posterior shoulder can restrict scapular mobility, hindering the upward rotation and posterior tilting necessary for overhead motion.

Yoga *asana* provides an opportunity to restore functional balance through mindful sequencing. Practices that alternate protraction and retraction (such as Plank to *Chaturanga* transitions), encourage scapular elevation and depression, and vary between internal and external shoulder rotation help reestablish this muscular equilibrium. Specific strategies include wall-assisted scapular mobilizations for releasing pectoralis minor and lengthening the anterior chest, serratus anterior engagement in weight-bearing transitions, and overhead arm variations in Bridge to access length in the latissimus dorsi.

## *Glenohumeral or Scapulohumeral Rhythm*

Optimal shoulder function, including the ability to lift the arms overhead (i.e., accessing full flexion and abduction) and circumduction of the arms, does not depend on glenohumeral motion alone. Rather, arm elevation, mobility, and circumduction arise from a coordinated rhythm involving the scapula, clavicle, thoracic spine, and humerus. These collaborative movements allow the arms to reach full elevation without compressing underlying soft tissues, particularly the supraspinatus tendon and subacromial bursa.

This kinetic relationship, commonly referred to as glenohumeral rhythm or (perhaps more accurately) scapulohumeral rhythm, describes how the upward and circular movement of the arm is created through a collaboration of multiple joints, muscles, and movements. It is helpful to remember that the glenoid fossa is on the scapula (many yoga professionals forget this anatomical fact). As such, movements of the humerus and scapula are always linked. When the arm is at the side in anatomical position, the glenoid fossa faces out to the side and slightly anterior. When the scapula rotates and elevates, this automictically moves the glenoid fossa upward and giving more freedom of movement to the humerus, especially in relationship to the acromion process. Given these relationships, the scapulohumeral rhythm can be understood as the following orchestrated collaboration:

- Engagement of four glenohumeral stabilizer muscles, namely, the rotator cuff muscles (supraspinatus, infraspinatus, teres minor, and subscapularis), alongside the deltoid
- Movement of the scapulae via four stabilizers, namely, serratus anterior, upper and lower trapezius, rhomboids, and levator scapulae
- Structural contributions from four bones, namely, scapulae (which rotate upwardly and tilt posteriorly), humeri (which externally rotate and may abduct), clavicles (which elevate and rotate posteriorly), and thoracic spine (which extends)

---

According to Judith Hanson Lasater (2009, 2020), the glenohumeral rhythm involves a collaboration of:

***Four Movements***:
1. Abduction or flexion of the humerus (depending on the arm's trajectory)
2. External rotation of the humerus
3. Elevation and rotation of the scapula
4. Extension of the thoracic spine

***Four Muscles*** (or muscle groups):
1. Rotator cuff (primarily supraspinatus, but all SITS muscles contribute to stabilization)
2. Deltoid
3. Trapezius (especially upper and lower fibers)
4. Serratus anterior

***Four Joints*** (or joint regions):
1. Glenohumeral joint (ball and socket joint of humerus and scapula)
2. Scapulothoracic articulation (functional joint between scapula and rib basket)
3. Acromioclavicular joint (between scapula and clavicle)
4. Sternoclavicular joint (between clavicle and sternum)

In yoga *asana*, this scapulohumeral interplay is activated in arm-lifting shapes such as Warrior 1, Extended Mountain, and Handstand. Restrictions in any element of this system (e.g., due to tight pectorals, limited thoracic extension, or poor scapular control) can disrupt the rhythm and shift excessive load onto the rotator cuff. Disruption of any part of this system, especially poor scapular mobility or thoracic extension, can result in compensatory strain, shoulder impingement, or reduced functional range of motion. Over time, compensations may lead to inflammation, degeneration, or rotator cuff injury. For instance, when thoracic extension is lacking, students often compensate by anteriorly tilting the scapulae and over-recruiting the upper trapezius, creating crowding at the acromion and risk for impingement.

Clearly, shoulder health in yoga *asana* requires more than isolated strengthening of the rotator cuff or simple cueing of external rotation to lift the arms. It depends on maintaining coordinated mobility through the upper back, developing eccentric control in transitions, and resisting the impulse to 'hang' in flexible joints. Cues that support scapular mobility, postural awareness, and gradual load adaptation are crucial for protecting the glenohumeral joint, especially in therapeutic yoga contexts. From a therapeutic perspective, supporting or perhaps restoring this rhythm means addressing both mobility and motor control. This may involve:
- Improving thoracic extension through supported backbends or foam rolling
- Releasing chronically tight anterior structures such as the pectoralis minor
- Strengthening scapular stabilizers such as the lower trapezius and serratus anterior
- Cueing active external rotation of the humerus while moving into overhead shapes and interior rotation at end range
- Avoiding excessive passive range of motion, especially in hypermobile students

Ultimately, the glenohumeral rhythm is less about individual muscle strength and more about coordination and timing across multiple systems. *Asana* practice benefits from emphasizing this synergy, ensuring that each joint, muscle, and structure has to contribute appropriately to the whole.

## *Stability and Load Management in the Glenohumeral Joint*

The glenohumeral joint sacrifices inherent stability for range of motion. Unlike the femur, which is grounded in the deep cup of the acetabulum, the head of the humerus rests against a shallow glenoid fossa (shaped like a shallow saucer) and relies heavily on soft tissue structures for containment (including many ligaments and the rotator cuff muscles). This architecture renders the shoulder joint particularly vulnerable to strain, especially during load-bearing in yoga. Biomechanically, the glenohumeral joint is least stable in positions of abduction combined with external rotation and flexion, the precise positions adopted in many yoga shapes requiring arm elevation while weight-bearing (e.g., Handstand, Downward Facing Dog). However, for the shoulder joint to be able to move into full flexion or abduction, it typically and automatically externally rotates and abducts for the majority of students. True, some individuals can access flexion abduction in the shoulder joint without external rotation; however, most cannot. What this means is that when the arms are lifted overhead, the glenohumeral joint is vulnerable. This is not a problem when the arms are lifted in upright positions; it becomes a challenge when this alignment in the shoulder joints occurs during load-bearing (i.e., during inversions and half-inversions). For these latter shapes, the alignment of the glenohumeral joint that is beneficial for mobility must be paired with neuromuscular strategies that promote stabilization in some situations, such as internal rotation once end range is reached.

This anatomical reality has direct implications for yoga *asana*, particularly in arm-standing shapes. For example, in Downward Facing Dog, Plank, Crow, and Handstand, joint integrity is improved by actively creating slight movement in the direction of adduction and internal rotation of the upper arms. These adjustments create a more stable joint capsule and enhance co-contraction of the surrounding musculature. It is essential for yoga teachers to understand this functional nuance: although external rotation may feel open or expansive, it renders the shoulder joint vulnerable under load. This is fine in upright shapes that lift the arms overhead, such as Warriors or Extended Mountain. However, this vulnerability must be addressed in yoga *asana* that involves load-bearing on the arms, such as during inversions and half-inversions. Actively internally *rotating and adducting* (understood as *actions*, not positions) during weight-bearing (i.e., while loading the arms and shoulder girdle) helps settle the humeral head into the glenoid fossa and can maintain optimal joint congruence in such cases of full shoulder flexion or abduction. This means that common adjustments, such as externally rotating a student's arm while in Downward Facing Dog, are not actually anatomically appropriate or helpful for most individuals.

This understanding has important pedagogical implications. External rotation may feel intuitively 'open' or appear aligned, but when performed under load without adequate rotator cuff engagement, it may destabilize the joint. Teachers best prioritize functional mechanics over aesthetic adjustments, avoiding habitual cues that encourage exaggerated external rotation or abduction of the upper arms in weight-bearing shapes. Nuanced guidance emphasizes external rotation during the active phase of moving the arms overhead and internal rotation and adduction to stabilize at end range.

## Forearms, Wrists, and Hands

The forearms, wrists, and hands form the distal end of the upper limbs, enabling precision, grip, and tactile feedback. These structures are highly adaptive, translating neural intention into fine motor control and expressive movement. In yoga practice, their engagement supports weight-bearing, balance, and sensory awareness, particularly in shapes where the hands serve as a base. Therapeutically, attention to this region can reveal patterns of overuse, strain, or compensatory tension originating elsewhere in the kinetic chain, especially in the shoulders and neck.

## Bones of the Forearms, Wrists, and Hands

Returning to the 1, 2, 3, 4, 5 arrangement of the limbs, the humerus was the singular bones at the most proximal location of the arms. The forearm is the next structure and consists of *two* long bones, the radius and ulna, which articulate with one another at both proximal and distal radioulnar joints. These bones work in tandem to allow pronation and supination – the rotational actions of turning the palm up or down. The radius, positioned laterally (thumb side), rotates around the ulna, which remains relatively fixed. The three major arm bones are shown in Figures 1.73 and 1.74.

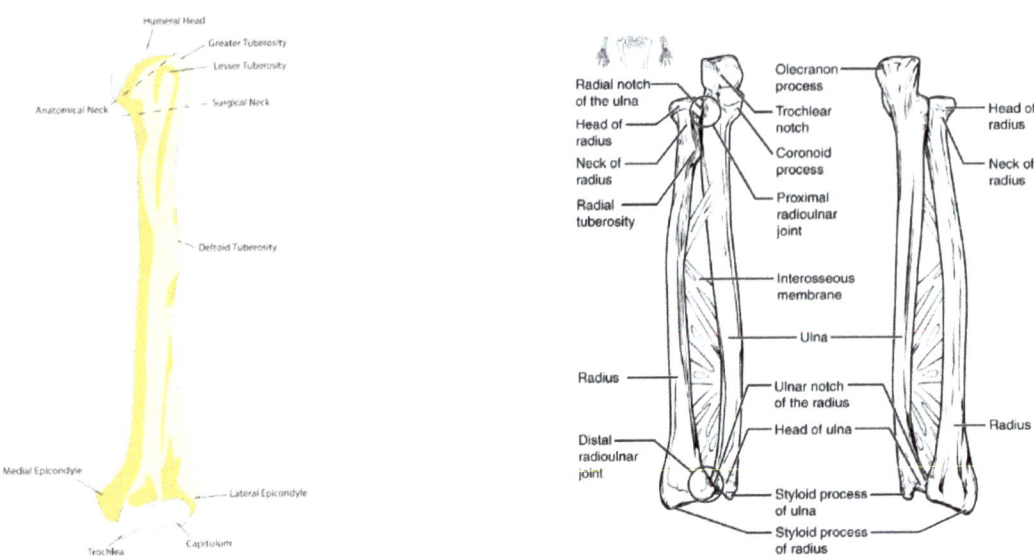

Figure 1.73 Humerus and its landmarks. (Data source: BDB; https://commons.wikimedia.org/wiki/File:HumerusFront.png; public domain)

Figure 1.74 Ulna and radius. (Data source: OpenStax; https://commons.wikimedia.org/wiki/File:805_Ulna_and_Radius.jpg; Creative Commons Attribution 3.0)

At the distal end, the radius connects to the carpal bones of the wrist (Figure 1.75), forming the primary articulation for wrist movement. The wrist proper comprises eight small, intricately arranged carpal bones in two rows that enable complex gliding and stabilizing motions. These, in turn, articulate with the five metacarpals of the hand, which form the skeletal framework of the palm, numbers as metacarpals 1 through 5 (starting from the lateral or thumb side of the hand and ending at the medial or little finger side). The metacarpals, in turn, articulate with the phalanges, or finger bones, organized into three rows in a proximal, middle (except in the thumb), and distal set of four (thumb) to five segments. Together, these bones support both fine motor actions in daily life, as well as weight-bearing during certain yoga shapes.

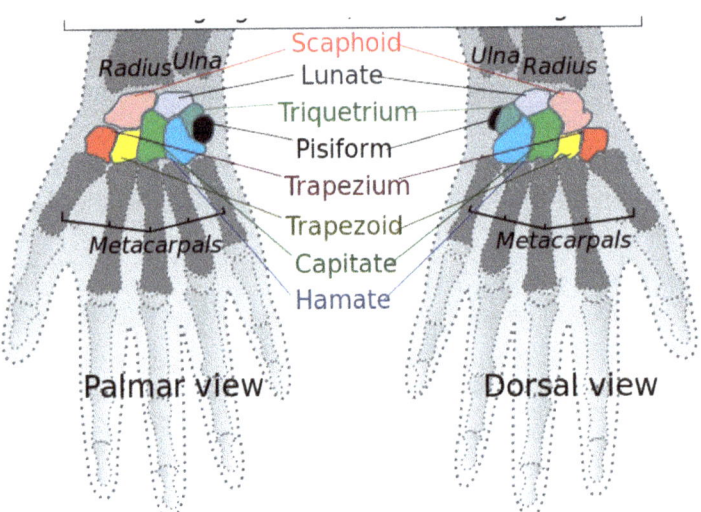

Figure 1.75 Carpal bones. (Data source: Source image by Arcadian and Mintz, derivative work by Mikael Häggström; https://commons.wikimedia.org/wiki/File:Carpals_-_english.svg; Creative Commons Attribution 3.0)

## Joints of the Forearms, Wrists, and Hands

The forearm's two long bones, the radius and ulna, articulate with each other proximally and distally to allow rotation of the forearm (including *pronation* and *supination*). These bones are connected by the interosseous membrane, a fibrous sheet that transmits forces between them. The elbow region includes three articulations (i.e., joints) within a single joint capsule (Figure 1.76). Although commonly referred to as the 'elbow joint,' anatomically it is a *compound synovial joint* composed of three articulations working together within one joint capsule:

- *Humeroulnar joint* – between the trochlea of the humerus and the trochlear notch of the ulna (primary hinge for flexion and extension)
- *Humeroradial joint* – between the capitulum of the humerus and the head of the radius (assists in flexion and rotation)
- *Proximal radioulnar joint* – between the head of the radius and the radial notch of the ulna (permits pronation and supination of the forearm)

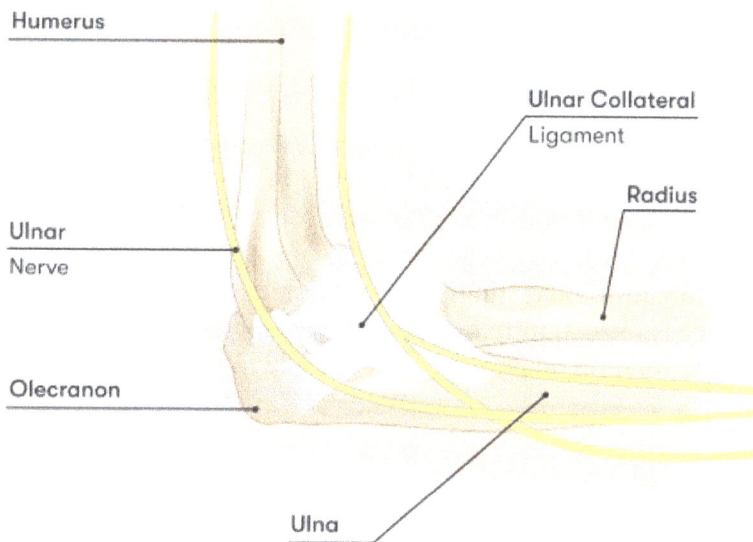

**Figure 1.76** Elbow joint – also showing nerves that cause the "funny bone" sensation. (Data source: InjuryMap; https://commons.wikimedia.org/wiki/File:Elbow_nerves.svg; Creative Commons Attribution 4.0)

The radiocarpal joint, commonly referred to as the wrist, connects the distal radius to the proximal row of carpal bones and allows flexion, extension, and deviation (radial and ulnar) of the hand. The wrist articulates with the eight carpal bones, which are arranged in two rows and named (from lateral to medial, proximal row first): scaphoid, lunate, triquetrum, and pisiform; trapezium, trapezoid, capitate, and hamate in the distal row. Distal to the carpals lie the five metacarpals, which form the palm and articulate at their bases with the carpals (carpometacarpal joints), and at their heads with the proximal phalanges (metacarpophalangeal joints). The fingers consist of phalanges, namely, three per finger (proximal, middle, distal; Figure 1.77) and two in the thumb, connected by interphalangeal joints that permit fine-motor flexion and extension. Together, these joints create the remarkable dexterity of the hand, essential in daily life and yoga *asana* requiring open palms, strong grips, or weight-bearing on the hands.

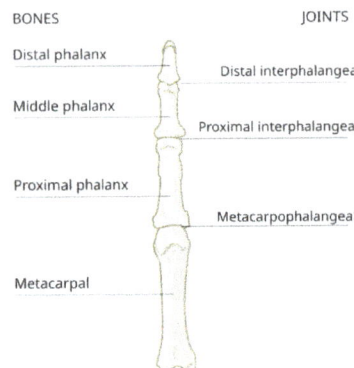

**Figure 1.77** Finger bones and joints – index finger shown. (Data source: Hariadhi; https://upload.wikimedia.org/wikipedia/commons/0/05/Bones_of_index_finger_svg_hariadhi.svg Creative Commons Attribution 4.0)

## Muscles of the Forearms, Wrists, and Hands

### *Muscles Around the Elbow*

The primary muscles responsible for flexion and extension at the elbow and shoulder include the biceps brachii, triceps brachii, and brachialis (Figure 1.78). Though these muscles act locally at the elbow, most also relate structurally and functionally to the shoulder joint via their scapular attachments. The biceps brachii, a two-headed muscle, originates on the scapula (the short head from the coracoid process and the long head from the supraglenoid tubercle) and inserts on the radial tuberosity of the forearm. Interestingly, it does not attach to the humerus, even though it spans its length. The biceps plays multiple roles: it flexes the elbow and shoulder joints and is a powerful supinator of the forearm, making it a key muscle in postural support and transitional control during yoga *asana*.

Opposing the biceps is the triceps brachii, which has three heads: the long head originates on the infraglenoid tubercle of the scapula; the lateral and medial heads originate from the posterior humerus. All three converge on a common tendon that inserts onto the olecranon process of the ulna. The triceps extends the elbow, and the long head additionally assists with shoulder extension. The latter is particularly relevant in shapes that involve shoulder extension with elbow flexion, such as in variations of arm placement in Cow Face. The third major muscle around the elbow is *brachialis*, a deep humeral muscle, originating on the anterior surface of the humerus and inserting on the coronoid process of the ulna. It is as elbow flexor, unaffected by forearm position, and often the strongest contributor to elbow flexion regardless of whether the palm is pronated or supinated. In yoga *asana*, understanding how these muscles interact can inform mindful transitions from shapes like Plank to Downward Facing Dog, optimization of load-bearing through the arms, and cultivation of balanced strength between the anterior and posterior kinetic chains.

### *Muscles of the Wrists and Forearms*

Although the forearm and wrist muscles are at times overlooked in yoga anatomy, their contribution becomes central in inversions and other shapes that create load-bearing on the hands. These muscles (shown in Figure 1.78), which originate along the radius and ulna and cross the wrist joint, include a complex array of flexors and extensors arranged along the medial (thumb-side) and lateral (little finger-side) forearm. Together, they create nuanced movements of the wrist and fingers, including flexion, extension, pronation, and supination, as well as providing isometric stabilization during load-bearing. In yoga inversions and half-inversions such as Downward Facing Dog, Forearm Balance, and Handstand, these muscles help transfer force from the ground through the hands and wrists, up along the fascial and muscular lines of the arms to the shoulders. Effective transfer of this force through the wrists and forearms contributes to creating a stable shoulder girdle and connects the effort of the hands with the postural support of deeper shoulder and back muscles (and related fascial structures), especially the rhomboids and lower trapezius.

Weakness or poor coordination in forearm musculature can contribute significantly to instability in inversions or load-bearing on the hands and wrists, manifesting as wrist discomfort or inability to maintain arm alignment. Additionally, if the pectoralis muscles are tight and the scapulae are pulled forward, the shoulder blades cannot fully stabilize on the posterior thorax. This combination of challenges can contribute to the excessive shoulder elevation (shrugging) that is so common in Downward Facing Dog, and even in Headstand. As will be explored further below and in Section 2, yoga *asana* that emphasizes strength and resilience in the wrist and forearm musculature, alongside length and mobility in the anterior shoulder, helps create a well-integrated foundation for stable inversions.

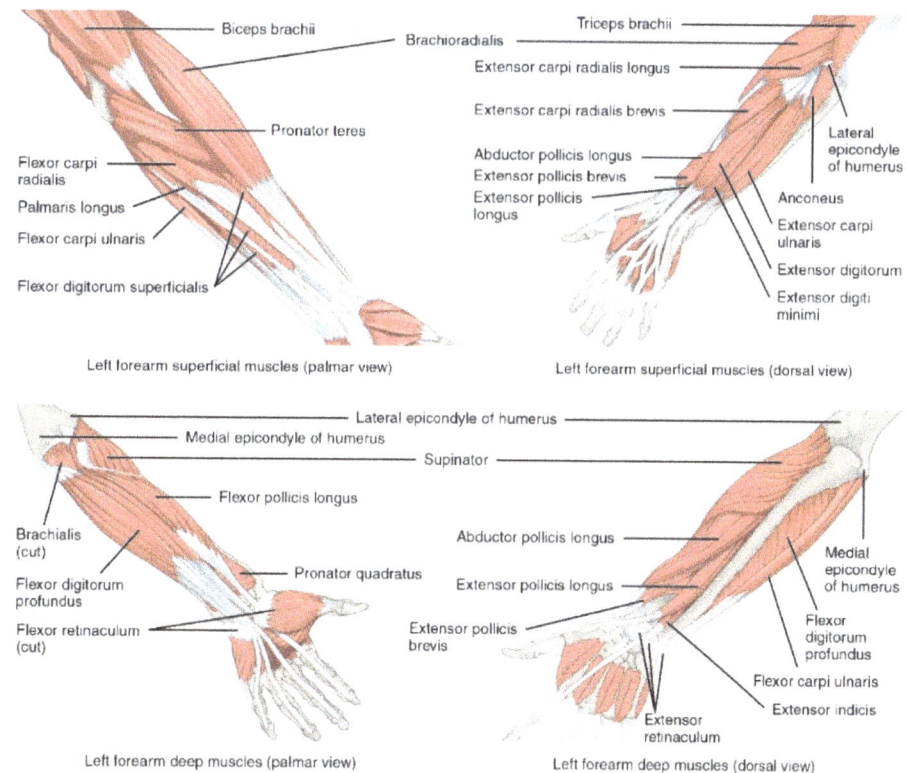

**Figure 1.78** Overview of major muscles affecting arm movement. (Data source: OpenStax; https://commons.wikimedia.org/wiki/File:1120_Muscles_that_Move_the_Forearm.jpg; Creative Commons Attribution 4.0)

## *Intrinsic Muscles of the Hands*

The *intrinsic muscles* of the hand, although super small in size, are essential for fine motor control, proprioceptive feedback, and adaptive grip. These muscles reside entirely within the hand itself, unlike the longer extrinsic muscles that originate in the forearm, discussed above. They include the thenar and hypothenar muscles (controlling the thumb and little finger), the lumbricals, and the palmar and dorsal interossei, which enable finger abduction, adduction, and coordinated flexion-extension across multiple joints. In yoga *asana*, these muscles contribute to the integrity during weight-bearing through the hands. Even subtle adjustments in finger engagement can alter the distribution of pressure across the wrists and support more stable joints and load transfer upward through the lower appendicular skeleton.

In shapes such as Plank or Handstand, conscious activation of the fingers (especially pressing through the pads of the index finger and thumb or isometric engagement of external rotation in the forearm and hands) creates muscular doming or arching in the palm that better distributes or even reduces load on the carpal bones (akin to creating an arch in the foot with similar movements in the lower limbs). Careful engagement also enhances proprioceptive input that informs the body's sense of balance. Mindful cueing of such intrinsic hand engagement and intelligent load distribution can support ease in load-bearing shapes and may prevent strain, even strain arising from repetitive stress that occurs during daily living. Therapeutic yoga practices integrate shapes and movements that promote full hand articulation, tactile feedback, and grip strength; this focus can be especially helpful for students or clients who present with hypermobility or joint laxity, especially in the elbows.

## Kinesiology of the Forearms, Wrists, and Hands

The primary kinesiological considerations offered here are about what happens in the shoulders, arms and hands during inversions and half-inversions (see Figure 1.79 for a review of the bony structures). The biomechanics of the upper limbs, with particular focus on the regions from the elbows to the fingertips, require a nuanced understanding of the journey of force and the transfer of load through this region when the body is up-side-down and relies on the upper appendicular skeleton for weight-bearing. The biomechanics are much more complex than the straightforward load-bearing mechanics of the lower appendicular skeleton.

Whereas the bones of the legs bear weight transferred from above directly through stacked joints into the pelvis and axial skeleton, the arms have to transmit force through a longer, more spiraled and complex *musculoskeletal* and fascial/connective tissue pathway. In yoga shapes with load-bearing on the hands or arms (or even during a simple fall onto an outstretched hand), the relevant kinetic chain and load transfer begins at the palm and continues proximally through a series of dynamic articulations. It is key to understand the journey of force and the myofascial and musculoskeletal dynamics to be able to teach inversions and half-inversions safely and effectively.

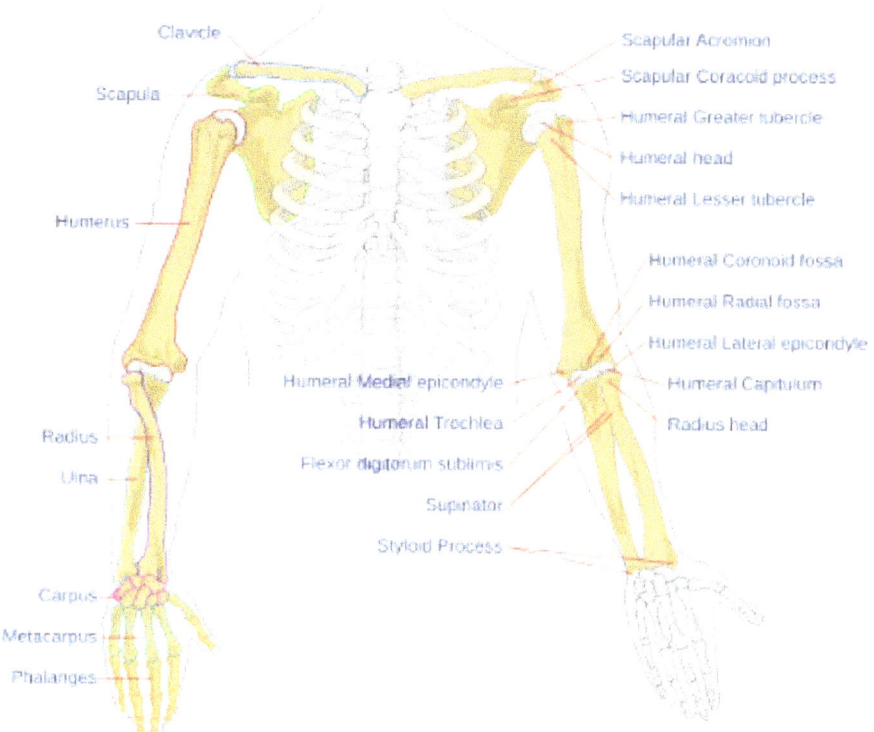

**Figure 1.79** Upper appendicular skeleton. (Data source: LadyofHats; https://commons.wikimedia.org/wiki/File:Human_arm_bones_diagram.svg; Creative Commons Public Domain)

### *Journey of Force During Load-Bearing in Inversions and Half-Inversions*

The journey of force travels first from the base of the hand through the carpal bones to the radius (the primary articulating forearm bone at the wrist). From there, force transfers across the interosseous membrane (the strong, fibrous sheet that bridges the radius and ulna), helping distribute load evenly through the forearm. The ulna then connects with the humerus via the humeroulnar joint, the anatomical elbow joint, which functions as a hinge to permit flexion and extension. At the elbow, the congruent fit between the trochlear notch of the ulna and the trochlea of the humerus provides mechanical stability, while the radial head articulates with the capitulum of the humerus to allow for rotational movements of the forearm.

Rotation of the forearm (i.e., pronation and supination) is controlled by the proximal and distal radioulnar joints. These actions are especially relevant in yoga *asana* in which the orientation of the palms and the alignment of the inner elbow creases can dramatically affect stability. For example, in Plank, Yoga Pushup, or Crow, subtle forearm rotation governs the degree of elbow flexion and the ability to maintain a stacked joint line from wrist to shoulder. The radiocarpal joint, where the distal radius meets the carpal bones, allows for wrist flexion, extension, and radial/ulnar deviation. This allows for the fine movements essential to distributing load in arm balances without overly compressing the carpal tunnel. Of great interest in the context of full or partial inversions is the fact that pronation of the forearm is mechanically linked to elbow extension, whereas supination is linked to elbow flexion. Additionally, neck extension triggers a reflex to extend the elbow.

This connection can be used to create more stability in the elbow during load-bearing in the arm:
- By pressing the inner hand into the earth (i.e., pronating the forearm) to create extension and lift through the elbow (firing up the triceps), and increasing stability in the shoulder joint
- By extending the neck when upside down and getting ready to lift into a head or handstand – for the latter, this means bringing the neck back and looking to toward the floor; for the former, it means pressing the back of the head into the hands that are placed anterior to the back of the head -- these mechanisms are explored further in Chapter 14 on Inversions.

The distal structures of the hand play a surprisingly significant role in stability and proprioception. The metacarpophalangeal (MCP) and interphalangeal (IP) joints, though small, must articulate freely to adapt to uneven pressure and support weight transfer during inversions. Intrinsic hand muscles and the flexors/extensors that originate in the forearm act to grip the mat and lift the arches of the hand. This doming action is not only protective for the wrist but also creates a crucial tension bridge from the palm all the way through the arm to the shoulder girdle.

To reiterate, the support of the shoulder girdle in contexts of load-bearing on the arms cannot come from bones alone. Unlike the pelvis and sacrum, which are stabilized by deep sockets and robust ligaments, the shoulder complex relies almost entirely on muscular and fascial coordination. From the scapula to the clavicle, and from the clavicle to the sternum, the upper limbs' force ultimately integrates into the rib basket through the sternoclavicular joint. This complex pathway in which force travels serves to highlight the combined importance of thoracic mobility, scapular stability, and clavicular alignment.

In practical yoga application, this means that alignment cues for the wrists and elbows account for the whole chain of action. Over-reliance on superficial arm muscles (like the deltoids or wrist extensors) can lead to compensatory strain; insufficient engagement of deep stabilizers (such as rotator cuff, serratus anterior, or intrinsic hand muscles) can reduce joint congruence. Teaching students to feel the whole line of force from palm to sternum fosters safety and sustainability in load-bearing shapes. Subtle shifts in alignment, such as engaging the fingertips, arching the palm, creating isometric engagement and deliberate directional movement, and tracking the inner elbow forward without collapsing the scapulae can make all the difference between creating muscular resilience versus cumulative strain.

## What's Ahead

Having established a thorough base of anatomical, structural, and kinesiological principles, the discussion can shift to applying these principles very concretely and tangibly in the practice, clinical use, and teaching of yoga *asana*. Section 2 explores major categories of yoga *asana* and weaves in the anatomy principles presented in Section 1. There will be redundant information; this repetition is intentional – it is offered to drive home the most important anatomical points for each type of *asana*, hopefully guiding yoga professionals toward an offering of movement that is well-grounded in sound anatomy and movement principles. It is also important to review Section 2 of *Integrated Holistic Yoga Psychology* to ensure a holistic and integrated approach that honors all aspects of the human experience, from the physical to the vital to the mental and emotional to the integration of wisdom and joy, as well as practices based in all eight limbs, from ethics to disciplined lifestyles, as well as breathwork and other practices.

# Section 2:

# Integrated Holistic Yoga Asana and Movement

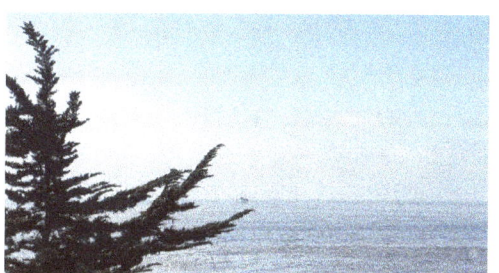

## Section 2 Introduction

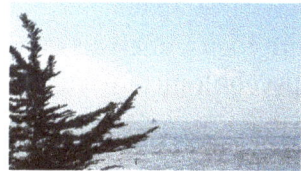

## Yoga Asana and Movement Overview

This section is dedicated to the foundations of the physical practices of yoga, including shapes, movement, and flow. The core competencies covered in Section 2 place heavy emphasis on the analysis of risk and benefits, intention and purpose, and contraindications for all covered shapes and movements. They identify essentials of yoga *asanas* via a range of pedagogical principles, optimal flow of an integrated yoga session, and appropriate planning for class composition and intention. Another strong content focus is accurately analyzing, selecting, and applying physical alignment principles (e.g., balancing effort and ease, creating a strong foundation, cultivating an engaged core, understanding lines of energy and healthful body mechanics, integrating yoga philosophy, and prioritizing safety) to maximize healthfulness and minimize risk. Strategies are covered for accurately discerning clients' need for, selecting, and demonstrating variations and adaptations of all yoga *asana* covered – with commensurate skill development for demonstration, observation, and attention to individuals' unique needs and resources. Particular emphasis is placed on alignment and practice instructions that honor human beings of all body shapes, conditioning, age, health status, backgrounds, and psychological wellbeing. Focus is placed on mindfulness in all layers of human experience (body, energy, mind, intuition, community), as well as on neuroception, interoception, proprioception, and exteroception during all movements and shapes. Integration of anatomical principles underscores the need for proper alignment and safety as well as healthful and functional movement. Integration of philosophical concepts underscores the need for thoughtful intention for and purpose of each selected practice in a given class.

With regard to shapes and movements presented, this Section anatomically, pedagogically, and didactically analyzes and provides examples in the following categories of shapes:

- *Upright standing*
- *Arm standing*
- *Upright seats*
- *Twists*
- *Forward folds*
- *Backbends*
- *Inversions*
- *Restoratives*

The first three categories are foundational in that they address shapes from the perspective of how individual practitioners are grounded on the earth – either through feet, hands, or seat (sitz bones and legs). The next three categories address shapes from the perspective of types of movements in various planes, with shapes in the sagittal, frontal, and transverse planes of movement. These three categories generally emerge from either standing, arm standing or seats; with some prone and supine shapes mixed in. The final two categories offer shapes that are psychologically or emotionally of great value, with inversions presenting shapes that can be supportive for emotional and mental resilience and restoratives offering practices that address affective and behavioral self-regulation as well as addressing specific nervous system states from a polyvagal theory perspective.

Given a healthcare and allied healthcare focus, analysis is encouraged to address unique and idiosyncratic physical, emotional, or psychological needs of the clients or students represented in the various types of setting in which yoga *asana* may be provided. All yoga *asana* teachings or clinical services addressed in this book are placed into the context of integrated holistic yoga, giving equal importance to all limbs of yoga, addressing all layers of human experience, and offering intentional and purposeful classes that are accessible and of benefit to all individuals and their unique biopsychosociocultural context and community. The deep grounding of yoga *asana* in a greater psychological and philosophical system of understanding the practice underscores that movement and movement practices are never divorced or separate from other layers of human experience (e.g., vitality, mind, emotions, actions, relationships), and their communal and collective applications.

In honoring the complexity that is yoga *asana*, it may be helpful to understand the study and practice of integrated holistic yoga as akin to committing to reading a complex novel with many plot lines, complex characters, and unexpected twists and turns. The study and practice of integrated holistic yoga is the very antithesis of scrolling through social media. It invites deep concentration and focus, rather than distraction and reaction. It invites cultivation of open awareness, profound insight, and dedicated compassion – all requiring curiosity, forethought, contemplation, humility, and passion. Practicing with commitment to integrated holistic yoga means understanding life as a complex web of relationships, as an intricate network of causes and conditions, with individual and collective impacts, applications, and implications. Depth of focus and openness to complexity – commitment to learning, unlearning, and relearning – are key to understanding how to provide yoga *asana* in the most therapeutic and auspicious manner.

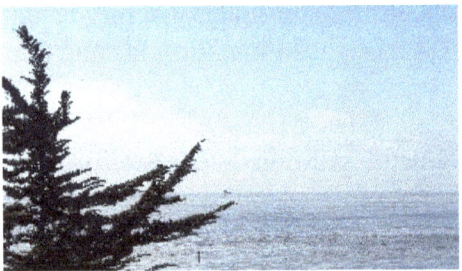

## Yoga Asana and Movement Learning Objectives

1. Understand, analyze, and discuss the implications of the benefits, potential risks, contraindications, and intentions of yoga asana practice, with the capacity to address each of these aspects within the following highly relevant human systems:
   a. anatomical, especially musculoskeletal, myofascial, and neuromuscular systems
   b. nervous system – emotional, energetic, self-regulatory
   c. nervous system – cognitive, mental, and memory
   d. other physiological systems (e.g., endocrine, immune)

2. Understand, analyze, and discuss issues related to working with physical pain and resistance:
    a. differentiating pain from discomfort and soreness
    b. understanding resistance in the context of physical contributors, neuromuscular factors, and emotional or mental influences
    c. apply appropriate guidance to support students as they work with pain, remaining within appropriate scope of practice
    d. apply appropriate guidance to support students as they work with resistance, remaining within appropriate scope of practice

3. Understand, analyze, demonstrate, and cue essential yoga *asana*, including competence in:
    a. demonstrated understanding the sequencing of an integrated holistic yoga class
    b. appropriate planning in the context of class composition and intention
    c. accurately analyzing, selecting, and applying alignment principles (e.g., balancing effort-ease, strong foundation, engaged core, lines of energy, healthful body mechanics, integration of *yamas*, assuring safety)
    d. accurately discerning the needs for, selecting, and demonstrating variations and adaptations
    e. proper cueing for mindfulness in all realms (body, breath/energy, mind, intuition, community)
    f. proper cueing for neuroception, interoception, proprioception, and exteroception

4. Be able to list, analyze, and provide examples of all categories of shapes covered; specifically, be able to define and provide guidance for:
    a. upright standing
    b. arm standing
    c. upright seats
    d. forward folds
    e. twists
    f. backbends
    g. inversions
    h. restoratives

## Yoga Asana and Movement Recommended Readings

Baginski, C. (2020). *Restorative yoga: Relax. restore. re-energize*. Alpha Books.
Bondy, D. (2020). *Yoga where you are*. Shambhala.
Heyman, J. (2024). *The teacher's guide to accessible yoga*. Rainbow Mind.
Lasater, J. H. (2020). *Yoga myths*. Shambhala.
Lasater, J. H. (2021). *Teaching yoga with intention*. Shambhala.
Lasater, J. H. (2017). *Restore and rebalance: Yoga for deep relaxation*. Shambhala.
Mitchell, J. (2019). *Yoga biomechanics*. Handspring.
Rountree, S. (2020). *The professional yoga teacher's handbook*. Bloomsbury.

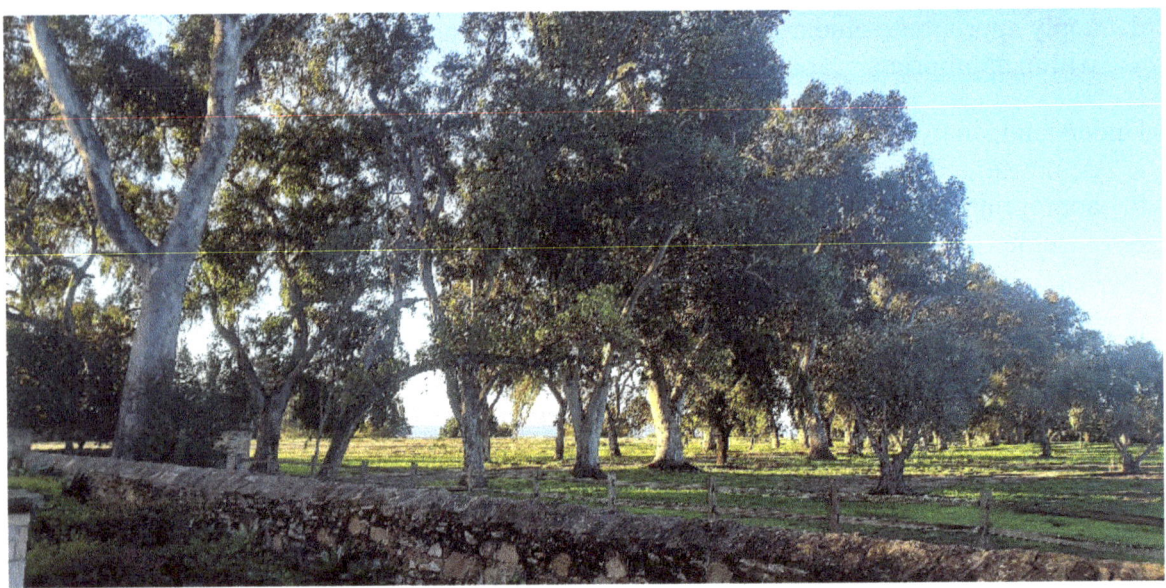

# Chapter 7: Principles of Integrated Holistic Yoga Asana and Movement

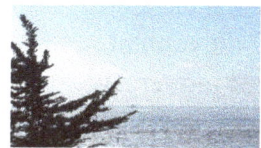

Yoga *asana* as practiced in integrated holistic yoga is always embedded in the greater context of all eight limbs and the biopsychosociocultural circumstances of students and teachers or clients and clinicians. It is important for yoga professionals to understand that they are not simply teaching people how to attain an outer shape, but instead, that they are teaching clients how to become wise practitioners who can make informed, empowered, self-efficacious, and knowledgeable personal choices about the practice of yoga. A wholesome yoga session includes not only instruction about how to move into and out of a shape, but empowers individuals to listen to feedback from their body, breath, and mind and to respect this information with truthfulness and non-violence. Successful engagement in yoga *asana* is more focused on cueing interoception, neuroception, proprioception, and exteroception than on attaining any outer shape. Cueing is focused more on inviting action and experimenting with movement than on embodying a pre-defined outer expression of a shape. This type of cueing invites agency and empowers students to discover their inner teacher and wisdom. It reminds clients again and again to move from the inside out – based on their interoception, neuroception, and proprioception – rather than striving for an outer goal.

## Intention and Purpose Related to Teaching Yoga Asana and Movement

Yoga professionals who have a clear intention or purpose for an offered practice tend to teach in a manner that is more integrated and holistic, and, as such more accessible, beneficial, and auspicious. Having intentionality for chosen shapes, breathwork, contemplations, and explorations means that the physical practice is not isolated from the other limbs of yoga and considers all *koshas* in the way yoga *asana* is taught. Selected intentions for the practice overall are effectively translated into intentionality and purpose in the practice *physically* (through proper cueing, demonstration, and adjustment), *energetically* (through creating appropriate sequences, environments, relationships, and breathwork), *cognitively* (through relevant verbal cues, contents, and information), and *emotionally* (through polyvagal co-regulation and instruction offered with compassion and kindness).

With regard to yoga *asana* per se, additional physical intentions – aligned with the intention for the practice overall – may include, but not be limited to, the following examples. These really are simply a few examples of *annamaya-kosha*-related intentions; actual possibilities are almost infinite and perhaps only limited by a teacher's or clinician's creativity and depth of knowledge.
- Core-strengthening shapes and movement
- Shapes and movement for physical strengthening and resilience
- Shapes and movement for balance and stability

- Physically restorative or energetically calming shapes and movement (e.g., moving individuals from *rajas* to *tamas* to *sattva*)
- Physically energizing or energetically uplifting shapes and movement (moving individuals from *tamas* to *rajas* to *sattva*)
- Mindfulness-focused and embodied movement
- Concentration- or meditation-focused movement
- Functional movement for life off the mat

## Beneficence Related to Teaching Yoga Asana and Movement

Much of modern yoga *asana* has its roots in relatively recent history that was strongly influenced by the colonization of India by the British (as well as other European body aesthetics and physical refinement movements). The colonization of yoga occurred most profoundly in the context of practice and monetization of *asana* (as separate from the other limbs) in Western culture. Modern postural yoga bias and stereotyping of *asana* has altered the definition and perception of yoga as being (almost) synonymous with pure *asana*. *Asana*, in this context, has been presented by Western yoga proponents as primarily an exercise or physical fitness practice. Yoga *asana*, thus extracted from the other limbs of yoga, is more prone to have risks and contraindications than engagement in shapes and movements that are integrated with the ethical and lifestyle limbs of yoga; that are engaged in along with supportive, optimal, and rejuvenating breathing practices; and that integrate the conscious practice of the inner contemplative work of yoga, grounding physical practice in mindfulness, awareness, concentration, compassion, and insight. Yoga a*sana* that is integrated and holistic is practiced as one of many yogic practices and naturally becomes more accessible, inclusive, equitable, humble, compassionate, kind, respectful, and beneficial not only to the practitioner, but also to the practitioner's community and relationships.

### *Benefits of Integrated Holistic Shapes and Movement*

It is helpful for yoga professionals to know and be able to communicate potential benefits of yoga overall as well as of offered shapes or movements, without overstating or overpromising particular possible positive outcomes of the practice. It is helpful to clarify that benefits of shapes and movements depend on the overall intention of a class or session and that different benefits may be highlighted at different times. A summary of documented benefits for integrated holistic *asana* practice follows. This summary does not imply that everyone will reap these benefits or that yoga *asana* is practiced to strive for these benefits. It is provided as a summary that can help yoga professionals design and verbalize potential positive impacts of yoga overall. This listing is offered as a general overview only; benefits for each specific shape are covered in each commensurate yoga *asana* chapter.
- *Anatomical (muscular system and skeletal system) benefits* include, but may not be limited to, postural effects, muscle strengthening or lengthening, maintained muscle and bone mass, fascial release, structural/skeletal alignment, enhanced physical balance, pain reduction, and more wholesome functional movement in day-to-day life, extension of healthspan (if not lifespan).

- *Nervous system impacts* include, but may not be limited to, stress reduction, increased resilience, top-down bottom-up integrations, enhanced mindfulness, entry into a state of flow, increased time spent in a ventral vagal state, and emotional regulation and co-regulation.
- *Other physiological benefits* include, but may not be limited to, positive impacts on organ systems, such as the circulatory system (e.g., improved blood pressure, increased heart rate variability), digestive system (e.g., enhanced digestion, decreased acid reflux), endocrine system (e.g., reduction in stress hormone production, increase in certain neurotransmitters, such as GABA), lymphatic/immune system (e.g., increased resilience to infectious disease; enhanced lymphatic flow), and respiratory system (e.g., more optimally functional breathing, greater lung capacity, smoother flow of breath that decreases symptoms of asthma).
- *Emotional and/or energetic effects* include, but may not be limited to, reduction of anxiety and depression, resolution of complex trauma, enhanced mood, enhanced sleep, greater coping capacity, and emotional resilience.
- *Cognitive and mental benefits* include, but may not be limited to, enhanced memory, concentration, and attention; improved learning capacity; neurogenesis in the hippocampus; neuroplasticity; improved recall; increased creativity; and sharpened concentration.

> *"...there is no such thing as a 'completed' or 'ideal' posture.*
> *Each posture is an ever-evolving,*
> *constantly moving energy phenomenon*
> *that is different from day to day,*
> *moment to moment, and person to person."*
> (Schiffmapossiblenn, 1996, p. 75)

## *Contraindications For Particular Shapes and Movements*

Yoga professionals need to understand contraindications for particular types of shapes and movements to support student and client wellness and health. This means having sufficient knowledge to assess and communicate which types of movements and shapes are most to least appropriate for which types of individuals or conditions. This knowledge is then applied in an individualized manner to each person who is present in the session through appropriate cueing, modeling, demonstration, variation, and attention to how people move and respond. Minimally, yoga professionals caution clients with the below-listed preexisting conditions as possible contraindications for a particular yoga session or given shapes or movements. Individuals with such conditions can be advised to seek guidance from a medical provider about how to vary and adapt their yoga *asana* practice to make it safe for their bodies and minds. Clients with significant challenges may best be asked to secure medical or psychological clearance before coming to a yoga practice designed for the general public (i.e., for students presumed healthy).
- Extant illness or medical condition
  - e.g., glaucoma, hyper- or hypotension, scoliosis, osteoporosis, cancer, herniated disk, sciatica, stenosis
- Extant injury
  - e.g., torn rotator cuff muscle(s), hamstring strain or sprain, sacroiliac joint dysfunction, carpal tunnel syndrome, ligaments tears (e.g., torn anterior cruciate ligament in the knee)

- Conditions of special considerations
  - e.g., hypermobility in joints, joint replacements
- Pregnancy by trimester
- Mental, emotional, or cognitive challenges (e.g., PTSD, panic disorder, depression, dementia, cognitive decline)

## *Potential Risks or Challenges of Some Shapes or Movements*

Yoga professionals need to be familiar with how particular shapes or movements may stress certain bodies and how they may result in injury or potential harm, especially if engaged in repetitively. Knowledge about potential risk or challenge is communicated openly and clearly in a manner that encourages safety and offers strategies for risk reduction. It is not offered in a way that over- or understates the risk, nor as a way of creating an excessive sense of vulnerability or fragility in students or clients. Through appropriate cueing, modeling, demonstration, variation, and attention to how individuals move and respond, risk can be ameliorated as healthy and functional movement patterns as well as inner or somatic awareness become the primary foci of instruction. In other words, language around potential risks is positive, emphasizing what people can do and how to engage in the most balanced variations and wholesome alignment options.

A few possible potential challenges or risks for a yoga session overall and some forms or movements in particular are listed below. It is helpful to stay mindful of these risks and to invite clients to listen to feedback from their *koshas* in making choices about how to engage with offered shapes and movements. It can be helpful for students to understand potential immediate, short-term, and long-term consequences of risks associated with particular practices. Yoga professionals can help by stressing that injury can result in the absence of significant pain in any given moment if shapes are engaged in in a way that creates repetitive stress in the practice over time (e.g., sacroiliac joint dysfunction due to excessive femoral leveraging as may happen in Pigeon or due to excessive spinal torquing as may happen in forced, bound twists with a fixed pelvis). The listing of potential risks and possible challenges that follows is a generic overview. Risks that are particular to specific shapes are covered in the context of these shapes and movements in later chapters. Some examples of potential risks of yoga *asana* practice include, but are not limited to:

- Hyperextension, hyperflexion, compression, or torquing of joints – e.g., ankles, knees, hips, elbows, wrists, facet joins in spine
- Compression of arteries – e.g., vertebral arteries, basilar artery at the base of the brain
- Sprain, strain, or tear to muscles, ligaments, or cartilage – e.g., hamstrings, Achilles tendon, plantar fascia, rotator cuff muscles, groin muscles, hip joint cartilage
- Nerve compression – beware of numbness, tingling, burning, pins and needles; beware of sharp or radiating (radicular) pain – e.g., prevent long-term nerve compression effects, such as sciatica, carpal tunnel syndrome, thoracic outlet syndrome
- Injury potential for sensitive areas – e.g., spinal discs, cervical spine, lumbar spine, sacroiliac joints
- Overheating and dehydration

## Practice Principles for Teaching of Yoga Asana and Movement

In teaching yoga *asana*, yoga professionals *explicitly* attend to a number of teaching elements as they develop and implement their classes or sessions. They remember that practice principles covered here are only one aspect of the overall teaching elements endorsed by integrated holistic yoga (see the *Teaching with Intention SANKALPA Spiderweb* in Section 2 of *Integrated Holistic Yoga Psychology;* Brems, 2025). Regarding yoga *asana* teaching per se, yoga professionals are encouraged to use all of the following practice principles to plan sessions carefully and offer appropriate adaptations and variations for each shape or movement to be taught. It is important to practice discernment and plan carefully which shapes and movements to include and in what order, especially given the context of student backgrounds and overarching intentions developed for a given practice.

It is helpful to remember the following broad guidelines for developing a yoga *asana* sequence:
- Have a clear intention for the session overall and each chosen shape, starting with the peak shape.
- Assess if all needed props are available and (re)plan physical forms and movements accordingly.
- Decide on variations and adaptations that will be offered and demonstrated.
- Understand and know how to verbalize the risks and benefits for each chosen shape.
- Be aware of contraindications and how they may apply to the students or clients who are expected to come to the class
- Be familiar with verbal and possible physical adjustments for all shapes and movements that are planned.
- Prepare to demonstrate the most accessible (not the extreme or 'advanced') versions of planned shapes.
- Think through language choices for cueing shapes and movements ahead of class time.
- Have proper cueing prepared in mind and notes, including for transitions from shape to shape. It is not enough to have a general idea; instead it helps to have specific notions about how to cue individuals from each preceding to the subsequent shape (e.g., it does little to know how to cue an individual into Downward Facing Dog from Mountain, when the planned sequence starts from Table Top.)

### *Sequencing with Focus on Yoga Asana and Movement*

Careful planning is essential to sequencing each yoga session as a whole, to honor the intention of the practice, to integrate principles of yoga psychology, and to build safely toward more challenging physical shapes and movements as sessions progress. Following is a quick reminder of sequencing suggestions that were covered in depth in *Integrated Holistic Yoga Psychology*. If this sequencing outline is not yet ingrained in memory, it may be helpful to double back to Section 2 of that first Volume (in the series of three) for a thorough review. Understanding sequencing is crucial to offering yoga in healthcare settings and with any vulnerable population of students and clients as it minimizes risk and maximizes beneficence, intentionality, and accessibility. The preparation that goes into careful sequencing is well worth the time investment as it creates a more client-centered and respectful practice offering.

*Preparation and Setting the Stage*

Three aspects of preparation can be offered in an adaptable order depending on intention, population, setting, and type of class (e.g., cohort versus new students each time). The order is less important than the idea that all of these aspects of setting the stage need to be addressed. The order can be varied even from session to session within a series, especially when dealing with a cohort of students. For example, if the same clients are present each week, setting stage may be less necessary in the later classes of a series.

- Opening comments
  - welcome participants
  - set the stage, especially as related to possible physical demands
  - introduce props that may be needed for the physical practice
- Conditioned stimulus for mindfulness to signal the start of the practice
- Presentation of the theme or intention for the session
  - ground the practice in an explicit aspect of yoga psychology and/or neuroscience that will be deliberately integrated into the shape and movement practice
  - carry the overarching psychological intention into teaching and cueing shapes and movements, both explicitly and implicitly
  - in a multi-class sequence, refer back and tie to prior times when particular shapes and movements were practiced

*Centering and/or Breathing Practices*

The below-listed practices can be chosen separately, in combination, sequenced as listed, or integrated with one another (e.g., the opening centering may be merged with a breath awareness practice; the intention may be embedded in the opening centering). The exact choice may depend on session length, client population, intention, or context. Two aspects could also be interwoven as one seamless practice (e.g., using breath as the centering).

- Opening centering to arrive in the present moment, space, and community
  - cue students into attunement of all *koshas* to bring all layers of experience into awareness – move through the *koshas*, starting with *annamaya*, then *pranamaya*, *manomaya*, *vijnanamaya*, and finally *anandamaya*
  - call forth attention and awareness to support interoception, neuroception, and proprioception as guides for movements and shapes
  - invite observation of the physical body for increased physical self-efficacy and self-understanding
- Breathing practice
  - practice a particular breath that may help support the planned physical practice
  - consider how the chosen breath may be used to accompany movement throughout the physical practice, and whether a different breathing practice may be indicated during particular phases of the practice (e.g., during cool-down)
- Intention setting for participants (individual *sankalpa*) – do not skip this offering
  - students' intention setting could instead be invited during the preparation phase – this choice depends on whether the teacher believes that the opening centering and breathing practice may support increased access to an intention

## Shapes and Movement Practice

### Choosing the Peak Shape(s)

Beyond setting a collective intention and creating a theme for the practice, choosing the peak shape(s) is the most crucial element that guides auspicious sequencing. All practices in the entire sequence need to align with session theme *and* serve a purpose vis-à-vis the intended peak shape(s). Choosing the peak, therefore, comes *before* planning specific physical warm-ups and preparations. To state this in another way, sequence *planning* is not done in the same order as sequence *implementation*. During implementation, of course, the peak shape(s) comes after warm-up and preparation. In choosing the peak shape(s),
- Have a sense of the needs and resources of the intended recipients of the practice
- Match the peak shape to class intention (or vice versa – the main point is to link peak and intention in a meaningful way)
- Have clarity about variations and adaptations for the peaks and all preparations that are possible in the context of participants and environment
- Be knowledgeable about adaptations that can be offered given available practice resources
- Have clarity which props will be necessary, available, and useful

The *asana* practice will, of course, invoke all *koshas*. Physical focus is offered to gain increased access to working with body, breath, mind, emotions, relationships, and action choices. All aspects of yoga psychology remain important. The following discussion highlights the physical practice choices and preparations. A more integrated holistic overview of sequencing (with a less specific focus on physical practice is offered in Section 2 of Volume 1).

### Warm-Up for the Peak Shape(s)

Physical warm-up is most efficiently and predictably offered via the six (or seven) movements of the spine. Specifically, healthy directions of warm-up motions in the spine include:
- *Flexion* (rounding or flexing forward)
- *Extension* (opening the heart – i.e., the front body)
- *Lateral flexion* (side-bending)
  - to the *right*
  - to the *left*
- *Rotation* (twisting)
  - to the *right*
  - to the *left*

Sometimes considered a seventh movement of the spine, there is also *axial spinal extension*. In this movement, the spine is elongated overall (e.g., as in Extended Mountain or Sun Breath). However, axial extension is due to a flattening of the spinal curves, not due to muscular action separating the vertebrae from one another (muscles separating the vertebrae to create *"length in the spine"* do not exist). Thus, some anatomy or movement professionals do not consider axial extension an active movement of the spine. However, axial extension is nevertheless useful as a warm-up.

Many variations are possible in each category of the spinal movements based on various orientations in space, such as engaging in them from quadruped, standing, seated, supine, or prone shapes, or in the context of yoga *kriya*. Choices of the specific orientation in space for the seven movements are guided by what is physically and psychologically appropriate for the chosen peak shape(s) to create a natural logical connection between the warm-up shapes and the pathway to the peak shape. The six or seven movements are a wonderful way to warm the body and invite blood flow, to gently engage all muscles and joints, and help shift mind states toward concentration, support vitality toward effort within ease and ease within effort, and encourage the emergence of wisdom and joy.

The following illustrations are offered as inspiration for the many ways in which the six or seven movements of the spine can unfold. From the base of the warm-up, preparation emerges to guide the practice further in the direction of the peak shape. Notably, if a practice runs longer than planned and needs to skip some of the sequenced practices, the recommendation is actually to stick to the warm-up and preparation and skip the peak shape, as the preparatory work does the real work of the practice emotionally, physically, and energetically.

*Warming Up with the Six Movements of the Spine*

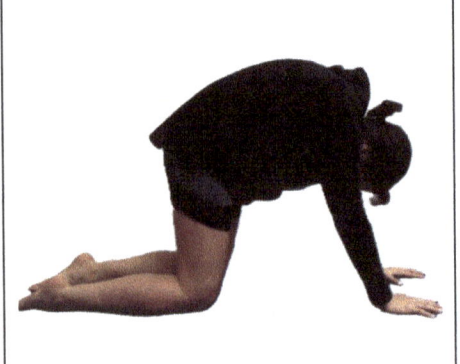
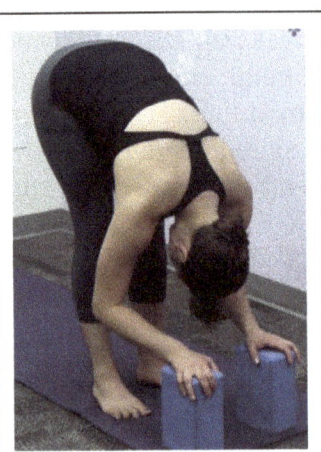
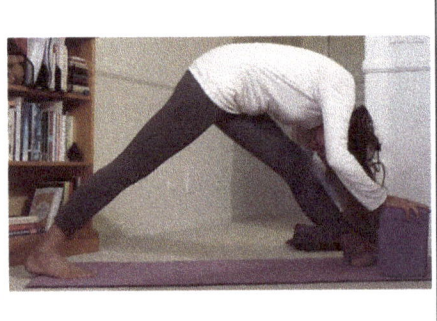

*Flexion – from various positions in space*

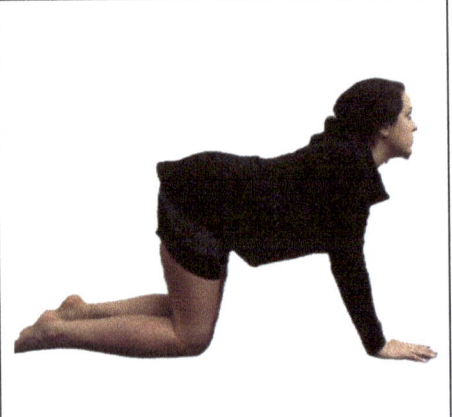
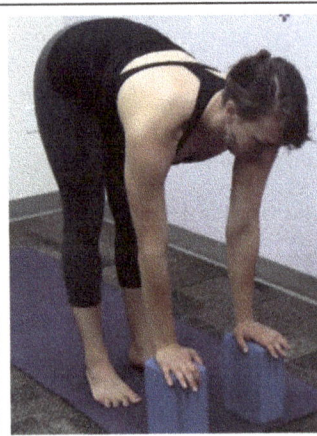
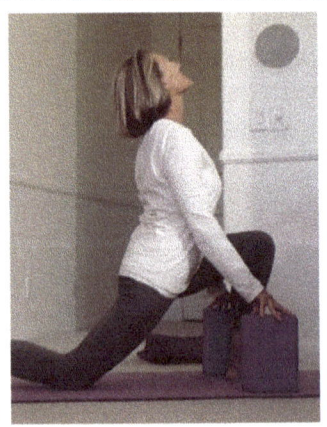

*Extension – from various positions in space*

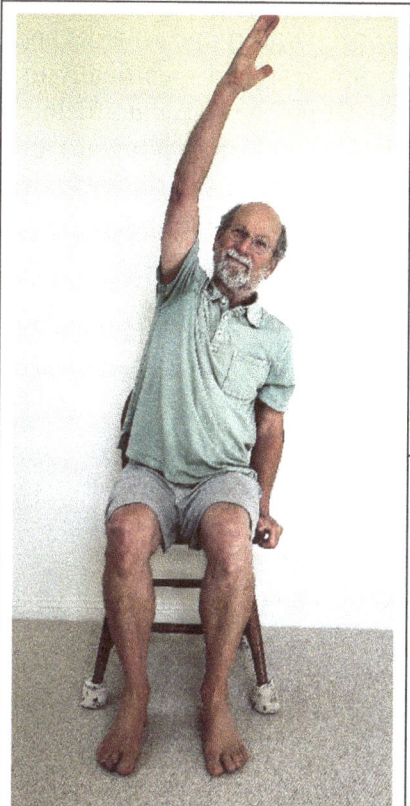
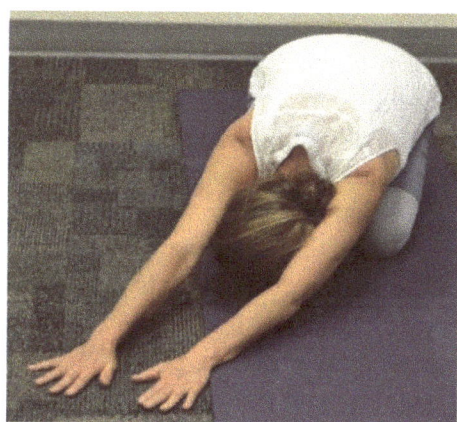
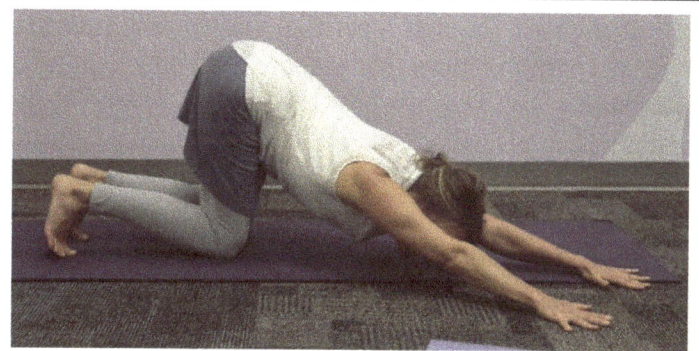

*Lateral Flexion/Extension Right and Left – from various positions in space*

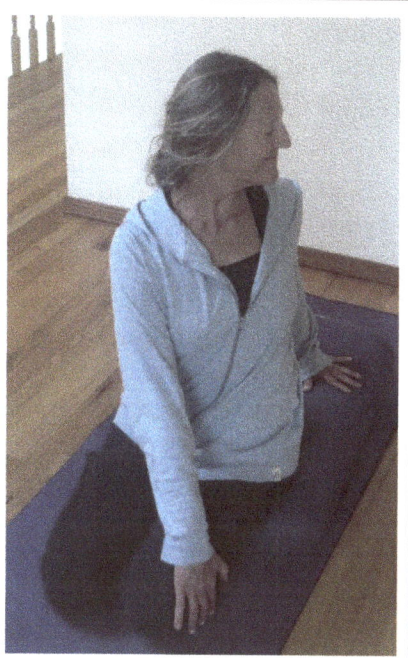
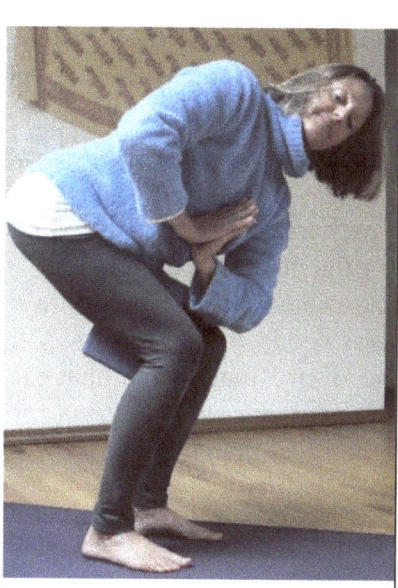
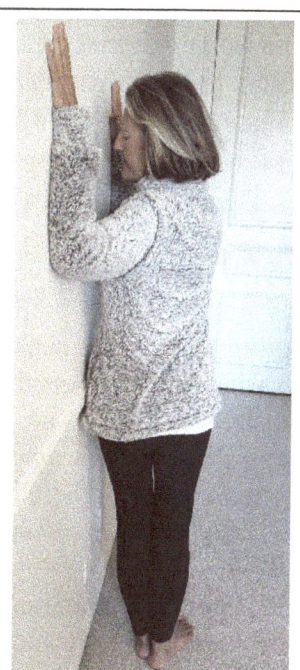

*Rotation Right and Left – from various positions in space*

### Preparation for the Peak Shape(s)

It is important to be intentional and purposeful about each choice of preparatory movements and shapes beyond warm-up via the six spinal movements. Preparations are designed specifically to lead students or clients into the direction of the peak shape – this is true physically/anatomically, energetically/emotionally, and mentally/ideationally. Preparations define a clear path toward an optimal experience of the peak shape in all layers of human experience – not just in the body. In other words, preparation is such that the peak shape needs to feel like a natural and logical outcome of the practices that preceded it, anatomically, energetically, psychology, mentally, and emotionally. As such, preparation meets the following purposes:

- Continue to warm the body and invite blood flow – with focus now on preparing the regions of the body most relevant to the peak shape (i.e., moving beyond the spinal movements), gently engaging relevant muscles, joints, and connective tissues
- Choose relevant dynamic and isometric stretching that progressively increases range of motion and ease through repetition in different muscular engagements and approaches
- Invite strength practices that prepare the body regions that need to create stability for the peak shapes
- Anatomically progress toward the peak shape: ground what needs to be grounded, open what needs to be opened, stabilize what needs to be stabilized for the peak
- Facilitate neuromuscular integration across a series of shapes that prepare the anatomy and nervous systems for new physical expressions and embodiment
- Energetically progress toward the peak shape by choosing a breathing pattern that can be maintained throughout and facilitates the peak shape
- Introduce or maintain breathing practices that are a logical link to the session and intention and peak shape
- Mentally and emotionally progress toward the peak shape – the peak is ideally never an emotional surprise, but rather more of an aha moment of recognition
- Relax the nervous system and invite a ventral vagal state
- Create curiosity, even joyful anticipation, for what is about to come

### Implementing the Peak Shape(s)

In moving through warm-up and preparation, yoga professionals ensure that their students or clients are thoroughly prepared for the peak shapes across all *koshas* before guiding them into it. When introducing the peak shape, teachers offer appropriate and tailored demonstrations along with variations that meet the diverse needs of their clients. Variations and demonstrations always emphasize that there is no 'advanced' or 'final' shape; that each variation and tailored expression the peak shape *is the shape that is accessible and healthful* for the individual in this particular moment and space. There is no other goal than to *be in the most person-centered and individually tailored embodiment of the shape.*

If time becomes a constraint in a yoga session, the best way to preserve the integrity of the sequence anatomically and psychologically is by omitting the peak shape rather than some of the preparatory shapes (unless deliberate redundancy has been incorporated in the preparation phase). This approach helps protect students from moving into the peak shape without the necessary support and readiness through all layers of experience. Once the peak shape is introduced, yoga professionals allow time for students to settle and reflect, facilitating an exploration of the shape's impact across the physical, energetic, mental, wise, and joyfully connected layers of human experience.

### Recovery Shapes

Recovery shapes are optional and often unnecessary when a sequence has been thoughtfully planned and skillfully delivered. Recovery shapes serve to neutralize any residual effects of previous shapes (whether anatomical, energetic, mental, or emotional) and ideally used only when a clear need arises, such as after particularly intense or demanding set of movements or shapes. In such cases, the best recovery is not another shape, but a moment at rest (in a logical physical position) to sense inward into the nervous system's reaction to the practice and the natural re-regulation that occurs automatically.

Similarly, rather than relying on counterposing to balance out a particular shape or movement, yoga professionals can emphasize transitions and pauses that help regulate the nervous system and support a shift into a ventral vagal state, fostering calm, safety, and integration. Introducing counterposes too early or too often in a sequence, particularly during the preparation phase, may disrupt the continuity of anatomical, energetic, emotional, mental, and relational intentions leading toward the peak shape. For example, in some heart-opening practices teachers alternate backbends with forward folds. This convention can be very counterproductive anatomically as well as energetically (in terms of arousal and affect) as these shapes can have very different physical or mental demands and emotional reverberations.

### Cool-Down and Calming Phase

The cool-down and calming phase offers an essential transition after the peak shape, allowing yoga professionals to help clients and students move toward re-regulation and re-grounding of the nervous system, managing arousal levels and settling emotional or physical exertion and challenge. Calming and gentle shapes, movements, and breaths at this point in the practice aim to reduce heart rate, cool the body, release unnecessary muscular effort, ease emotion and affect, and support gentle awareness and focus, thus creating conditions for deeper rest and integration of the practice. By facilitating neuromuscular settling and softening of the breath, teachers can guide students toward a more balanced energetic state, fostering *sattva* (or a ventral vagal nervous system state) and emotional steadiness. This calming phase of the session provides an opportunity to remain aligned with the communal and personal core intentions that were set at the beginning (and that were expressed in the other prior phases of the practice) while gently preparing for the stillness and receptivity of a silent *Savasana*.

### Inner Practices and Silent Savasana

Inner practices and a long, silent, and carefully supported *Savasana* offer a culminating space and moment for students to absorb the full arc of the practice and experience in all *koshas*. Yoga professionals can guide students into a resting or relaxation shape that emerges naturally from the physical and energetic trajectory of the session (i.e., the peak shape), ensuring that the body is fully supported (with physical props) and at ease psychologically. This closing phase may include a guided meditation or focused concentration that echoes the communal intention, allowing for a gentle recapitulation across the dimensions of body, breath, mind, intuition, and joy.

*Savasana* is the *pratyahara* of nothing – which means no outer or inner stimulation. Clients are invited to release the body to earth, the breath to the flow of *prana*, the mind to inner wisdom to rest in complete silence. Resting in silence completes the yoga journey, offering space for integration, spacious awareness, and deep restoration. Resting in *silence* means exactly that – there is no more talking (not even readings, quotes, or ponderings – this could happen before or after *Savasana*), no music, no intentional sound (e.g., no sound bowl, no simulated nature sounds), no interruptions. It is helpful to let clients know beforehand about how long the silence will last and how the yoga professional will cue the end of Savasana (e.g., noting something like "*now rest in silence for about 3 minutes until my voice brings you back*"). A deliberate process is then used to cue clients back to alertness and a seat, ready for a session closing.

## Closing Comments and Gratitude

Closing comments provide a meaningful opportunity for yoga professionals to bring the arc of the practice full circle by reconnecting to the communal class theme and each individual's personal guiding intention. The final reflection can invite students to identify conscious takeaways, recall their personal or shared intention, and dedicate the benefits or merits of their practice with a sense of purpose beyond the self and toward community wellbeing. Linking the work done on the mat to daily life and relationships reinforces functional movement insights and encourages emotional integration off the mat or outside the clinical office. A sincere expression of gratitude by the teacher or clinician – toward the practice, the group, and the individual efforts made by each student – adds a beautiful conclusion to the experience with a tone of presence, connection, and reverence for what the yoga has to offer. Such expression of gratitude is not performative; to be meaningful, it is authentic and comes from the heart.

> ### Why no Namaste at the End of Class
>
> Increasing numbers of yoga teachers are choosing not to use the word namaste to end their classes, out of a growing awareness of its cultural and linguistic origins and concerns about cultural appropriation. In its original context, namaste is a respectful greeting in several South Asian languages, most notably Hindi and Sanskrit, used in both daily life and spiritual settings. While it is often loosely translated as "I bow to you" or "the divine in me honors the divine in you," these interpretations are frequently romanticized or oversimplified in Western yoga contexts. Ending class with namaste can reflect a superficial or decontextualized borrowing from Indian culture, especially when used without a full understanding of its roots. Furthermore, some South Asian practitioners have expressed discomfort with the commercialization and misuse of the term in the global yoga industry. In response, many teachers are opting for more inclusive or culturally respectful ways to close practice, such as a simple bow, a moment of silence, or a heartfelt expression of gratitude. The Integrated Holistic Yoga lineage has chosen not to close practice with namaste, in recognition of the term's cultural complexity and as an expression of cultural humility.

## *Optimization of Opportunities for Physical Safety*

Auspicious teaching integrates optimized opportunities for safety very explicitly in all teaching methods and interactions with students without scaring students. Humans are resilient; we do not want to discourage exploration and growth. As humans, we can and must expand beyond our comfort zone eventually – we simply do not want to push too far too fast. This auspicious pacing can be recapitulated in a movement practice by encouraging clients to play at their edges, slowly expanding them or pulling back (e.g., if there is a tendency to overdo) as needed. Sometimes, the comfort zone that needs expanding is not in the body – it may be emotional or mental aversion, attachment, or confusion that need to flex and stretch more. In such cases, expanding the comfort zone may mean accepting that it is more healthful to do less rather than more, to let shapes emerge from the inside out rather than to force the body into outer shapes that do not serve.

Speaking anatomically and physiologically, teaching strategies honor physical safety by working within healthful physical boundaries and wise application of body mechanics, especially when working in healthcare and mental healthcare settings, where yoga professionals may encounter greater vulnerability in students or clients. The offerings of a yoga session are made with attention to how the practice reverberates physically and energetically for the individuals who are present with clear invitations to create a practice that serves the bioindividual physical needs of each client. A few physical safety guidelines include, but are not limited to the following:
- Maintain healthful range of motion to protect muscles, ligaments, and joints
- Safely work at the edges or boundaries of flexibility: maximum edge, intermediate edge, and minimum edge (White, 2007)
- Understand and make healthful use of extant physical reflexes
- Learn how to differentiate discomfort from pain
- Coordinate movement with breath
- Honor and understand pain signals

Teaching also honors physical safety by working within yogic principles of ethics and commitment to an integrated holistic, and therefore often emotionally and psychologically transformative, yoga *asana* practice. Especially when working in mental healthcare or behavioral health, it is important to remember that teaching yoga is not primarily about the body, but also about energetic wellness, emotional resilience, and mental health. Sometimes, the practice seeks to change students' emotional relationship to a particular *asana* to find physical safety. A few safety guidelines related to teaching *asana* within the context of the *yamas* and *niyamas* include, but are not limited to the following:
- Honor the *yamas* by working with the discernment of non-violence, truthfulness, abundance, moderation, and non-grasping for a deeper shape
- Integrate the *niyamas* by inviting purity in the work, discipline, introspection, contentment, and devotion to a purpose beyond physical exercise
- Reground into the philosophical and anatomical intentions for the practice
- Work with patience, consistency, and regularity to create an environment that optimizes the opportunity for students to feel safe, supported, and properly challenged
- Cultivate a sense of personal responsibility for your teaching and for your practice
- Always bring compassion, joy, lovingkindness, and patience to the offered practice and invite the same emotions in clients or students

Physical safety often also rest on the discerning use of supports. This does not simply mean offering yoga props to students, but also means that the teacher uses props, integrates such supports into demonstrations, and is very explicit and clear that the use of supports and prop may be the most obvious sign of an advanced practice – a practice that honors inner needs, not outer shapes. A few helpful suggestions follow but by no means are these the only strategies for this particular teaching caution. More cautions are provided throughout, as individual shapes are discussed; it is helpful to learn as many of these hints as possible.

- Use props freely, especially in demonstrations
- Always offer choices, variations, and options
- *Invite*, do not demand or direct, and generally defer to students' or clients' judgment about their own body, breath, energy, and mind
- Be thoughtful about which shapes and variations to demonstrate and how to demonstrate them
- Default to verbal adjustment cues whenever possible
- Never use physical adjustment without consent
- Never use physical adjustment with force (review Section 2 in Volume 1 about the ethical and respectful use of physical adjustments and interventions)

## General Movement and Alignment Principles and Cues

Physical alignment and movement principles and cues are relevant to all *koshas*, although *annamaya* and *pranamaya* may be most explicitly invoked. It is helpful in cueing physical alignment to pay particular attention to functional movement skills and transferable activation skills that bring strength and stability into daily activities. It is more helpful to students to realize how *asana* can support their physical wellbeing in daily life than to strive for a complicated outer shape that has no relevance to daily movements off the mat. Some common yoga forms and movements have no direct applicability to healthful physical movement and yet hold much inherent risk. It is important to consider the risk-benefit ratio for such shapes. A few examples may include (especially the extreme versions of) Shoulderstand, Plow, Triangle, Pigeon, and Twists with a fixed pelvis. Following are several sets of cueing suggestions that serve to invite an integrated holistic yoga practice that optimizes the opportunity for the whole person to show up in the yoga *asana* practice. Offering diverse strategies and approaches to yoga *asana* supports the notion of creating intentionality, facilitating accessibility, and supporting beneficence.

### Emphasizing Action, Not Shape in Cueing and Explaining Asana

Attuned and experienced yoga professionals emphasize cueing *actions* rather than prescribing outcomes or outer alignment, focusing on how a movement is initiated and experienced rather than how an embodied shape looks from the outside. In this approach, instructions highlight dynamic stability and movement over static holding of shapes, and encourage students to attune to internal sensations via interoception, proprioception, and kinesthetic awareness, rather than aiming for external aesthetic standards. Teachers may guide clients to enter shapes from the inside out, using activation cues that support dynamic, isometric, or active engagement as appropriate. Demonstrations and verbal instructions are used to communicate principles of skillful movement and muscular engagement (e.g., scapular mobilization, shoulder stabilization, or spinal alignment), offering clients tools for the practice on the mat and for daily life. This way of teaching helps bridge the gap between mat-based exploration and real-life application. For example, it might help translate spinal and hip mechanics in yoga *asana* to practical movements such as lifting objects or reaching while twisting.

### *Balancing Effort and Ease for Responsiveness in Asana*

*Effort* represents the commitment to work toward wholesome physical expressions; as humans, we cannot relax our way to wisdom. We have to work to apply yogic values, to remain clear and focused in our motivations, and to remember that each moment is important. Equally important, *ease* represents the commitment to stay playful and honor safety amidst physical effort; as humans, we cannot force our way to enlightenment either. We have to stay light-hearted, open-minded, and easeful to be able to find wisdom, compassion, and awareness without becoming attached to the fruits of our labor. Cueing ease and effort in a yoga *asana* practice can be accomplished in a variety of ways. Following are a few ideas for cues and concepts:

- In annamaya kosha
  - balance strength and mobility
  - balance grounding and expansion
  - move with compassion
  - play at the edges, neither giving up too early nor pushing too hard
  - release stressful (excessive) physical effort (i.e., trying too hard) to reduce risk for injury
  - avoid zoning out or blissing out (i.e., not trying enough) and losing attention or integration
  - engage muscular power rather than hanging in the joints
  - draw inward and upward rather than losing tone
  - invite a sense of easeful rebound and expansiveness from a strong foundation
  - ground down with strength to expand up with ease
  - create some challenge within ease to support the building of physical strength and power
- In pranamaya kosha
  - balance exertion and rest
  - soften the breath and expand the exhalation to find ease
  - focus on the inhalation to invite more vitality
  - balance cooling and heating
  - balance the nervous system or *gunas* to find *sattva* and ventral vagal presence
  - create sympathetic mobilization to overcome fatigue or sluggishness
  - invite restful letting go to counter anger or aversion
  - balance control and surrender to find ease in effort or effort in ease
- In manomaya kosha
  - release stressful mental expectation and judgment
  - invite concentration to overcome zoning out
  - be spacious, not space
  - invite compassion in the face of harsh expectations
  - find lovingkindness during perceived failure
  - release any forcing of outer shapes and embrace the inner experience of the practice
  - temper wanting with letting be

*Working from Edges to the Center Versus Working from the Center to Edges*

While working on and cueing for all of the above principles related to working with the body, it is very useful to make discerning choices about whether to invite students to work from the periphery toward the center or whether to work from the center to the periphery. A few helpful hints are offered here; yet, as is true for all skills, observation of students is crucial to guiding cueing.
- Finding the most auspicious direction can be helpful especially for beginners
    - some have less awareness at the center than at the edges – for these students, cues are best focused on the center to help maintain attention at the places that count for stability
    - while this is the less common scenario, some students have more sensitivity to their extremities – for these students cueing may start at the edges, and then moves to center
    - for many students, distal parts of the body tend to stay put once the core is settled
    - for many students focus at the end on the distal edges can mean losing integration at the center; this is true especially for less experienced students
    - for some students focus on the center means a loss of control at the extremities
- Examples of distal to proximal cueing – that is, cueing from the edges inward or upward to the core or torso
    - from the feet to the calves to the knees to the thighs to the hips
    - from the hands to the elbows to the upper arm to the shoulder to the chest
- Examples of proximal to distal cueing –cueing from the core or torso downward or outward
    - from the hips to the thighs to the knees to the calves to the feet
    - from the chest to the shoulders to the upper arms to the elbows to the hands
    - from the belly to the hips to the legs

*Proximal stability trains distal athleticism*
Stuart McGill

*Creating Physical Grounding, Expansion, and Stability*

Teaching *asana* skillfully means helping students create somatic, energetic, and mental awareness and wisdom. This intention means working with grounding and settling, building a sturdy and reliable foundation; expansion and freedom, inviting lightness, playfulness, joy, and exploration; and stability and adaptability in body (e.g., core, foundation), breath (e.g., optimal functional breathing), and mind (e.g., soft focus, mindful attention). A few ideas related to grounding, expansion, and stability follow here. Many more are offered for each type of *asana* in this Section and it is recommended to use as many of these strategies as possible. A table of cueing for grounding, expansion, and stability for all *koshas* is included in *Integrated Holistic Yoga Psychology* (Section 2). Cueing tips for grounding, expansion, and stability by categories of shapes is offered below in Chapters 8 to 14.

*Physical Grounding*

Physical grounding emphasizes a strong foundation – or downward, strengthening lines of energy – wherever the body meets the floor. Possible physical (and energetic) cueing includes, but is not limited to the following ideas:

- Firmly ground through the body parts that meet the floor
- Imagine growing roots into the earth to ground deeply
- Use the exhalation to support a sense of settledness, a grounding energy
- Find a bounce-back of uplifting energy through pressing into the ground, combining opposite lines of energy
- Ground the limbs in line with gravity
- Anchor the limbs or the core or any other body part
- Ground through healthful alignment
- Anchor into inner awareness of sensation (interoception)
- Ground and steady the mind with focus and mindfulness

### *Physical Expansion*

Physical expansion involves upward or uplifting lines of energy through the limbs and the crown of the head. It is about creating space without losing engagement and strength. Expansiveness can arise out of groundedness through gravitational rebound. Expansiveness can manifest in the body (a rising upward or outward), in the breath (especially on the inhalation), and in the mind, both emotionally (being receptive to whatever feelings may arise) and mentally (being open to new possibilities). Possible physical (and energetic) cueing includes, but is not limited to the following ideas:

- Find spaciousness, expansion, and openness wherever possible – through the crown or the extremities
- Once grounded and stable, invite joyful extension at the edges
- Invite a sense of energy flowing from the core to the edges, allowing that energy to guide the edge of the shape (sometimes finding flow means backing away, sometimes it means dancing or playing at the edge, and sometimes it means exploring reaching farther)
- Maintain a light-hearted focus and soft attention, using *drishti* (not laser-like gaze), especially in balancing shapes
- Be mindful not to hyperextend or overstretch – be careful not to abuse any physical propensity for flexibility
- Continuously monitor the balance of strength or engagement (groundedness) and flexibility or extension (joyfulness)

### *Physical Stability*

Stability refers to the ability to withstand force. Stability is *adaptability;* that is, it is not forceful or rigid but dynamic and ever-evolving based on inner and outer stimuli and conditions. Stability is not the same thing as strength. Stability is more strongly related to *resilience* – the ability to dynamically receive and efficiently transmit and transform force. It incorporates strength with fluidity, agility, mobility, and balance. Having stability protects all joints in the body as it is a responsive way of being in the world, able to make use of all aspects of the human experience to be adaptable, to move dynamically and naturally, to remain injury-free, and to grow and evolve.

Possible physical (end energetic) cueing includes, but is not limited to the following ideas:

- Use the breath as a stable yet dynamic anchor, deepening core resilience and muscular responsiveness through allowing the breath (exhalation is easiest) to support engagement of the deep abdominal muscles, especially the transverse abdominis
- Look for healthful breathing by exploring the low ribs (should neither be flared outward nor strongly drawn inward) and their freedom of movement outward and upward with the inhalation and downward and inward with the exhalation
- Find stability through the base of the body, especially when the base is simply the feet – explore the corners of the feet – avoid pronation or supination and create resilient arches instead (see fancy footwork in Chapter 8)
- Maintain natural alignment in the spine – neither braced nor collapsed – and notice how breath and breathing interact with spinal alignment; use one to affect the other in a wholesome way – a natural spine is key to stability
- Find engaged action in all movements and lean into active, rather than passive, range of motion (the latter results in more injury than the former)
- Engage the core and other muscles needed to achieve and maintain the shape or movement
- Identify the deep core muscles and ways/tricks/hints to engage them (e.g., laughter or coughing to find the deepest layers that are often 'asleep')
- Work from the edges to the core, encouraging strength at the center
- Engage muscles before lengthening, moving, or opening

> *"Your hand opens and closes and opens and closes.*
> *If it were always a fist or always stretched open, you would be paralyzed.*
> *Your deepest presence is in every small contracting and expanding.*
> *The two as beautifully balanced and coordinated as birdwings."*
> Rumi

### Incorporating Breathing and Energy in Asana

In applying integrated holistic principles, yoga professionals emphasize breath awareness as a key aspect of guiding students through yoga *asana* practice, particularly within more demanding shapes, flow sequences, and *kriyas*. Breath cues are auspiciously used as a feedback mechanism to help clients explore the relationship between effort and ease, and to observe when they may be operating from nervous system states of depletion, agitation, or balance (i.e., from *tamas* or dorsal vagal collapse, *rajas* or sympathetic upregulation, or *sattva* or balanced ventral vagal connection. By weaving breath awareness into *asana* instruction, cueing can facilitate interoceptive awareness and neuroception, inviting clients to sense and respond to their internal physiological and energetic states as they unfold during practice. Integrating optimal functional breathing supports functional breath off the mat and self-aware and compassionate breath on the mat. Attention to over- or under-breathing among clients can help them guide back to subtle, gentle, nasal, and diaphragmatic breathing that invites healthful states of arousal and easeful yet engaged affective states.

### Integrating Mindfulness and Awareness in Asana

The role of mental and emotional awareness within yoga *asana* practice is highlighted, offering cues that draw attention to how mind states and contents can either support or distract from embodied engagement and somatic presence. Teachers can helpfully invite clients to notice habitual mental patterns (such as preconceived ideas about how a shape ought to look or feel) that may influence physical effort or alignment from a place of attachment, aversion, ego, or confusion. Rather than tuning out mentally or dissociating emotionally during movement, individuals are encouraged to remain mentally present and focused, cultivating a sense of integrated concentration or awareness throughout practice. Such clear and lucid mental and emotional presence includes observing the narratives and assumptions that the mind generates during the practice, and noticing how these internal stories may shape movement choices, alignment strategies, or attitudes toward specific shapes and ideas.

As teaching skills refine, cueing will naturally increase to invite students to attune to their inner sensations in all *koshas*. This issue was addressed in *Integrated Holistic Yoga Psychology* and is reiterated here with emphasis on attunement specifically to the physical body or somatic experience (though this is sometimes hard to differentiate from other layers of experience). Clients are invited again and again to sense into their needs and to begin to understand their physical edges and reactions through mindfulness, attention, and awareness. Physically, the attunement focus is on somatic mindfulness – the capacity to read the body from the inside out, to draw attention to particular parts of the body and to maintain awareness of the body as a whole. Interoception, neuroception, and proprioception are crucial skills that can be encouraged and honed in students through attunement and mindfulness cueing.

### Somatic Attunement and the Four 'Ceptions

Attunement and somatic mindfulness-related cueing may change and vary depending on what is observed in specific individuals in class. Creating accessibility through cueing attunement is complex, especially when the same class includes clients with differing needs. This teaching skill is strongly linked to skillful observation of students' physical (and energetic) bodies and tends to find refinement over time as teachers' capacity to observe and read bodies improves.

Cueing that encourages safely-titrated interoception, somatic mindfulness, and attunement to a felt sense in the body can be helped along by the following suggestions:
- Use cues that help students become mindful of their inner physical states – sensations and perceptions – via learning to pay attention to signals that come from the body
- Use cues that help students recognize how they interpret this information from the body and if there is self-protective reactivity that may suggest that a particular body signal triggers a sense of danger or threat
- Use cues that help students learn to differentiate sensation from the body that truly signals danger versus sensation that has a conditioned danger (trauma) response – student may begin to realize that their associations with particular body signals are conditioned by prior experiences and challenges and do not actually pose a threat in the present moment; this may help them transform their relationship with particular body states from fear to acceptance to health
- Use cues that invite practices that help students tune into their capacity to self-regulate, to self-soothe, and to self-calm – for example, after a particular activity that may result in nervous system arousal, invite attunement with the reality that heart rate, breathing, and arousal reregulate automatically

- Titrate cueing for interoception and neuroception based on the reactions, reactivities, and responses noted in students; this is true especially in healthcare settings where more students may present with trauma histories
- Titrated cueing can start small (and always in a context of having established environmental and relational safety) and carefully, alternating challenge with ease, arousal with calming, exploration with predictability

*A Caution*: Remember that attunement means that students stay safely connected to themselves and their physical being. They may also need to stay connected to the teacher and can co-regulate through the teacher's stability, groundedness, and capacity to remain in a ventral vagal space. This means that if the teacher has a day of dysregulation and distress, less invitation for student interoception and vulnerability may need to be cued so that teacher and student do not dysregulate together. Much more information about this process as relevant to all *koshas* is provided in *Integrated Holistic Yoga Psychology*. As a quick review, cueing and encouraging the following 'ceptions can be encouraged to help students (re)gain access to their physical experience.

Specifically:
- *Neuroception* – cueing the evaluation of current level of safety that results in a felt sense of safety, danger, or life threat, followed by a commensurate nervous system response that activates either the ventral vagal complex (safety), the sympathetic nervous system (danger), or the dorsal vagal complex (life threat)
- *Interoception* – cueing to help develop the capacity to attune to, receive, process, and integrate signals about the internal and affective state of the body, including the capacity to sense the physiological state of the body from within via sensations arising from various physiological systems of the body, including but not limited to the respiratory, cardiac, gastrointestinal, thermoregulatory, and nociceptive systems
- *Proprioception* – cueing to help cultivate the ability to assess and refine the body's alignment and positioning in space
- *Exteroception* – cueing for the ability to attune to stimuli from outside the body, to perceive and take in stimulation from the outside world – conscious and mindful perception of these stimuli can then be integrated with stimuli arising from inside the body (i.e., interoception) and help inform neuroception of safety, danger, or life

Finally, following is a table with vocabulary for helping clients find language for their somatic or inner physical experience. This listing is offered to increase the repertoire of understanding how sensation in the physical layer of experience can manifest. It is not offered as a listing that is a complete representation of possible sensations – nor as a listing that is to be used at length in any one session or with any one client. The listing certainly is not offered a way to tell students what or how to feel. Often, it is not necessary for individuals to name their sensations – they can simply be in the sensation or experience without words. However, at times it becomes appropriate to name an experience. The listing is for those moments when a client is struggling for words and the yoga professionals has an inkling of what might help the individual come closer to being able to share their experience or sensations verbally in a safe and supportive therapeutic relationship with a co-regulating other.

| Possible Physical Sensations – A Partial List To Get Started ||||| 
|---|---|---|---|---|
| achy | dull | joyful | satisfied | tearful |
| adaptable | dense | lax | sensitive | tender |
| agile | easeful | light | shaky | tense |
| agitated | elastic | lifeless | shivering | throbbing |
| alive | energetic | limber | silent | tickly |
| antsy | expansive | limited | slack | tight |
| at ease | exposed | limp | smooth | tired |
| blocked | firm | lively | soft | tranquil |
| bound (up) | flexible | loose | solid | trembly |
| braced | fluttery | loud | sore | twitchy |
| bright | fulfilled | nauseous | spacious | unbending |
| breathless | fuzzy | numb | spacy | uncomfortable |
| calm | healthy | open | stable | unhappy |
| choked | hearty | painful | startled | unhealthy |
| clear | heavy | pleased | sticky | unstable |
| clogged | hungry | prickly | stiff | unyielding |
| cold | fluttery | quiet | still | vibrant |
| coarse | hot | queasy | stretchy | vigorous |
| comfortable | hurting | relaxed | strong | vulnerable |
| congested | ill | restricted | sturdy | warm |
| constricted | inflexible | rigid | suffocating | weak |
| content | intense | robust | supple | wiggly |
| contracted | itchy | rough | sweaty | wobbly |

## Troubleshooting Physical Discomfort and Physical Resistance

Students encounter many physical sensations in yoga sessions and daily life that affect their comfort or ability to move with ease. Having precise, supportive language helps guide safer and more empowering choices related to practice on the mat and functional movement off the mat. In therapeutic yoga settings, especially when working with individuals managing physical or mental health challenges, it is essential for yoga professionals to clearly understand and be able to articulate to clients the distinctions between pain, discomfort, and soreness and to work with the emergence of physical resistance, recognizing its likely sources and possible explorations.

### *Working with Physical Pain, Discomfort, and Soreness*

*Note*: This section offers guidance about working with *physical* sensations – not emotional or mental discomfort, suffering, or resistance (that is a different topic). Physical sensations of pain, discomfort, and even soreness can have strong emotional and mental overlays. These are not explored here – the focus is on how to manage the physical sensation in the moment. This does not mean that the client or student will not also have an emotional response – especially with pain, this can happen. The guidance here is about how to manage the physical reaction. Emotional support may also be necessary as students encounter physical challenges. Teachers need to understand and have the capacity to explain how to differentiate between pain that warrants immediate withdrawal from physical sensation versus uncomfortable physical sensation that may invite mindful exploration. If this understanding and guidance is present in a yoga session a therapeutic practice can become trauma-informed, interoceptively oriented, and variation-rich with guidance for clients that fosters autonomy and resilience in practice and life.

## Physical Pain: A Signal to Pause and Reassess

Pain is a protective mechanism of the nervous system and is often described as *sharp, burning, electric, stabbing,* or *radiating*. It typically provokes a reaction of alarm and/or an immediate desire to stop or change a movement or yoga shape. Pain signals the potential for or presence of tissue injury or inflammation and can emerge during or after an activity. If a student continues to engage in the action that causes pain without adjusting in some way, the pain usually intensifies, indicating a lack of physiological or anatomical safety. Care needs to be taken not to add harm to pain by persisting with sensations (i.e., physical signals) that alert the individual that something is not safe or helpful.

Yoga professionals working in healthcare-focused environments need to understand that pain may require medical evaluation, especially if it is persistent, severe, or unexplained. It is outside the professional scope of most yoga professionals (unless they are also medically trained and in a provider-client relationship with the client) to diagnose or treat pain. Thus, the appropriate response in a therapeutic yoga context when pain arises is to invite the student to pause the practice, adapt or eliminate the triggering movement, and encourage the student to consult a licensed healthcare provider if symptoms persist for more than one to two weeks. In the realm of pain, exploration and curiosity are delayed as shifting and changing is necessary to ameliorate the immediate danger signals. Cautious exploration may be possible if pain dissipates quickly – however, the first course of action is to *alleviate pain*, not to push through pain.

## Physical Discomfort: A Space for Reflection and Adaptation

Discomfort is subtler than pain and may arise during or after a movement. It might feel *achy, tight, annoying,* or *odd*, but not sharp or alarming. Students often describe discomfort as a set of experiences or sensation they can linger with or explore – this is unlike pain, which usually triggers a need for immediate change or discontinuation of the activity at hand. Discomfort can serve as a helpful feedback mechanism, alerting clients to the need for tailored and adaptive alignment, gentler effort or more supportive engagement, or a different type of breath support.

In therapeutic yoga contexts, students can benefit from being cued to notice and sense into discomfort, increasing interoceptive and neuroceptive awareness to facilitated exploration and self-regulation. However, if left unattended or repeatedly pushed through with lack of compassion or honesty, discomfort can escalate into pain. A helpful approach to discomfort encourages curiosity (rather than endurance or worse yet, ignoring) to become familiar with physical sensations that are present, to note how sensation evolves and changes with shifts in body position or breathing patterns, and to stay carefully attuned to what is unfolding.

The key is to helping students explore their physicality and somatic experiences with compassion and lovingkindness, curious about how to be with sensation, how to tend to sensation, and, perhaps most importantly, how to prevent harm without backing away from all physical exploration. It is in the realm of discomfort a fragility and vulnerability mind sets can develop if physical sensation is treated as dangerous when it is not. It is helpful to support clients in discovering the difference between discomfort and pain so they can avoid a sense of vulnerability when it is not needed and rely the validity on their internal signals of threat when they do arise.

## Physical Soreness: A Natural Part of Recovery

Soreness is sensation not in the moment, but a physical experience that usually develops 12 to 72 hours after an unfamiliar or effortful activity. It typically presents as a dull ache or tenderness in muscles and fascia, especially when touched or moved. Unlike pain, soreness is not sharp or radiating and typically resolves on its own within a few days. Mild muscle soreness can indicate appropriate muscular engagement and adaptation. In therapeutic yoga, it is important to normalize delayed onset muscle soreness (DOMS) as a possible but not necessary outcome of practice. In fact, it may be helpful to note that soreness is actually most typically a sign of a muscle healing – and through this healing becoming stronger. Soreness may become especially likely when students are rebuilding strength, improving posture, or re-engaging with movement after injury, illness, or prolonged stress. Soreness, in other words, is not typically encountered *in* a session but *after* a session. Giving clients a heads-up about the possibility of soreness developing later can be helpful to their capacity to respond positively and compassionately to its experience. Gentle movement, breath awareness, hydration, and adequate rest can support recovery.

## Guidance Related to Pain and Discomfort for Therapeutic Contexts

A few supportive tips and a summary of the physical sensation spectrum are offered; these are simple offerings and not guidance about how to work with students with chronic or acute pain conditions. These tips are about how to manage the emergence of physical sensations within a therapeutic yoga session; they are not meant to imply that yoga professionals actively work with students on pain. Scope of practice considerations need to remain foremost on the mind of yoga teachers as they manage classroom situations.

| | Overview of the Physical Sensation Spectrum | | |
|---|---|---|---|
| | *Pain* | *Discomfort* | *Soreness* |
| *Timing* | During or after movement | During or after movement | 12–72 hours after activity |
| *Quality of the Sensation* | Sharp, burning, stabbing, electric, radiating | Achy, stuck, irritating, odd, annoying | Tender, achy, tight (not sharp or radiating) |
| *Typical Response* | Immediate desire to stop; worsens if ignored | May linger or explore; can meet with curiosity and compassion | Improves with gentle movement and rest |
| *Therapeutic Guidance* | Stop the activity; refer to healthcare provider if persistent | Cue interoception and neuroception; modify to prevent escalation | Normalize; support with movement and recovery |

- *Support clear communication about sensation*
    - use language that helps students differentiate between types of sensation without inducing fear or a sense of fragility
    - offer metaphors for clear and quick communication (e.g., 'yellow light' for discomfort and 'red light' for pain)
    - role model appropriately descriptive and accurate language related to physical sensations – offer a variety of descriptors if students struggle to name their experience
- *Foster interoception, neuroception, and self-regulation*
    - integrate physical awareness development in opening centerings, breathing practices, and meditative contexts that develop interoception and neuroception in the absence of physical movement
    - cue students to notice how they feel physically *before*, *during*, and *after* movement
    - invite students to notice their sense of safety and ease with the practice *before*, *during*, and *after* various shapes
    - encourage rest or shifts in movement and realignment within shapes based on students' in-the-moment experience and inner sensation – not based on external form
- *Invite self-inquiry, agency, and autonomy*
    - regularly invite students to skip shapes, pause, or choose alternative movements
    - create an atmosphere of honest self-exploration and agency to create change or do things in a personalized manner
    - avoid language that may imply that students should 'push through' sensation
    - avoid directive or prescriptive cueing, emphasizing curiosity and responsiveness instead
- *Be available for emotional co-regulation (with care not to overstep scope of practice)*
    - understand that for students with trauma, chronic pain, or anxiety, even the experience of discomfort can be emotionally dysregulating
    - reinforce that all sensations and response choices to sensations are valid
    - reflect that avoiding pain is not a sign of failure but of resilience and self-trust
    - support exploration and plays at the edges in situations that do not involve pain, risk, or danger to work with students' windows of tolerance
- *Collaborate with and refer to other care providers*
    - when working in healthcare settings, it helps to stay in communication with referring providers (when appropriate)
    - understand and respect scopes of practice
    - refrain from interpreting, diagnosing, or advising students or clients on symptoms

## *Working with Physical Resistance*

Clients may encounter various aspects of physical resistance that impede comfort or ability to move easefully through shapes or flows, either because of inability to recruit muscles that are needed for the movement or because of limitations in range of motion. It is helpful to develop an understanding of causes for physical resistance. The first set of causes that can be explored is tensile resistance (arising from soft tissue) and compressive resistance (arising from bony structures). Both are *physical causes* of tissue resistance that leads to access to certain ranges of motion, restrictions, or movement patterns. In addition to tensile and compressive resistance, there are also *neuromuscular, emotional, or mental causes* that may limit range of motion or muscular recruitment. For some students, resistance may be multifactorial, with fear perhaps combining with tissue tightness and mental attitudes that lead to hesitation, aversions, or fear.

Helping students or clients understand these possible relationships between body, mind, emotions, and nervous system can be transformative for their yoga practice, functional movement in daily life, and self-understanding. It can deeply inform the focus and compassion of cueing for teachers, inviting students into the practice in their own way and at their own pace. That said, it remains important to be clear about scope of practice, not to transgress across professional boundaries, and not to expose clients' vulnerabilities to peers in the same class.

*Tensile and Compressive Causes of Physical Resistance*

*Tensile resistance* arises from soft tissue, such as muscle and fascia. Several forms of tensions or tensile resistances can occur:
- Surface tension
- Myofascial tension
- Muscular tension
- Tendinous and ligamentous tension

Some tensile resistance may yield over time as function follows form. Nevertheless, no force or power is used to through this resistance; the work proceeds with compassion, mindfulness, and patience to find greater yield over time. However, tendinous and ligamentous tension is not necessarily tension we want to reduce. Tendons and ligaments may become more resilient through yoga practice; however, they do not lengthen (if they do, they are strained and slack – no longer do their job). On the other hand, skin or surface tension and fascial tension may release in time as fascia reshapes and realigns. Muscles likely will increase in resilience. Some research suggests that new cell growth in muscles replaces tendinous tissue and creates more flexibility in the region where muscle becomes tendon. Others argue against this idea.

*Compressive resistance* arises from structural barriers, including from soft tissue as well as from the shapes of bones and joints. Several forms of compression can occur:
- *Soft*: flesh on flesh (e.g., belly flesh on thigh flesh in twisting)
- *Medium*: flesh on bone
- *Hard*: bone on bone (e.g., carpal compression in wrist flexion; external rotation in hip joint; lumbar spinous process compression in spinal extension)

Whereas soft compression can be worked with to create more ease over time, hard compressive resistance has to be accommodated. There is no goal or expectation for change over time related to hard bony limits as yoga does not remodel joints or bones.

On the other end of the physical spectrum related to range of motion and muscular recruitment, some students may encounter too little resistance and present with hypermobility. With these students, it is important to understand that we do not want to cue them to the end range of their comfort as this actually reinforces their less than stable joints. There are many joints that can be hypermobile. Particular attention can be paid to elbow and knee joints. If hypermobility is noted

in these (or other) joints, cueing centers on creating *less* range of motion and *more* strength and muscular engagement around these joints. The following cueing guidelines can help:
- Avoid overstretching – this increases instability
- Engage and strengthen the muscles around the joint to increase stability
- Use alignment cue to prevent hyperextension of joints
- Teach interoceptive and proprioceptive awareness of hyperextension as students with hypermobility are typically not aware that they are hyperextending a joint

*Neuromuscular Causes of Physical Resistance*

Neuromuscular activation can play a crucial role in both range of motion and the capacity to effectively recruit muscles during movement. This relationship hinges on the integrity of neural pathways that connect the central nervous system with specific muscle groups. When these pathways are clear and responsive, as seen in well-conditioned neuromuscular patterns, muscles are more readily recruited, contributing to both stability and functional range of motion. Conversely, conditions like *gluteal amnesia*, a phenomenon where the gluteal muscles are under-activated due to prolonged sitting or poor movement habits, illustrate how disrupted neural connections can limit effective muscle engagement. In this example, nervous system signaling to the gluteal muscles is weakened, reducing both the muscles' capacity to activate and their contribution to movements such as hip extension, rotation, and stabilization. Over time, such diminished neuromuscular communication not only affects movement efficiency but can also contribute to compensatory patterns and restricted range of motion. Intentional practices that stimulate neuromuscular activation, such as targeted strength training and proprioceptive exercises, can help reestablish these pathways, enhancing both muscular recruitment and joint mobility.

*Emotional and Mental Causes of Physical Resistance*

Emotional and mental factors significantly influence neuromuscular activation, range of motion and even strength or stability, often serving as unseen barriers to effective movement. Fear of certain movements ( e.g., going upside down into a full inversion or opening the heart space in a backbend) can create unconscious bracing patterns or inhibiting fears that get in the way of necessary muscular engagement. Emotional barriers can become particularly evident among individuals in healthcare settings who are recovering from injury or those who have developed protective habits due to chronic pain. Similarly, in mental healthcare settings, anxiety, trauma, depression, or aversion may derail attempts to move into shapes that kindle fear or other emotional challenge. When fear or anxiety is present, the nervous system might trigger a guarded response, restricting range of motion and reducing the capacity for muscles to fully activate, as the body prioritizes perceived need for safety over functional movement. Trauma triggers (e.g., such as the use of a yoga strap or invitation into a shape such as butterfly that creates emotional vulnerability) can also lead to reactive withdrawal or disengagement, both physically and psychologically.

At times, simple cognitive expectations or misunderstandings about muscular actions can lead to inefficient recruitment patterns. For example, if individuals believe that backbending is purely about spinal extension in the lumbar rather than balanced extension through the entire kinetic chain, they may over-recruit the lumbar region while neglecting support from the gluteal muscles, hamstrings, or pelvic floor. This belief about how to engage the shape not only limits range of motion but can also perpetuate imbalanced neuromuscular activation. Addressing psychological and educational barriers through information, awareness, mindful practice, and accurate anatomical understanding can help reframe movement as safe and accessible, gradually restoring confidence, muscular recruitment, and fluidity in range of motion.

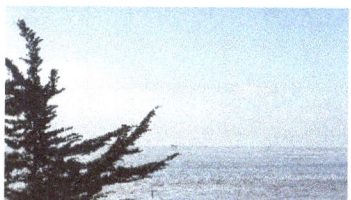

## Biomechanics Related to Teaching Shapes and Movement

Biomechanics are about the
*"effects of force on the human body in the context of anatomical position, placement, posture, and movement (p. 3)"*
(Mitchell, 2019)

Biomechanics explore the effects of force or load on the human body along a variety of dimensions, including but not necessarily limited to, effects on movement, anatomy, physiology, energetics, contraindications, risks, and benefits. Biomechanics work with the idea of adaptation of the organism onto which force is applied, that is, the increased ability of the organism's capacity to bear load or force under optimal stress conditions. In other words, working with biomechanics means utilizing (optimal) stress to create resilience. Since resilience depends on the right amount of stress, rest and recovery are best integrated into physical practice for adaptation to be cultivated successfully. Biomechanics are utterly relevant to the teaching of yoga *asana*, which is a method of applying force to the body to create strength and resilience.

### *Understanding Force and Load*

Human organisms (i.e., tissues) evolved to withstand load – *and* human bodies are subject to *wear-and-repair principles.* The fact that human tissue consists of living, changing cells means that human tissue (as opposed to human-made or other materials) is adaptable and changes according to the demand characteristics of a given situation or habits across time. Tissues are marvelously capable of adapting to the loads placed on them, an essential adaptation since gravity places us under the constant influence of force. Each type of tissue responds differently to different force and load variables; therefore, the same level of internal or external force may create different loads depending on the type of tissue (i.e., muscle, bone, fascia, ligaments, tendons) that is being challenged. Because the human body is a biotensegrity, placing force on any place in the body reverberates throughout the entire tensegrity structure. Weight distributes throughout the structure and different angles in movements and shapes make themselves felt in various places in the body, not necessarily only the regions actively moving or under load.

> **What is Load?**
>
> **Load = force applied to the body**
>
> In other words, the effect of force on the body is called **load**.
> Weight is not equal to load – though this is often a proxy variable; instead, load is the experience created by weight or other types of force.

Force or load on a human structure is not good or bad in and of itself; it simply has to be auspicious for and perhaps adapted to the needs of the individual who has to endure it. The dosage of load that is tolerable varies greatly across individuals based on their experiences and training. A load or force that would be an overdose that causes injury for one individual may be perfectly fine for another, just at the edge of tolerable for a third, and an underdose that does not foster any progress for a fourth. In other words, outer parameters of force and load cannot predict the reaction of the organism who has to endure this force; it is just as important to understand the inner structure, readiness, and preparedness of the individual. This has clear implications for a yoga session. As clients are invited to place themselves under various forces and loads when they attempt yoga shapes and movements, they are encouraged to attune to their bioindividuality to adapt and vary the offered practice according to their own needs and resources. Students need to develop sensitive interoceptive, neuroceptive, and proprioceptive skills to receive and understand feedback from their own body about the load or force they experience in a given yoga shape to make personal decisions about how to interact with the practice.

It is important to recall in embarking on teaching yoga *asana* (in the context of our focus on the physical aspects of the practice) that the biomechanics of movement are not simply about the anatomical structures involved but also about all other *koshas*, including the human nervous system. Muscles, as noted in Chapter 3, may be better labeled as neuromuscular tissue. This becomes particularly relevant in yoga *asana* that is integrated and holistic, practice that attends to all layers of experience. The function of the nervous system (e.g., polyvagal states) has a direct effect on the expression of yoga *asana* in individual bodies. In fact, research has demonstrated that gains in muscular strength or power cannot exclusively be attributed to changes in muscle fibers and in their contractility (Gross, 2025). Instead, changes in physical capacity occur also due to enhanced muscle activation via changes in the nervous system (Enoka, 2025). Gluteal amnesia is an excellent example of the interaction of muscle action and neural activation. For many human beings, an inactive, often seated lifestyle has alienated the gluteal muscles (which are meant to be very powerful and set human anatomy apart from other animals) from the nervous system, to the point that these muscles no longer activate naturally as they should (Gross, 2025). Effortful movement (e.g., squat and kicks such as in found in some yoga shapes and vinyasas) appears necessary to reawaken the neural activation and bring the gluteal muscles back on line. Further, not surprisingly to most yoga professionals and underscoring the involvement of all *koshas* during physical movement, even attentional focus – what an individual is thinking about or focusing on – can affect physical performance, including strength and power (Wulf, 2013). These neuromechanical realities may help explain why yoga *asana* can be such a powerful intervention; by its very nature, it addresses not only anatomy, but also nervous system states (e.g., via working with the *gunas* or polyvagal states) and the involvement of the mind and emotion (via mind states, mindfulness, and concentration).

> *We have to take the time to ... take muscles seriously*
> *not merely as an instrument of the soul,*
> *but as the vital, inextricable, and effective partner of the soul.*
> (Gross, 2025; p. 357)

### *Definitions and Concepts Related to Force and Load*

Mass is the amount of matter that makes up an object and is measured in kilograms. Human bodies have mass, composed of the sum total of our four types of tissues [neural, muscular, connective, and epithelial] that organize themselves into organs and organ systems, including our musculoskeletal system). In terms of defining mass, it is important to understand that mass is independent of gravity, compared to weight, which is not. A human body in outer space maintains its mass, but not its weight (because there is no gravity). On earth, mass is affected by load, which in turn, is created by force. Force can be applied to our bodies via pushing on them or pulling them. Force can vary in terms of magnitude (*how strong is the force?*), direction (*where is the force coming from?*), and point of application (*where on the body does it make impact?*). We make use of these concepts, which are elaborated upon in Newton's laws (see Box), in yoga *asana* by using changes in orientation, adding weights (or resistance bands), and moving creatively in space.

In yoga *asana*, we want to understand how the application of force affects movement and resilience, adaptability, and strength of tissues. When force, and thus load, is applied to a human tissue, internal resistance occurs as a reaction to that load to prevent tissue deformation. This internal reaction to load is called *stress*. The ability to withstand the load is called *tolerance*. When load exceeds tolerance, injury results. Tolerance can be increased through progressive and variable loading (more about this below).

---

#### *Newton's Laws of Motion*

- Newton's 1st Law of Motion is the law of *inertia*: Unless a force acts on an object, that object will either stay at rest or stay in motion at the same rate of speed (however the object started out) – in other words, *to start, stop, or change motion requires force*
- Newton's 2nd Law of Motion is the law of *momentum* (or the changes force can produce in the movement of a body) and defines force as follows: *Force = mass\*acceleration* (where acceleration = change in velocity)
- Newton's 3rd Law of Motion is the law of action and reaction and is about *ground reaction forces* (GRF): when an object exerts force on another object, that object exerts an equal and opposite reaction on the first object
- Gravity is a constant force on our body at an acceleration of 9.8 meters/second$^2$

Load on the body changes as we change position, direction, and/or acceleration (e.g., jumping). Extra force can come from muscle action (i.e., when a muscle contracts, it creates force throughout our biotensegrity) or external sources (see factors below, e.g., kettlebells, dumbbells, resistance bands). This can be referred to as internal versus external load, where *internal load* is load emanating from within the body (e.g., muscle contraction puts mechanical forces on the involved tendons and bones; contraction of the diaphragm changes pressure in the lungs) and *external load* is load due to force applied from outside the body, that is, load that is in addition to your body weight (e.g., a bolster on our back in Plank; a weight in our hand as we abduct the arm; a resistance-band-supported row in Staff).

It is interesting to note an individual's *rate of subjectively perceived effort* while engaging in movement. While this is not really an aspect of load per se, rate of perceived effort acknowledges that the same amount of load may be perceived very differently at different times, depending on how we feel in the moment and what we bring to the practice physically, emotionally, and mentally (i.e., the personal or bioindividual factors mentioned above) and what our environment throws our way (i.e., the external or biopsychosociocultural factors noted above).

## *Types of Loading*

Various types of loading emerge from different ways of applying force. When we load an object, it deforms in response to the stress that is created. How the object deforms and recovers defines how much stress is experience based on the load it is receiving. "*Human musculoskeletal connective tissues are able to maintain structural integrity because they have the ability to undergo large deformations while simultaneously absorbing force at a capacity similar to that of stainless steel*" (Mitchell, 2019, p. 21). In other words, the human body is made to withstand stress – tremendous amounts of stress. It is truly resilient and adaptable.

The following types of loads can be exerted on a body and result in deformation accordingly (Mitchell, 2019). The first two of the following loads are the unique; the last three are simply combinations of the first two.
- *Tensile loading* (tension) – stretches or pulls the object apart via tension – this happens in all our muscles as we bear weight
  - tension injuries can happen in the tendons if we overload the muscle, that is, if the force is greater than the body can tolerate (e.g., a bicep tension may separate from the bone if excessive weight is lifted)
- *Compressive loading* (compression) – squeezes or pushes the object together; for example, there is compression force through the spine that compresses the intervertebral discs; through the knee at the point where tibia and femur meet
  - compression injuries can result from excessive compression force (e.g., a compression fracture in the vertebrae, especially with osteoporosis)
- *Shear* – slides the surfaces parallel to each other
  - shear injuries can happen if the ligaments around a joint are torn or sprained and do not provide enough stability anymore to the bony articulation (e.g., shear can happen at the

articulation of the tibia and femur in the presence of an ACL tear – the knee surfaces have too much side-to-side movement and lack stability at the joint)
- *Side-Bending* – curves the object; essentially, this represents asymmetrical loading that creates compression on inner side of the side-bend and tension on the outer side of the bend
    - injuries that may happen here are breaks of bones deformed beyond their capacity to bend; in young kids these can be green stick injuries, where the bone does not break through but cracks a bit on the tension side of the bend
- *Torsion* – twists or rotates the object along the transverse plane
    - torsion injuries to the bone can lead to spiral fractures when the rotational force is too strong (e.g., might see this in domestic violence or child abuse where torsion is applied to the humerus)

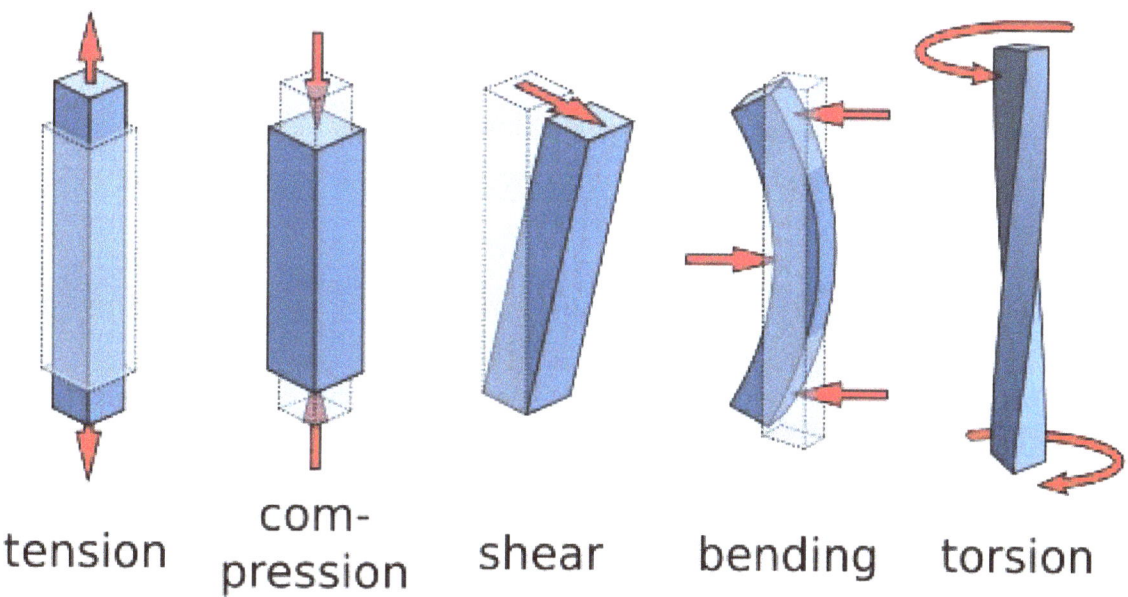

**Figure 2.1** Types of loading. (Data source: MikeRun; https://commons.wikimedia.org/wiki/File:Different-types-of-mechanical-stress_EN.svg; Creative Commons Attribution 4.0)

Elasticity of a tissue is defined by the relationship of stress to strain (*elasticity=stress/strain*). Different types of tissues have different levels of elasticity – some can regain their shape easily after being deformed by load (e.g., muscle); others not so much (e.g., ligaments). The more stress a particular type of tissue can tolerate without strain, the greater its elasticity. In response to load that is within tolerance, deformation can occur in terms of length, width, or shape. The amount of deformation that happens in the tissues (relative to their starting shape or position) despite their resistance to it is called *strain*.

Overload is essentially an excessive deformation of (i.e., strain on) the tissue in question (whether bone, ligament, or tendon) that exceeds the tissue's elasticity and results first in injury and finally in ultimate failure beyond which repair may require surgery as the tissue can no longer heal itself. This progression can be shown in the form of a deformation curve for human tissue as shown below.

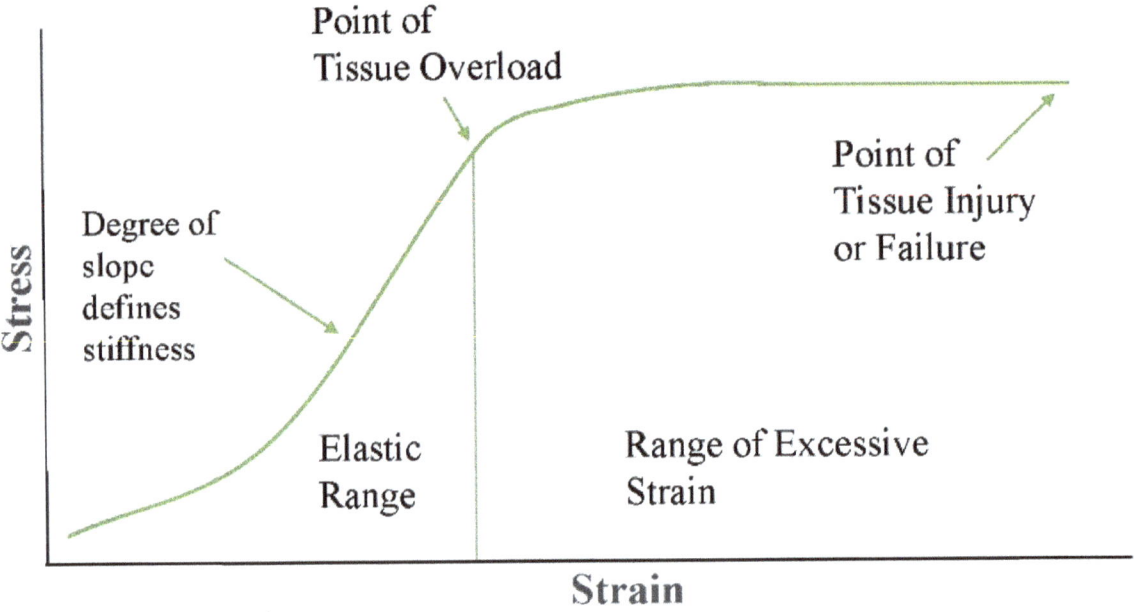

## Variations within Types of Loads

Compressive and tensile loads can vary by many factors, all of which take place in yoga *asana* and demonstrate that any one yoga shape can have tremendously different impacts (very different load characteristics) depending in how it is executed. We cannot ever talk about a given yoga shape and define how it might load the body. Too many factors affecting load can vary in a particular *asana* depending on its specific expression in a given human body. This is the great thing about yoga; we can create tremendous load variety for the body by shifting any of the following factors for any given shape (to create endless variation):

- *Magnitude* – pounds of weight lifted (body weight and added weight)
- *Location* – where the load is felt (e.g., in Plank the greatest load might be on the shoulders; or if taken with knees on the ground, load may be more equally distributed)
- *Direction* – orientation in space changes load (e.g., Side Plank versus regular Plank; Half Handstand versus Downward Facing Dog at the wall – same shape, different orientation in space)
- *Duration* – amount of time under load (i.e., how long we hold a shape)
- *Frequency* – how many times the same load is exerted onto the body (e.g., how many squats)
- *Velocity or Rate* – the rate of speed at which the load is exerted (e.g., how fast or slow we move in a particular yoga shape like *Chaturanga*)
- *Acceleration or Variability* – the rate of change in the speed of the load (e.g., maybe we start with very quick *Chaturangas* and then slow them down more and more); maybe we hold a shape for a long time with equal load or we hold for a long time but at variable loads

It is helpful to explore repetitive versus acute loading (basically a *combination of magnitude and frequency*). Repetitive stress refers (generally) to loading that, if applied once, might not do harm. However, if applied over and over again (a *samskara*), can lead to injury. Acute overload is a single event of force that results in an injury (of the types already referenced above).

## Effects of Load on Human Bodies

Bony, soft, and muscle tissue have mechanobiological stability and adaptivity. They can change in mass, adapt to lines of imposed demand, and maintain equilibrium under new demand characteristics. In the absence of imposed demand, human bodies will maladapt or atrophy. This ability of cells and tissues to adjust to various demand characteristics (i.e., types of load and factors) is called *mechanotransduction*, where mechanical signals are used by cells to change their chemistry, structure, and function. Because of this process, human bodies, over time, reflect the sum total of all loads applied to the cells.

| *Examples of Mechanotransduction* | | |
|---|---|---|
| *Action* | *Mechanisms of Change* | *Relevance* |
| Resistance training or weight-bearing activities (e.g., walking, jumping) | Osteocytes detect strain from loading → trigger osteoblasts to deposit bone matrix → bones become denser and stronger | Bone remodels to adapt to the load under which it is placed (Wolff's law) |
| Lifting weights or engaging in weightbearing yoga *asana* such as Plank, Yoga Pushup, Handstand, and more | Mechanical load stretches muscle fibers → activates mechanosensitive pathways (e.g., mTOR signaling) → increases protein synthesis → muscle growth | Muscles build strength and bulk (hypertrophy) |
| Long-held yoga shapes or physical therapy stretches | Fibroblasts in fascia and tendons sense sustained mechanical stretch → modify extracellular matrix production → increase elasticity or realign collagen fibers | Connective tissue develops resilience that supports mobility and injury prevention |
| Aerobic exercise, including yoga *kriya* and *vinyasa* | Endothelial cells detect fluid shear stress on blood vessel walls → increase nitric oxide production → vasodilation and improved vascular function | Endothelial changes occur in blood vessels that support cardiovascular health and the prevention of atherosclerosis |

## Compressive Tissues

Compressive tissues, such as bone and articular cartilage, are specifically adapted to respond to and absorb compressive forces. These structures possess high compressive strength, enabling them to resist deformation under load, and this mechanical loading actually enhances their capacity to tolerate such stress over time. The process of adaptation is load-dependent: regular, optimal compressive force increases stress tolerance, while sudden or excessive loading (particularly in the context of already weakened tissues, such as in osteoporosis) may result in injury, such as a vertebral compression fracture. Wolff's law articulates this adaptive mechanism clearly, stating that bone tissue remodels in response to the mechanical demands placed upon it.

When compressive or tensile forces are applied, osteoblast activity increases, leading to greater bone formation and improved density. As a result, bones subjected to regular loading become stronger, while those that are not (e.g., astronauts in zero-gravity environments) progressively weaken due to decreased stimulation.

### Tensile Tissues

Tensile tissues, including ligaments, tendons, fascia, joint cartilage, and aponeuroses, are structurally designed to respond to and adapt under tension. While many of these tissues also possess compressive strength, their primary function is to withstand tensile force without deforming. Tendons, for example, have one of the highest tensile strengths of any soft tissue, an essential feature given their role in transferring the force of muscle contractions to bones, thus affecting movement in joints. In general, tensile strength of connective tissue varies with form: longer structures tend to have less tensile strength and are more pliable, whereas larger or thicker tissues are stiffer and more resistant to stretch. With consistent, appropriate loading, tensile tissues adapt by becoming more resilient and increasing their tolerance for force. According to Davis's Law, soft tissues remodel in response to direction and magnitude of mechanical stress.

When tensile loads exceed a certain threshold, tissues elongate along the line of force; when tensile load is reduced or absent, such as during prolonged rest, long periods of sitting, or immobility due to injury or illness, tissues tend to shorten. This remodeling reflects a broader principle of physiological adaptation: specific adaptation to imposed demand (SAID), in which the structure and function of a tissue evolve in direct response to the mechanical environment. This principle also helps explain how range of motion (ROM) may increase with stretching. In part, improvements in ROM arise from increased sensory tolerance and the development of new neural pathways that reduce the nervous system's resistance to stretch. Muscles themselves can become more pliable, yielding more readily to tensile forces, while the surrounding connective tissue adapts over time, increasing both resilience and functional length. In these ways, both neural and structural factors contribute to enhanced flexibility and joint mobility.

### Variable Loading for Health and Resilience

Yoga *asana* can help facilitate greater resilience, remodeling, and adaptation via optimal progressive overloading and variable tensile loading. Variable loading of tissues means loading them in ways they do not expect (that are different from current typical patterns), breaking habits (or changing physical *samskaras*) to help create resilience. Variable loading provides novel stimuli, prevents repetitive stress, and creates resilience. It can be accomplished via progressive overload to strengthen and/or changing tensile loads to create resilience (typically creating more mobility and range of motion).

### Progressive Overload

Progressive overload is a foundational principle of tissue strengthening and adaptation. It refers to the gradual and deliberate increase of mechanical load on a tissue beyond its current baseline capacity. This increase in demand, if applied strategically and consistently, stimulates adaptive remodeling processes in muscles, tendons, bones, and connective tissues. Over time, tissues become stronger, more resilient, and better able to tolerate mechanical stresses. The central idea is that the body adapts to what it regularly experiences; if the stimuli or inputs never change, neither will the tissue.

Compressive loading supports the maintenance of humans' strength (the amount of force that can be created) and power (the speed with which force can be applied) to be able to maintain functional movements, such as being able to get out of chair, to respond quickly and strongly to a dangerous stimulus that requires a quick sprint or a forceful strike, to lift heavy grocery bags out of a car trunk, walk briskly out in nature, or to pick up a puppy or a grandchild. Strength and power decrease over the course of the lifespan if not actively maintained. For example, without regular strength and power training, adults may:

- lose 4-6 pounds of muscle per decade starting as early as in their 30s
- lose muscle strength starting around age 50 at a rate of 1.5 to 5% per year
- lose 30-50% of their peak strength between the ages of 20 and 80
- lose grip strength starting by age 40

This decline is an unfortunate development as muscular strength and power are strongly associated with the following lifelong benefits:

- *Functional independence*
    - preservation of mobility and self-care abilities into older age (e.g., dressing, bathing, rising from the floor)
    - ability to perform daily tasks such as lifting, carrying, bending, and climbing stairs without assistance
    - reduced risk of dependence on others for basic movement or care
- *Injury prevention and resilience*
    - improved joint stability and postural control, reducing the likelihood of falls and related injuries
    - greater tissue tolerance and load capacity, lowering the risk of musculoskeletal strain or trauma
    - faster physical recovery after accidents, surgeries, or illness due to maintained strength reserves
- *Bone density and structural integrity*
    - stimulation of osteogenesis (bone formation) through weight-bearing and compressive forces
    - slowed progression or prevention of osteoporosis and osteopenia, particularly in postmenopausal populations
    - improved joint alignment and support through strong surrounding musculature
- *Metabolic and cardiovascular health*
    - increased resting metabolic rate due to higher lean muscle mass
    - improved glucose regulation and insulin sensitivity, lowering risk of Type 2 diabetes
    - support for healthy blood pressure and lipid profiles through active muscle engagement
- *Cognitive and neurological benefits*
    - enhanced neuroplasticity and motor learning, especially through complex strength-based movements
    - improved cognitive function and memory, particularly in aging adults, linked to regular strength training

- greater emotional regulation and stress resilience, with strength training shown to lower symptoms of depression and anxiety
- *Psychological and emotional wellbeing*
  - increased confidence and perceived competence in physical and social environments.
  - improved body image and self-efficacy, especially as strength gains are measurable and empowering
  - greater capacity to engage in joyful, physically demanding activities, such as dancing, sports, or playing with children
  - enhanced relationships dynamics given greater capacity to be physically present and accountable

Loading can be varied in various ways to achieve progression. One of the most direct methods is increasing the magnitude of the force, such as adding more weight or increasing resistance. Other variables include the direction of the force (e.g., changing the angle of load on a joint or limb), the rate at which force is applied (e.g., transitioning from slow to faster, more dynamic movement), or the duration and volume of exposure (e.g., holding a shape longer or increasing repetitions). Each of these variables contributes to the cumulative mechanical challenge presented to the tissue and can be adjusted according to the needs and current capacity of the individual.

Within a yoga *asana* context, progressive overload can be seamlessly integrated through thoughtful sequencing, sustained holds, repetition of shapes, and the use of props to vary leverage and resistance. For example, holding a Lunge for longer periods, moving through Plank and Yoga Pushup transitions more slowly, or using a resistance band in a Warrior 2 shape to increase tension can all progressively challenge the neuromuscular and myofascial systems.

Crucially, progressive overload plays an essential role in rehabilitation and healing. Injured tissues, if left unloaded, weaken and atrophy. A common mistake is to avoid moving or loading an injured area altogether. However, when done with care, progressive loading of injured tissue can stimulate repair processes, restore strength, and prevent compensatory overuse of surrounding areas. Load must be introduced in a dose that the healing tissue can tolerate, then gradually increases as capacity improves. This approach not only supports recovery but also prevents re-injury by ensuring that the tissue regains its stress tolerance.

An optimal yoga *asana* practice for strengthening does not avoid challenge, it invites it gradually and with intelligence. When progressive overload is applied mindfully, it enhances not only muscular strength but also joint stability, connective tissue resilience, and long-term movement capacity. In this way, yoga becomes not just a tool for flexibility or mindfulness, but a robust framework for building physical durability and adaptability over time.

### *Variable Tensile Loading*

The human body is best understood not as a rigid compression-based structure, but as a dynamic tension-based system, a *tensegrity* structure, in which stability arises from a balance of continuous tension and discontinuous compression. Bones provide localized compression, but it is the tensile network of muscles, tendons, fascia, and ligaments that primarily maintains structural integrity and enables movement. From this perspective, the ability to respond effectively to changing loads depends on how well our tissues adapt to varying kinds of tensile force. Yoga *asana* supports this adaptability by offering diverse opportunities for *variable tensile loading*, the strategic application of different types of stretch stimuli to challenge and enhance tissue responsiveness, resilience, and balance across the body's tensegrity system.

Tensile loading supports the maintenance of humans' ability to stretch and respond resiliently with healthy ranges of motions in joints, and by extension in the limbs and spine. Flexibility in the sense of range of motion decreases over the course of the lifespan if not actively maintained. For example, without regular flexibility and range of motion training, adults may:
- Experience a 25 to 30% reduction in overall flexibility by age 70, compared to their younger years
- Be subject to significant range of motion in important joints such as shoulder and hip joints, with declines of 6° of ROM per decade from age 55 to 85
- Lose 30% of spinal flexion between the ages of 20 and 70
- Experience significant loss of ankle dorsiflexion (and thus have shorter stride lengths and more falls)
- Have a decrease of 20 to 30% of hip extension capacity as they age

These changes are a regrettable development as flexibility and healthful range of motion are associated with the following (sample) benefits:
- *Enhanced functional movement*
    - improved coordination and movement efficiency across daily and athletic activities
    - better balance and proprioception, reducing the risk of falls and movement errors
    - greater ease in completing functional tasks such as walking, reaching, squatting, and lifting
    - enhanced resilience in the breath, including better access to the rib movements that are crucial to resilience breathing and optimal functional breathing.
- *Injury prevention and recovery*
    - reduced risk of strains, sprains, and soft tissue injuries due to improved tissue elasticity and joint mobility
    - more efficient neuromuscular recovery following injury, surgery, or periods of immobility
    - improved lymphatic circulation which supports the healing process and reduces inflammation
- *Musculoskeletal health*
    - maintenance of fascial integrity and hydration, especially in response to varied tensile loading
    - balanced muscular tension across joints, reducing wear and tear and joint degeneration
    - sustained bone and connective tissue resilience through mechanical stimulation
- *Nervous system and brain health*
    - stimulation of afferent sensory feedback, enhancing body awareness and neural integration
    - improved cognitive function through movement-linked neuroplasticity (e.g., via the cerebellum and motor cortex)

- reduced sympathetic arousal (i.e., less chronic stress), as mobility work often co-activates parasympathetic tone
- enhanced capacity to access a parasympathetic nervous system state and its positive effects on restoration and healing
- *Emotional and psychological benefits*
  - increased sense of agency and confidence in movement
  - support for mood regulation, since physical movement and stretching are linked to endorphin release
  - reduced anxiety and tension, as mobility practices often engage breath and mindfulness

The degree of loss in flexibility over the lifespan is greatly affected by movements and resilient responsiveness to momentary demands in daily living as well as by formal physical exertion related to creating or maintaining flexibility. Stretching and resilience practices in general, and – of focus here – via the practice of yoga *asana* can be of great benefit in maintaining resilient tissue and the capacity to stretch and flex creatively late into the lifespan.

Modulating tensile load is a prime way to maintain flexibility and can be accomplished in multiple ways (all included within the practices of yoga *asana*). Understanding the various types of creating variable tension in the body and their distinct effects allows yoga professionals to apply them purposefully. The following stretching methods can be recruited in yoga *asana*:

- *Ballistic stretching*, which involves bouncing or rapid rhythmic movements (such as hopping or jumping in yoga), imposes sudden tensile forces that can stimulate a strong stretch reflex. While this form of loading may have limited use in traditional yoga practice, it does appear in more dynamic expressions, such as jumping transitions or certain athletic-style flows. These movements require advanced proprioceptive control and are to be approached with caution, particularly for individuals with limited mobility or joint instability.
- *Dynamic stretching* consists of controlled, repetitive movements that gradually increase range of motion and load without the abrupt force of ballistic methods. This includes yoga *asana* sequences that build gradually in complexity and intensity, or forms of yoga pulsing where the practitioner rhythmically moves in and out of shapes, often with the flow of breath. These techniques increase tissue temperature, enhance blood flow, and prepare the body for deeper loading. Dynamic stretching is particularly useful as a warm-up, helping to prime the neuromuscular system for more intensive activity.
- *Static stretching*, by contrast, involves maintaining a position for a longer period, allowing tissues to experience sustained tensile load. Holding tensile load encourages gradual release of tension in connective tissue structures. Within yoga *asana*, static stretching is valuable for both recovery and re-patterning of physical *samskaras* (or pattern locks). When practiced after repetitive or high-intensity movement (such as after a long run), it may help tissues release accumulated tension. It is also effective for addressing habitual holding patterns (or physical *samskaras*), encouraging the plastic (long-term) deformation of tissues and improving elasticity. Static stretching can be subdivided into two forms:
  - *Active static stretching* is produced by internal force. This often involves co-contraction of antagonist muscle groups to stabilize and deepen the stretch. In yoga, this might be cued as '*hugging muscle to bone*' or engaging an opposing muscle group to influence range of motion, such as activating the hamstrings while stretching the quadriceps.

Isometric stretching falls under this category and has been shown to strengthen muscles as well as working on creating resilience.
- *Passive static stretching* relies on an external force to create the stretch, such as a wall, strap, prop, or another person. This method often seems accessible and inviting in terms of allowing for relaxation into the stretch, which can facilitate nervous system downregulation and greater receptivity to tissue lengthening. However, as noted elsewhere, passive stretching can lead to overstretching as it may override inner signal that stretching has become excessive. Caution and mindfulness are necessary.

- *Resistance stretching* offers another dimension to tensile loading by engaging the muscle in an *eccentric contraction*, that is, lengthening under tension (or stretching a muscle amidst its activation). This method strengthens tissues while they are stretched and builds resilience, endurance, and strength, especially at end ranges of motion. In yoga *asana*, this type of stretching, which essentially involves extension during flexion, might be incorporated through slow, resisted transitions, such as slowly lowering from Warrior 1 Lunge to Warrior 3 with control or pulling against a resistance band while maintaining length.

By integrating diverse forms of tensile load into yoga *asana*, the practice can create an environment in which tissues adapt intelligently to a wide spectrum of demands. The easeful effort or effortful ease of such practices not only improves flexibility and mobility, but more importantly, enhances tissues' functional strength and resilience across various ranges of motion. In this way of engaging in it, yoga *asana* becomes as a beautiful and healthful expression of the body's biotensegrity, one in which form continuously responds to function, and movement becomes a means of maintaining structural integrity and easeful strength. The principles of understanding pain, resistance, load, and ways to create strength, power, and resilience in all tissues are also reflected in the final general yoga *asana* guidance of this chapter: the understanding and use of reflexes in yoga *asana*.

### *Understanding Open- Versus Closed-Chain Movement*

Understanding the distinction between open-chain and closed-chain movements provides a powerful lens through which to analyze movement strategies and load distribution in yoga *asana* practice. These kinesiology and biomechanics principles describe how limbs interact with a fixed versus moving base during movement. Often applied in strength training and rehabilitation contexts, these concepts have direct application to how we understand movement in yoga *asana*. Incorporating open- and closed-chain movements can refine how yoga *asana* is taught, cued, and sequenced. Their use allows for precise assessment of student needs, helps individualize level of challenge or demand, and offers creative variations that can tailor the engagement of stability versus mobility as appropriate. These principles help ensure that practice develops with anatomical integrity and functional intelligence.

### *Closed-Chain Movements: Creating Grounding and Stability*

In closed-chain movements, the distal end of the limb (i.e., hand or foot; in yoga, we might even include the head in this category) is fixed against a stable surface, such as the ground or a wall, creating a feedback loop between the body and the environment. Closed-chain movements tend to be integrated and simultaneously engage multiple joints and muscle groups. When the hands or feet are grounded (e.g., feet in Mountain or hands and feet in Downward Facing Dog), movements in that limb occur in a closed chain. Closed-chain movements co-activate multiple muscle groups, improving joint stability and proprioception. For example, in Plank, the closed-chain, grounding contact of the hands on the mat recruits stabilizers in the shoulder girdle, core, and even feet.

Closed-chain movements are excellent in the context of developing grounding, stability, and load-bearing capacity, especially in foundation-based shapes, such as standing, arm-standing, and seated shapes. Closed-chain actions provide immediate feedback from the environment (such as a mat, wall, floor, or chair), enhancing proprioceptive awareness and supporting careful alignment principles. This is particularly important in therapeutic yoga contexts that focus on healthful alignment and overcoming habitual movement patterns (or physical *samskaras*). Further, in closed-chain positions, load is transmitted through the kinetic chain from the ground upward or from the limbs inward toward the spine. Such tangible biofeedback supports whole-body alignment and integration. This effect can be heightened further via cueing of rooting and pressing actions (e.g., grounding firmly through the palm of the hands) to harness the stabilizing, yet expansive, upward energy of gravitational rebound forces.

Closed-chain movements are typically more stable and are foundational for teaching safe load-bearing and core integration in yoga *asana*. They are especially helpful for building strength and grounding. However, they can create compensatory patterns if alignment or strength are not yet optimized (e.g., evident when students collapse into the wrists in Downward Facing Dog).

## *Open-Chain Movements: Inviting Expansion, Creativity, and Play*

In open-chain movements, the distal end of the limb is free to move in space and is not fixed to an external surface. The movement typically isolates a single joint or muscle group for action and therapeutic attention. Classic examples in gym or rehabilitation settings include leg extensions (acting on the muscles and tissues around the knee) or bicep curls (acting on the muscles surrounding the elbow). Yoga *asana* involves many open-chain movements. When standing with one raised leg out in front of the body, either with knee straight or bent (as in preparation for Tree), the lifted foot is neither on the ground, nor placed against the other leg. In that moment, the practitioner is in an open-chain position for that leg. All Warrior arm movements (i.e., reaching up to the sky in Warrior 1, to the side in Warrior 2, or forward in Warrior 3) are open-chain positions for the arms.

Open-chain movements isolate or bias certain sets of muscles or joints, which can be useful for awareness or therapeutic work, but may require careful control to avoid joint strain. Open-chain movements are helpful for cultivating coordination, mobility, and expansiveness, such as in hip or shoulder circles, even open-swing twists and side-bends. Open-chain movements require great internal awareness and balance, as there is less external and biofeedback to guide alignment and proprioception. It is helpful in many yoga *asana* contexts to enhance proprioception in closed-chain contexts before using open-chain variations. For example, in a Half Lift, we may teach grounding the hands firmly on a block before inviting a rag doll variation. Open-chain actions can introduce shearing forces or increased demand for control at specific joints, which can be used intentionally to develop mobility or assess functional range of motion.

Compared to closed-chain movements, open-chain movements are more variable and offer opportunities for dynamic exploration, mobility training, and expressive range. Because of this, they can expose vulnerable joints to instability if engaged in without adequate strength or awareness (e.g., high-leg lifts without core engagement can stress the lumbar spine). Open-chain *asana* may appear in creative and exploratory sequences, are to be used with great attention and mindfulness, and can have targeted purpose and value in therapeutic contexts.

## *Understanding and Making Use of Reflexes*

As noted previously, we sense the world from the outside in via *exteroception* and ourselves from the inside out via *proprioception*, *interoception*, and *neuroception*. In the current context, we are interested in proprioception, the body's ability to sense itself in space – a key capacity that gives us continuous access to information about how our various body parts are oriented in space, are moving relative to one another, and are positioned. This capacity supports complex and coordinated movement with ongoing subtle (automatic) adjustments that keep us balanced and safe within an optimal range of motion in joints and extensibility of the musculotendinous region being moved (i.e., lengthened or contracted); Biel & Dorn, 2019; Coulter, 2001).

Several types of receptors are built into our musculoskeletal system for this purpose and link to various types of reflexes that allow for ongoing and quick adjustment that is necessary for the many complex physical actions we engage in all day long. Of particular importance to proprioception are mechanoreceptors called muscle spindles, Golgi tendon organs, and joint receptors. For head position, proprioceptors are also embedded in the vestibular system. Further contributing to skeletal movement are signals from nociceptors that result in self-protective motor reflexes.

Most importantly in a yoga *asana* context, muscle spindles are mechanoreceptors (i.e., support proprioception) in all skeletal muscles, interspersed with muscle fibers. They sense increases in muscle length and the rate of change in muscle lengthening (i.e., they sense excessive or sudden *stretch* or lengthening in a muscle). Their protective function is to send an alert signal to the spinal cord that activates lower motor neurons to inhibit stretch of a muscle in danger of being overstretched via provoking contraction in that muscle and inhibiting contraction in the antagonist muscle. Muscle spindles underlie stretch reflexes (e.g., myotatic stretch reflex) and, if triggered repeatedly, can contribute to excessive muscle tightness, with implications for yoga that are explored in more detail below.

Golgi tendon organs are mechanoreceptors embedded in the tendons of all skeletal muscles at the muscle-tendon junction. They monitor skeletal muscle/tendon load and rate of increase in muscle/tendon load. Their protective function is to monitor excessive load on the tendon and may signal imminent injury due to excessive load that may threaten to sever the muscle from its bony attachment. Such load triggers an alert signal from the Golgi tendon organ to the spinal cord that activates motor neurons to promote stretch or a sudden release of contraction in a muscle being loaded. Specifically, this motor signal inhibits tension in the contracted agonist and initiates tension in the antagonist. Golgi tendon organs underly autogenic inhibition (i.e., Golgi tendon reflex or inverse stretch reflex) and proprioceptive neuromuscular facilitation (all described below).

## Role of Reflexes in Yoga

As shown above, reflexes play a role in dealing with compressive and tensile loads on the body; yet, their importance goes way beyond that. Reflexes are hardwired because they are important to guaranteeing our physical survival and reactivity in response to perceptions of danger or threat. Relevant to the musculoskeletal system and thus yoga *asana*, there are two types: short latency and medium or long latency reflexes. These reflexes draw on the actions of the muscle spindles and Golgi tendon organs.

*Short latency reflexes* are mediated in the spinal cord (i.e., sensory signals travel from the proprioceptors in the muscle to spine; the motor signal travels back from the spine via lower motor neurons to create a reflexive action in the muscle). These reflexes are not cerebral and not under voluntary control. They occur through sensory and motor neurons, sometimes very directly and monosynaptically; at other times, polysynaptically via a connection of a sensory with a motor neuron through an associative, relay, or inter-neuron. Because the sensory signals only travel to the spine (not all the way to the cortex) and the motor signal is initiated at the level of the spinal cord, these reflexes are extremely fast. At the somatic level (i.e., related to skeletal muscle), we have them for purposes of injury prevention in response to (perceived) excessive load (either compressive or tensile). At the autonomic level (including smooth and cardiac muscle), they occur in reaction to pain, temperature, or similar sudden stress, danger, or threat perceived by the nervous system.

*Longer latency reflexes* have supraspinal control. The sensory signal travels above the spinal cord to the brain and then back down (via upper motor neurons). This pathway is in action for medium or long latency reflexes. As alluded to above, autonomic reflexes affect the inner organs. Somatic reflexes, of interest in the yoga *asana* context, affect the muscles. Interestingly, some reflexes (especially flexion reflexes) can be induced by non-physical stress, acting similarly to reflexes induced by pain or threat (Payne & Usatine, 2002). We all know this when we say things like '*I carry my stress in my neck*'. It is essentially a part of the fight-flight sympathetic nervous system response (i.e., *rajas* or sympathetic arousal that has solidified into a particular *samskara* in the body). This means that stress and trauma can decrease muscle resilience or increase continuous muscle tension. Affected muscles begin to hold their tension without being able to release it on their own. Yoga can reteach muscles their more optimal function through slow and mindful movement as well as subtle, nasal, and diaphragmatic breathing. Diaphragmatic breathing counters the fight-flight response; slow movement combined with subtle breathing relaxes the nervous system. As we teach students to move while in their ventral vagal state, with patience, muscles can reset (Schwartz, 2024).

Understanding reflexes can help yoga professionals better predict what may be happening in students' bodies and facilitate greater resilience and adaptation in their bodies through deliberate cueing. This is so because reflexes are triggered by sensory receptors that influence muscle tension – either via releasing tension or creating it in response to sensory inputs (Coulter, 2001). An exploration of relevant reflexes and their applicability in yoga *asana* follows. However, a little detour into another brain-related issue is helpful first. Understanding reflexes also needs to include an understanding of the fact that humans have unique wiring in their brains that sets them apart from other mammals, in that it allows humans to make conscious decision about how they move, in essence being able to override reflexes if circumstances demand. For example, plenty of stories exist of yogis being able to walk across hot coals. This capacity is grounded in this ability to use higher cortical activation to override the reflexes that would under typically circumstance trigger an escape from such a dangerous stimulus.

*Brief Detour to the Anterior and Posterior Insula*

The section of the brain that allows for this overriding control of hard-wired reflexes is in the insula. The insular cortex, often referred to simply as the *insula*, plays a crucial integrative role in how we perceive bodily states and regulate our movement responses. Functionally, the insula can be divided into anterior and posterior regions, each with distinct contributions to movement coordination and sensory interpretation.

The *posterior insula* serves as a primary hub for the integration of *interoception* (internal bodily sensations), *proprioception* (positional awareness of the body in space), and *neuroception* (the subconscious evaluation of safety or threat). It registers the physiological reverberations of movement – stretch, load, breath, and internal rhythm – and classifies these sensory experiences in affective terms: positive, negative, or neutral. This evaluative process is essential for generating split-second somatic decisions: whether to continue a movement, stop it, or remain indifferent. For example, the posterior insula helps determine whether a stretch is beneficial, potentially injurious, or inconsequential. In this sense, it functions as the neuroanatomical seat of *vedanas* – the feeling tones that, in traditional frameworks, precede attachment, aversion, or confusion (*kleshas*). The posterior insula makes these implicit value judgments rapidly, shaping our ongoing motor behavior and influencing our memory of bodily experience. The *anterior insula*, by contrast, is more involved in processing exteroceptive stimuli such as taste, smell, and tactile input. These sensory cues contribute to our emotional and behavioral responses by linking external sensory information to internal states. Together, the anterior and posterior insulae form a bridge between raw sensory data and complex emotional-motor decisions.

A particularly significant feature of the insula's functional capacity is its population of *von Economo* neurons (sometimes referred to as VENs). These large, spindle-shaped neurons are relatively rare in the animal kingdom and are more abundant in humans and great apes. They are located primarily in the anterior insula and the anterior cingulate cortex and are thought to support rapid, high-level decision-making in uncertain or complex social and somatic situations. *Von Economo* neurons play a direct role in overriding reflexive responses to pain, discomfort, or perceived threat. For instance, during a stretch that activates the muscle spindle reflex, *von Economo* neurons can support a discernment-based override: deciding that the context is safe, the movement is controlled, and parasympathetic regulation can be maintained. This enables individuals (such as yoga students) to consciously downshift into a relaxed state and explore a range of motion that might otherwise trigger protective withdrawal. In essence, it is this human capacity that allows us to play at the edges in a yoga *asana* practice.

In effect, the insula, through the function of *von Economo* neurons, grants humans a remarkably refined capacity to modulate movement intentionally. It enables humans to pause at the edge of physical limitations, assess internal signals, and choose the next action based not solely on instinctual reflexes but on contextual awareness and conscious judgment. This capacity is foundational to somatic practices such as yoga *asana* that emphasize mindful movement, self-regulation, and nervous system adaptation. The discussion that follows relies on understanding the interaction between the reflexive and deliberate movement actions that can be applied in a yoga *asana* context, especially in its therapeutic and deliberately mindful applications.

## *Myotatic Stretch Reflex*

The myotatic stretch reflex, also known as stretch reflex or muscle stretch reflex, is a monosynaptic (the only one of its kind), somatic, ipsilateral spinal reflex. It is mediated by muscle spindles, specialized proprioceptive receptors located within skeletal muscle fibers that detect changes in muscle length and the speed of that change. Although commonly referred to in clinical practice as the deep tendon reflex, this label is anatomically misleading. The response originates in the muscle spindles, not the tendons themselves. The stretch reflex is the fastest somatic reflex in the body due to the direct (monosynaptic) communication between the sensory neuron and the motor neuron. The reflex helps regulate muscle tone, maintain posture, and protect muscle integrity. Here is how the reflex works:

- Muscle spindles detect a rapid or excessive stretch in a muscle, activating Type Ia afferent sensory neurons.
- These sensory neurons carry the signal to the spinal cord, where they synapse directly onto alpha motor neurons that innervate the same (agonist) muscle.
- The motor neurons trigger a contraction of the stretched muscle in order to resist further lengthening and protect the muscle from potential tearing.
- Simultaneously, inhibitory interneurons are activated to relax the antagonist muscle, a process known as reciprocal inhibition, which enhances the efficiency of the reflex.
- A classic clinical example is the patellar reflex, where a tap on the patellar tendon stretches the quadriceps and triggers an immediate contraction (causing the leg to kick forward).

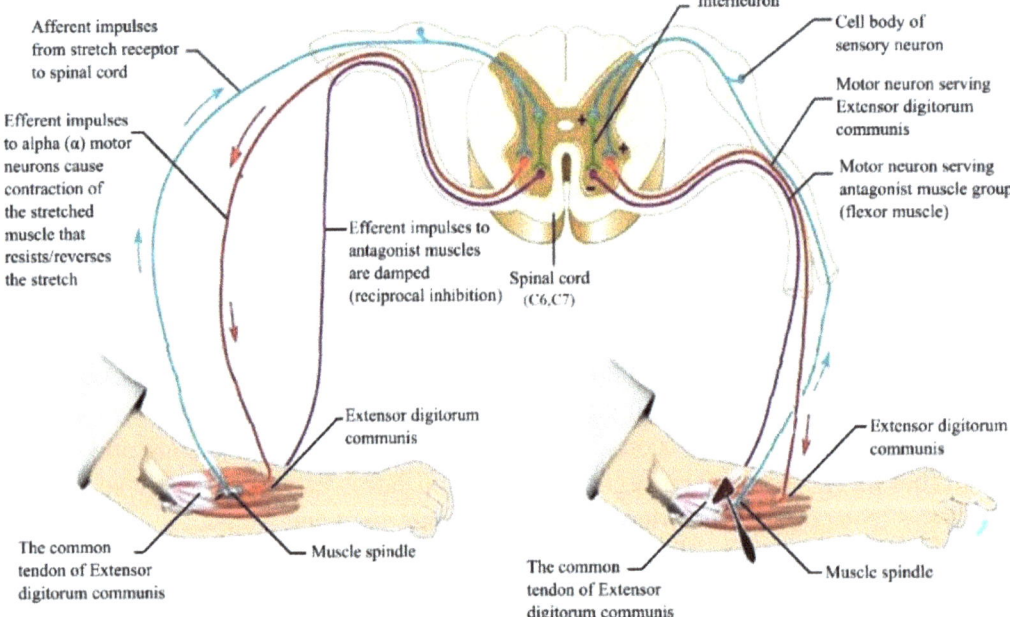

**Figure 4.2** Sample of a stretch reflex. (Data source: Zhang MJ, Zhu CZ, Duan ZM, Niu X.; https://upload.wikimedia.org/wikipedia/commons/2/22/The_extensor_digitorum_reflex.jpg; Creative Commons Attribution 4.0)

*Relevance to Yoga: Slow Mindful Movement Into and Out of Shapes*

In yoga, it is important to understand the myotatic stretch reflex because it governs how the body naturally responds to sudden or intense stretching. When a muscle is lengthened too quickly or too far, the embedded muscle spindles send signals to trigger contraction of that same muscle. This protective reflex prevents overstretching and potential tearing; if provoked suddenly during practice, it can also lead to muscle guarding, which inhibits the very release we may be seeking.

For example, in a forward fold, if a practitioner suddenly drops into the shape without adequate preparation, the hamstrings may reflexively contract in response to the perceived threat of rapid stretch. This involuntary contraction creates resistance and tension, which can feel like tightness or stuckness and increase the risk of strain. In contrast, when we move slowly and with awareness, we give the nervous system time to interpret the stretch as safe, allowing the spindles to adapt and reducing the likelihood of triggering the reflex. This is one reason why gradual progression into a shape, with mindful breathing and attentive transitions, can lead to a more effective and sustainable range of motion.

Repetitive high-impact actions like jumping into or out of yoga shapes can lead to habitual activation of this reflex. Each time a muscle undergoes rapid eccentric lengthening (such as the hamstrings during a jump), the reflex triggers a contraction to prevent overstretch. Over time, this repeated contraction response can condition the muscle to remain in a slightly shortened or more guarded state, ultimately reducing its elastic capacity and resilience. Some practitioners, like Coulter (2001), caution against bouncing in yoga poses for this very reason, suggesting it may repeatedly activate the stretch reflex. Others, such as Mitchell (2019), argue that bouncing may not be intense enough to consistently trigger it. Likely, the response varies depending on the individual's level of conditioning, neuromuscular patterning, and tissue health.

What is more universally agreed upon is that slow, mindful movement into and out of shapes helps minimize unnecessary activation of the stretch reflex. When a shape is entered gradually, with control and breath awareness, the muscle spindles have time to adapt to the stretch. This builds neurological trust, reducing reflexive contraction and allowing the muscle to lengthen more safely and effectively. Holding a shape with endurance further supports this adaptation, helping the muscle settle into its lengthened state, increasing flexibility over time. Importantly, the stiffer or more resistant a student's muscles are (whether due to training, stress, or structural imbalances), the longer it may take for the stretch reflex to release during a pose. Patience is key. Only once the reflex calms and the muscle begins to relax can the fascia begin to deform and remodel, contributing to more lasting change in range of motion. In this way, yoga becomes a tool not for overpowering the body's protective systems, but for working with them by inviting gradual, intelligent adaptation rather than abrupt force.

Sustained holds with gentle muscular engagement can help recalibrate the muscle spindle response, encouraging more elasticity and responsiveness over time. Thus, reciprocal inhibition can be used strategically: gently activating the antagonist muscle group can create reflexive relaxation in the muscle being stretched. For example, engaging the quadriceps during a hamstring stretch signals the hamstrings to soften and facilitates deeper access to the shape without forcing. Ultimately, working with the stretch reflex requires building trust between body and nervous system. Rather than forcing range of motion, it is invited via gradual transformation through slow, gentle, intelligent movements that honor the nervous system's protective role.

## Golgi Tendon Reflex

The Golgi tendon reflex, also called autogenic inhibition, inverse stretch reflex, or clasp-knife reflex, is a polysynaptic, ipsilateral reflex mediated by Golgi tendon organs (GTOs), sensory receptors located at the junction of muscles and tendons. These receptors monitor tension rather than length (unlike muscle spindles) and function to prevent damage to the muscle and tendon from excessive force. Here is how the reflex works:

- When excessive tension is detected in a muscle-tendon unit, the Golgi tendon organs send afferent signals via Type Ib sensory fibers to the spinal cord.
- These afferents synapse interneurons, which then inhibit the alpha motor neurons of the same muscle, resulting in reduced contraction (muscle relaxation).
- Simultaneously, excitatory signals may be sent to the antagonist muscle to promote contraction, a phenomenon called reciprocal facilitation.
- This mechanism helps protect tendons from injury by reducing the muscle's force output when strain becomes too high.
- 'Clasp-knife reflex' refers to the sudden collapse of resistance in a muscle, often observed in sudden muscular release (e.g., during arm wrestling) or neurological conditions (when it may be considered pathological).
- Isometric or active isotonic contractions can stimulate GTOs, making this reflex clinically and functionally useful for increasing range of motion.
- Manual stimulation (e.g., massage) at the musculotendinous junction can also increase GTO firing and enhance release of muscular tension.

### Relevance to Yoga: Proprioceptive Neuromuscular Facilitation

In yoga practice, the Golgi tendon reflex can be leveraged to facilitate deeper, safer muscular release—particularly when working with tight or overactive muscles. This principle underlies techniques such as Proprioceptive Neuromuscular Facilitation (PNF), where a muscle is intentionally contracted prior to a stretch to trigger its relaxation response. For example, if a student struggles with adductor tightness that limits external rotation in the hips (such as difficulty entering half lotus), they can apply this reflex as follows:

- Begin by lying on the back with the legs opened into a comfortable wide-legged position.
- Using a yoga strap looped around one leg, a helper gently pulls the leg outward while the student actively contracts the adductors – as if trying to draw the leg toward the midline.
- This isometric effort against resistance activates the GTOs in the adductor tendons.
- After holding this contraction for several breaths, the helper releases the outward pull, and the student stops contracting.

This brief, deliberate effort sends a strong signal through the GTOs, which triggers an inhibitory response, allowing the adductors to release more fully. To further support this release, gentle massage at the inner groin (near the musculotendinous junction of the adductors) can stimulate the same reflex pathway, encouraging relaxation through sensory input.

After repeating this process on both sides, students often experience a noticeable improvement in range of motion, making entry into shapes like half lotus more accessible and more comfortable. This use of contraction to facilitate release reflects a broader yoga principle: sometimes we must engage with resistance in order to let go.

## *Flexion Reflexes*

The flexion reflex, also called the pain reflex or flexor withdrawal reflex, is a polysynaptic, protective spinal reflex that causes the body to flex away from danger, such as a painful stimulus or mechanical threat. It is mediated by nociceptors and other somatic sensory receptors that detect pain, temperature, or tissue damage. This reflex helps prevent or limit injury by producing rapid muscular responses that pull the affected body part away from the source of harm. Because it involves coordination between multiple muscle groups, the flexion reflex is antagonistic and polysynaptic: a single sensory signal triggers multiple motor outputs, exciting one muscle group simultaneously and inhibiting its antagonists. Here is how the reflex works:

- A sensory signal indicating potential harm (e.g., from nociceptors in the skin or fascia) is sent to the spinal cord.
- This signal activates interneurons, which coordinate two motor responses:
  - An excitatory signal causes the agonist muscle to contract, pulling the body part away.
  - An inhibitory signal is simultaneously sent to the antagonist (extensor) muscle, allowing it to relax and lengthen so that flexion can occur efficiently.

A classic example is withdrawing a hand from a hot stove. However, this reflex is not limited to physical stimuli—it can also be triggered by neuroceptive danger, a term coined by Stephen Porges to describe unconscious detection of threat. In these cases, tissue tension may arise in response to emotional, environmental, or psychological stress, activating a flexion pattern that readies the body for protective responses like fight, flight, or collapse. In some cases, the reflex also includes a crossed-extension component: when one leg flexes to withdraw from harm (such as stepping on a sharp object), the contralateral leg extends to stabilize and support the body's weight. This is known as the crossed extensor reflex.

### *Relevance to Yoga: Reciprocal Muscle Inhibition*

In yoga, the flexion reflex provides a functional neurological basis for reciprocal muscle inhibition, a principle that can be actively harnessed in yoga *asana* cueing and practice to promote safer, more effective release. Specifically, reciprocal inhibition refers to the process in which contraction of one muscle (the agonist) leads to reflexive relaxation of its opposite (the antagonist). This is rooted in the same neural circuitry as the flexion reflex. For instance, when the quadriceps are activated, the hamstrings naturally receive a signal to reduce their contraction. Instead of asking students to stretch or lengthen the hamstrings (a concept that is difficult to act on neurologically), active contraction of the quadriceps can be cued (e.g., *lift the kneecaps* or *draw the kneecaps toward the hips*), prompting the body to release tension in the back of the legs through reflexive pathways. This neurological insight changes how yoga professionals can help students approach tight or painful areas. If an individual has a tight lower back, a direction or cue inviting the student to try to stretch the back may simply provoke more guarding. Instead, the invitation can be for flexion elsewhere, such as making fists with the hands or flexing the knees, to invite reflexive release in the spinal extensors. This mechanism can be helpful in *savasana*: if low back discomfort is present, placing a rolled blanket under the knees encourages knee flexion, which can help downregulate hypertonic spinal muscles through the same mechanism.

Crucially, the reflex works across muscle groups and not just isolated muscles, and sometimes even across sides of the body. In the crossed extensor reflex, for example, if one foot steps on something painful, the opposite leg's extensors engage to support the body's withdrawal. This means that in some yoga *asana*, contralateral activation (engaging muscles on the opposite side) can provide unexpected support or release on the targeted side. Though the flexion reflex is automatic, it is also subject to conscious modulation (see above).. Skilled yoga practice builds awareness and control over movement patterns that are normally reflexive. However, in conditions of heightened stress, trauma, or altered states (such as fatigue or intoxication), the flexion reflex may override conscious control, manifesting as muscle tension, protective postures, or limited mobility. A trauma-informed or mindful approach to yoga recognizes these reflexes not as blocks, but as signals that may indicate where and how the body is seeking safety and self-protection. By working with the nervous system, not against it, neurologically intelligent cueing can help soften tension, prevent reactivity, and invite muscular and emotional release.

| *Understanding Reflexes in the Context of Cueing in Yoga* | | | |
|---|---|---|---|
| | *Golgi Tendon Reflex* | *Myotatic Stretch Reflex* | *Flexion Reflexes* |
| *What it senses:* | Strong or sudden muscle contraction leading to excessive tension in a tendon (e.g., lifting too heavy of a weight) | Strong or sudden muscle lengthening (e.g., like when we jump off a height and the quads are stretched) | Threat or danger of injury as well as threat or danger to survival (e.g., via nociception or neuroception) |
| *What results:* | Release the contraction in the agonist and cause contraction in the antagonist (e.g., the sudden collapse of contraction in the biceps that happens in arm wrestling) | Cause contraction in the stretched muscle and cause lengthening in the reciprocal muscle (e.g., quads strongly contract and the hamstrings release) | Safeguards against injury by promoting muscular collaboration that facilitates movement away from a source of danger or threat |
| *Also called:* | Autogenic inhibition → an inverse stretch reflex | Muscle stretch reflex or stretch reflex → shock-absorbing reflex | Pain reflex or flexor withdrawal reflex |
| *Mediated by:* | *Golgi tendon receptors* at the musculotendinous junction that sense stretch in a muscle tendon | *Muscle spindles* in muscles that sense change and rate of change in muscle length | Receptors, including nociceptors and neuroceptors, that signal danger to the organism |
| *Type of sensory signal sent:* | A sensory signal of *excessive or sudden tension on a tendon due to strong contraction of a* | A sensory signal of *excessive or sudden stretch or lengthening in a muscle* is sent to spinal cord | A sensory signal of danger is sent to the spinal cord to safeguard the area of body under threat against injury |

| **Understanding Reflexes in the Context of Cueing in Yoga** | | | |
|---|---|---|---|
| | *Golgi Tendon Reflex* | *Myotatic Stretch Reflex* | *Flexion Reflexes* |
| | *muscle* is sent to spinal cord | | |
| *Type of motor signal received:* | A motor signal is sent to the muscle fibers to *inhibit contraction (i.e., to lengthen the muscle)* and release tension on the tendon; Another motor signal is sent to *cause the antagonist muscle to contract* | A motor signal is sent to muscle fibers to *contract to protect the muscle from over-stretching or tearing*; another signal is sent to *cause the antagonist to lengthen* (to inhibit contraction) | *Two motor signals* are sent back to *different locations* in the body to produce two simultaneous but opposite effects *in response to the single sensory signal*; *agonist(s) flex(es) away*; *antagonist(s) relax(es) contraction and lengthen* |
| *Yoga applications:* | • Use this reflex by holding isometric contraction for a while in a muscle we seek to stretch, until the muscle gives<br>• Actively contract a muscle to be stretched before lengthening it (e.g., against a force such as a strap)<br>• Proprioceptive neuromuscular facilitation | • Slow movement (as rapid movement triggers the reflex to tighten) into and out of shape and holding them to increase flexibility and resilience<br>• Fascia is hypothesized to stretch when the myotatic stretch reflex lets go and muscle begins to lengthen (to return to its usual state)<br>• Avoid sudden or jerky loading | • We can release a muscle via contraction of the antagonist: the muscle on one side of a joint relaxes (releases its contraction somewhat) to accommodate contraction of the reciprocal muscle<br>• Cue strengthening (concentrically contracting) the antagonist rather than lengthening or stretching the agonist |
| *Other implications:* | • Can add self-massage to the tendon of a contracted muscle (targeted for stretching) to create even more tendon stretch and hence a faster or stronger signal to release the contracted muscle to protect the tendon | • High-impact yoga jumping may serve to decrease resilience of involved muscles due to repeated reflexive contraction in suddenly lengthened muscles<br>• Some argue that bouncing activates the myotatic stretch reflex and hence recommend against this practice; others say bouncing is not strong enough to trigger this reflex – this may depend on student conditioning | • Realize that often agonists and antagonists are actually not individual muscles but whole muscle groups<br>• They are not always obvious agonists and antagonists, e.g.: a tight back can be released by making fists with the hands because flexion here results in relaxation/extension in the back muscles |

## What's Ahead

Having explored sequencing, practice principles, pedagogy, biomechanics, and principles for understanding and working with physical pain and resistance, load and force, and reflexes, it is time to delve into the specifics of the various categories of yoga *asana*. All major categories of shapes are included in integrated holistic yoga, always with a focus on teaching from a therapeutic lens that emphasizes clear intention, optimized accessibility, access to information about risks, contraindications, and realistic assessment of potential benefit, as well as clarity about prop use, individual variation, patient-centered adaptation, and an invitational and empowering style. All shapes and movements are offered in a manner that addresses all five layers of human experience (i.e., all *koshas*), while integrating all limbs, from yoga ethics to lifestyle and discipline, breathwork, and contemplative practice, into the yoga *asana* practice. The following categories of *asana* are covered in the chapters that follow, with emphasis on the most accessible, beneficial, and intentional forms and movements – always offered in the context of all eight limbs and five layers of human experience.

| Upright standing – Chapter 8<br>• Warrior 1, Warrior 3, Eagle<br>• Warrior 2, Side Angle, Triangle, Tree | Forward folds – Chapter 12<br>• Standing: Legs together and wide-legged<br>• Seated: Legs together and wide-legged<br>• Head-of-Knee, Child |
|---|---|
| Arm standing – Chapter 9<br>• Table Top, Downward Facing Dog<br>• Plank, Side Plank | Backbends – Chapter 13<br>• Camel<br>• Cobra, Locust<br>• Bridge and related |
| Seats – Chapter 10<br>• Easy Seat, Bound Angle<br>• Hero, Staff, Cow Face | Inversions – Chapter 14<br>• Handstand, Half Handstand<br>• Headstand, Tripod Headstand<br>• Candlestick |
| Twists – Chapter 11<br>• Standing<br>• Seated<br>• Supine<br>• Prone | Restoratives – Chapter 15<br>• Seats<br>• Folds<br>• Twists<br>• Backbends<br>• Inversions |

For each category, several issues are addressed, first for the category of shapes overall and then for select, but representative and foundational, individual shapes in that category:
- Helpful anatomical foci, with reference back to relevant chapters in Section 1
- Sample cueing related to grounding, expansion, and stability
- Benefits and cautions related to specific shapes or categories of shapes
- Preparations that will optimize the experience of the practice
- Key alignment invitations for each specific shape
- Variations and suggestions for explorations to deepen the experience within each shape
- Recovery guidance

## Important Disclaimer – Please Read

In using the remainder of this book, as the focus shifts to teaching and practicing specific yoga *asana*, a few disclaimers are important to hold in mind:

- Whenever there is reference to a specific muscle, please understand that the reference is really to the entire complex of connective tissue, muscle, and bone in the region identified with (i.e., connected to) to that muscle – the specific muscle label is a shortcut word for the entire myofascial and bony structures connected to the muscle; it will also tend to include additional muscles directly surrounding or collaborating with this muscle (including perhaps as an antagonist).

- Please remember the concept of anatomy trains; the physical structures around referenced muscles connect to other structures around other muscles below, above, and otherwise adjacent to that muscle. The concept of anatomy trains reminds us that everything is always connected to everything else in the body and it is impossible to spell out the entire chain of events and experience in one cue or sentence.

- The reverberation of a shape or movement always happens throughout the entire physical, vital, mental and emotional organism, not just the specific muscles or structures under close observation. Body is not separate from breath or mind. Every shape and movement is not just physical; it is also vital and psychological

- Reverberations and mutual influences can also <u>arise</u> from other *koshas*; shapes and movements may be profoundly affected and influences by energetic, emotional, or mental factors that are habitual or acute. It is important always to keep an open mind in observing muscles as simply a symbolic representation of the entire human being in motion when teaching movements and yoga *asana*.

- For some shapes, emotional and mental contributions, in fact, may be more powerful than the physical capacity or preparedness. These effects of contributions can cut in multiple ways:
  - sometimes emotional or mental strivings or attachments lead students to force themselves into a shape that is not actually auspicious for them
  - sometimes emotional or mental fears and preconceptions prevent students from even considering the possibility that a shape may be accessible to them
  - in either situation, well-attuned and co-regulating teachers can help create access to a shape that is most auspicious for the given client by remembering to draw on all *koshas*, or layers of experience, that are expressed by the individual in the context of their lifetime, their biopsychosociocultural context, and their present moment experience

*Knowledge is only a rumor until it lives in the muscle.*
Asaro tribe of Indonesia and Papua New Guinea

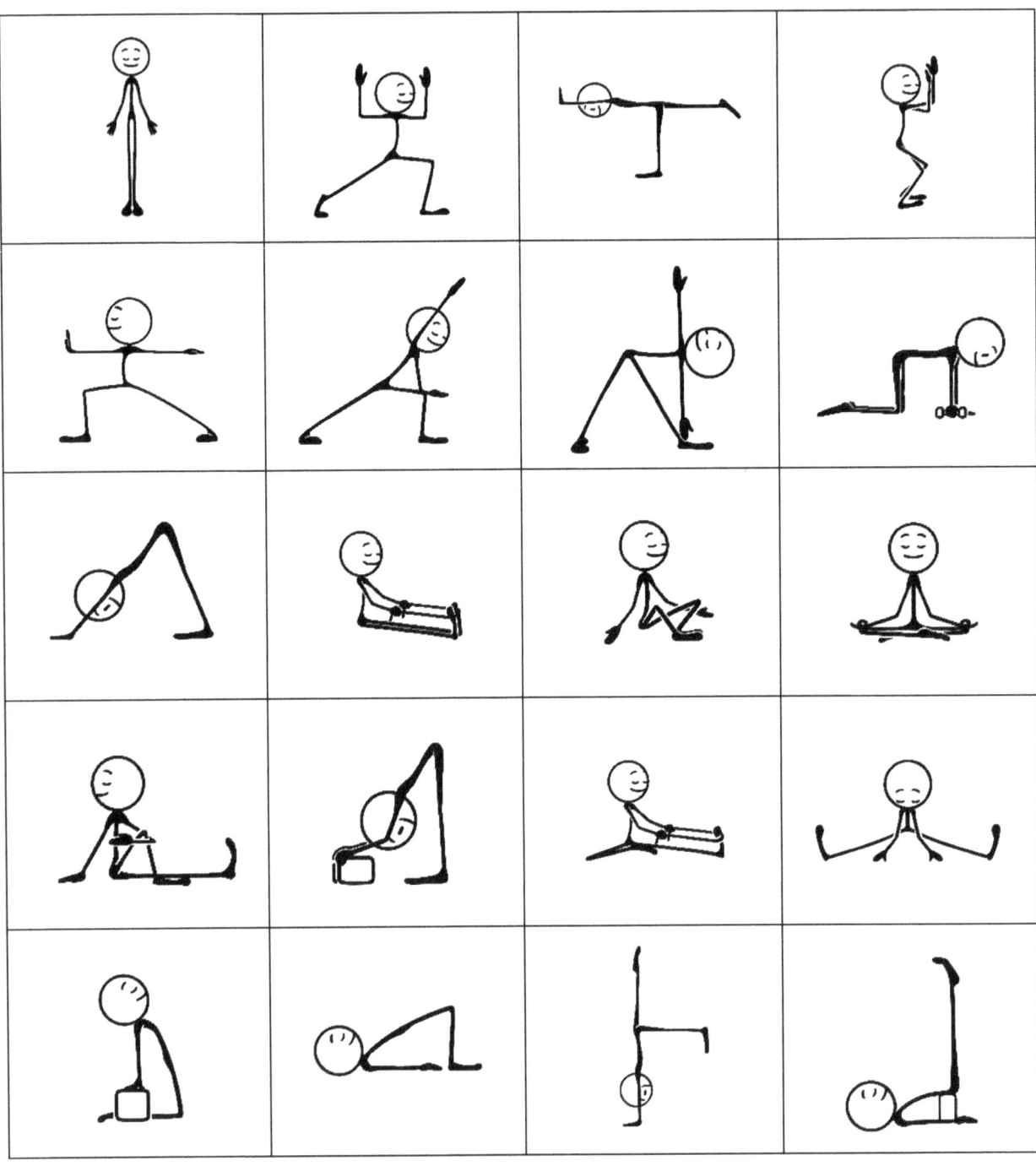

# Chapter 8: Upright Standing Shapes

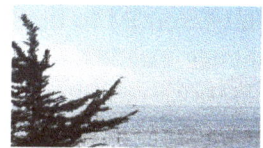

This chapter covers foundational standing shapes, offering optimized teaching strategies that allow for individual tailoring and careful discernment about how and which shapes to offer, as well as about how to cue alignment informed by interoception, proprioception, exteroception, and neuroception. General principles for this category of yoga *asana* are provided and apply to most if not all upright standing shapes. Specific follow-up guidance is added for the chosen sample shapes.

## Anatomical Foci for Upright Standing Shapes

Standing shapes serve as the foundation for understanding postural alignment and load distribution in yoga and yoga therapy. A well-aligned standing shape reflects the natural architecture of the spine, the dynamic stability of the pelvis and hips, and the integrated engagement of the feet, legs, and core. Teaching standing shapes well lays the groundwork for all upright shapes and for cultivating functional postural resilience off the mat. Important issues in teaching upright standing include, but are not limited to, cultivation of a natural spine, stabilization of the core, and assembly of the shape from the bottom up, with careful attention to feet, knees, and pelvis (especially hip and sacroiliac joints), in that order. Foot work can be a great preparatory practice that awakens the feet, enhances balances, and can serve to support individuals with peripheral neuropathy or other balance or proprioceptive challenges. Understanding natural spinal alignment spine is key, along with all its reverberations into the pelvis, legs, and feet.

### *Understanding and Recruiting the Natural Spine*

A natural spine is both a structural and functional concept – referring not only to the anatomical curves of the vertebral column but also to the dynamic balance, postural tone, and intersegmental relationships that support upright orientation. In standing yoga shapes, the integrity of these spinal curves is a central contributor to postural ease, balanced effort, and musculoskeletal health. A review of Chapter 4 will be useful before working with this material, as it details the axial skeleton's structure and developmental curves.

In standing, healthful and stable posture arises from being anchored in grounded feet, strong ankles, and resilient knees aligned with hip and shoulder joints. The pelvis is the foundation of strength and resilience for the entire spine above it – regardless of whether standing or seated. A resiliently anchored pelvis that can support a resilient and dynamic spine is in its natural position, neither tucked posteriorly, nor tilted (excessively) anteriorly. An anchored pelvis invites the spine to move with the pelvis as a dynamic unit that is adaptable and resilient – neither braced nor collapsed. In its natural curves, a spine invites diaphragmatic breathing that unfolds optimally at the mid-torso with gentle movements of the abdomen and low rib basket.

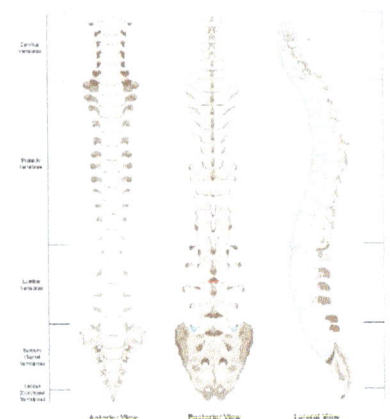

**Figure 2.3** Human spinal anatomy. (Data source: istock)

The natural curves of the spine are central to upright posture and essential to the structural intelligence of standing shapes. As described in Chapter 4, the axial skeleton is composed of alternating primary (kyphotic) and secondary (lordotic) curves. These curves form developmentally sequentially and move in sympathetic relation to one another. The thoracic and sacral curves emerge in utero and are associated with the flexion-dominant shapes of early life. The cervical and lumbar curves arise later as the infant begins lifting the head and moving upright against gravity. These alternating curves provide the spine with its structural balance, allowing for both mobility and stability.

In standing shapes, preserving and refining the natural spinal curves enhances the body's ability to bear weight efficiently while maintaining a sense of energetic lift and spatial orientation. Rather than thinking of the spine as a rigid column, it is useful to envision it as a responsive, three-dimensional structure with vertebrae stacked to allow for load distribution, shock absorption, and subtle adjustments. The natural spine positions the head directly over the pelvis with the ears aligned vertically above the shoulders and a gentle inward curve at the neck. This alignment supports engagement of the deep spinal stabilizers, especially the postural, endurance-based muscles that prevent fatigue during sustained upright shapes. A simple stability test to assess this alignment is offered in the Box below.

> *Spine Stability Test*
> 
> - Ask the student to stand in Mountain with arms by the side of the body
> - Ask permission to touch; if granted, proceed; if not, stop
> - Press straight down on the tops of the student's shoulders
> - Note if the student buckled or swayed – especially in the knees
> - If no, the student is already well aligned and stable
> - If yes, ask the student to realign according to the principles noted elsewhere (natural spine and pelvis; soft knees; etc.)
> - Upon realignment, retest; continue realignment until the student is aligned and stable

When teaching spinal alignment in standing shapes, it is helpful to cue and help clients or students understand each spinal curve distinctly:
- The *sacral curve* is naturally kyphotic and sits in the pelvis, which in its natural position is slightly anteriorally rotated. Over-cueing a posterior pelvic tuck flattens this curve and can negatively affect spinal and pelvic stability. However, it is also necessary to recognize excess anterior rotation of the pelvis (as may be present in hypermobile individuals) to help them find a less extreme position for the pelvis. In such cases, it may be helpful to invite a tucking of the tailbone to actually achieve a natural position for the pelvis. Finding the sweet spot of

anterior pelvic rotation is key for the rest of the spine as natural alignment of all superior spinal sections depends on such natural positioning of the pelvis.
- The *lumbar curve* is lordotic, characterized by a gentle inward curve. Maintaining this curve, without exaggerating it, is crucial for load-bearing in standing shapes. It is important to understand the difference between hyper- and hypolordosis to adjust cueing that is student-centered and tailored to the individual presentation of the spine in standing.
- The *thoracic curve* is kyphotic, and although many students present with excessive rounding here, it is important not to overcorrect by flattening the curve. The thoracic spine is meant to be convex and flexible. It is helpful to learn to differentiate natural versus hyperkyphosis in the thoracic spine to optimize cueing and adjustment.
- The *cervical curve* mirrors the lumbar spine in its lordotic shape. The head ideally rests effortlessly atop the spine, with the chin gently tucked and the gaze level.

The spinal curves operate as an integrated system that is = collaborative and influential upward and downward along the entire length of the spine. Altering one region (e.g., flattening the lumbar spine by tucking the pelvis) can initiate a cascade of changes and compensation, in the other sections of the spine, from the tailbone to the skull. Yoga practitioners and professionals are well served to understand these interrelationships and to find access to a balanced, whole-spine organization.

> *Avoiding Inauspicious Cueing Related To Pelvic Positioning*
>
> One common indiscriminately-used cue in yoga instruction is the invitation of pelvic tucking. Although pelvic tucking can serve a specific purpose in certain shapes (e.g., arm standing, backbending), in standing shapes it may disrupt the sacral angle, flatten the lumbar curve, and inhibit the recruitment of core stabilizing musculature. Pelvic tucking in standing shapes is only invited for students who are hyperlordotic and whose pelvis is too far anterior. It is helpful to cue students to explore the angle of their pelvis instead, letting them find their own way of creating the most auspicious anterior tilt that supports grounding and uprightness.
>
> In other words, rather than cueing indiscriminately, teach students how to recognize their pelvic angle and to adjust toward the middle sweet spot – students with too much anterior tilt learn to tuck slightly; students with too little anterior tilt learn to roll the pelvis forward. This tailored cueing is educational for clients and preventive of misaligning the pelvis to either extreme.

When the spine is in its natural curves, the deep postural muscles, including but not limited to the multifidi, rotatores, and spinalis groups, are engaged in the most auspicious manner for posture, core strength, and spinal health. These slow-twitch muscles are made for endurance and their engagement invites steadiness and ease rather than bracing or strain versus collapse or loss of integration. A wobbly or collapsed standing shape signals interference with natural alignment and suggests the presences of dysfunction or misalignments that could possibly addressed through subtle repositioning based on careful proprioception and interoception.

*Understanding the Spinal Curves in the Sagittal Plane*

Spinal alignment is most readily assessed in the sagittal plane, which reveals the anterior-posterior relationships between spinal segments and the orientation of the spine relative to the pelvis, head, and legs. A plumb line or visual reference tool such as a dowel or yoga strap suspended from the ceiling can help students perceive vertical alignment. Chapter 4 offered additional detail; a brief summary follows.

A well-aligned vertical line typically passes through the following anatomical landmarks:
- External auditory meatus (center of the ear)
- Midpoint of the acromion (shoulder)
- Lateral waist (around L3)
- Center of the greater trochanter (hip joint)
- Anterior to the midline of the knee joint
- Anterior to the lateral malleolus (ankle)

Observation can focus on the following questions:
- Are any spinal curves natural, flattened, exaggerated, or shifted?
- Is the pelvis in a natural anterior tilt, or tipped anterior or posterior to an extreme?
- Is the head carried forward or sitting well-aligned above the spine?
- Are the knees hyperextended, and if so, how does that affect spinal positioning?
- Is there excessive dorsi- or plantar flexion in the ankle?

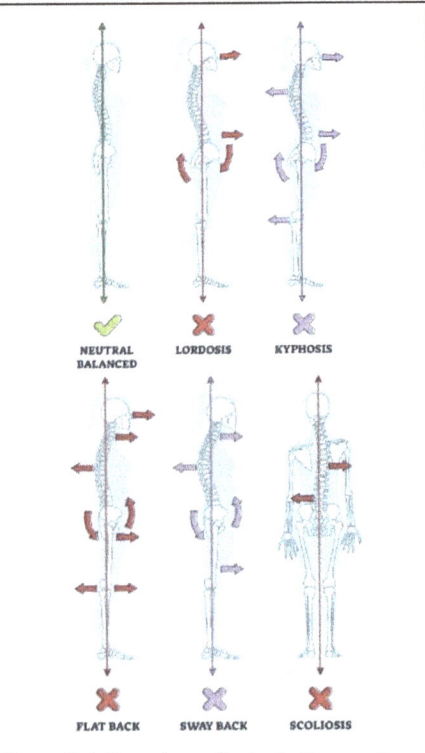

Observations may help identify the more common spinal misalignments seen in students or clients, and can be used to enable clients to sense their alignment proprioceptively and interoceptively. Students can learn to create dynamic balance through active, self-initiated micro-adjustments. Some of the more common patterns include, but are not limited to, the following (a more detailed discussion can be reviewed in Chapter 4):
- *Forward head position*, often paired with cervical hyperextension at the base of the neck and hyperflexion at the joint with the skull
- *Exaggerated thoracic kyphosis,* often combined with a posterior pelvis
- *Exaggerated lumbar lordosis*, often associated with tight hip flexors and anterior pelvic tilt
- *Flattened lumbar lordosis*, often accompanied with slumped posture and misaligned neck and head
- *Flattened thoracic spine*, often resulting from scapular retraction or a misapplied desire to stand up straight
- *Pelvic displacement due to knee hyperextension*, often causing the pelvis to shift forward of the plumb line and disrupting the spinal curves above

**Figure 2.4** Overview of spinal alignments – sagittal view. (Data source: istock.com)

*Understanding the Spinal Curves in the Frontal Plane*

While the sagittal plane gives insight into spinal curves, the frontal plane reveals side-to-side asymmetries and compensatory patterns that may be structural or functional. These can be viewed well from the front or the back and may be more visible and felt in weight-bearing shapes such as Downward Facing Dog. Observation from the front and back helps identify lateral deviations, scoliosis, and imbalances in limbs. Chapter 4 offered additional detail; a brief summary follows.

A well-aligned spine side-to-side typically creates the following anatomical landmarks *across both sides of the body*:
- Equal lift and openness across the rib basket and abdomen
- Horizontal positioning of the clavicles and acromion processes
- Symmetry in the waist, flanks, and obliques
- Even hip height –uneven iliac spines may signal scoliosis, pelvic torsion, or leg length discrepancy
- Alignment of the knees – neither valgus (knock-knee), nor varus (bowlegged) tendencies
- Equal weight distribution across the medial and lateral foot
- Centered ankles – neither inversion, nor eversion

From the back, it is useful to notice the presence or absence of the following:
- A spinal curve to one side
- Difference in rib flare or resilience between the two sides
- Uneven positioning of the scapulae, including winging, elevation, or rotation
- Asymmetries in muscle development side-to-side
- Uneven weight distribution across the feet
- Uneven patterns of compression and tension in the two sides of the body

Mild lateral curves are common and often do not present significant challenges in yoga or daily life. If significant spinal deviations exist, it may be necessary to inform the yoga *asana* practice through referral for structural assessment and guidance about contraindications and supports. Referral can help identify the type of scoliosis (e.g., C-shaped versus S-shaped curves) and commensurate compensation patterns. It can clarify which side is convex (bulging outward) versus concave (drawing inward), helpful to know in yoga *asana* because often the concave side has tighter, shorter musculature and the convex side tends to exhibit weakness and lengthening.

Over time, these patterns can influence limb length perception, foot loading, and even the capacity for balance. Yoga *asana* cannot change bony structure, but asymmetries in muscle tone, resilience, or load distribution may be addressed through thoughtful yoga movement practices emphasizing proprioception, strength, and balance – all with guidance from an appropriately-trained healthcare professional.

Some of the more common patterns that emerge in the presence of side-to-side spinal deviations include, but are not limited to, the following:
- *Lateral deviations* in the spinal midline, especially in the thoracic and lumbar regions
- *Uneven flanks*, due to shortened or overactive muscles (e.g., quadratus lumborum, obliques, or psoas)
- *Uneven pelvic leveling* with one iliac crest higher than the other
- *Uneven scapular movements* notable in rotation or protraction; habitual rounding of one side
- *Lower limb misalignments* (external or internal knee rotation, ankle inversion or eversion, unequal weight distribution of across the feet)

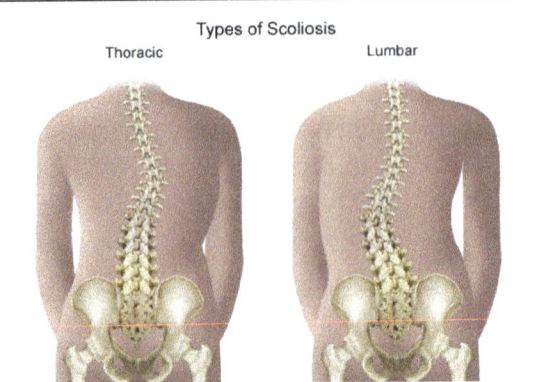

**Figure 2.5** Overview of spinal alignment – frontal view. https://commons.wikimedia.org/wiki/File:Ei_0417.jpg; Creative Commons Attribution 4.0).

### Recruiting Core Stabilization and Engagement

Effective standing shapes are not created and maintained by the axial skeleton alone. They are supported by a responsive and integrated core musculature that stabilizes the trunk by creating natural tone that is neither tense or hard, nor collapsed or buckled, but *supportive and yielding*. The abdominal muscles, pelvic floor, psoas complex, diaphragm, and deep slow-twitch spinal muscles form a dynamic, multilayered support system that provides excellent stability and resilience while optimizing intraabdominal pressure. When properly engaged, these muscles and their connective tissues preserve the natural curves of the spine, protect against shear and compression, allow breath to remain subtle and gentle, and create movement that is flowing and effortless, even graceful.

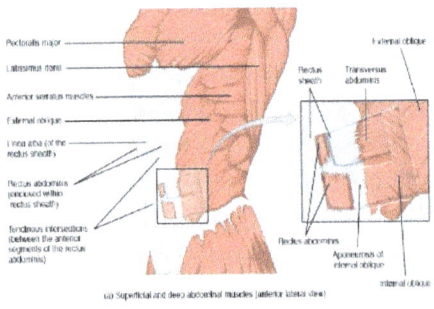
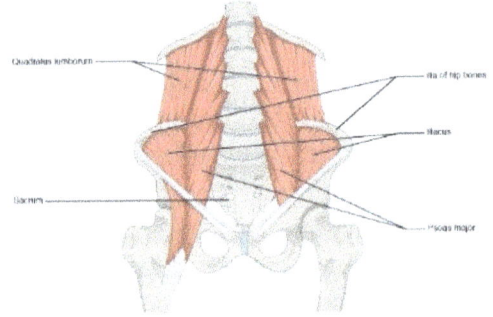

**Figure 2.6** Stabilizer muscles. (Data source: OpenStax; https://commons.wikimedia.org/wiki/File:1112_Muscles_of_the_Abdomen.jpg, Creative Commons Attribution 4.0)

Core stabilization is deeply grounded in the actions of the *transverse abdominis* (TA), the deepest abdominal layer of muscles. The TAs act like a corset, drawing the abdominal wall inward and supporting the vertebral column, especially at the L4-L5 region (which is particularly prone to instability). Engagement of this set of muscles can be felt most easily on the exhalation, especially a forceful exhalation, such as during a cough, laughter, or Lion's Breath. Interestingly, the tongue can be recruited for supporting core engagement as it is fascially strongly connected to the core musculature. Sticking out the tongue (as in Lion's Breath) can be a great way for clients to access deep core engagement.

The *internal and external obliques* support rotation and lateral flexion. These muscles are especially active in standing shapes that involve twisting or side bending, and are engaged in a balanced way to maintain spinal stability in more complex transitions. The *rectus abdominis* muscles play a less central role in spinal stability during standing shapes but are secondarily involved when flexion or stabilization against gravity is needed (such as in arm standing). Notably, the abdominal wall as a whole supports the vertical positioning of the abdominal organs, referred to as the *organ column*, and stabilizes our body during movement. The abdominal muscles act as a container, holding the viscera in place and allowing upright movement and standing without collapse or excessive pressure on the pelvic floor.

Although abdominal engagement is essential, it is not the primary means by which we remain upright. In standing shapes, the hips and legs are main load-bearing structures. The gluteal muscles, hip rotators, and deep lateral stabilizers of the pelvis play a primary role in postural integrity. Overemphasizing abdominal strength in standing shapes can lead to unnecessary bracing and gripping, a sign of over-efforting that needs to be balanced by ease. Overall, ideal core engagement is responsive rather than rigid; gently anchored in the breath cycle, felt in the deepest layers on the exhalation and as a sense of softness on the inhalation; and coordinated with natural spinal alignment, as well as dependent on healthful natural anterior rotation of the pelvis. On the inhalation, the abdominal wall remains soft, allowing for easeful diaphragmatic movement and its effects on the organs. Even when engaging the core, students are well served to maintain natural and soft tone rather than forcefully bracing the abdomen. For tricks and movements for discovering core engagement, see *Practice and Teaching Tips for Core Stabilization* in Chapter 9.

Cueing can focus on the core as a central point of support that is dynamic, responsive, and connected to breath and movement. In challenging standing shapes, such as one-legged balances or rotational shapes, the core helps stabilize the spine against gravitational or rotational forces. In foundational shapes, such as *Mountain*, it contributes to the sense of grounding, expansion, and steadiness. Targeted exploration of core engagement that is gentle and dynamic, yet powerfully supportive and stabilizing is an excellent preparation for a sequence that is centered on standing shapes (and even more so for arm standing and arm balancing). A sample of a class that invites interoception of core engagement and strengthening of all involved muscles (from the pelvis to the abdomen to the spine) is offered in this integrated holistic yoga core stabilization class: https://youtu.be/We6gIj-EWJw

## *Assembling Standing Shapes from the Bottom Up*

A review of Chapter 5 is helpful to recall the main movement principles related to the lower appendicular skeleton. Cueing from the bottom upward means starting with attention to the feet, knees, legs overall, and hips – linking this entire assembly to the curves of the spine, and even the alignment of the shoulder girdle. It is crucial to avoid cueing that lines up any aspect of the feet, legs, or hips with outer parameters, such as edges of a yoga mat or 'ideal' outer shapes. Instead cueing emphasizes students' bioindividuality and the notion that how the limbs and other body parts are placed depends on each student's anatomy.

It helps to support standing shapes with *alive and grounded feet with strong ankles*. Awakening the feet with foot work (e.g., ball rolling, toe twining, toe grasping) and strengthen the ankles (e.g., ankle rolls, unilateral squats) can be great preparation.

**Fancy Foot Work**

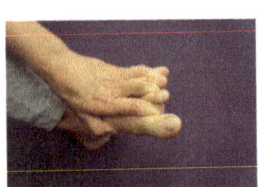
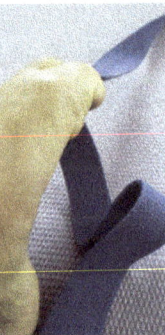
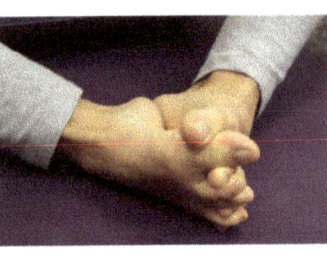
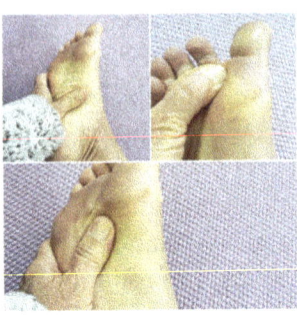
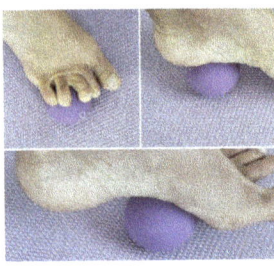
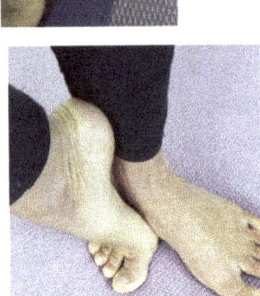
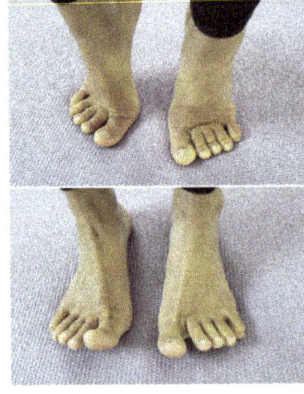
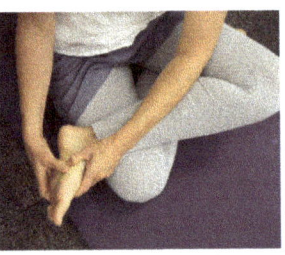

**Foot Work Class**:
https://youtu.be/eV4EHsesRIg

During work in standing shapes, it can help to integrate the following general concepts in cueing:
- Cue the corners of the feet, acknowledging that some students feel three corners (big toes and little toe ball mound, and heel as a whole) and other students feel four corners (big toe and little toe ball mounds and inner and outer heel) – this helps with grounding and rooting
- As relevant, *mention the four arches*, though it is not essential to cue all of them each time
  - medial (primary shock absorber)
  - lateral (super stabilizer – our outrigger)
  - distal transverse (helps with weight distribution)
  - proximal transverse (a great weight bearer)
- emphasize that grounding is not a flattening; the medial and lateral longitudinal arches remain responsive
- Encourage subtle doming of the arches and a soft spread through the toes
- Note that over-gripping the toes is counterproductive and often reflects instability upstream

Moving power upward through the extremities, cueing focus shifts to *engaged legs healthful alignment of the knees*. Integrating the following cueing guidance may be helpful:
- Cue awakening the leg muscles with props, such as block squeezes between legs and/or strap presses with strap around thighs; both could be combined in same shape
- Cue drawing knee caps toward the hips to help students feel the stabilization of the patella, the engagement of the quads, and the responsiveness of the hamstrings

- Look out for hyperextension of the knee joints as well as valgus and varus shifts and offer remedial cueing that is tailored to individuals
- Cue foot, knee, and hip alignment that maximizes knee health, not foot position – emphasize the fact that the knee is a joint between two joints and thus prone to torquing to make up for any missing range of motion above (in the hip joints) or below (in the ankle joints)
- Once the knee is aligned to optimal position, cue letting the feet follow in the direction of the knee cap by either turning out, in, or neutral

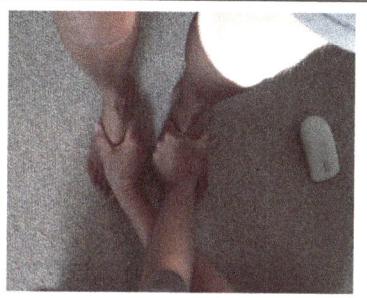

*Medial Arch Resonance Test*

To be able to walk well, the medial arch has to collapse when we step down; it then reestablishes itself when we press up in walking (collapse = weight acceptance).

You can feel this by placing your hands under a student's arches while they simulate walking by crossing the arms and swaying side to side slowly.

*Knee and Foot Alignment Test*
- Look for an isosceles triangle between the lateral and medial superior edges of the patella to the tibial tuberosity
- If there is no isosceles triangle (i.e., if one side of the triangle is longer than the other), the knee is rotated
- If this is the case, do not parallel the feet or you will risk harm to the knee
- That means: for students with a rotated knee, the instruction is to face the knee caps straight forward (rather than cueing parallel feet), aligned with the hip joint; make sure the knee hinge is aligned and not torqued

Next in the upward assembly is finding a *natural pelvis*, which means a slight anterior tilt with a focus on stability. The slight anterior tilt preserves the lumbar curve and optimized load transfer. Common cueing related to tucking the tailbone does not serve (all) students in standing shapes, as it interferes with natural assembly of the spine for many individuals. Tailbone cueing is not typically necessary in standing shapes; it can be of utility in forward folds and backbends. From a natural alignment in the pelvis and lumbar, emphasis moves upward to the natural thoracic curve. A few useful cues may address the following points:
- Note the position of the low ribs, ensuring they are neither tucked too far into the body nor flaring out; it can be helpful to cue drawing the low ribs toward anterior superior iliac spine
- A slight kyphotic curvature of the upper back will be visible and is natural
- Let the head rest naturally on top of the cervical spine, assuring a slight lordosis of the cervical spine and a very slight anterior rotation of the head
- The chin is tucked ever so slightly and then drawn back to align the openings of the ears with the center of the tops of the shoulders

> ***Potential Downsides of Tucking the Pelvis in Upright Standing Shapes*** *(Lasater, 2020, pp. 9-13)*
>
> *(Note: These downsides likely do not apply to hypermobile individuals, who may benefit from a slight tucking as it will decrease any possible hyperlordosis in the lumbar spine)*
>
> - Flattens lumbar lordosis
> - Flattens the cervical spine (due to lumbar-cervical sympathetic movement)
> - Distorts the sacroiliac joints
> - Drops the weight of the trunk onto the discs, increasing compression
> - Drops the weight of the organs onto the pelvic floor
> - Weakens the pelvic floor
> - Disengages the abdominals
> - Interferes with freedom of movement of the diaphragm and hence the breath
> - Results in a shape that fights gravity

### *Creating Tailored Foundations for Standing Shapes*

To refine knee and foot placement and gain a deeper understanding of standing shapes, it is helpful to recall the various movements and positions that can occur in the joints of the pelvis, especially the hip joints and sacroiliac (SI) joints. A review of *Kinesiology of the Pelvic Girdle and Thighs* in Chapter 5 is helpful to refresh the memory about movements, cautions, and challenges in this region of the body that is so key to healthful standing shapes in yoga and functional movement in daily life.

Yoga professionals can help protect the hip and sacroiliac joints (and often, by extension, the knee joints) by cueing in a manner that empowers students to:
- Avoid femoral leveraging – e.g., choosing a Warrior 1 Lunge over a Warrior 1 that forces the back foot into a grounded and angled placement on the mat
- Beware of spinal leveraging – e.g., allowing the pelvis to move freely and naturally toward a diagonal orientation in Triangle rather than forcing the body to sidebend 'as if between two panes of glass'
- Prevent lumbar or sacral corkscrewing – e.g., let the pelvis move as a whole unit when moving into rotations within standing shapes such as Warrior 2; or make sure the rotation is exclusive to the thoracic spinal section
- Differentiate pelvic and femoral movement in standing (and seated) shapes – e.g., tune into the reverberations of movements by the femur into the pelvis, noticing excess strain in the SI joints and backing away rather than persisting in extreme femoral positioning
- Avoid extreme end positioning of the limbs to avoid compromising the integrity of the hip joint – e.g., allow the lifted leg to land in a natural diagonal position rather than forcing it outward to be completely in the frontal plane in Tree
- Work within individual anatomical limits, rather than outer idealized shapes – e.g., choosing a diagonal placement of the pelvis in Warrior 2, rather than forcing the hips parallel with the sides of the mat

> *Related Anatomy Refreshers*:
>
> *Spinal leveraging* refers to spinal movements and alignments (whether intentional or inadvertent) that create shearing or rotational forces into the lumbar spine or the connection between the sacrum and ilia (essentially torquing the sacrum inside the ilia). In yoga such a situation occurs most commonly in asymmetrical or unsupported spinal shapes. Standing shapes such as Triangle, Side Angle, and Half Moon are common culprits.
>
> *Femoral leveraging* occurs when movement of the femur in the acetabulum exceeds the natural range of motion and essentially forces a bypassing of the hip joint – movement is continued, instead of ending at maximum healthful range, and quite literally pries excessive movement into the SI joints. This stress on the SI joints occurs most commonly when a practitioner pushes beyond available range of hip abduction or external rotation, especially in standing shapes such as Warrior 2 or Triangle, and possible in Warrior 1 with the back foot angled and the heel forced to the ground.
>
> *Lumbar or sacral corkscrewing or torquing* is the most insidious risk to the SI joints. This phenomenon occurs when rotational forces are directed into the lumbar spine, which has very limited capacity for axial rotation (10–15 degrees across all segments). When the pelvis is rigidly fixed during standing rotational movements (e.g., in Warrior 2 or Triangle), the lumbar spine is forced to absorb the rotational demand. This stresses the intervertebral discs and creates a corkscrewing effect where the sacrum is twisted inside the ilia, destabilizing the SI joints.

By reinforcing healthy hip joint and SI joint mechanics through cueing and awareness, the practice of standing shapes can become therapeutic, supporting structural integrity rather than undermining it. When pelvic orientation is rooted in interoception rather than aesthetic, and when joint actions are grounded in anatomy rather than assumption, the hip and sacroiliac joints remain resilient and functional over time. All the actions on and cautions about that is happening in the pelvic joint leads to the final general consideration that is essential to all standing shapes, namely, understanding the primary foundations of these shapes.

In teaching standing shapes, a grounded understanding of both hip joint function and the planes of movement is essential to intelligent sequencing. As students move into these complex shapes, they benefit from a logical anatomical progression that honors the structural demands of each shape and minimizes joint stress, especially across the hips, knees, and sacroiliac joints. The orientation of the hip joints (whether they are primarily in flexion, extension, or rotation) determines the directional and muscular emphasis of the shape. What is happening in the hip joints is strongly related to the plane in which the shape emerges and is embodied. Some standing shapes occur primarily in the sagittal plane (with the stance relying on hip flexion and extension); others occupy mostly the frontal plane (with the stance involving abduction or adduction) and/or the transverse plane (with the shape requiring rotational movement in the hip joint). Once planes of movement (and the commensurate demands on the hip joints) are understood, standing shapes can be logically grouped and sequenced in a way that no unnecessary strain in the joints. The most basic standing shapes arise from anatomical position. All joints are in their natural position. All other standing shapes evolve from this Mountain shape. They can be grouped into two categories: shapes that use a Warrior 1 Lunge foundation and shapes that use a Warrior 2 foundation.

## Sagittal Plane Standing Shapes (Warrior 1 Foundation)

Standing shapes that involve both hips primarily in flexion or extension unfold mostly in the sagittal plane. These shapes emphasize forward and backward action in the hip joint and are biomechanically less complex and demanding than their multiplanar counterparts. Students tend to find these shapes easier to stabilize and can focus on organizing their pelvis and spine without the added complexity of rotation or abduction. These shapes offer an excellent place to begin, particularly in therapeutic or beginner contexts, because clients can focus on a single orientation in space. This fact reduces neurological and muscular complexity and creates more accessible somatic learning.

Examples of sagittal plane standing shapes include:
- *Warrior 1 Lunge* (i.e., with the back heel lifted)
- *Warrior 3*
- *Eagle*
- *Lunge* variations (with or without props)

In sequencing these shapes, it is important to emphasize grounded alignment and healthy spinal curves. It is helpful to guide students toward maintaining a natural lumbar curve rather than moving into a backbend through the thoracolumbar junction. Often this alignment requires conscious moderation of shoulder flexion to avoid anterior rib flare and unnecessary spinal extension. Cueing a slight movement of the low ribs toward the anterior superior iliac spine can greatly facilitate such natural alignment. Warming up the psoas supports this way of accessing Lunge shapes, as the lumbar spine will be in its natural position which requires a resilient psoas complex. Detailed teaching considerations for each of these shapes is provided below.

## Multiplanar Standing Shapes (Warrior 2 Foundation)

Standing shapes that unfold from a Warrior 2 foundation are significantly more complex, as they typically involve a combination of hip flexion, extension, abduction, and rotation. These movements happen across multiple planes (sagittal, frontal, and transverse) and require greater joint differentiation and neuromuscular coordination. This reality introduces significantly more neuromuscular integration, movement, and mental complexity, as body parts must move and stabilize in multiple directions at once. *Warrior 2* foundation shapes place higher demands on balance, proprioception, joint range, and integrated support systems.

Examples of multiplanar standing shapes include:
- *Warrior 2*
- *Extended Side Angle*
- *Triangle*
- *Tree*

Because these shapes distribute movement across several joints and axes, engaging in them requires greater attention to the interplay between the pelvis, sacrum, femurs, and knees. It is especially important to maintain sacroiliac integrity. This involves ensuring that femoral rotation does not drive torque into the pelvis and that the lumbar spine does not compensate for limited hip mobility by side-bending or rotating excessively. Care needs to be taken to address sacral torquing and femoral leveraging. Perhaps most importantly, these shapes place various rotational forces on the pelvis, making it essential to focus careful attention on stable sacroiliac alignment, hip range of motion, possible torquing at the knee, and pronation at the foot. Detailed teaching considerations for each of these shapes is provided below.

| | *Tips for Grounding, Expansion, and Stability in Standing Shapes* |
|---|---|
| Grounding | • Develop a strong and balanced foundation through the feet, legs, and pelvis<br>• Create grounding awareness through the feet<br>• Engage the legs, perhaps lifting the knee caps toward the hips and feeling the engagement of calf and thigh muscles<br>• Feel the restful presence of the torso on the pelvis, especially the sacrum<br>• Use the outbreath to ground physically and emotionally<br>• Anchor the mind to a focus of attention or concentration<br>• Find a gaze point or *drishti* |
| Stability | • Access your natural spine and pelvis; find the center of gravity for your head<br>• Engage the core with soft awareness and ease, especially the deep layers of core muscles<br>• Root and stabilize through the feet while lifting the toes and finding lightness in the arches<br>• Engage and lift the pelvic floor<br>• Notice how the exhalation supports an engaged, strong core; notice how the inhalation welcomes lightness and space<br>• Lift the rib basket away from the hips while drawing in the floating ribs<br>• Lift the limbs out or up with the integration of power and ease<br>• Settle the shoulder blades on the back (retraction and depression) to access power and stability; let them soften to find ease when appropriate<br>• Find grounding, expansion, and stability in combination to support yielding<br>• Find stable responsiveness to the demand characteristics of the *asana*<br>• Create a natural spine with vertebrae stacked so as to yield natural curves |
| Expansion | • Find length in the spine – lifting the ribs away from the hips (hands at low rib basket to help it move upward)<br>• Reach up through the crown of the head<br>• Feel energy traveling outward through the extremities<br>• Feel lightness in lifted limbs or lifted rib basket<br>• Feel spaciousness/openness in the chest – lift the manubrium<br>• Feel spaciousness or space in body and breath<br>• Find an open-hearted expression of the *asana*<br>• Let the breath lighten the shape or movement<br>• Find space and lightness with the inhalation<br>• Let the mind be light and open to whatever is unfolding in the moment, not holding on to preconceived notions about the shape or movement |

## Analysis and Experience of Sample Upright Standing Shapes

The following standing shapes are analyzed in detail below:
- *Mountain*
- *Warrior 1 Lunge*
- *Warrior 3*
- *Eagle*
- *Warrior 2*
- *Side Angle*
- *Triangle*
- *Tree*

The cueing guidance offered for each shape needs to be considered in the context offered in the *general principles for upright standing shapes.* The basics discussed above need to permeate the cueing for all these shapes. The additional cueing, shape by shape, offered here is icing on the cake. Always integrate integrated holistic yoga cueing that addresses the following teaching principles:
- *Accessibility* – creating access through variation, adaptation, affiliation, individualization, and person-centeredness
- *Intentionality* – embedding the practice of each shape in the overall arc of the session, grounding in the theme for the class and the meaning of the practice
- *Beneficence* – honoring the wellbeing of each student and always making sure to first do no harm
- *Holism* – cueing all *koshas* or layers of experience in all shapes, never forgetting that each shape has reverberations into and is affected by all *koshas* – it is not enough to cue anatomy; also address energy and vitality, thoughts and emotions, behavioral and action choices, even community and interbeing
- *Integration* –in teaching *asana*, integrate breathwork, concentration and mindfulness, as well as the ethical principles and lifestyle practices of yoga

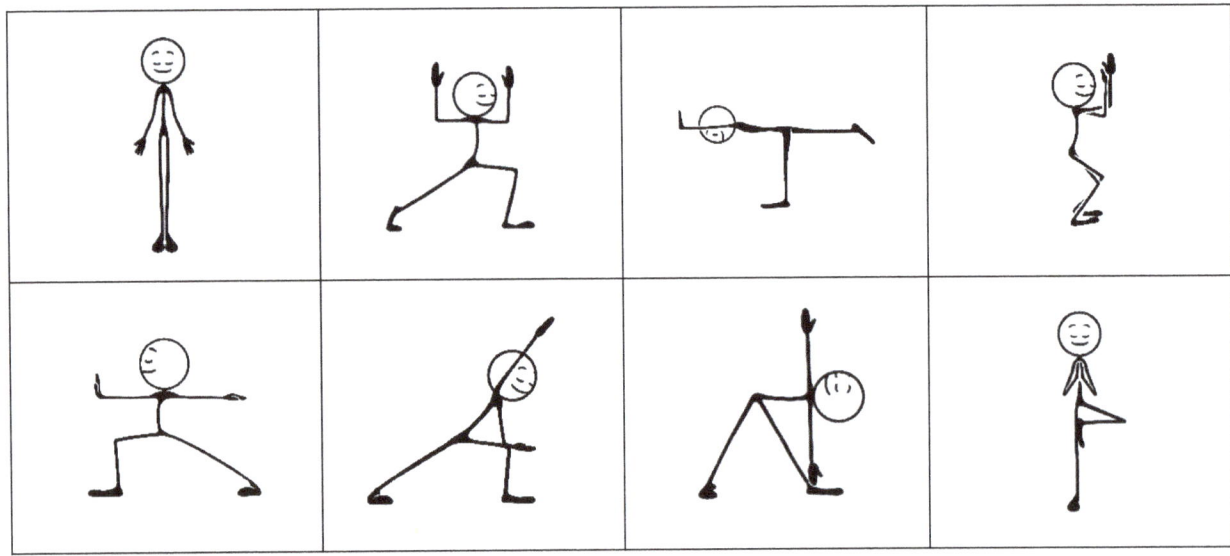

## Mountain or Tadasana

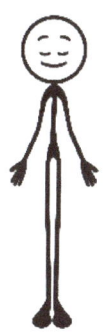

Mountain is a foundational yoga shape that allows for a great introduction to the concepts of expansion, stability, and grounding. It is versatile and can be used as a warm-up, resting, or cool-down position during a yoga practice, providing stillness and connection between more dynamic sequences. The primary variations are traditional Mountain with the arms by the side, Extended Mountain with the arm lifted, and Seated Mountain for anyone who cannot stand. The shape's seeming simplicity makes it an excellent shape for cultivating awareness, including interoception, neuroception, proprioception, and exteroception. The shape is also a wonderful base position from which to establish a focus on creating a profound connection between body, breath, and mind. Mountain can be an excellent opportunity for a moment of stillness, recalibration, and self-assessment between other shapes and after *kriyas*.

### Benefits

In addition to its calming and awareness-enhancing effects, Mountain offers a wide range of physical, energetic, emotional, and mental benefits. For example, it has been shown to:

- *Improve breathing*: By encouraging an open heart and engaged alignment of the shoulders, Mountain helps increase lung capacity and improves overall breathing efficiency. This can be particularly beneficial for reducing stress and enhancing breath resilience during physical activity or meditation.
- *Strengthen the lower body*: Maintaining stability in Mountain requires engaging the muscles of the legs, including quadriceps, hamstrings, and calf muscles. Over time, this engagement strengthens and tones the lower body.
- *Enhance mental focus*: This shape can be an effective tool for grounding and centering the mind, which is useful both in yoga practice and daily life. The stillness and focus required in Mountain help develop concentration and mental clarity.
- *Establish body awareness:* Mountain encourages practitioners to tune into their bodies, notice imbalances, and make adjustments to achieve more wholesome and sustainable alignment. Such increased body awareness can translate into improved posture and functional movement patterns in daily life off the mat.
- *Reduce muscle tension:* By actively aligning the body and lengthening the spine (into axial extension), Mountain can release tension in shoulders, neck, and low back. Emphasis on gentle engagement without bracing allows for a relaxed yet active shape with enhanced head placement.
- *Support joint health:* By emphasizing person-tailored alignment and uniform weight distribution through the feet and legs, Mountain helps support joint health in ankles, knees, hips, and spine. It promotes equal engagement of the muscles around these joints, reducing risk of injury or strain.
- *Prepare for balance shapes:* Mountain is an excellent preparation for balancing shapes, as it helps establish the connection between the feet and the ground while activating the core stabilizers. Its cultivation of equanimity in body, breath, and mind prepares students to access

balance in more challenging shapes and in daily life – not just physically, but also energetically and emotionally.
- *Improve circulation:* Standing with healthful alignment and an engaged core in Mountain facilitates blood circulation throughout the body, supporting cardiovascular health.

## Cautions

Generally speaking, there is little risk associated with Mountain per se. Challenges may arise from fast or non-mindful transitions into or out of the shape, more so than the shape itself. The following considerations can be held in mind:
- For individuals with low blood pressure, there can be a risk of fainting during Mountain, especially when transitioning from forward folding or reclining positions.
- For individuals with uncontrolled high blood pressure, lifting the arms into Extended Mountain can raise blood pressure excessively, especially with a fast lift.
- Practitioners with acute headaches best proceed with caution, as the upright position and emphasis on elongation can exacerbate symptoms. It is advisable to take breaks or modify the shape as needed.
- Individuals with foot, ankle, or knee injuries may need to move with caution as inauspicious weight distribution may exacerbate these conditions.
- Students with sciatica may need to explore different stances to avoid aggravating symptoms, ensuring the pelvis remains in its natural alignment to reduce strain on the low back.
- Individuals with balance challenges may consider using a wall or other supports (e.g., touching the back of a chair with one hand) until they feel confident in their ability to maintain stability.
- Practitioners are cautioned not to lock the knees, as hyperextension can lead to joint strain. This caution may be particular helpful to individuals who are hypermobile and need to maintain vigilance about not hyperextending the knees in standing shapes.

## Preparations

No specific preparation is required for Mountain, as the shape itself can serve as a warm-up and grounding practice. If preparations are desired for Mountain, these involve gentle movements that awaken the spine, enhance physical awareness, invite cultivation of balance, and connect movement with breath. Since Mountain focuses on grounding, expansion, and stability through the axial body, the following sample warmups may prove particularly helpful:
- *Six movements of the spine:* Seated or standing, move the spine in its six directions – forward flexion, back extension, lateral flexion to each side, and rotation to each side. This helps gently awaken the spine and prepare for optimal posture, balanced movement, and awakened experience in all layers.
- *Ankle and foot exercises:* Rolling the ankles, flexing, and pointing the feet, as well as spreading and lifting the toes, can prepare the feet for grounding and balance.
- *Pelvic tilts:* Gentle pelvic tilts help establish awareness of the natural pelvis position. This will assist in aligning the hips and reducing strain during Mountain.
- *Hip openers:* Simple hip-opening exercises, like seated or standing hip circles, help bring awareness to the hip joint and promote balance. This also encourages healthful placement of the femur in the acetabulum.

- ***Leg and shoulder warm-up***: Light leg stretches or gentle knee lifts activate the muscles of the lower body, while shoulder rolls or arm stretches can release tension in the shoulders, allowing the shoulder blades to settle into alignment in Mountain.
- ***Standing Cat-Cow***: Engaging in a Cat-Cow flow in a standing position can help activate the spine and establish a feeling of spinal resilience. It helps set the foundation for the upright, natural spine required in Mountain.

## Key Alignment Invitations

In Mountain, the hip joint is in a neutral position, meaning that the femur sits evenly within the acetabulum. This alignment allows the hips to be balanced, reducing strain on surrounding muscles and supporting a natural, upright posture. To achieve healthful alignment in Mountain, compassionate attention can be given to each part of the body, starting from the feet and moving up toward the head. Not every instance of teaching Mountain needs to address each of the covered invitations, as this will likely overwhelm students and may interfere with their natural embodied wisdom. Alignment suggestions are offered as carefully applied and selected guidance based on what teachers observe in students.

- *Invitations related to the feet*: Begin by standing with the feet hip-width apart or together, whichever feels more stable.
  - Press evenly through the corners of each foot. Some students feel four corners (the ball of the big toe, the ball of the little toe, the outer heel, and the inner heel); others feel three corners (ball of the big toe, ball of the little toe, and heel). Create equality in cueing for both ways of perceiving the feet.
  - Lift and spread the toes, then gently lower them to the ground, creating a strong foundation. Feel the arches of the feet lifting naturally to avoid collapsing inward.
  - Shift body weight forward and backward, and side to side, to find an even balance point. This exploration helps develop awareness of auspicious weight distribution between both feet.
- *Invitations related to the legs*: Engage the quadriceps (front of the thighs) by lifting the kneecaps without locking (i.e., hyperextending) the knee joints. Keeping a micro-bend in the knees avoids hyperextension. To engage the legs, imagine drawing energy upward from the feet through the thighs, creating a sense of length and strength through the lower body.
- *Invitations related to the hips and pelvis*: In Mountain, the pelvis is in its natural alignment, meaning it is neither tucked posteriorly, nor excessively tilted anteriorly.
  - *Create natural pelvic alignment*: To find a naturally aligned pelvis, imagine leveling the upper line of the hip bones (the ASIS) and stacking the hips above ankles. Engage the lower abdominal muscles gently to support this pelvic positioning without tightening or tucking. The hip joints are wholesomely positioned if they feel natural and stable, allowing the femoral heads to sit evenly in the acetabulum, creating balance and stability.
  - *Check pelvic alignment*: Ask students to find their natural pelvis by tilting the pelvis slightly forward and back, and then finding a balanced middle position. This movement helps them understand what their natural pelvis feels like and how it supports their spine.
- *Invitations related to the spine*: Maintain the natural curves of the spine – the cervical (neck), thoracic (upper back), and lumbar (low back) regions are in their natural alignment without

exaggeration. Imagine growing taller from the tailbone to the crown of the head, creating space between vertebrae.
- *Invitations related to the core*: Lightly engage the lower abdomen by drawing the navel inward and upward. This core engagement helps support the spine and maintain balance. Avoid sucking in the stomach too tightly; instead, focus on a gentle activation that maintains both stability and freedom of breath.
- *Invitations related to the chest and shoulders*: Lift the sternum slightly to open the heart, while keeping the rib basket drawn gently inward to prevent overarching the low back. Allow the shoulders to relax down and back, with the shoulder blades drawing slightly toward each other without pinching. This action keeps the heart open while maintaining space between the shoulders and the ears.
- *Invitations related to the head and neck*: The head is balanced over the shoulders, with the chin tucked and drawn slightly posterior to align the head in line with the neck. Avoid jutting the chin forward or tucking it too much. The gaze is soft, either directly forward or slightly downward, keeping the eyes relaxed. For some students it helps to imagine lifting the crown of the head toward the sky, moving from the posterior aspect of the skull.
- *Invitations related to the arms and hands*: Keep arms relaxed by the sides, with palms naturally facing inwards or slightly forward. Fingers are relaxed, with a gentle sense of expansiveness through the fingertips. If arms are raised, maintain length without locking the elbows, keeping the shoulders relaxed and away from the ears.

## *Variations and Explorations*

Mountain can be adapted in numerous ways to challenge balance, increase flexibility, or deepen awareness. Variations include side-bending, placing the arms in different positions (e.g., at the sides, at heart center, extended upward), or moving the arms up and down through an imagined viscous substance for isometric muscular engagement. Practicing against a wall provides feedback for alignment, while experimenting with feet at different distances apart can explore stability. For an additional balance challenge, practitioners can rise onto the balls of their feet or close their eyes. Weight shifting from foot to foot also encourages dynamic stability and builds awareness of the body in space.
- *Wall assistance:* Ask students to practice with their back against a wall to feel auspicious alignment. The back of the head, shoulder blades, and sacrum touch the wall while maintaining a natural curve in the low back and neck. This helps students develop a better sense of where their body is in space.
- *Arm placement:* Explore extended Mountain with arms lifted up and overhead, calibrating the distance between the hands to explore different ranges of motion and reverberations. Another option is to have elbows bent, placing the arms into a cactus or goalpost shape.
- *Balancing exercises*: Have students lift one foot slightly off the ground to help improve balance and body awareness. This small adjustment challenges their stability and helps them engage their core and leg muscles more deeply, which enhances balance.
- *Adjust foot position*: Encourage students to experiment with the distance between their feet. While traditional Mountain might call for feet together (with toes touching and heels slightly apart), some students may find it more stable and comfortable to stand with feet hip-width apart. This variation can help with balance and allow for better alignment in the hips and spine. A prop between the legs can be helpful for adjusting the width of the stance.

*Recovery*

Mountain can serve as its own form of recovery, providing a natural reset for the body during practice. It can also be followed by gentle forward folds, shoulder rolls, or hip circles to release any residual tension in related body parts. Inviting students into intuitive movements, little shakes and wiggles, even light jogging in place, can release tension in the spine, in particular, and in body, breath, and mind overall after a period of standing.

*Additional Teaching Tips*

A few additional tips are offered here as possible means to help students achieve a deeper understanding of alignment and stability in Mountain. These are suggestions are the cherry on top of the icing on the cake – they offer additional explorations that can guide the student into a deeper relationship with the shape. They would not all be applied all at the same time – just as we do not overuse the basic cues for the shape.

- *Use props for feedback:* Place a yoga block between a student's thighs and ask them to gently press the thighs into the block. This can help create awareness of engaging the inner thighs and maintaining alignment in the legs and pelvis.
- *Invite the imagination for refinement*:
    - imagine roots growing from the feet into the ground, providing a stable foundation
    - imagine a string drawing the crown of the head gently upward
    - create a sense of lightness and expansion in the spine – upward and outward
    - think of a plumb line running through the center of the body, from the crown of the head to the feet – this visualization helps ensure wholesome stacking of the joints, promoting stability and reducing unnecessary strain
- *Cue the four 'ceptions:* Help students attune to interoception, exteroception, neuroception, and proprioception; for example:
    - notice the subtle differences in muscle engagement with small adjustments (e.g., lift and lower the toes to notice how the arches of the feet adjust and the leg muscles engage differently)
    - invite awareness of interoceptive changes in response to small actions that may refine alignment
    - explore how outer distractions may intrude on stability or focus
- *Integrate breath awareness*: Remind students to breathe mindfully and consistently throughout the shape. Encourage them to sync breath with body awareness, inhaling as they lengthen the spine and exhaling as they relax the shoulders. Breath awareness helps keep the shape calm and meditative.
- *Integrate body scanning*: Guide students through a body scan, moving from the feet upward. Ask them to make small adjustments, such as engaging the thighs, lifting the chest, and relaxing the shoulders. A step-by-step scan helps reinforce awareness and fine-tune alignment.
- *Work with partner feedback*: If students are comfortable, partner them up so they can provide each other with feedback. One student can gently press down on the other's shoulders or guide their alignment based on the cues given. Partner work can help students understand their body positioning more clearly.

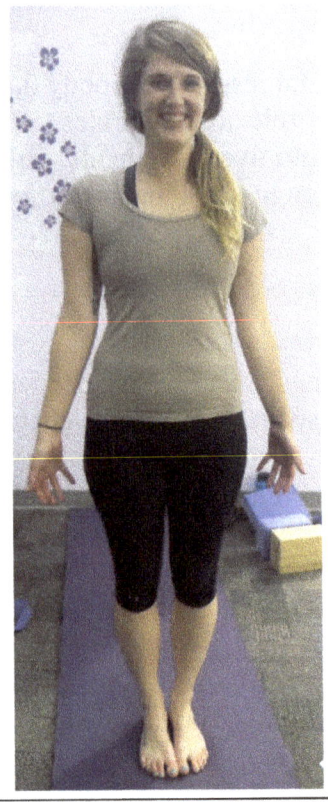

*Mountain – or anatomical position* ←

*Extended Mountain - with props for leg and arm stability* →

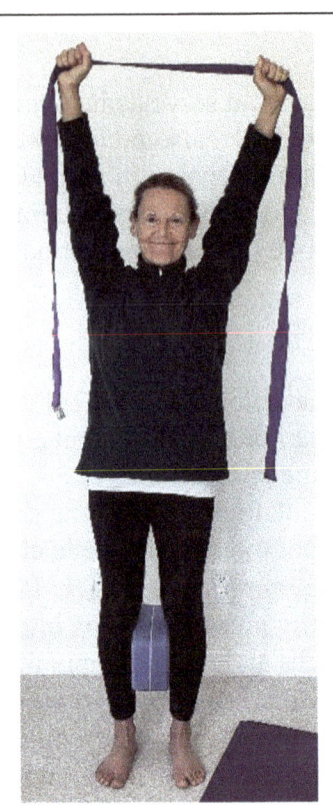

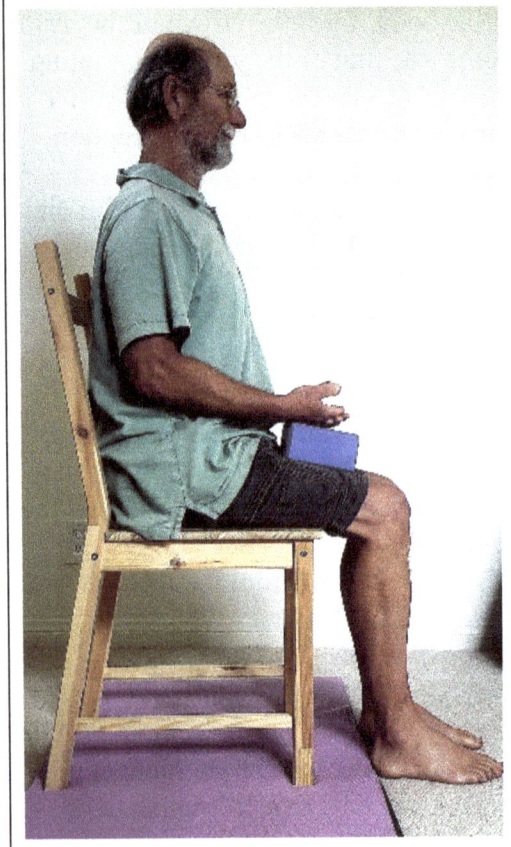

*Seated Mountain - embracing ease and stillness* ←

*Mountain with Cactus Arms – enagaging the scapulae on the back* →

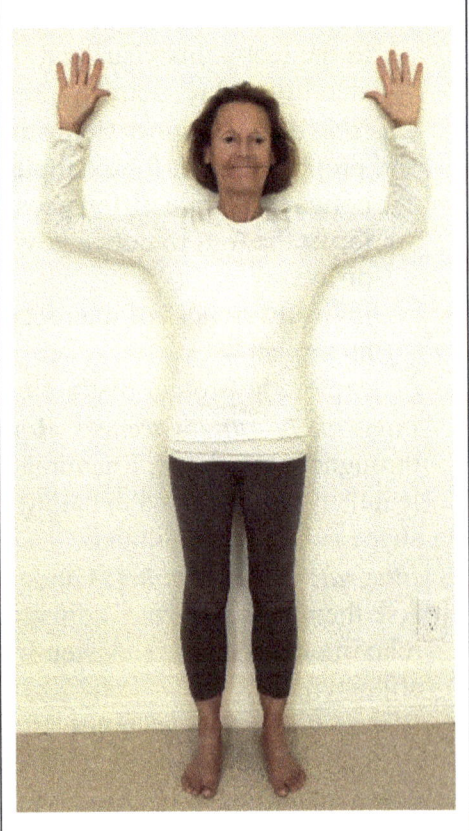

## Warrior 1 Lunge or Virabhadrasana I Lunge

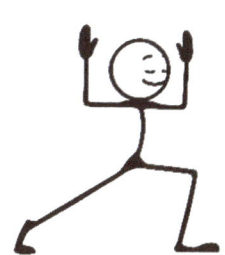

Warrior 1 Lunge is a powerful standing shape emphasizing balance, stability, and dynamic internal hip rotation. Unlike in traditional Warrior 1, the back heel in Warrior 1 Lunge remains lifted, creating an active and balanced stance that requires strong engagement through the legs and core. It promotes strength, focus, and resilience. This Lunge helps build muscular endurance and stability while energizing mind and body. Unlike Warrior 2, which involves external hip rotation, Warrior 1 Lunge focuses on internal rotation or neutral femur placement, making it better suited for sequences that include other shapes involving such hip joint alignment or engagement. Notably, Warrior 1 is *not* covered in *Integrated Holistic Yoga Movement* because the traditional shape with the back heel dropped and the back foot angled tends to create challenges for many human beings, most of whom do not have the hip range of motion demanded by this shape (see Chapter 5, especially the pelvic girdle kinesiology section).

### Benefits

Warrior 1 Lunge offers numerous benefits that contribute to overall wellbeing, enhancing physical, vital, emotional, and mental strength. The shape:
- *Promotes balance, focus, and willpower*: The asymmetrical stance enhances balance and focus, fostering a sense of empowerment and willpower.
- *Strengthens legs, ankles, and feet*: The deep lunge engages multiple muscle groups in the lower body, promoting strength and endurance.
- *Supports sacroiliac (SI) joint health and stability*: Maintaining level hips and an engaged core helps improve SI joint health and stability.
- *Energizes and mentally stimulates*: The dynamic nature of Warrior 1 Lunge can uplift energy and promote concentration, especially if combined with a *drishti* (or gaze point).
- *Improves muscular endurance*: Holding this shape helps develop stamina in leg, core, and hip musculature over time.
- *May provide relief to sciatica*: Maintaining proper alignment and core engagement can alleviate pressure on the sciatic nerve, making it beneficial for those with sciatica.

### Cautions

When teaching and practicing Warrior 1 Lunge, it is helpful to keep in mind and observe students related to the following cautions:
- *Knee or low back injuries*: Auspicious alignment deliberately protects knees and low back. Shortening the stance or bending the back knee may help alleviate strain.
- *Pregnancy (6+ months):* Pregnant students may practice this lunge with support, such as a wall or a chair, to maintain stability and ease.
- *Poor balance*: Practicing near a wall or using props can help students who present with balance challenges maintain stability.
- *Sacroiliac joint instability*: Students experiencing sacroiliac instability need to be mindful of hip, knee, and foot placement to avoid unnecessary stress on the SI joints. If engaged wholesomely and in an individualized manner, this shape can actually support SI health

because it strengthens the musculature around this joint. Inappropriately engaged, it can worsen existing SI instability.

## *Preparations*

To prepare for Warrior 1 Lunge, it is helpful to focus on mobilizing the hips, warming up the legs, and engaging the core. The following preparatory practices, in addition (of course) to a warm-up that uses the six movements of the spine (see above for description), can be particularly helpful to preparing students for this shape.
- *Low Lunge*: Opens the hip flexors and helps prepare the legs for this powerful stance.
- *Lizard*: This low Lunge, with the forward foot at the outside of the forward hand, increases resilience for hip opening and prepares for hip engagement in Warrior 1 Lunge.
- *Wide-legged Standing Forward Bend*: Challenges the hip joints and stretches the legs.
- *Tree*: Engages the core stabilizers (from pelvic floor to abdominals, back muscles, and hip flexors) while incorporating balance and alignment awareness.

## *Key Alignment Foci*

Warrior 1 Lunge is characterized by an asymmetrical stance, internal to neutral hip rotation, and a strongly lifted spine (with or without spinal extension; also see variations). Maintaining a sense of curiosity and adaptability in alignment helps students explore what feels most supportive in their bodies. Following are key alignment invitations to guide students. Again, not all of these invitations are to be made each time and for every student. Being selective based on observation is key to not over- or under-cueing any and all shapes. Like all asymmetrical shapes, Warrior 1 Lunge is engaged in on both sides.
- *Invitations related to stance*
  - *Stance width and length*: The width of the stance (side-to-side) is ideally aligned with the hips but can be wider to enhance balance and stability. Length of the stride (front to back) is determined by individual flexibility and strength – some students may shorten their stance to avoid excessive backbending (a common occurrence in this shape); others may lengthen it to deepen engagement.
  - *Back foot position*: The back heel is lifted, and the foot is positioned in line with the leg and knee. This angle of the foot optimizes comfort in the hip and SI joints. Avoid cueing (unfortunately commonly heard cues) about angled foot or heel alignment and about fully grounding the back foot; neither serves most students.
  - *Micro-bend in back knee*: A gentle bend in the back knee can help protect the low back from overextending and prevent hyperextension in the knee joint.
- *Invitations related to forward knee*
  - *Alignment with ankle*: The front knee is aligned above the ankle, without collapsing inward or outward (which may torque the knee joint). It is fine for the knee to be slightly ahead of or behind the ankle. Encourage students to use their hands to press gently on the sides of the knee to ensure stability.
  - *Stability in front knee*: Proper knee alignment is crucial, particularly if an individual has a lack of balance between the external hip rotators and adductors, which can cause misalignment and instability (with the knee either collapsing inward or outward).

- *Invitations related to pelvis and spine*
  - *Hips remain level*: The hips remain level, with a slight internal rotational movement in the hip joints to promote stability in pelvis and sacroiliac joints. Note any side-to-side asymmetries that may require different muscular engagement depending on which leg is forward.
  - *Alignment of pelvis in relation to spine*: The pelvis aligns naturally above the spine without any torquing in the region of the SI joints. It is in a natural position, neither overly tucked (posterior), nor tilted (anterior).
  - *Maintain natural spinal curves*: Students with tight psoas muscles tend to tilt the pelvis forward and create an excessive lumbar arch. Encourage them to neutralize the pelvis, which may require a shorter stance and/or flexion in the back knee.
- *Invitations related to shoulder and arm position*
  - *Shoulder relaxation*: As the arms extend overhead with an inhalation, students may choose to keep palms facing each other or turn them slightly outwards. Avoid scrunching the shoulder girdle towards the ears; instead, create space by allowing the shoulder blades to move naturally down the back.
  - *Arm variations*: Arms can also be placed in cactus position, on the hips, or adjusted to explore different levels of intensity and engagement.
- *Invitations related to head position*
  - *Natural position for head and neck*: Encourage students to keep the head facing forward, with a slight tuck and posterior movement of the chin to align naturally with the spine.

## Variations and Exploration

Warrior 1 Lunge offers many variations to support health and wellbeing for different bodies. The following suggestions are just that – they can be used creatively to create more access to a joyful expression of the shape. Many other possibilities exist and can be allowed to emerge organically.
- *Arm variations*: Place hands on the hips, take cactus arms, extend one or both arms overhead, or explore different hand positions or gestures.
- *Backbend exploration*: Invite a gentle and comfortable backbend into the thoracic or cervical spine, while ensuring core engagement and preventing hyperlordosis or hinging in the lumbar spine.
- *Adjusting the stance*: A wider side-to-side stance provides enhanced stability, while a shorter stance can reduce strain on the low back or hips.

## Recovery

Following Warrior 1 Lunge, it can be helpful to release tension in the low back, sacroiliac joints, and legs. The following are options for recovery, but many more possibilities exist.
- *Mountain*: Helps reset alignment, balance, and breath
- *Forward fold* or *Half-lift* (i.e., 90° angle at hips with arms on block, chair, or legs): Releases tension in the hamstrings and relaxes the low back, while relaxing quadratus lumborum
- *Gentle twist*: Releases the spine and helps reset alignment in the hips and low back
- *Downward Facing Dog*: Lengthens the spine and releases tension in the legs
- *Shaking or gentle jogging*: Releases residual tension, promoting relaxation
- *With prop supports*: Invites interoception and self-compassion

## Additional Teaching Tips

To help students access natural and tailored alignment for optimal engagement and ease in Warrior 1 Lunge the following additional suggestions can be considered.

- *Use props for support and feedback*: Place a chair under the front thigh for stability or an angled block under the back foot to explore adjustments in alignment.
- *Imaginative cues for refinement*:
  o Invite students to imagine placing their outstretched arms and shoulder girdle on a shelf to release tension in the neck and shoulders.
  o Encourage visualization of energy extending through the arms and out the fingertips, creating a sense of expansion, power, and playfulness.
- *Cue the four 'ceptions*: Help students attune to interoception, exteroception, proprioception, and neuroception:
  o Interoception: Guide students to notice sensations in the hips, knees, and back, making adjustments as necessary.
  o Proprioception: Invite students to explore balance by adjusting their foot placement or experimenting with closing their eyes.
  o Neuroception: Encourage awareness of how internal or external stimuli might affect stability or focus during the shape.
  o Exteroception: Invite students to notice how external stimuli may affect balance, concentration, and mindfulness.
- *Integrate breath awareness*: Remind students to maintain light nasal breathing while experiencing Warrior 1 Lunge, using breath to explore body and mind in this shape.

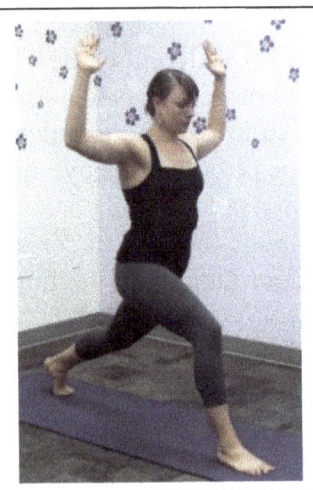

*Warrior 1 Lunge with Cactus Arms – engaging the scapulae*
←

*Warrior 1 Lunge with Props → creating support*

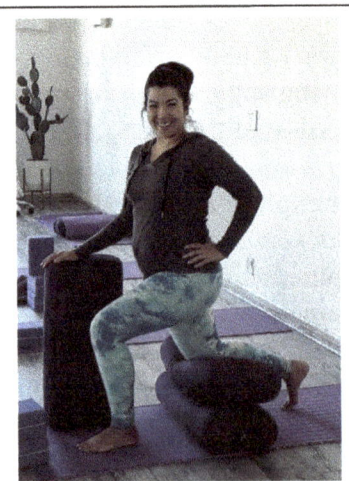

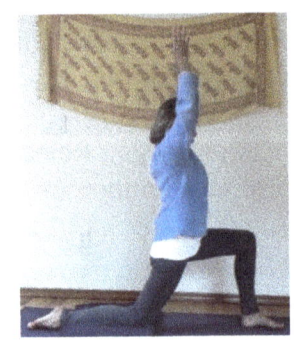

*Warrior 1 Lunge on One Knee – inviting ease into effort*
←

*Warrior 1 with Side Bend – adding challenge and balance*
→

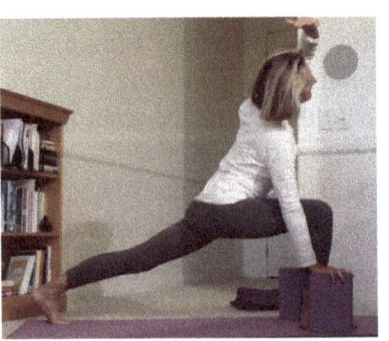

## Warrior 3 or Virabhadrasana III

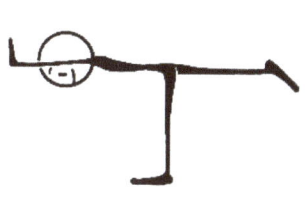

Warrior 3 is a dynamic standing shape that challenges coordination, stability, and focus, while emphasizing slight internal rotation and adduction in the hip joints. With the entire body hinging forward from the hip of the standing leg, and extending parallel to the ground, this movement cultivates strength through legs, core, and upper body. Warrior 3 is a powerful expression of focus and perseverance, designed to enhance muscular endurance while promoting mental clarity and resilience. Warrior 3 requires balancing and stabilizing alignment, along with physical strength and mental fortitude. It is ideally sequenced with other movements that include internal hip rotation and adduction (e.g., Warrior 1 Lunge and Eagle) to develop a healthfully sequenced practice that supports joint stability, muscular strength, and courageous concentration as well as balanced emotions.

### Benefits

Warrior 3 offers numerous benefits that contribute to overall wellbeing, enhancing both physical and mental aspects of the practice. Given its many dimensions in all layers of experience, Warrior 3 can help:

- *Improve balance, focus, and mental resilience*: The balancing nature of the shape enhances mental clarity, fostering a sense of determination and willpower.
- *Strengthen the legs, core, and glutes*: Engaging the entire posterior chain, Warrior 3 strengthens muscles of the legs, glutes, and core, promoting overall stability and strength, while requiring resilience.
- *Support postural alignment and spinal lengthening*: Extending through the crown of the head and the lifted heel, Warrior 3 encourages postural awareness and spinal elongation.
- *Enhance circulation and muscular endurance*: The full-body engagement in Warrior 3 promotes increased circulation, develops stamina in muscles, and creates stability in concentration.
- *Cultivate a sense of self-efficacy and confidence*: By maintaining balance and focus, this shape fosters a sense of self-efficacy, confidence, and empowerment.

### Cautions

When practicing Warrior 3, it is helpful to keep in mind the following cautions. These are not invitations to impart to students a sense of fragility – quite the opposite. Being mindful of where attention and care are indicated can be empowering and supportive of a sense of agency.

- *Ankle, knee, or low back issues*: Moving into Warrior 3 gradually and with attention to alignment can help prevent unnecessary strain on the ankles, knees, and low back.
- *Balance concerns*: For individuals with balance challenges, practicing near a wall or using a chair for support can provide added stability and a sense of security.
- *Sacroiliac joint sensitivity or instability*: Moving in and out of Warrior 3 with control helps protect the SI joints, particularly for individuals experiencing SI joint instability or sciatica.
- *Pregnancy (6+ months)*: Practicing with support from props or reducing the range of motion may help pregnant students maintain balance and comfort.

*Preparations*

To prepare for Warrior 3, it is auspicious to focus on building strength in the legs, creating stability in the core, and preparing physically and mentally for balance. Incorporating the following preparatory movements, integrated into the sequence after a warm-up that includes the six movements of spine, can be empowering and invites all layers of experience to be prepared for the challenge that is about to come.

- *Warrior I Lunge*: Strengthens the legs and prepares for the balance and engagement needed in Warrior 3.
- *Eagle (see below)*: Improves balance and strengthens the stabilizer muscles, enhancing proprioception and stability. Other standing balancing shapes with neutral hips and adduction are also helpful.
- *Lunges and pyramid*: Mobilize the hips, stretch the legs, and prepare the body for the slight internal rotation and adduction of the hips required in Warrior 3.
- *Concentration practice:* The opening centering and breathing practices can be used to begin to bring stability and balance to mind and emotions in an effort to find physical steadiness. Clear focus and concentration greatly support the capacity to engage this shape physically.

*Key Alignment Foci*

Warrior 3 requires strong alignment and awareness from head to heel, creating a dynamic and lengthening line of energy throughout the body and into the other layers of experience. Maintaining adaptability is key to finding comfortable and stable balance in body, breath, and mind. Following are key alignment invitations that can be offered and selectively applied as appropriate. Almost all cueing offered for Warrior 1 Lunge will also be helpful to finding an auspicious expression of Warrior 3. It is most balancing to repeat Warrior 3 on both sides, as it true for all one-side or asymmetrical shapes.

- *Invitations related to stance*
  - *Foot placement of standing leg*: Ensure that the standing foot is rooted into the ground, with even weight distributed across the balls and inner and outer heels of the foot. A slight micro-bend in the knee helps maintain joint health and prevents hyperextension.
  - *Engaging the back leg*: The lifted leg extends straight behind, with toes pointing towards the floor. Provide reminders about leveling the hips and creating stability in the pelvis. Invite pressing through the lifted heel.
  - *Stability in the standing leg*: Encourage students to check the alignment of their standing leg to ensure proper internal hip rotation, with the ankle, knee, and hip stacked and facing forward. Let knee alignment guide foot alignment (not vice versa).
- *Invitations related to hip alignment*
  - *Internal hip rotation*: Both hips are slightly internally rotated and adducted, with particular attention to keeping the pelvis level side to side to prevent tilting. A sense of adduction (drawing both legs toward the midline) is very helpful to creating a sense of stability.
  - *Engaging the core*: All core muscles in the broad sense are engaged to stabilize the pelvis. Low ribs can be drawn in and down toward the anterior superior iliac spine (ASIS) consciously, preventing arching or hinging in the lumbar spine.

- *Invitations related to upper body and spine*
  - *Spinal lengthening*: Extend the spine from the tailbone to the crown of the head. Avoid rounding the back by maintaining length through the chest and a lifted heart.
- *Invitations related to arm placement*
  - Arms may be extended forward alongside the ears, in line with the body, brought to the hips, or pointing to the floor with the possibility of hands resting on a block. Arm positioning is chosen by the students based on their perception of personal strength, balance, and comfort to support stability.
- *Invitations related to head and neck position*
  - *Natural alignment*: Keep the gaze downward or slightly forward, maintaining a natural neck position that is comfortably in line with the spine. Avoid hyperextension of the neck by keeping it relaxed and aligned.

## Variations and Exploration

Warrior 3 can be explored with many variations to suit different body types and needs in all layers of experience. Following are a few ideas; many more variations and experimentations are possible and encouraged.
- *Arm variations*: Place hands on the hips, extend arms forward or out to the side, bring them to prayer position, or rest hands on blocks for added stability.
- *Using props*: Practice with a wall, chair, or yoga ball to hold onto for support, or place the lifted foot on the wall or a chair to explore balance with less intensity.
- *Standing on both legs*: Experimenting with standing on both legs can help practitioners get familiar with the alignment of the upper body and hips before moving into a full one-legged balance. This is essentially a Half Lift – a great preparation or substitution for Warrior 3.
- *Adding rotations or side bends*: From a stable base stance in Warrior 3, creative play can be added through motions in the torso that further challenge balance, such as rotations or side bends in the upper spine. Various arm positions are also possible to explore, with arms out to the side, forward, or resting on the back of the hips.

## Recovery

After practicing Warrior 3, the following options may help release tension and allow for a transition into a grounded ventral vagal nervous system state.
- *Child*: Helps calm the nervous system and bring the body back into a relaxed state.
- *Mountain*: Resets alignment and allows for observation of the effects of Warrior 3.
- *Forward fold or half lift*: Releases tension in the hamstrings and low back.
- *Figure four stretch*: Reduces tension in the hips and gluteal muscles.
- *Shaking, wiggling, or gentle jogging*: Helps release residual tension physically and emotionally, promoting a sense of ease and relaxation.

## Additional Teaching Tips

To help students find healthful alignment and ease in Warrior 3, many additional invitations can be offered and explored. These types of cues invite students into their own inner wisdom and to bring in all layers of experience to support mindful embodiment.

- *Use props for stability*: Practicing with a wall, chair, or blocks can provide feedback on balance and alignment, helping students stabilize their movement. Placing the lifted heel on a wall can be very helpful in creating stability in the shape. Resting one hand or both hands on blocks or the back of a chair can create grounding and balance.
- *Imaginative cues for refinement*:
  - Invite students to imagine they are extending from the base of the spine through the crown of the head and out through the lifted heel.
  - Encourage students to visualize rooting down through the standing foot while reaching out through the lifted leg.
  - Invite students to imagine that the hands are reaching forward toward something, while the back heel moves in the opposite direction to create a counterweight.
- *Cue the four 'ceptions*:
  - *Interoception*: Guide students to notice sensations in the core, standing leg, and lifted leg, and to breathe calmly and lightly to support core stability and mental balance.
  - *Proprioception*: Invite students to explore various arm placements or shifting their weight slightly to identify positions of greatest balance for all layers of experience.
  - *Neuroception*: Encourage awareness of how internal or external stimuli may affect perceptions of safety versus fear in the shape.
  - *Exteroception*: Notice how distractions from the environment affect balance and stability. Alternatively, create external foci (such as *drishtis*) can be used to create a visual point of stability.

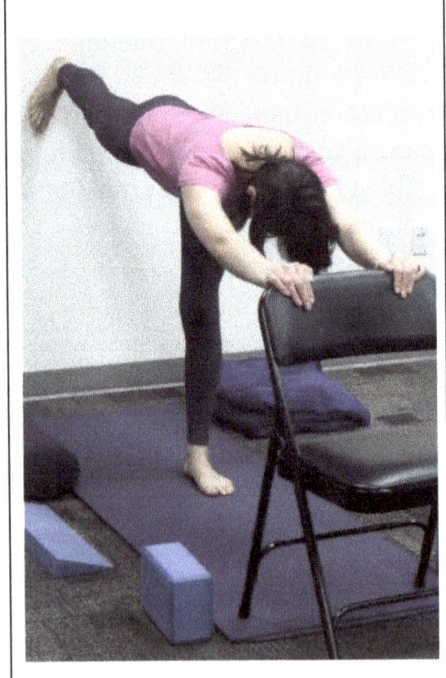
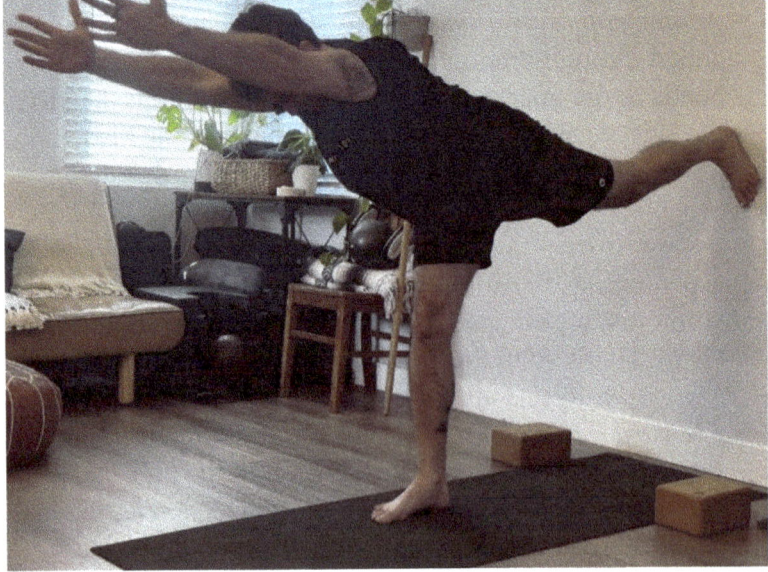

*Warrior 3 with Wall and Chair Support*

*Warrior 3 at a Wall for support and balance*

## Eagle or Garudasana

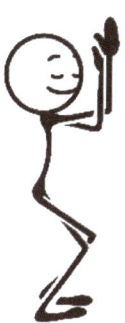

Eagle is an asymmetrical standing balancing shape that involves wrapping the limbs, creating both slight internal rotation and adduction in the hip and shoulder joints. Eagle encourages deep focus, concentration, and equanimity to maintain a sense of balance in the various layers of experience. The compression of the limbs invites a sense of stability and grounding within the balance challenge. In addition to this drawing inward for stability, it is equally essential to maintain spaciousness in the breath and body to prevent the shape from feeling restrictive. Eagle invites tangible balance between effort and ease, stability and mobility, contraction and openness. By focusing on mindful alignment, breath awareness, and individualized exploration, Eagle invites practitioners to deepen their physical, mental, and energetic experience while developing balance, strength, and coordination.

### Benefits

Eagle offers a multitude of physical, vital, and psychological benefits, related to the comingling of balance, coordination, and mindfulness. The shape serves to:
- *Promote mental focus and endurance*: Eagle requires intense concentration, fostering an undistracted mind and developing physical and vital endurance as the body sustains a wrapped, compact shape that can have a profound effect on how breath moves through the body.
- *Improve balance and coordination*: This shape challenges balance by narrowing the base of support and intertwining the limbs; it enhances proprioception and creates coordinated engagement throughout all layers of experience, tangibly connecting body, breath, and psyche.
- *Move lymph and improve circulation*: The wrapping of the arms and legs promotes lymphatic movement, enhancing detoxification and energizing physical and energetic vitality and wellbeing.
- *Create spaciousness in the body*: Though the shape may feel restrictive at first, Eagle creates the potential for finding spaciousness within contraction by encouraging students to release unnecessary tension and find ease in the breath, especially in the areas of the hips, shoulders, and rib basket.

### Cautions

Several important considerations support safety and ease when practicing Eagle. Many other cautions may exist; this list simply inspires awareness of what may need special attention and mention.
- *Knee and shoulder injuries*: Eagle places significant demand on several joints, including knees, wrists, shoulders, hips, and more. Students with knee or shoulder challenges are invited to work with gentler, less restrictive variations of Eagle, such as partial wraps of arms and legs. They may keep both feet on the ground or lightly cross the arms without binding.
- *Tight hips and piriformis concerns*: Internally rotating the hip joints is key to avoiding excessive strain on the knees or tightening the piriformis muscle, which could exacerbate

sciatica. It is helpful to focus on internal rotation and explore gentler leg positions if the hips feel constricted.
- *Balance disorders*: Practicing near a wall or using a block under the lifted foot can offer stability for individuals who need additional support. Allowing the body to find balance gradually enhances confidence and stability in mind and emotions over time.
- *Breathing restrictions*: The wrapping of the limbs may cause breath restriction and with that a sense of anxiety, even panic, especially if the body feels overly compressed. Invite students to maintain spaciousness in the chest and soften into the shape, ensuring that breathing remains smooth and quiet, not labored or fast.

## *Preparations*

Eagle requires strength and flexibility in the legs, shoulders, and core. Preparing the body with grounding, stretching, and balancing makes Eagle more accessible and stable. Specific preparations for Eagle follow a warm-up via the six movements of the spine.
- *Leg engagement*: Work with shapes such as Chair to build leg strength and stability, which is essential for the deep flexion and adduction in the legs during Eagle.
- *Shoulder opening*: Cow Face arms or Eagle arms (shown in Chapter 10) in a seated or standing position can help open and prepare shoulders, making the wrapping action of the arms less anxiety-provoking and more comfortable.
- *Balancing practice*: Integrating balance work, such as exploring standing on one leg or engaging with Mountain on tiptoes, helps activate the stabilizers in the legs and core and develop mental focus before moving into Eagle's more complex alignment.

## *Key Alignment Invitations*

Eagle encourages exploration of internal rotation, adduction, and stability while staying curious and open about breath and alignment. By working from the inside out, practitioners can create space within the compactness of the shape. A few invitations that can be offered follow; many more options exist. As always, be cautious not to offer too many of these cues at once, instead selecting those with the greatest relevance to the students in class. Like all asymmetrical shapes, Eagle is best practiced in on both sides.
- *Invitations for the feet and legs*:
  - *Standing leg*: Ground through the corners of the standing foot, feeling a strong connection with the earth. Start with a soft micro-bend in the knee to protect the joint and avoid locking.
  - *Lifted leg*: Cross the lifted leg over the standing leg, allowing the thighs to press against each other. The wrapping of the legs ideally feels stable and supported. The toes of the lifted leg can rest on the ground or a chair; the foot can hook behind the calf if that alignment is accessible without forcing or passive stretching – be especially cautious of torquing the knee joint for the sake of wrapping the foot.
  - *Adduction and internal hip rotation*: Focus on gentle internal rotation, as well as adduction of the hips (i.e., moving the thighs of the legs toward each other and slightly inward). These actions stabilize the legs and protect the knees, ensuring the rotation happens in the hip joints rather than the knees. Honor the natural range of motion in the hip joints to protect the knees.

- *Invitations for the arms and shoulders*:
  - *Arm wrap*: Cross the arms at the elbows, bringing palms or backs of the hands together or using a prop to connect them, if desired. Press the arms into each other to create stability, but avoid sacrificing the alignment of the shoulders. Allow the shoulder blades to remain resting lightly on the back.
  - *Relax the shoulders*: Find a balance between stretching and strengthening the shoulders. Avoid excessive pulling down of the shoulder blades, which can compress the chest and restrict the breath. Create a spacious, light feeling in the upper back and invite the shoulder girdle to relax away from the ears.
- *Invitations for the spine and core*:
  - *Engage the core*: Gently engage the core muscles to support the spine and maintain balance. This action creates stability without inducing excessive tension.
  - *Natural spine*: Maintain the natural curves of the spine, avoiding rounding or overarching. The spine ideally feels long and centered, balancing the energetic engagement of the upper and lower body.
  - *Level hips*: Keep the hips level side-to-side, even as the legs wrap. Watch for excessive tilting or twisting in the pelvis, which can lead to imbalance or strain in the low back and the sacroiliac joints.
- *Invitations for drishti* (gaze):
  - *Find a steady gaze*: Establish a *drishti*, or steady gaze, on a fixed point ahead to anchor the mind and support emotional and physical balance. Focused attention can stabilize the entire experience of the shape, including in body, breath, and psyche.

## Variations and Exploration

Eagle is an adaptable shape with many variations that allow for personalization and playful exploration. The following invitation can be made; many other possibilities exist and are limited only by the creativity of teachers and students.

- *Foot placement variations*: The lifted foot can rest on the ground, block, or chair; for some students, it may be able to hook around the calf. Experimenting with different foot positions can help students identify their most stable and supported shape in their various layers of experience.
- *Arm height variations*: Arms can stay at shoulder height, or students can explore raising or lowering the wrapped arms to adjust the experience of the shoulder stretch. Ensuring that the breath remains smooth can help guide students to their most auspicious arm position – when the breath is dysregulated, the students are over-efforting.
- *Wall assistance*: Practice near a wall to support balance and alignment without the added challenge of being in the middle of the room or mat. This balance support allows for a focus on healthful alignment before adding the balance challenge.
- *Forward fold variation:* Once stable, some students may want to explore folding forward while maintaining the wraps, deepening the engagement in the legs and stretching the spine. Mindful awareness of the four 'ceptions is key.
- *Chair variation:* Sit on a chair and find café legs. Play with arm variations (see illustrations below) to find an easeful and joyful variation of this challenging shape.

*Recovery*

After Eagle, if can be helpful to create spaciousness in the body and calm the nervous system through a few more expansive shapes. The following possibilities are offered to inspire additional ideas.

- *Extended Mountain*: Invite students to reach upward and create length in the spine, bringing calm and balance after the intense focus of Eagle.
- *Wide-legged forward fold*: A gentle forward fold with legs wide apart can release tension in the hips and shoulders, while still drawing on the internal rotation in the hip joint. Beware of hyperextension in knee joints in very flexible students.
- *Mild backbend*: A soft backbend opens the chest and heart space, countering the contraction of the arms and upper body. For example, draping the body in a supine position over a large yoga ball can bring inspiration and release.

*Additional Teaching Tips*

Healthful alignment can be inspired by several added teaching tips, based on observation of students in the moment. Such additional cues are offered to attune students into their inner wisdom in all layers of experience.

- *Breath awareness*: Encourage students to stay attuned to their breath throughout their time moving into and out of Eagle. The wrapping or hugging motions can restrict breathing; it typically serves well to remind students to soften unnecessary tension and create space for the breath, particularly in the low rib basket and abdomen.
- *Props for feedback*: Invite the use a block or chair under the lifted foot for stability, and/or practice near a wall for balance support. Supports help students feel more secure emotionally while exploring the alignment in the legs and hips and arms and shoulders.
- *Balance through engagement*: Give reminders to press legs and arms into each other to create stability, without sacrificing alignment in the joints, especially the knees and glenohumeral joints. Mindful engagement fosters strength and spaciousness, balancing ease and effort.

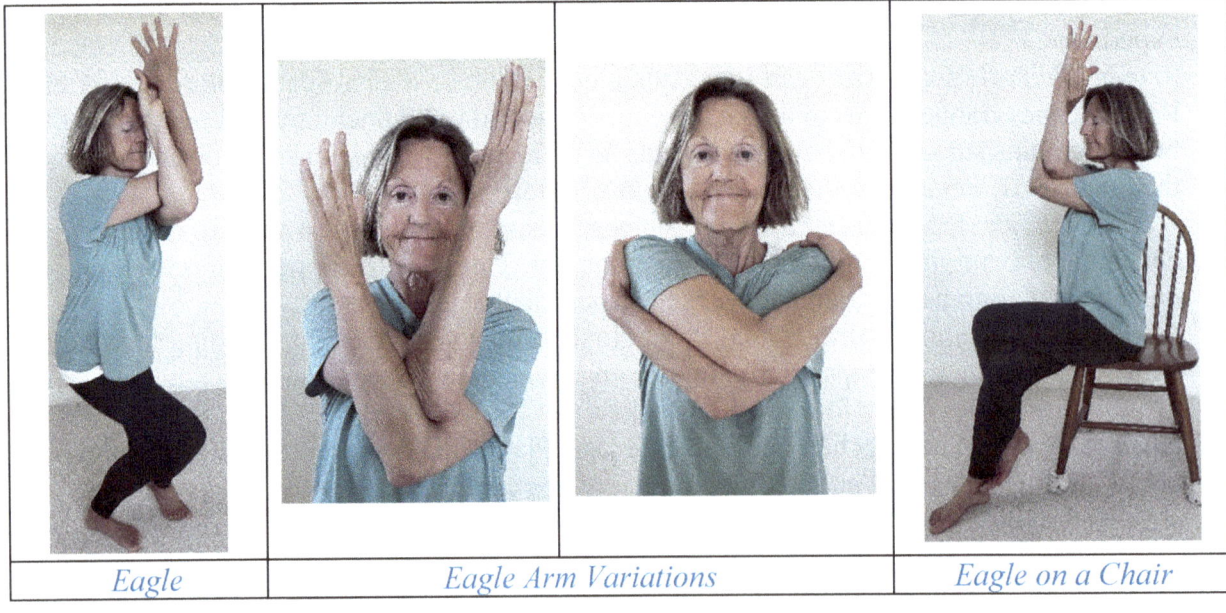

*Eagle* | *Eagle Arm Variations* | *Eagle on a Chair*

## Warrior 2 or Virabhadrasana II

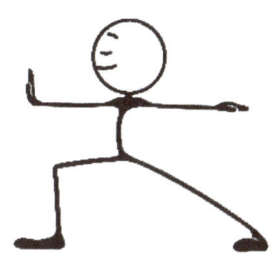

Warrior 2 is a powerful standing shape that emphasizes external hip rotation and dynamic asymmetry. This shape encourages strength, stability, and a sense of resilience throughout body, breath, and mind. It is commonly practiced to build leg strength, increase stamina, and improve focus. The external hip rotation in the front leg complements other shapes involving external rotation, making it an excellent addition to sequences with other hip-opening shapes. Although Warrior 1 and Warrior 2 are often taught one after the other, it is important to recall that anatomically, this sequencing may not be ideal due to differences in hip rotation and alignment (for a review see Chapter 5 and the General Principles for Standing Shapes in the current chapter). Warrior 2 offers an opportunity to explore stability, grounding, and openness while fostering willpower and determination in a complex, multiplanar shape.

### Benefits

Warrior 2 offers numerous physical, mental, and energetic benefits that contribute to overall wellbeing in body, energy, mind, emotions, and relationships. The shape can serve to:
- *Develop willpower and alertness*: The strong and open stance of Warrior 2 creates focused attention, cultivates mental resilience, and invites a sense of empowerment.
- *Strengthen feet, ankles, knees, and legs*: Warrior 2 engages multiple muscle groups, promoting strength and stability throughout the lower body.
- *Improve endurance in leg, hip, and buttock musculature*: Holding Warrior 2 helps build stamina in the legs and hips, increasing endurance over time.
- *Enhance shoulder alignment*: Holding the arms outstretched at shoulder height encourages healthful alignment and strength in the shoulder girdle.
- *Improve balance and stability*: The asymmetrical nature of Warrior 2 challenges balance and helps improve stability through focused engagement and rooting into the earth.

### Cautions

There are a few important cautions to consider when practicing Warrior 2. Cueing around these cautions invites care while avoiding inducing a sense of fragility or vulnerability, so as not to undo or undermine the empowerment function of the shape.
- *Knee injuries or issues*: Warrior 2 can be challenging for the forward knee joint due to the weight-bearing bend in the front knee. It is essential to focus on healthful side-to-side alignment to minimize the risk for strain and injury.
- *Sacroiliac instability:* Warrior 2 can be a very risky shape for students with SI instability and needs to be approached with caution to cue inner experience rather than outer alignment.
- *Balance disorders*: Individuals with balance disorders can be advised to practice near a wall or use a chair for added stability.
- *Pregnancy (6+ months):* Pregnant students can practice this shape with caution, ideally near a wall or using other supports to maintain stability and reduce the risk of becoming unbalanced or unsteady.

- *Neck injuries*: Students with neck injuries are advised to avoid turning the head to look forward over the front hand. Instead, they can keep the head in line with the spine and shoulder girdle (i.e., facing most likely diagonally forward).

## Preparations

Preparations for Warrior 2 involve strengthening the legs, opening the hip joints, and preparing the shoulders for the strength required to keep the arms extended out to the side at shoulder height. The following preparatory shapes and practices are offered in a meaningfully sequenced manner after the standard warm-up that includes the six movements of the spine.
- *Leg strengthening*: Shapes like Mountain on tiptoes or with arms raised help establish stability in the legs, providing a strong foundation for Warrior 2.
- *Hip openers*: Shapes like Lizard are helpful for gently preparing for externally rotating and opening the hip joint.
- *Shoulder alignment*: Preparing the shoulders for Warrior 2 can be facilitated through stretches like Eagle arms or stretches at the wall (see the various preparations for heart opening covered in Chapter 13), ensuring openness and stability, along with strength, when extending the arms out to the sides.
- *Tree variation balance work*: Practicing variations of Tree (see below) can help activate the stabilizers in the legs while incorporating external hip rotation, preparing for the stance and balance required in Warrior 2.

## Key Alignment Invitations

Warrior 2 is characterized by a wide stance and long stride, external hip rotation in the front leg, and a naturally upright spine. It is healthful to approach alignment with a sense of curiosity and respect for the body's unique tendencies and abilities. The following alignment invitations provide guidance, but each individual is encouraged to adapt movements based on what feels most appropriate in their own body, engaging in the shape on both sides in sequence:
- *Invitations related to stance*: Stance has two reference points: Width and length. Width refers to the distance between the two feet in the frontal plane (i.e., how wide apart are the feet side-to-side). Length (also referred to as stride length) is the distance of the stride in the sagittal plane (i.e., how far ahead from the front foot is the back foot).
  - Width between the two feet in this shape is ideally calibrated to the width of the hips and needs of the joints in the pelvis and legs – there is no one size fits all, A common cue for width is to align the arch of the back foot with the heel of the front foot. The challenge with this is that not all bodies are the same and for many, the stance may need to be much wider apart that this cue requires.
  - Stride length is determined by flexibility and strength. For some students, length will be such that the forward thigh is parallel to the ground; for others the stride is short and the thigh is angled upward, with the hip joint higher than the knee joint. Again, there is no one size (or length) fits all. Resist providing cues that require students to strive for a standard outer shape and instead commit to helping each individual find the shape that fits best for their body.

- *Invitations related to front knee*: Encourage students to develop interoception and proprioception in the front knee, tuning into the sensations and adjustments as needed to create stable, supported flexion in the joint, without torquing or forcing.
    - In the sagittal plane, the knee can be ahead of or behind the ankle, as feels more appropriate to the individual student.
    - In the frontal place, the front knee is placed directly above the ankle (i.e., neither medial nor lateral to the ankle) to protect the joint and maintain stability.
    - The front knee tracks in line with the ankle, neither collapsing inward or outward. If the knee is observed to collapse one way or the other, this can put strain on the joint. It can be helpful to invite the student to place their hand on the opposite side of the knee and to press the knee into the hand while the hand presses into the knee.
- *Invitations related to back leg and foot:* It is very important (and counter to much conventional cueing) <u>not to be</u> prescriptive about the placement of the feet.
    - The back foot is positioned at an angle that honors the shape of the student's hip socket, shape of the head and neck of the femur, and stability in the SI joints. The back leg is extended and strong but does not overpower the needs of the joints for the sake of a standardized outer shape.
    - It is helpful to encourage students to experiment with adjusting the back foot until they find comfort in the hip and sacroiliac joints.
    - *Watch for hyperextension in the back knee*: Ensure that students keep a gentle micro-bend in the back knee to avoid hyperextension, which could strain the joint. This is especially important for hypermobile students.
- *Invitations related to external rotation in the hip of the forward leg:* The front hip is externally rotated, creating openness in the hip and ensuring proper alignment in the pelvis.
    - Avoid collapsing into the hip; instead, actively lift through the front thigh.
    - Honor the shapes of the acetabulum, femoral head and neck, and their union in the hip socket.
    - In other words, do not force an inappropriate degree of external rotation for the sake of a standardized outer shape, but instead allow the opposite hip to move forward and the back foot to pivot in such ways that all joints involved in the shape feel well supported, not torqued, and able to bear weight. This means the pelvis will likely never point to the side (as is often incorrectly cued – more below).
- *Invitations related to working optimally with pelvis and spine:* The pelvis remains level and natural, allowing the spine to rise upward in its natural curves. It might help to imagine lifting through the crown of the head to elongate through the spine. The pelvis likely is in a diagonal line relative to the edges of the mat. This alignment runs counter to what is often cued, that the pelvis should be aligned with the long side of the mat. The challenge with this cueing is that such a wide opening is not compatible with most human acetabula or femur shapes (especially the neck and head of the femur) and, if followed, can cause SI joint disruption for many individuals.
    - *Protect the sacroiliac joints*: Pay attention to the rotation of the back hip and adjust the alignment of the foot and leg as needed to prevent stress in the SI joints. There is no prescribed foot placement either for the front or back foot. Instead, comfort in the SI joints and ease in the knee joints determine where the feet are placed.
    - *Develop lumbar curve awareness*: Guide students to explore the natural curve of the lumbar spine and avoid overarching, which could cause discomfort. A gentle activation

of the stabilizer muscles may help support this natural alignment in the low spine and sacrum.
- *Invitations related to explore shoulder alignment:* Encourage students to be mindful of shoulder positioning, avoiding impingement by keeping shoulders relaxed and heart open.
  - The arms are extended at shoulder height, with palms facing up or down and with the shoulder girdle relaxed.
  - Avoid scrunching the shoulders up towards the ears, and instead invite the shoulder blades to move naturally down the back.
  - Invite the student to imagine placing the entire shoulder girdle on a shelf to help facilitate ease and release in the neck and shoulder muscles.
  - Align the shoulders above the hips, rather than reaching too far forward or too far backwards – yoga lore is that students who reach toward the front of the mat, are living in the future; those who reach to the back of the mat, live in the past (check out what modern science has to say in the "*Fun Facts*" box).
- *Invitations related to natural head position:* Begin with the head looking straight ahead and the chin slightly tucked and drawn back to place the head in its natural position above the spine. Encourage students to experiment with turning the head to gaze over the front hand only if it feels comfortable and safe for their neck.

---

*Fun fact from modern science …*

Chronesthesia (i.e., mental time travel) and Body Alignment

When individuals fitted with motion sensors were thinking about the past, they swayed backwards. When they were thinking about the future, they swayed forward. So – when yoga teachers joke about Warrior 2 alignment reflecting preoccupation with past, present, or future, they may not be joking after all. ☺

Miles, L. K., Nind, L. K., & Macrae, C. N. (2010). Moving through time. *Psychological Science, 21,* 22-223. DOI:10.1177/0956797609359333

---

*Variations and Exploration*

Warrior 2 offers many variations and explorations. These can be adapted to suit each practitioner's needs and to create new challenges as well as joyful ways of embodying the power and strength of this shape.
- *Arm positions*: Experiment with different arm placements such as placing hands on the hips, choosing a cactus arms position, extending one or both arms overhead, or taking a Peaceful Warrior variation (see photo below) to stretch the side body.
- *Adding a forward fold*: Invite a hinging in the forward hip to bend the torso over the forward leg into a Humble Warrior (see photo) to find humility and reverence.
- *Wall assistance*: Practicing with the back heel at a wall can help provide feedback for healthful alignment, allowing students to feel a sensation of grounding and stability.
- *Play with balance*: Add gentle swaying or intuitive movement; experiment with the rotation of the head to explore balance and proprioception; or try closing the eyes (only of the student feels stable and grounded).

- *Internal vs. external rotation in back hip*: Encourage students to experiment with rotating the back hip internally or externally to understand how this affects foot placement and overall alignment, especially in the sacroiliac joints. This is a very gentle exploration appropriate only for students with adequate interoceptive awareness and the ability to use inner sensation to guide alignment and variation.

*Recovery*

After Warrior 2, it can serve students well to consciously release accumulated tension in the hips, shoulders, and back. Consider practicing the following recovery possibilities; many more exist.
- *Downward Facing Dog*: This shape may help release the hips, lengthen the spine, and alleviate tension in shoulders and back.
- *Wide-legged Forward Fold*: This shape can help relax the low back, stretch the legs, and release residual tension in the body.
- *Seated Forward Fold*: Gently stretches the hamstrings and relaxes the back, offering a soothing recovery after the effort of Warrior 2.
- *Intuitive movement*: Little shakes and wiggles, or gentle jogging in place can be helpful releases after Warrior 2.

*Additional Teaching Tips*

To help students find a deeper sense of stability and alignment in Warrior 2, consider the following additional suggestions that touch more directly on the psychological benefits of the shape. Many other explorations exist and creativity can be invited.
- *Use props for feedback*: Placing a chair or yoga ball under the front thigh can be a challenging or easeful variation. Placing a block under the back foot can help students explore how to feel more or less grounded.
- *Invite the imagination for refinement*:
  - Image placing the entire shoulder girdle on an imaginary shelf to help facilitate ease and release in the neck and shoulder muscles.
  - Imagine sending energy outward through the arms, hands and finger tips as a way to feel the power and energy of this shape.
  - Imagine offering up a peaceful heart when moving into Reverse Warrior 2.
- *Cue the four 'ceptions*: Help students attune to interoception, exteroception, neuroception, and proprioception; for example:
  - Notice the subtle differences in muscle engagement with small adjustments in foot, knee, or hip positioning.
  - Invite awareness of interoceptive changes, such as sensations in the front knee as the shape is held. Invite commensurate ongoing changes and adjustments to maintain a compassionate and wholesome alignment and experience.
  - Explore how external distractions from the environment may influence stability or focus.
  - Invite exploration of inner distractions, such as thoughts or emotions that arise during the shape.
  - Notice how changing position and focus affects the nervous system and its perception of safety and presence within the shape.

- *Integrate breath awareness*: Remind students to maintain steady and light breathing while holding Warrior 2. Encourage them to connect their breath with their physical experience, using inhalations to expand and lengthen the spine and using the exhalations to stabilize and ground into the shape.

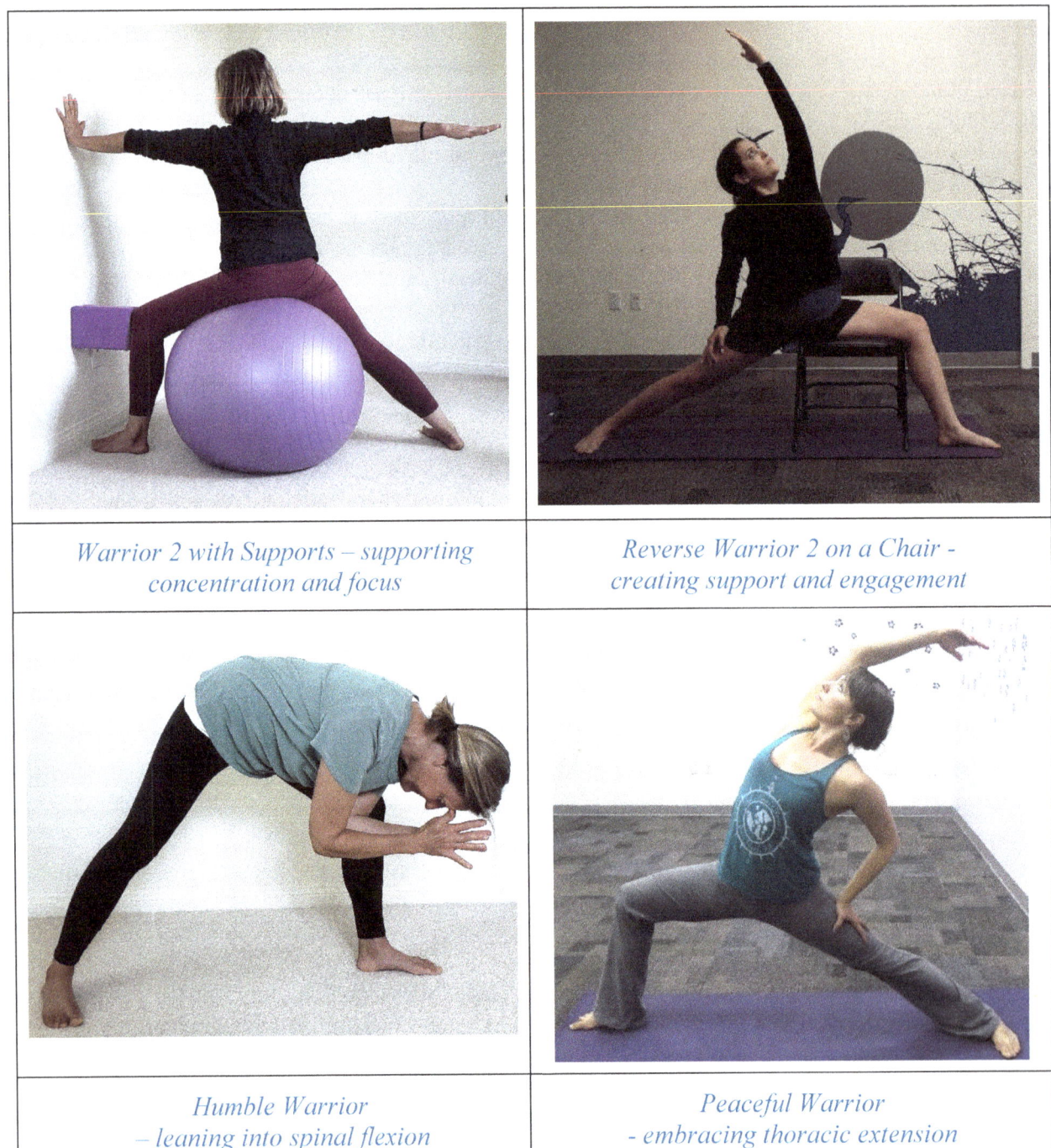

*Warrior 2 with Supports – supporting concentration and focus*

*Reverse Warrior 2 on a Chair - creating support and engagement*

*Humble Warrior – leaning into spinal flexion*

*Peaceful Warrior - embracing thoracic extension*

## Side Angle or Utthita Parsvakonasana

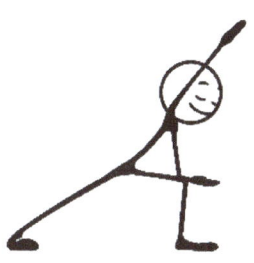

Side Angle is a dynamic standing shape that encourages lateral extension and grounding. This shape is designed to promote strength, length, and openness throughout the body while cultivating a sense of fluidity and stability. It can help students explore their hip joint range of motion, spine elongation, and conscious integration of the upper and lower aspects of the body (namely, the upper and lower appendicular parts of the skeleton). Often taught after foundational standing shapes such as Warrior 2, Side Angle complements hip sequences that revolve around external hip rotation and adduction (i.e., occur in the sagittal, transverse, and frontal planes) and encourages awareness of the connection of body, breath and nervous system response, and psyche, with its mental and emotional reactivities and stories.

### Benefits

Side Angle offers a wide range of physical, energetic, and psychological benefits that contribute to an overall sense of wellbeing. Although the following benefits are highlighted here, there are no doubt many others. Side Angle has been documented to:
- *Lengthen the side body*: The extended side body creates resilience in the rib basket, facilitating a more easeful breath and promoting a sense of emotional openness.
- *Strengthen the legs and hips*: The bent forward leg and grounded back leg work together to build strength in the pelvic and thigh muscles, increasing stability and vitality.
- *Encourage balance and integration*: Side Angle challenges the entire organism to find equilibrium – physically, through weight distribution while maintaining an expansive shape; vitally, through an even and gentle breath within challenge; and psychologically by inviting emotional and mental ease in the midst of great effort.
- *Create resilience in the chest and shoulders*: The upper arm reaching overhead helps create an opening of the heart space that promotes greater freedom in the shoulder joint and awakens resilience in the rib basket.
- *Cultivate focus and awareness*: Balancing the strength of the lower body with the openness of the upper body emphasizes focused attention and mindful awareness.

### Cautions

Given the complexity of Side Angle, it is not surprising that there are several important considerations and cautions that can be explored and noted as appropriate when teaching this shape. The following issues need to be tracked and addressed commensurate with student observation and needs. Cautions noted about Warrior 2 also apply.
- *Knee injuries or issues*: The bent front knee is weight-bearing, which can place pressure on the knee joint. It is crucial for students to practice with mindful alignment of the knee side-to-side to reduce risk of undue strain, torquing, or injury, especially over time.
- *Shoulder injuries or limited range of motion*: If a student experiences shoulder discomfort or experiences restricted range of motion, Side Angle can be practiced with the upward hand resting on the hip or pointing straight upward to the sky, rather than extending it forward.

- *Low back concerns*: Twisting or collapsing into the low back can create tension or strain in the lumbar and sacroiliac joints. It is important to guide students to maintain natural length and supportive engagement in the spine to reduce risk of discomfort. Place focus on natural movement into the rotation for the pelvis rather than cueing to an artificial outer alignment.
- *Balance challenges*: Side Angle can present issues for students who have limited stability (e.g., due to strength or neurological issues). Such individuals are encouraged to practice near a wall or to use a chair for support as they build capacity and strength.

## Preparations

Preparations for Side Angle involve leg strengthening, hip mobilization, and awareness across all layers of experience. Preparatory shapes are offered after a standard warm-up that includes the six movements of the spine. All preparations for the other standing shapes based on external hip rotation and abduction (e.g., Warrior 2, Tree) are useful for Side Angle as well.
- *Leg strengthening*: Shapes like Mountain and Warrior 2 help establish stability and strength in the legs, preparing the body for the deep bend required in the front knee.
- *Hip openers*: Lizard or Tree can assist in awakening the hip rotators, flexors, and abductors, creating a foundation for increased stability and mobility in the hip joint.
- *Shoulder and side body lengthening*: Extended Puppy or Cat-Cow movements can help prepare the shoulders and side bodies, or flanks. Standing lateral flexion is also excellent.

## Key Alignment Invitations

Side Angle is characterized by a Lunge-like shape, with the forward hip joint in external rotation and both hips in abduction (the legs are wide apart). Its alignment also involves lateral elongation (or extension), and a sense of openness throughout the heart space and flanks. Side Angle arises most helpfully out of the same alignment in the lower body as in Warrior 2, with the same care not to torque any joints in the pelvis, low back, and legs, with particular care for the knee and SI joints. The following alignment suggestions can help students explore the shape with mindfulness. These cues are applied based on observation and not all offered at once to make sure students can absorb and apply cueing in a targeted and healthful manner. Ideally, the shape is practiced on both sides, as is typical for all one-sided shapes.
- *Invitations related to stance*: As noted above, a stance has two reference points: width and length. Width refers to the distance between the two feet in the frontal plane (i.e., how wide apart are the feet side-to-side). Length is the length of the stride in the sagittal plane (i.e., how far ahead of the front foot is the back foot).
    - The width between the two feet in this shape is ideally calibrated to the width of the hips and needs of the joints in the pelvis and legs – there is no one size fits all (forget about cues that encourage aligning the arch of the back foot with the heel of the front foot; many individuals' stance may need to be much wider than that). Artificial cueing based on attaining a standardized outer shape has the risk of torquing knee and/or SI joints and can become counterproductive and harmful.
    - The length is determined by flexibility and strength. For some students, length will be such that the forward thigh is parallel to the ground; for others the stride is short and the thigh is angled upward, with the hip joint higher than the knee joint. Again, there is no one size (or length) fits all.

- *Invitations related to front knee alignment*:
    - Encourage students to keep the front knee aligned side-to-side directly above the ankle, with the foot pointing in the same direction as the knee. This alignment protects the knee joint and promotes stability.
    - There is little risk to the knee being forward or behind the ankle front-to-back. In other words, the knee does not have to be exactly above the ankle in the forward or backward direction. However, it is best placed neither to the inside nor the outside of the knee (i.e., it is aligned with the ankle in the frontal plane).
    - Awareness of sensations in the knees supports healthful stability in a potentially vulnerable position. If the knee tends to collapse inward or outward, encourage the use of a gentle press of the arm against the knee for support on the opposite side of the collapse (i.e., if the leg collapses inward, place the hand to the outside of the foot and press the leg outward into the arm).
- *Invitations related to back leg and foot positioning*:
    - The back leg remains strong and engaged, with the back foot planted at an angle that feels comfortable for the student's hip and sacroiliac joints. Avoid artificial cueing about a particular alignment of the back foot along dimensions of the mat – inner experience aligns the foot, not the quest for a standardized outer shape.
    - Encourage a gentle micro-bend in the back knee to avoid hyperextension, which can strain the joint.
- *Invitations related to working optimally with pelvis and spine*: The pelvis remains level and natural, allowing the spine to rise upward in its natural curves. It might help to imagine lifting through the crown of the head to elongate through the spine. The pelvis is likely to settle in a diagonal line relative to the edges of the mat – not aligned with the long side of the mat as is often and inauspiciously cued. Such wide opening is not in line with most human acetabular or femoral shapes (especially as related to neck and head of the femurs and the depth and orientation of the acetabula).
    - *Protect the sacroiliac joints*: Pay attention to the rotation of the back hip and adjust the alignment of the foot and leg as needed to prevent stress in the SI joints. There is no prescribed foot placement either for the front or back foot. Instead, comfort in the SI joints and ease in the knee joints determine where and how the feet are placed (the back heel is likely even lifted or may rest on a prop).
    - *Develop lumbar curve awareness*: Guide students to explore the natural curve of the lumbar spine and avoid overarching (hyperextension and/or hinging), which could cause discomfort. Gentle activation of the stabilizer muscles may support natural alignment for the low spine and sacrum, especially relative to the ilia of the pelvis.
- *Invitations related to side body length and spinal elongation*:
    - Encourage students to open through the side body, creating length from the outer edge of the back foot all the way to the extended fingertips. Avoid collapsing into the bottom side; instead, create spaciousness and upward lift.
    - Avoid spinal leveraging by moving mindfully and slowly based on interoception.
    - The spine remains elongated without excessive effort or lengthening
- *Invitations related to heart space and shoulder opening*:
    - The heart space is open, and the shoulder gridle remains relaxed. The upper arm may extend upward or alongside the ear.

- If reaching the arm overhead is uncomfortable or leads to collapse in the heart space, the hand can rest on the hip or the low back.
- *Invitations related to bottom arm placement*:
  - The bottom hand can rest lightly on the inside of the front foot, a block, or the shin. The most healthful choice allows the heart space to stay open and prevents the side bodies from collapsing downward or forward.
  - Avoid placing excessive weight into the bottom arm; rely on legs and core for support.
- *Invitations related to head position*:
  - Invite students to experiment with their gaze. They may look straight ahead, towards the top hand, or down at the ground, depending on what feels most auspicious and healthful for their neck, breath, and physical and psychological balance.

## *Variations and Exploration*

Side Angle can be explored and varied in many ways to suit each practitioner's needs or to create ease or complexity to the practice. The following ideas are just that – invitations to be creative. Many more options for exploration exist.
- *Arm placement variations*:
  - The top arm can extend directly upwards, reach overhead, or rest on low back, depending on needs within any layer of experience. For example, although a students may be physically able to reach the arm forward alongside the ear, their nervous system in a given moment may be better served by a more grounded and supportive placement of the hand on the back body.
  - The bottom arm can rest on a block or other support to reduce or adjust the lateral flexion, create more stability in the body, or provide more accessibility emotionally.
- *Wall and other prop support:*
  - Practicing with the back heel or side of the foot against a wall offers additional support and grounding, helping students find stability and alignment, especially if there is a sense of worry or anxiety about this shape in the middle of the room (or for any other reason).
  - The back knee can be on the ground to provide a lower profile and more physical stability and emotional accessibility in the shape.
  - Using a chair under the bent front thigh or bottom hand can help students maintain the shape while offering additional support, allowing them to focus on easeful alignment and a vital and gentle breath.

## *Recovery*

The following recovery shapes may serve to release tension and transition into a more relaxed state. Many other possibilities exist, depending on what comes next in the overall sequence.
- *Downward Facing Dog*: Helps release the side body and lengthens the spine.
- *Wide-legged Forward Fold*: Offers a release for hamstrings and spine.
- *Child*: Creates a sense of grounding while releasing tension that may have crept into the hip region or back from excessive bracing in the shape.
- *Reclined Twist*: Helps release the spine and gently relaxes the hip joints.
- *Intuitive movement*: Gentle shaking, wiggling, or jogging in place can help release residual tension all over the body.

## Additional Teaching Tips

To support students in experiencing the full benefits of Side Angle, additional suggestions can be offered based on observed need and self-expression. Use these additional cues with discernment and, as always, be careful not to overwhelm students with excess verbiage.

- *Use props for feedback:*
  - Blocks can help bring the ground closer to the student, ensuring that the heart space remains open and that they do not collapse into the lower side body.
  - A blanket under the lowered back knee can transform the shape.
  - Placing the back heel or side of foot against a wall can create lift and ease.
- *Invite visualization or imagery:*
  - Encourage students to imagine lengthening through upward-facing side of the body, as though they are creating space in the rib basket.
  - Invite the student to visualize energy radiating out through the extended top arm and the back heel, creating a sense of active expansion and joy.
- *Cue awareness of sensations:*
  - Encourage interoception and proprioception by inviting students to tune into sensations in the front knee, side body, or spine as they hold the shape, making subtle adjustments from the inside out to enhance comfort and stability.
  - Invite awareness of how breath affects the shape, perhaps exploring the inhalation as a support to lengthen and the exhalation to ground with ease.
- *Integrate breath with movement:*
  - Guide students to connect breath with movement, using the inhalation to expand and create length and the exhalation to settle in while maintaining integrity and engagement in muscles around the major joints that need attention for healthful alignment.

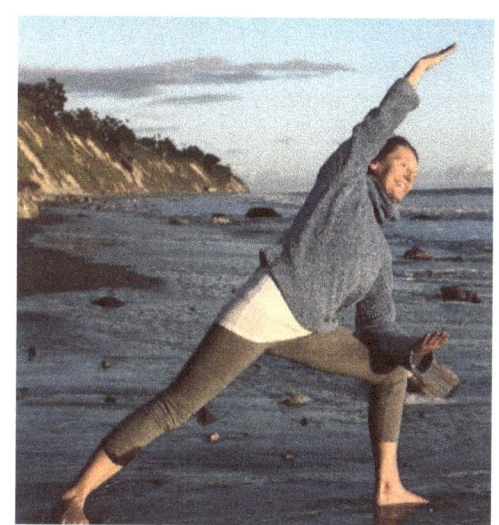

*Extended Side Angle – finding expansiveness*

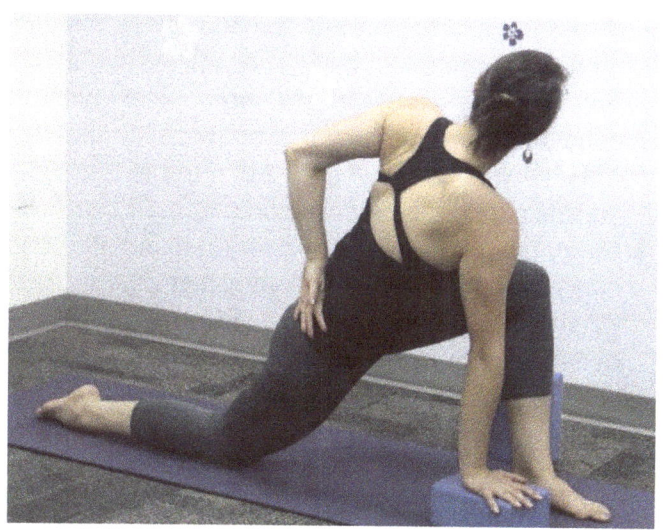

*Side Angle with Rotation – exploring with curiosity and grace*

## Triangle or Utthita Trikonasana

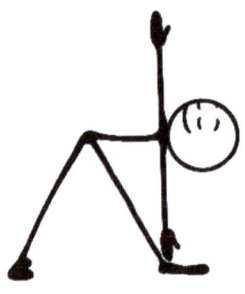

Triangle is another asymmetrical standing shape that arises in concert with other standing shapes that involve external rotation and abduction in the hips. Triangle encourages a combination of grounding and lateral elongation, promoting a sense of spaciousness and strength. Practicing Triangle helps lengthen the side body, strengthen the legs, and open the heart space, making it a possible addition to standing sequences that focus on balance and flexibility. It is often taught following foundational shapes such as Warrior 2 and Side Angle (i.e., shapes that share the same hip joint demands). Although often promoted as a quintessential yoga shape, Triangle is not actually all that accessible in a healthful manner for first-time students or students who do not yet have easy access to interoception and proprioception. Its functional movement value is limited. It is not appropriate for inexperienced students or students with (yet) limited interoception.

### Benefits

Triangle offers a few physical, energetic, and mental benefits. It has been documented that Triangle may:
- *Invigorate the side body*: The extended torso creates space in the rib basket, facilitating breathing into the midriff and supporting diaphragmatic breathing as opposed to thoracic breathing.
- *Strengthen the legs and core*: Both legs remain actively engaged throughout the shape, promoting stability and strength in thighs, hips, and core.
- *Open the heart space and shoulders*: The expansive or radiant shape encourages openness across the heart space and freedom in the shoulder joints. It may bring the same openness to mind and emotions.
- *Improve balance and coordination*: The balance between grounding through the legs and extending through the upper body may improve coordination and body awareness.
- *Build focus and willpower*: Attention to balance, alignment, and breath encourages focus, presence, and mental resilience.
- *Open the hips*: External hip rotation and abduction can promote greater hip mobility, balanced by strength and engagement.
- *Create flexibility in the spine*: Elongation through the spine encourages resilience and dynamic stability along the vertebral column.

### Cautions

When teaching Triangle, consider the following cautions:
- *Pregnancy (6+ months)*: The shape may require significant variations to avoid compressing the abdomen. It is not recommended.
- *Low blood pressure*: Reread all cautions related to femoral leveraging, sacral corkscrewing, and spinal leveraging. All can co-occur in this shape.

- *Hypermobility and sacroiliac joint instability*: Pay attention to the alignment of the pelvis and back leg to avoid placing undue stress, torque, or mobility on the SI joints. Watch for hyperextension in the knees in students who tend toward hypermobility.
- *Knee issues*: Hyperextension of, or torquing in, the knee joints can lead to strain. Encourage students to engage the quadriceps to stabilize the knees and invite a micro-bend to prevent locking this important joint.
- *Neck injuries or discomfort*: Turning the head to gaze upward can put pressure on the cervical spine and compress the many structures that wind through it (such as veins, arteries, and nerves). Students are encouraged to keep their gaze in a direction that feels comfortable.
- *Low back concerns*: Collapsing into the low back, torquing, or excessive rotation can create strain. Encourage students to maintain natural length and alignment and to allow the pelvis to pivot naturally into the shape to avoid discomfort, especially in the SI joints.
- *Balance disorders*: Triangle requires balance, which can be challenging for some individuals. Students may benefit from practicing near a wall or with a chair for support.

## *Preparations*

Preparation for Triangle focuses on leg strength, hip mobility, spinal lengthening, and heart opening. Preparatory shapes are typically introduced after a general warm-up, including the six types of spinal movements. All preparations for the other standing shapes based in external hip rotation and abduction are useful, as are all of those shapes in and of themselves.
- *Quadriceps engagement*: Practicing kneecap lifts in Mountain helps activate the quadriceps and prepare the legs for strong engagement in Triangle.
- *Leg strengthening*: Mountain, Warrior 2, and Side Angle help prepare the legs by establishing stability and grounding through the feet and legs.
- *Hip openers*: Low Lunge, Lizard, and Tree assist in creating resilience in the hip joints and dynamic stability in the pelvis.
- *Shoulder and side body lengthening*: Extended Puppy and flowing through lateral flexion prepare shoulders, rib basket, and side body for the required lateral extension in Triangle.

## *Key Alignment Invitations*

Triangle is characterized by lateral extension through the spine, with both legs extended at the knee joint and leg muscles strongly engaged. It arises most helpfully out of the same stance as Warrior 2 or Side Angle, with similar attention to maintaining integrity of the joints, especially in the knee and sacroiliac regions. The following alignment suggestions can help students explore Triangle safely. Triangle is practiced on both sides of the body as is true for all asymmetrical or one-sided shapes. Nearly all instructions offered for Warrior 2 and Side Angle also apply, making those shapes excellent precursors to Triangle. Not all instruction for Warrior 2 and Side Angle that apply to Triangle are repeated here. It is helpful to re-read those instructions and integrate the information.
- *Invitations related to stance width and length*:
  - *Width of the feet*: The stance's width is based on individual hip width and comfort in the pelvis. The feet are positioned to allow for stability and an even weight distribution between both legs.

- *Length of the stance*: The distance between the front and back foot can vary depending on flexibility and balance. A shorter stance can help maintain stability and support, while a longer stance requires more strength or may result in strain.
- *Invitations related to front knee and foot engagement*:
  - *Front knee and ankle*: Encourage students to keep the front knee extended without locking it. The toes points in the same direction as the kneecaps.
  - *Anchor through the feet*: The front foot points forward, and the back foot is turned in to the optimal degree that honor the uniqueness of each student's hip socket and femoral head and neck. Both feet remain grounded with relatively even distribution of weight.
- *Invitations related to back leg engagement*:
  - *Engaged back leg:* The back leg remains strong and actively engaged, with a gentle lift of the kneecap to avoid hyperextension. Encourage a strong contraction of the quadriceps to lift the kneecaps and stabilize the knees, without locking or hyperextending them.
  - *Foot positioning*: The back foot is planted in a way that maintains a sense of grounding. Allow the back hip to roll forward to protect the SI joints.
- *Invitations related to working optimally with pelvis and spine*: The pelvis remains in its natural slight anterior tilt, allowing the spine to express its natural curves. It might help to imagine lengthening through the crown of the head to invite a natural expansiveness throughout the spine. The pelvis likely aligns naturally and intuitively in a diagonal line relative to the edges of the mat – not aligned with the long side of the mat as is often and inauspiciously cued. Wide opening is not in line with most human acetabula or femur shapes (especially the neck and head of the femur). Use props freely to support the spine and protect the pelvis.
  - *Protect the sacroiliac joints*: Pay attention to the rotation of the back hip and adjust the alignment of the foot and leg as needed to prevent stress in the SI joints. Just as there is no prescribed alignment of the pelvis (with the arbitrary edge of the mat), there is no prescribed foot placement either for the front or back foot. Instead, comfort in the SI joints and ease in the knee joints determine where the feet (and pelvis) land. Prevent sacral corkscrewing.
  - *Develop lumbar curve awareness*: Guide students to explore the natural curve of the lumbar spine and avoid overarching and hinging, which could cause discomfort. A gentle activation of the stabilizer muscles may help support this natural alignment in the low spine and sacrum.
- *Invitations related to heart space and shoulder opening*:
  - *Open the heart space*: The heart space is resilient, with the top arm extending upward. Encourage students to rotate the torso open by <u>first</u> placing the hand of the lifting arm on the sacrum to assist with diagonal hip alignment (to an appropriate and individually-determined range of motion) before extending the arm. Give students the agency to decide whether to lift the arm skyward or leave it resting on the side body or sacrum.
  - *Relax the shoulders*: Relax the shoulder girdle away from the ears, drawing shoulder blades gently toward each other to create a sense of openness across the heart space. Invoke the shelf imagery offered in Warrior 2 (though this shelf is tilted 😊 ).
- *Invitations related to bottom arm placement*:
  - *Hand placement*: The bottom hand rests lightly on a block or chair <u>*not the floor*</u>, whichever allows the shape to stay open without collapsing. Emphasize that the hand is used for balance rather than weight-bearing. Avoid spine leveraging.

- *Invitations related to head and neck position*:
  - *Head position*: Invite students to experiment with the head position – looking upward towards the top hand, looking forward, or looking down towards the ground. The choice depends on what feels best for students' cervical spine and physical or emotional balance. Turning the head is not important and only used if it is comfortable, even joyful, for the experience of the shape.

## Variations and Exploration

Triangle can be varied in many ways to suit individual needs or add complexity. As always, additional cueing is offered based on observation, need, and appropriateness in terms of not overwhelming students with too much cueing or exploration.
- *Arm placement variations*:
  - The top arm can start with the hand on the sacrum to help roll the heart space open,.
  - The bottom hand ideally always uses a block or chair for support, whichever helps maintain stability and alignment.
- *Knee variations*:
  - Students can explore a slight bend in either or both knees to avoid hyperextension or to accommodate tight hamstrings or balance challenges.
- *Wall support*:
  - Practicing with a portion of the back or side body against a wall can help with alignment and provide a sense of support for balance.
- *Neck placement*:
  - Experimenting with different neck positions (e.g., looking up, forward, or down) can help find a comfortable alignment for the cervical spine. Accompanying this exploration with finding a gaze point or *drishti* can add mental focus and emotional stability.
- *Revolved Triangle*:
  - For students ready to explore twisting, Revolved Triangle offers a variation that engages the core and increases spinal mobility. It is advisable to read up on specific cueing for this variation as it adds significant nuance to the shape. It is notable, that for many individuals, Revolved Triangle feels more accessible that Triangle. In Revolved Triangle (pictured below), the arm opposite the forward leg is placed on the ground and the arm on the same side as the forward legs is lifted up to create the revolution in the upper spine.

## Recovery

After practicing Triangle, recovery shapes can be offered as needed to release tension and rebalance to body, breath, and psyche. Recovery is best offered in a way that honors sequencing of the session overall. In other words, it leads naturally to the next aspect of the practice – in all layers of experience, not just the body.
- *Release the low back*: Transitioning through Side Angle to Low Lunge, and then to Downward Facing Dog may release tension in the low back.
- *Wide-Legged Forward Fold*: Finding a forward-facing, wide-legged stance that releases the rotation in the hips may release unnecessary bracing in the hamstrings and low back.

- *Child*: Creating a sense of grounding with this restorative forward shape may allow the hips and back to relax. However, for some students this shape is too tight to feel like a release; thus, use it with discernment.
- *Shaking, wiggling, and jogging*: Gentle shaking or light jogging can help release residual tension in the legs and elsewhere in the body (e.g., shoulders) as well as in any pent-up energy (such as stress apnea that may have crept in), or emotional bracing.

## Additional Teaching Tips

Instructing Triangle can be explored by using different approaches to make the shape accessible, engaging, or more wholesome depending in client needs. A few additional teaching tips are shared here; many others exist. Discerning and calibrating use of these cues is key, as always.

- *Use metaphors or imagery*: Encourage students to imagine themselves expanding like a star, radiating energy outward from their center through both the hands and feet. This helps emphasize length and openness while maintaining grounding.
- *Activate grounding and stability*: Remind students to stay rooted physically and energetically. Encourage them to imagine growing roots into the floor that create a stable base for the expansive side body opening.
- *Invite breath awareness*: Guide students to synchronize their breathing with movement for wholesome alignment. On an inhalation, students may find length through the spine; on an exhalation, they may draw inward for emotional and physical stability.
- *Empower customization of the shape*: Remind students to find the expression of the shape that meets their needs. This could mean keeping a slight bend in the knee, choosing a different hand placement, practicing with their back against a wall for stability, and more.
- *Offer gentle reminders about joint safety*: Remind students to remain attuned interoceptively and to avoid strain or stress related to femoral leveraging, spinal leveraging, and sacral or lumbar leveraging.

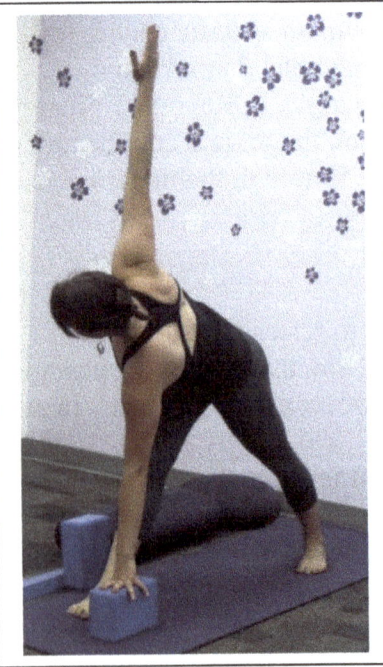

*Revolved Triangle – embracing strength* ←

*Triangle with Supports – accessing ease* →

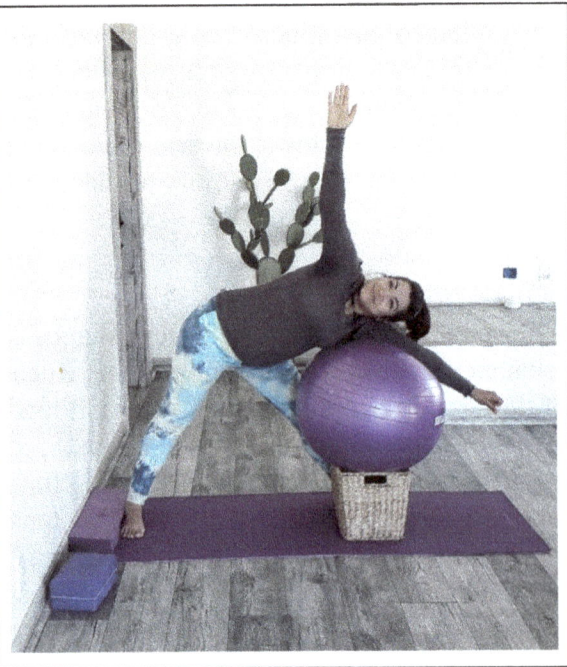

## Tree or Vrksasana

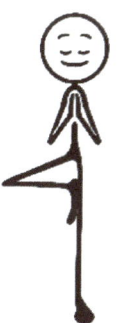

Tree is a foundational standing balancing shape that emphasizes external hip rotation (in the lifted leg) and asymmetry. It encourages stability, focus, and a sense of grounding in all layers of human experience. Tree is commonly practiced to build balance, strengthen the legs, and improve mental focus and concentration. The external hip rotation of the lifted leg provides a hip-opening effect that complements other shapes in a sequence involving external hip rotation (and abduction). Tree allows for exploration of grounding through the standing leg while inviting calmness of emotion and clarity of mind.

### Benefits

Tree offers numerous physical, mental, and energetic benefits that contribute to overall wellbeing in body, energy, mind, emotions, and relationships. Tree has been documented to:
- *Calm the mind*: Tree encourages focused attention on alignment, balance, and breath, helping calm the mind and bring it into a meditative state. The physical stability required in this shape is mirrored by calmness in the breath and stillness in the mind.
- *Improve posture and spinal alignment*: By establishing a strong connection with the ground through the standing leg and lifting through the crown of the head, Tree helps cultivate tall, aligned posture. This promotes spinal health and supports a more upright and balanced daily stance.
- *Improve balance*: Tree challenges and strengthens proprioception, the body's awareness of its position in space. Practicing Tree helps improve balance, beneficial not only in other yoga shapes but also in activities of daily living.
- *Tone the arches of the feet*: Pressing down evenly through the foot of the standing leg helps lift and tone the arch of the foot, making Tree useful for those who may have weak, less toned, or collapsed arches. Enhanced tone in, and experience of, the arches of the feet increases a sense of collaborative connection with the earth, enhancing stability and balance.
- *Open the heart space*: Lifting the arms or keeping the hands at heart center in Tree encourages a natural opening of the chest musculature. This helps create a sense of expansiveness and opens the heart space physically, energetically, and emotionally.
- *Improve circulation*: Standing on one leg while maintaining an aligned shape helps improve circulation throughout the body, especially in the lower extremities.

### Cautions

A few important cautions are helpfully considered when offering Tree in a yoga class. These considerations can ameliorate risk, increase the benefits of the practice, and help students work with discernment and care. They are not offered in a way that increases perceptions of fragility, but as empowerments through knowledge.
- *Headache or dizziness*: Students who experience headaches or dizziness approach Tree cautiously to prevent falls or disorientation. They can be invited to move slowly and

mindfully while focusing on a calm breath and mental stability. They may be encouraged to practice with the support of a wall for greater physical and emotional ease.
- *Pregnancy (6+ months):* Pregnant students, especially those past the sixth month, ideally practice Tree near a wall or other use supports to accommodate changes in balance. Keeping one hand lightly touching a wall or the back of a chair can help maintain stability without excess strain or effort.
- *Balance disorders:* Individuals with balance disorders are advised to practice using a wall for support. They can practice Tree with their back grounded on the wall until they feel comfortable balancing increasingly independently.

## *Preparations*

Preparation for Tree involves externally rotating the hips, strengthening the legs, and preparing the mind for balance and focus. Following are several preparatory movements that can support the practice, all in addition to the standard warm-up that includes the six movements of spine.
- *Hip openers:* Shapes like Lizard are helpful to externally rotate and abduct the hip joint, providing more comfort in the externally rotated hip during Tree.
- *Strengthening the standing leg:* Mountain helps establish stability in the legs and a strong foundation, which is essential for maintaining balance in Tree. Warrior 2 is equally strengthening – not just physically, but also emotionally and mentally.
- *Pre-Tree leg work:* Moving through one-legged balances such as standing knee lifts (with the knee pointing forward) helps activate the stabilizers in the standing leg without involving external hip rotation.
- *Working with drishti (gaze points for the eyes):* Establishing a stable *drishti*, or gaze, is extremely supportive for finding stability and ease in standing balances. Practicing a soft, unwavering gaze while standing on both feet prepares the mind for the single-leg balance practiced in Tree.
- *Working with stability in mind and emotion:* Attending to the *gunas*, *kleshas*, and *vrittis* during the opening centering and throughout the practice that precedes Tree creates optimal emotional balance and awareness.

## *Key Alignment Invitations*

In Tree, the hip joint of the standing leg remains in a neutral position, while the femur of lifted leg rotates externally and abducts. It is important to approach alignment with a sense of curiosity and respect for the body's unique tendencies. The following alignment invitations provide guidance; students are continuously reminded to adapt and vary movements and embodiments based on what feels healthful and appropriate in their body. Practicing Tree on a firm surface supports stability. Stepping off the yoga mat, especially if it is thick, can provide a better sense of grounding. Like all asymmetrical shapes, Tree is engaged in on both sides.
- *Invitations related to the feet:*
  - Grounding evenly through the corners of the standing foot, including the heel, base of the big toe, and base of the little toe ensures a stable foundation. Some students perceive four corners (inside and outside of heel, little toe and big toe mounds), whereas others experience three (heel as a single unit, and the two toe mounds). Cueing ideally considers this uniqueness of perception.

- Lift the arch of the standing foot without scrunching the toes, creating an active yet relaxed connection with the earth.
- If the lifted foot is connected to the standing leg, press the lifted foot and standing leg into each other with equal force, creating balance and engagement in both legs.
- Strongly encourage students to experiment with placing the lifted foot on different parts of the standing leg, finding the height that feels most comfortable and stable for them. A block under the toes of the lifted foot can be helpful some individuals. Although it is often cautioned not to place the lifted foot against the standing knee, newer science suggest that the knee has adequate stability to tolerate this placement without worry. However, for hypermobile individuals or individuals with knee injuries, this caution may be appropriate.

- *Invitations related to the legs:*
  - Cue a gentle micro-bend in the standing knee to avoid hyperextension, especially for students who tend toward hypermobility or hyperextension. Such active engagement invites the muscles to support the knee joint and contributes to balance.
  - Remind students to avoid locking the knee of the standing leg, especially if they are hypermobile.

- *Invitations related to the pelvis and hip joint:*
  - Ensure the pelvis remains level side to side. To achieve this, students may need to slightly drop the hip on the lifted leg side to maintain equilibrium and reduce strain.
  - Do not passively force external rotation in the hip joint of the lifted leg (e.g., by using a hand to move the leg outward). The lifted leg does not have to move out to the side very far. Instead, its positioning authentically expresses the shape of the student's acetabulum and the angles of neck of the femur.

- *Invitations related to the core:*
  - Engage the lower abdominals to support the spine, gently drawing them inward and upward. This helps maintain balance without tensing excessively.
  - Invite the breath to support physical balance by staying connected to the stabilizing influence of the exhalation and the expansive nature of the inhalation in the midriff of the body, especially notable in the slight lifting and lowering of the low ribs.

- *Invitations related to the spine and chest:*
  - Keep the spine in its natural curves, neither arching excessively nor rounding. Imagine a string gently pulling upward through the crown of the head, encouraging axial extension.
  - Open the heart space by allowing the shoulder blades to relax down the back and widen across the chest. The shoulder girdle is comfortably released downward, rather than braced toward the ears.

- *Invitations related to the arms:*
  - Arms can be positioned in various ways to create different levels of challenge in this shape. They may be nestled at heart center, placed on the hips, extended overhead, or swaying overhead – increasingly adding balance challenge. Students can choose to explore a variety of arm position to express and self-assess their sense of dynamic stability and balance physically and emotionally.

- *Invitations related to drishti:*
  - Developing a *drishti*, or focused gaze, on a fixed point ahead can calm mind and emotions as it tends to support balance.

## Variations and Exploration

Tree can be offered with great variety and opportunity for exploration and accessibility. In fact, only creativity limits the options that can make Tree more or less challenging, increasingly creative and joyful, or a greater expression of mental and emotional balance and stillness. Following are some ideas for variations; many additional explorations are possible.

- *Arm positions:* Try different arm placements such as palms together at heart center, arms extended overhead, or arms out to the sides to explore stability.
- *Wall assistance:* Practicing with the back or one side of the body lightly touching a wall helps with finding proper alignment before adding the balance component. This is true especially for finding a wholesome degree of external rotation in the hip joint of the lifted leg. The leg does not have to reach the wall, but more likely will be at a diagonal between the sagittal and frontal planes.
- *Forward fold variation:* Explore folding forward from Tree, bringing the torso towards the ground and placing the foot into a half-lotus position, with the top of the lifted foot resting in the groin of the standing leg, if accessible. This can deepen the balance and flexibility challenge. Use this variation with caution.
- *Foot positions on the leg:* Experiment with placing the lifted foot on different parts of the standing leg (e.g., calf, thigh, or with a block underfoot).
- *Swaying and playing:* Add a gentle sway from side to side or forward and back, allowing for exploration of dynamic balance. Try closing the eyes to test balance and deepen awareness of the body's ongoing micro-adjustments that happen naturally in this shape.
- *Extended knee:* Extend the knee of the lifted leg in front, perhaps using a strap for support. This adds strengthening to the shape.

## Recovery

After Tree, it helps to take time to relax the standing leg and release tension in the low back. This can occur through the following possible movements and shapes; however, many other options exist. As always, recovery needs to be blended with overall purpose and sequencing.

- *Release the erector spinae muscles*: Invite a gentle follow-up with a compassionate forward fold (using blocks under the hands) or a half-lift to release the spine in particular and relax body, breath and mind.
- *Ease tension in the neck*: From a standing or seated (in a chair) forward fold, gently release the head and neck via an easeful swaying motion.
- *Let go of bracing everywhere*: Gentle jogging or shaking and intuitive wiggling of the legs, arms, and torso can help release residual tension in all layers of experience and helps reset muscles and joints, as well as vitality and emotions.

## Additional Teaching Tips

To help students find a deeper sense of stability and alignment in Tree, additional suggestions can be offered. These additional tips invite accessibility and exploration; they can support students' creativity and self-awareness.

- *Use props for feedback:* Place a yoga block under the foot of the lifted legs so the toes have a support while the foot presses against the calf. This support can create awareness of engaging adduction in the legs and maintain level alignment in the pelvis.
- *Invite the imagination for refinement:*
  - Imagine swaying in the wind as the arms move in an intuitive pattern to challenge balance.
  - Imagine the axial body as the trunk of a Tree and the arms as branches that can either hug in tight to the axis (less challenge) or can reach out to the side (like a balance bar).
  - Create a sense of lightness and expansion in the spine – reaching upward toward the sky like a Tree.
  - Imagine growing roots through the foot of the standing leg.
- *Cue the four 'ceptions:* Help students attune to interoception, exteroception, neuroception, and proprioception:
  - Notice the subtle differences in muscle engagement with small adjustments (e.g., lift and lower the toes of the standing foot to notice how the arches of the feet adjust and the leg muscles engage differently).
  - Invite awareness of interoceptive changes in response to small actions that may refine alignment, such as pressing the sole of the lifted foot to the inner edge of the standing leg.
  - Explore how outer distractions may intrude on stability or balance.
  - Explore how inner distractions in the form of thoughts or emotions may intrude on stability or balance.
- *Integrate breath awareness:* Remind students to breathe gently and lightly while in the shape. Encourage them to synchronize breath with body awareness, inhaling as they lengthen the spine and reach out through the arms and hands; exhaling to create stability and poise, feeling a sensation of grounding and rooting.
- *Work with partner feedback*: If students are comfortable, partner them up so they can balance each other. They can stand back-to-back; they stand side to side, each with the outer leg lifted so that the two standing legs are side by side; they can clasp hands –with opposite legs lifted.

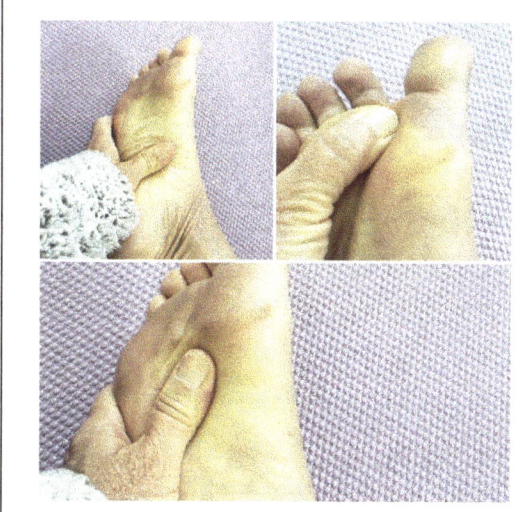
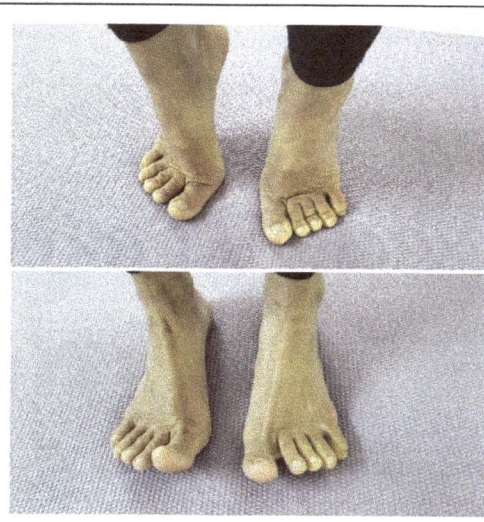

*Preparing for Tree – enlivening the feet*

| | |
|---|---|
| 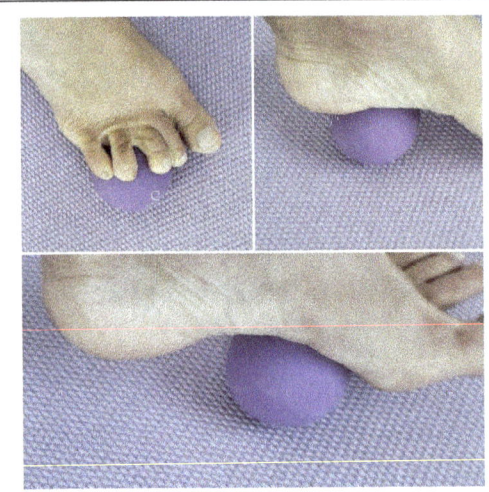 *One more helpful prep ….* | 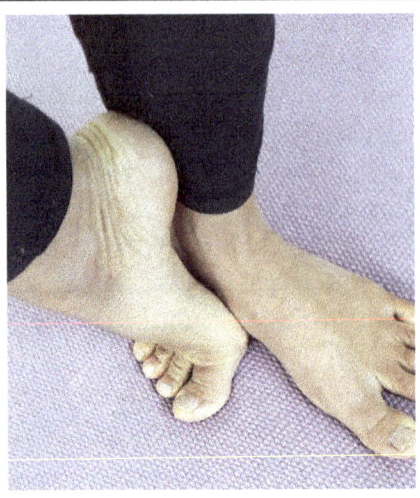 *Foot Variation for Tree – grounding and rooting* |
| 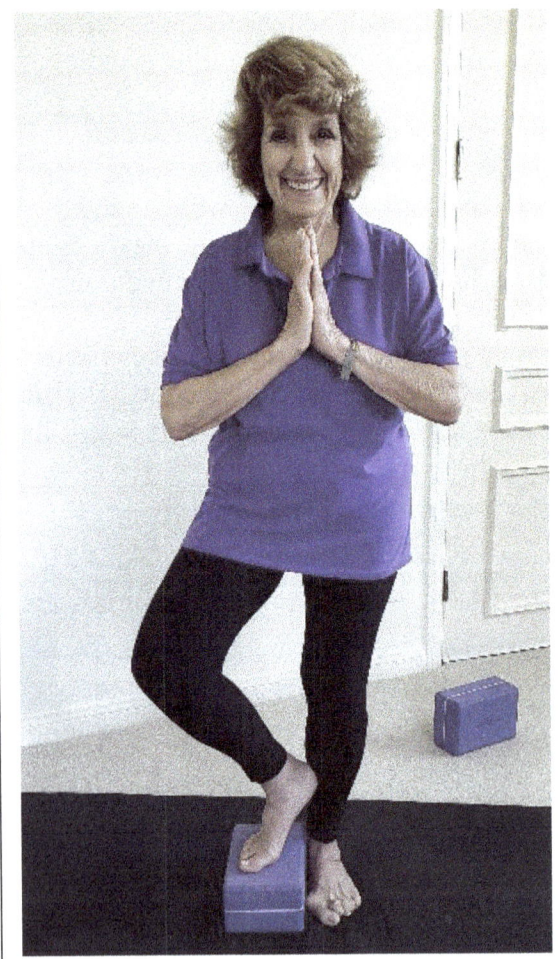 *Tree with Foot Support – drawing inward with ease* | 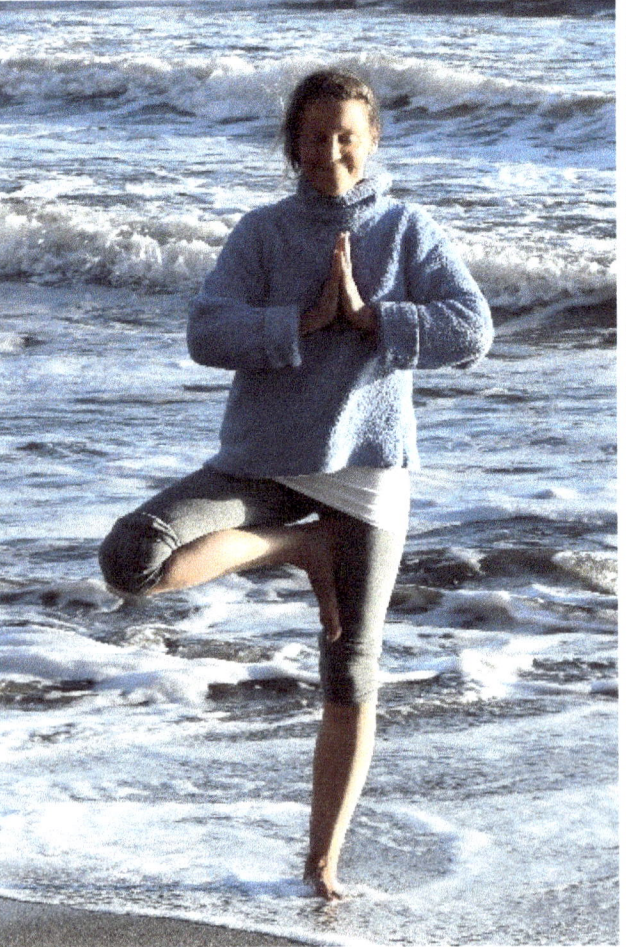 *Tree – finding a steady focus within distraction* |

# Chapter 9: Arm Standing

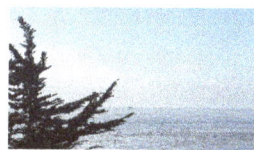

This chapter covers foundational arm-standing shapes, offering optimized teaching strategies that allow for individual tailoring and careful discernment about how and which shapes to offer, as well as about how to cue alignment informed by interoception, proprioception, exteroception, and neuroception. General principles for this category of yoga *asana* are provided and apply to most if not all arm-standing shapes. Specific follow-up guidance is added for the chosen sample shapes.

## Anatomical Foci for Arm Standing

Arm-standing shapes (in this context *not* including full inversions) demand a sophisticated interplay of stability and mobility within the upper extremities, balanced with the lower extremities which are also grounded in these shapes and share the weight-bearing burden. Unlike the structural path of force transmission in the lower limbs (which is relatively direct from the feet to the pelvis), the arms rely more strongly on a trajectory for force that traverses multiple soft tissue networks rather than mostly bony articulations. Understanding the nuanced pathway of force in shared weight-bearing on the arms and pectoral girdle is crucial to well-informed cueing and safe alignment in this category of yoga *asana* practices.

The arm's architecture for bearing weight is highly reliant on muscular engagement and fascial integrity, particularly within the shoulder girdle. Unlike the pelvis and legs, which are deeply stabilized by the bony structure, the shoulder complex derives its primary support from dynamic muscular stabilization. This anatomical reality places unique demands on practitioners, requiring not only strength but also fine-tuned proprioception and alignment awareness. The discussion of these shapes starts with this basic premise and then integrates foci and principles on how core and trunk engagement can be invited to collaborate to support arm-standing shapes.

### *Understanding the Journey of Force through the Arms*

Successful arm-standing shapes depend on teachers' and students' understanding of the strange and unusual path of forces through the arms when a body is in a shape that shares weight-bearing between the upper and lower appendicular skeleton (e.g., Downward Facing Dog, Plank, Yoga Pushup, or Table Top). Although this discussion also applies to full inversions such as Tripod Headstand, Handstand (covered in Chapter 13) or Elbow Balance, the current chapter is focus on shared weight-bearing across arms *and* legs. The pathway of force in arm-standing shapes a is long and winding road (my apologies to the Beatles), unlike in the legs where the path of force is straight and essentially ends at the hip joint. It relies heavily on soft-tissue networks to relay force and necessitates conscious recruitment of muscles, tendons, and ligaments and is heavily influenced by the myofascia and distribution of force through anatomy trains and the entire biotensegrity structure of each individual. The support and stability of the shoulder girdle, in others words, has to come largely from muscles, fascia, and other connective tissue and less so from the bones along this path (despite the fact that bones are used as the primary landmarks in the path's description that follows). Following is the outline of the specific path of force through the upper appendicular skeleton:

- *Hand and wrist to radius*: Ground reaction force begins at the hands and wrists, transmitting upward through the radii
- *Radius to ulna via the interosseous membrane*: a fascial structure called the interosseous membrane shuttles force laterally to the ulnae, creating a balanced distribution between the two forearm bones
- *Ulna to the humerus*: the ulnae articulate with the trochleas of each humerus, further transmitting force proximally
- *Humerus to the glenoid* (shoulder socket): force is then received by the glenoid fossa, stabilizing the arms within the shoulder joints
- *Glenoid to the scapula and clavicle*: force continues medially along the scapulae, distributing outwards along their spines to the clavicles
- *Clavicle to the sternum and rib basket*: at the end of the chain, the clavicles articulates with the sternum, grounding the entire kinetic chain into the axial skeleton at these very small joints at the anterior portion of the rib basket

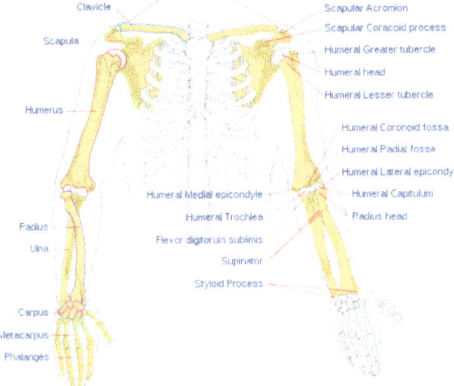

**Figure 2.7** Upper appendicular skeleton with connection to the axial skeleton. (Data source: LadyofHats; https://commons.wikimedia.org/wiki/File:Human_arm_bones_diagram.svg., public domain)

### *Understanding and Recruiting the Shoulder Girdle*

Once this pathway is understood, it becomes clear that the integrity of the shoulder girdle is key to this category of yoga *asana*. Both stability and mobility are needed in the shoulder girdle and need to be cued with wise discernment and ongoing invitation of interoception, neuroception, and proprioception. To recap from Chapter 6, the shoulder girdle includes the scapulae, clavicles, and sternum, and serves as the primary stabilizing structure for arm standing. The scapulae are the key to moving the entire upper axial skeleton (i.e., the hands [phalanges, metacarpals, carpals]), arms [radii, ulnae, humeri], and shoulder girdle [clavicles, sternum, scapulae]). The shoulder blades have several key joints and relationships, namely:

- To the thoracic spine via the scapulothoracic junction
- To the humerus via the glenohumeral joint
- To the clavicle via the acromioclavicular joint

Important to arm standing is the understanding that the only connection between the shoulder girdle and axial skeleton is via the sternoclavicular joint. Thus, unlike the hip joint, which gains stability from deep bony articulation, the shoulder complex has to be stabilized almost entirely by muscles and connective tissues. This muscular reliance allows for significant mobility but also demands precise engagement for safe load-bearing.

---

*Joint Stacking Versus Hanging in the Joints: Structural Integrity and the Art of Support*

*Joint stacking* refers to the intentional alignment of bones such that mechanical load is transmitted through the central axis of each joint, allowing for structural integrity, stability, and more efficient muscular engagement. In contrast, *hanging in the joints* is a passive collapse, where weight is transferred into non-contractile tissues (such as ligaments, joint capsules, or tendons) possibly leading to discomfort, instability, and, over time, potential degradation of joint integrity.

Why stack the joints?
- *Stability*: Load is borne through bone architecture, reducing strain on surrounding soft tissues.
- *Control*: Muscular engagement becomes dynamic and responsive rather than reflexive or compensatory.
- *Sustainability*: Repeatedly stacking joints builds patterns that support joint longevity and minimize overuse or wear and prevent buckling or collapse.

*Stacking the Joints in Asana: A Functional Blueprint*
In Downward Facing Dog:
- Hands press firmly through the inner palm and finger pads to activate the arch of the hand
- Elbows are neither hyperextended nor splaying inward; they maintain a soft engagement, aligning in a clean vector between the wrists and shoulders. The arms internally rotate and adduct slightly to stabilize the shoulder girdle.
- Shoulders integrate into the same diagonal plane as the spine, distributing force through a continuous vector from hands to hips
- The pelvis lifts back and up, so weight is not jammed into the shoulders.

In Side Plank:
- The supporting hand aligns under the shoulder with the elbow and wrist stacked in a vertical column, minimizing torque at the shoulder
- The upper arm externally rotates, broadening the collarbones and Stabilizing the scapula against the posterior rib basket
- The hips lift actively to engage lateral line musculature, preventing collapse into the lower shoulder or waist
- The neck stays long, with ears aligned between arms to create a supportive line of load for the head

Leaning into joint stacking is an active practice; it requires muscular engagement and proprioceptive refinement. Rather than collapsing or gripping, practitioners cultivate balanced effort and structural clarity. Over time, this fosters healthful answers to questions such as:
- *Where is the weight landing?*
- *Is the load traveling through skeletal support or sinking into soft tissues?*
- *Can I sense support without excessive bracing or tension?*

Tactile feedback (such as pressing into a wall or block) can help students feel the difference between passive hanging and aligned support. Such embodied awareness enhances proprioception, supports injury prevention, and builds long-term functional integrity.

---

The key muscles that connect the scapulae to the spine and are involved in shoulder stabilization include the trapezius complex (upper, middle, lower) and rhomboids in the back and the pectoralis and serratus anterior in the front. These posterior and anterior muscles need to be in a balanced relationship for arm standing. Here is a refresher about their actions:

- *Trapezius muscles:* Elevate, rotate, retract, and depress the scapulae, contributing to both movement and stabilization.
- *Rhomboids*: Retract and stabilize the scapulae

The rhomboids are counterbalanced by the serratus anterior. Pectoralis minor and the lower trapezius interact to help to position the scapulae optimally during weight-bearing. Stability in the shoulder girdle is achieved through coordinated movements of the scapulae, with associated reverberations into the thorax and humeri. The primary actions to know about in cueing arm standing are:

- *Scapular retraction and depression*: Drawing the shoulder blades toward the spine and downward helps anchor the scapulae against the ribs.
- *Scapular Elevation and Rotation*: Certain shapes, like *Downward Facing Dog*, require upward rotation of the scapulae to accommodate full shoulder flexion.

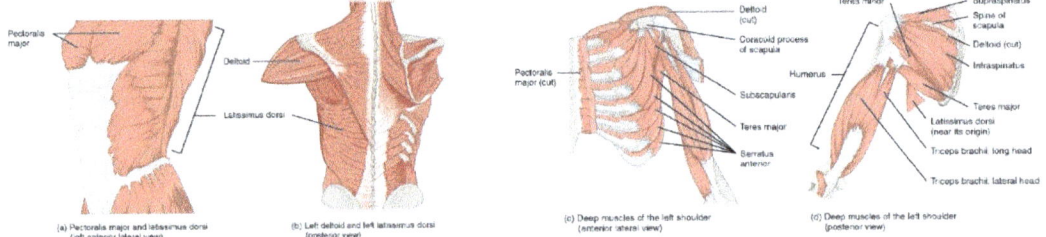

Figure 2.8 Muscles associated with movement of the shoulder girdle and humerus. (Data source: OpenStax; https://commons.wikimedia.org/wiki/File:1119_Muscles_that_Move_the_Humerus.jpg., Creative Commons Attribution 4.0)

## Shoulder Girdle Stability

Stability in the shoulder girdle is a multifaceted process that relies heavily on the scapulae and the glenohumeral joints. The *scapulae*, in particular, serve as the foundational elements of shoulder stability, functioning as dynamic platforms for arm movement. Proper scapular stabilization is primarily achieved through retraction (drawing the shoulder blades toward the spine) and depression (drawing them downward along the rib basket's surface).

Anchoring the scapulae onto the back of the rib basket is not a static action but rather a dynamic engagement facilitated by a network of muscles that work in balanced opposition. Specifically, rhomboids and serratus anterior play essential roles. Imbalances between these muscles are common: yogis who emphasize heart-opening shapes often overly concentrically load the rhomboids and trapezius, leaving them locked short, whereas weightlifters may excessively strengthen serratus anterior, leading to rhomboid weakness and lengthening. This imbalance disrupts scapular stability, affecting the shoulder's capacity to support arm-standing shapes and inversions. It is crucial to maintain isometric balance between serratus anterior and the rhomboids. This means not letting the shoulder girdle drop forward or collapse, a capacity that relies on flexion and extension in the elbow and the glenohumeral joint. For this action to work easefully, the scapulae need to be stabilized on the back. If destabilization is noticed, such as via shoulder blade winging, two sets of cues can be helpful. First, cueing to draw in the low ribs can activate serratus anterior (it will also stabilize the core – always a good thing in arm standing). Second, to kick in the rhomboids, a cue to broaden the collarbone bones can be very helpful.

Further stability is derived from the intricate relationship between the lower trapezius and pectoralis minor, along with the surrounding clavipectoral fascia. The lower trapezius aids in drawing the scapulae down and back, while pectoralis minor opposes this action by tilting the scapulae forward and down. For arm-standing shapes, this opposition must be delicately balanced. If pectoralis minor is overly tight or short, it can inhibit scapular stabilization, diminishing the structural integrity needed for weight-bearing through the arms. Open and well-aligned pectoral muscles are crucial for allowing the scapulae to remain stable and flush against the rib basket during inversions and arm balances. This interplay between muscle groups, coupled with core engagement, fortifies scapular positioning, enabling a stable base for the glenohumeral joints to articulate with precision.

The *glenohumeral joints*, while inherently more mobile than the scapulae, also require intentional stability, particularly during arm-standing shapes. Unlike the scapulae, which rely on muscular coordination for their positioning, the glenohumeral joints' stability is reinforced by strategic alignment and muscular engagement. The joints are most stable when the arm is in adduction, internal rotation, and extension, positions that encourage the humeral heads to nest securely within the glenoid fossae (Lasater, 2009, 2020). However, many arm-standing shapes place the arms in full flexion and abduction (either in the final shape and/or in the movement toward the shape), which reduces this inherent stability.

To counter the required destabilization to move into a fully flexed shoulder joints (e.g., in Downward Facing Dog; and, if we also think about full inversions, in Handstand), engagement of an internal rotational movement and isometric adduction at the end range of these movements or shapes helps reestablish a sense of stability in the joints, even while the humeri are externally rotated to achieve the shape. To be really clear, at end range in arm-standing shapes that require full flexion of the glenohumeral joints, it is very auspicious to emphasize internal *not external* rotation while cueing alignment in the arms.

In arm-standing shapes that place the body horizontal to the ground (e.g., Table Top, Plank, Side Plank, Yoga Pushup) stability is attained via placement of the glenohumeral joints directly above the wrists, optimizing weight-bearing for the glenohumeral joints and brings the greatest sense of ease to these joints. Finally, it is worth noting that shoulder stability is also supported by core engagement and in some shapes (namely those when the whole body is horizontal to the ground) by tucking the tailbone. For example, Plank requires the following actions to achieve healthful alignment in the pectoral girdle:
- Scapular stability (i.e., retraction and depression) via the large back muscles and rotator cuff along with an engaged core and pelvic floor
- A lifted thoracic spine (higher than the scapulae)
- No arch in the lumbar (i.e., slightly tucked pelvis) to prevent the thorax from dropping drop down between the shoulder blades (which would create excess load in the glenohumeral joints)
- Low ribs drawing toward the anterior superior iliac spine (shortening the distance between them in the front body to create length in the back body)

It is noteworthy that stabilization in certain half inverted yoga shapes may first require mobilization. For example, to fully flex or abduct the arm as is necessary for moving into

Downward Facing Dog, the scapulae have to mobile (they have to elevate and rotate). Once full flexion has been achieved, stability can once again be attended to, achieved via internal rotation of the humerus and a settling in of the scapulae, balanced by the back and front muscles. Thus, the next step in preparing for teaching arm standing is to create an understanding and discerning application of shoulder mobility.

## Shoulder Girdle Mobility

Mobility in the shoulder girdle is largely facilitated by the capacity of the scapulae to elevate, rotate, and protract in synchrony with the movements of the arm. This mobility is not merely a matter of local movement but a product of coordinated functioning across multiple joints and fascial connections. Central to this coordinated movement is the glenohumeral rhythm, discussed in detail in Chapter 6. This rhythm describes the intricate coordination between humerus and scapula during shoulder flexion and abduction, which allows the arm to lift overhead smoothly and without impingement. In arm-standing shapes such as Downward Facing Dog and Dolphin, this rhythm is crucial for achieving alignment without strain, as the scapulae must rotate upward and elevate to accommodate full shoulder flexion against gravity.

During full flexion or abduction, the scapula must upwardly rotate and elevate because it houses the glenoid fossa, the shallow socket that receives the head of the humerus. As the arm moves upward, the scapula has to move to position the glenoid fossa in a direction that supports the trajectory of the arm. Attempting to lift the arms without scapular movement is anatomically impossible (for most people), as the glenoid would no longer face the correct direction to accommodate the humeral head. This concept is especially relevant in shapes like Downward Facing Dog, where effective weight-bearing in the hands requires upward scapular rotation to allow the humerus to flex fully without restriction. A common misalignment in these shapes occurs when practitioners depress and retract the scapulae excessively, inhibiting necessary upward rotation and compromising both range of motion and joint integrity.

Thoracic extension also plays a role in enhancing this needed mobility. At the end range of shoulder flexion and abduction, the thoracic spine must move into slight extension to permit the scapulae to glide upward and outward along the *scapulothoracic junction*. This subtle backbend enables the scapulae to slide freely, preventing restriction in the shoulder girdle. When the thoracic spine is slumped or rounded, this coordinated mobility is compromised, making full overhead reach nearly impossible. This is a consideration in Plank to Downward Facing Dog transitions, where thoracic extension allows for fluid scapular movement and optimally stacked alignment. When this extension is neglected, students may experience shoulder binding or excessive load on the wrists due to inauspicious weight distribution.

Another important consideration during end-range flexion and abduction is the prevention of *supraspinatus tendon entrapment*. The supraspinatus tendon, which traverses the superior aspect of the humeral head near the acromion process, is particularly vulnerable during these movements. Entrapment occurs when the humerus remains externally rotated and the scapula is retracted and depressed rather than elevated and rotated. This positioning narrows the subacromial space, potentially compressing the tendon. Effective cueing to allow upward scapular rotation and slight internal humeral rotation at full overhead flexion can prevent this.

*Balancing Shoulder Girdle Mobility and Stability*

Arm standing yoga shapes require a precise balance between shoulder mobility and stability. The ability to bring the arms into full overhead flexion or abduction, as seen in Downward Facing Dog (and in Handstand), depends on flexibility and strength in the shoulder girdle. Mobility allows the arms to reach overhead, whereas stability ensures that the humeral head remains securely seated in the glenoid fossa. This intricate balance is further supported through the coordination of the *SITS* muscles (also known as the rotator cuff). These four muscles (Supraspinatus, Infraspinatus, Teres Minor, and Subscapularis) wrap around the head of the humerus, stabilizing it within the shallow glenoid cavity. Their role is analogous to the way the extraocular muscles direct the eye balls in the direction of what needs to be seen: the rotator cuff directs and stabilizes the humeral head, ensuring it tracks in the direction of the desired movement.

As noted previously, the glenohumeral joint is most stable in extension, adduction, and internal rotation because here the head of the humerus is snug within the glenoid cavity, with maximum surface area contact and supportive tension from surrounding ligaments and muscles. The least stable (most mobile) position occurs during flexion, abduction, and external rotation, the very configuration required for arm-standing shapes like Downward Facing Dog or Dolphin. These shapes rely on external rotation at the glenohumeral joint to move the arm into full flexion and abduction, placing considerable demand on the rotator cuff muscles and supporting ligaments. This is a vulnerable moment for weight-bearing, and needs to be followed with the creation of stability. This means that once the arms are at end range, the scapulae must upwardly rotate and elevate to accommodate shoulder flexion and abduction. This coordinated movement creates the necessary space for the humerus to align overhead without impingement or strain. However, the movement cannot not stop at mobility. For structural stability, the bottom tips of the scapulae must draw toward the spine, though not excessively. This action, combined with internal rotational movement of the humerus to stabilize the glenohumeral joint.

Additionally, the overall structure of the chosen shape plays a significant role in facilitating shoulder mobility and stability. In Downward Facing Dog, the length between the hands and feet needs to be optimized. A stance that is too short may compresses the shoulder girdle and compromises the thoracic extension needed for optimal scapular rotation. Conversely, a stance that is too long may pull the scapulae too far forward, destabilizing the shoulder girdle and placing undue strain on the rotator cuff. Finding the 'Goldilocks spot' in stride length allows the spine to lengthen and the scapulae to rotate upward without restriction, supporting both stability and freedom of movement. Optimal width between the hands can also contribute suspicious ease within stability (see Box).

> *Life is like riding a bicycle.*
> *To keep your balance, you must keep moving.*
> Albert Einstein

> **Auspicious Width of Hand Placement**
>
> Measure the optimal distance by reaching the arms out in front and assessing the quality of alignment in the clavicles:
>
> - If they feel scrunched open the arms a bit wider
> - If they feel too loose, bring hands close together
> - This measurement will result in the chest region being open, yet able to strengthen –
> - Remember that the pec muscles support arm adduction which supports strength in arm standing
>
> **Do not forget the possibility of bringing more ease into the hands and wrists with a prop under the hands – such as a wedge or blanket**

*Helpful Preparations Related to Shoulder Girdle Stability and Mobility*

*Rows*: Seated and quadruped rows (on hands and knees) are a great choice for the creation of strength and resilience in the thoracic spine to support scapular stabilization. Rows create strength in the back body while opening the front body. They are a great practice that can be done daily and as a warm-up for breathwork, yoga, or other physical activity.

Seated Row Version
- Sit on the floor with both legs outstretched in Staff
- Wrap a resistance band around the balls of the feet and hold one end of the band in each hand
- Draw the bands back, bringing the elbows as far behind the back as possible
- Repeat 10 to 20 times
- Can be done without the resistance band depending on the needs of the individuals

Quadruped Row Version
- Come to Table Top (on hands and knees)
- Take a small hand weight (or other weighted object such as a bag of rice) into your right hand
- Lift (or row) the right elbow up toward the ceiling and then down toward the floor, to lift and lower the weight
- Alternatively, place one end of a flexible band under the left hand, and grab the other end with the right hand; row the right elbow up toward the sky as high as possible, then release back down
- Repeat a few times; then switch sides and repeat on the other side

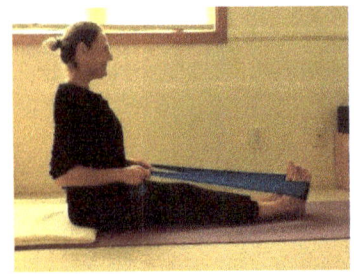

*Seated row*
←

*Row in Table Top*
→

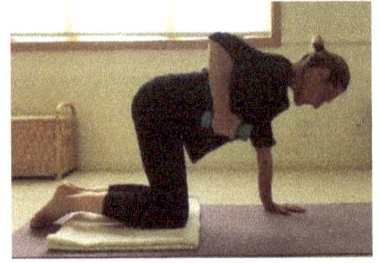

*Shoulder Vs:* Working with a Shoulder V mobilizes the shoulder blades and scapulothoracic junction. It strengthens several sets of back muscles (including mid-trapezius and rhomboids) while encouraging resilient opening of the clavipectoral fascia. Creation of strength and mobility around the rib basket translates into better resilience and endurance during arm standing.

Scapular Squeezes – the Shoulder V
- Come to standing or sitting with a natural curve in the spine
- Bring the arms to goal post
- Draw the arms toward the back plane of the body, careful not to overdo
- Draw the shoulder blades toward each other and down the back
- Pulse gently with the breath, opening the heart with the inhalation and releasing the stretch with the exhalation; or inhale to open and hold for a few breaths, release with the exhalation
- Repeat 5 to 20 times

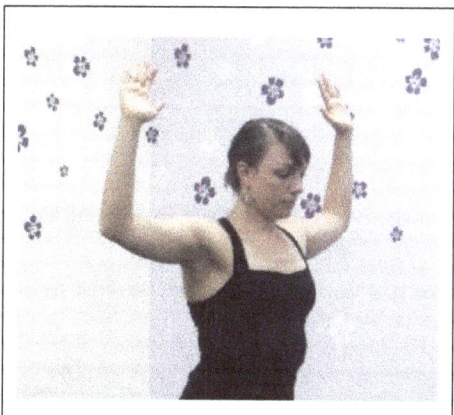

*Scapular squeezes with cactus arms ←*

*with alternative arm placement →*

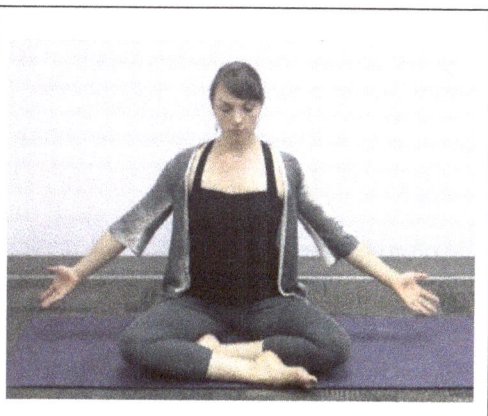

Cat-and-Cow Flow with Shoulder V
- Come to Table Top to move through Cat-Cow with the following variations:
- Extension and flexion occur high in the shoulder girdle
- In Cow, make a strong V with the shoulder blades drawing them toward each other and down the back
- In Cat, move into flexion drawing the shoulder blades outward and slightly upward
- The low back and neck stay relatively still
- Repeat 5 to 10 times

Elastic Band Pull-Apart with Shoulder V
- Stand or sit with a natural curve in the spine
- Take one end of the elastic band in each hand
- Stretch the arms out wide, stretching the elastic band across the front of the body
- Maintain a strong V in the shoulder blades, drawing them toward each other and down
- Either open and close the arms (loosening the band) with the breath (opening while inhaling; closing while exhaling) or open the arms (tightening the band) with an inhalation and then hold for a few breaths; release with an exhalation

*Working with Arms and Shoulders*: These preparations work especially well with scapular mobility in several directions.

Cow Face Arms
- Opens the chest and mobilizes the shoulders; may require a strap
- Reach one arm forward and supinate the wrist to face the palm upward, thumbs pointing out (external rotation of shoulder)
- Reach the arm up and overhead; bend the elbow and bring the palm to the upper middle back
- Bring the other arm forward and turn thumb in and down (internal rotation of shoulder)
- Reach the arm behind and slide the hand up the back
- Connect the two hands directly or with a strap – the latter is highly recommended
- Pressing the lifted hand and/or arm into the back of the head, shoulder, or back adds strength and stability

Eagle Arms
- Opens the upper back and shoulders while promoting shoulder stability; may use a strap as needed to connect the hands.
- Reach both arms forward at shoulder height and cross one arm over the other at the elbows (e.g., right over left). Bend both elbows so the forearms point upward.
- Wrap the forearms around each other, aiming to bring the palms to touch or the backs of the hands together.
- If palms do not meet, press the backs of the hands together or use a strap held between the hands.
- Lift the elbows to shoulder height and gently draw the hands away from the face to deepen the stretch.
- Press the forearms together to engage the shoulders and build strength and stability in the shoulder girdle.

Shoulder Flossing
- From Table Top, invite auspiciously spaced hand placement – not too narrow and not too wide
- Invite the sternum to move between the arms, toward the floor with control, on the exhalation – retracting the scapulae through contraction of the rhomboids
- Invite the sternum to rise upward away from the floor with the inhalation – protracting the scapula through contraction of serratus anterior

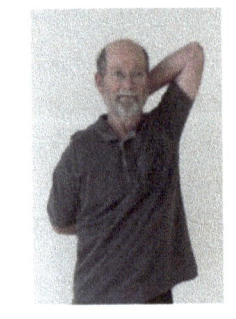
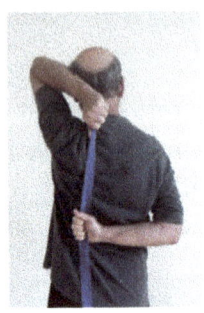

*Cow Face Arms, front and back*
←

*Eagle Arms*
→

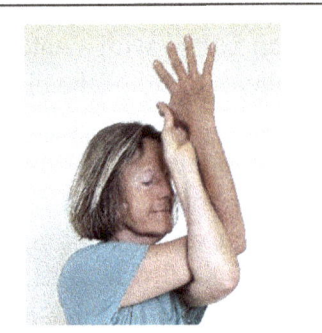

> *Sample Cueing for Shoulder Stability and Mobility*
>
> *Stability*
> - Draw the shoulder blades down the spine
> - Push the floor away with the hands
> - Draw shoulder blades together toward the spine
> - Plug/settle/nestle the arm bones into the shoulder sockets
> - Create openness in the chest/heart
> - Release the shoulders down
> - Inwardly rotate the humerus bones once the arms are fully overhead
> - Feel energy moving from the ground up to your shoulders through your hands and arms
> - Rotate eyes of the elbows or elbow pits forward
>
> *Mobility*
> - Create space between shoulders
> - Allow the shoulder blades to move up and out
> - Invite freedom for the shoulder blades to elevate and rotate
> - Externally rotate the upper arm outward while reaching up
> - Broaden your back
> - Draw arms/biceps towards one another
> - Create length in the spine

## Core/Trunk Engagement and Stabilization

While stability in the shoulder girdle forms the foundational support for arm-standing shapes, core engagement and stabilization are equally crucial. Effective arm standing is not simply a matter of upper body strength; it relies on the integration of deep core musculature that provides the necessary stability. In arm-standing shapes such as Plank, Side Plank, Downward Facing Dog, and Table Top, engagement of the deep core muscles, pelvic floor, and deep spinal stabilizers (including the erector spinae [multifidi, semispinalis, rotatores] and transversospinalis group [spinalis, longissimus, and iliocostalis]) creates a robust core from which the limbs can extend with control and balance. These muscles, primarily composed of slow-twitch fibers, are endurance-based and designed for holding postural alignment. Their role in maintaining structural integrity during weight-bearing is essential for stability and protection of the spine.

### Stabilization of the Trunk in Arm Standing

The primary function of the core muscles in arm-standing shapes is to stabilize the spinal column, trunk, ribs, and pelvis. This stabilization allows the body to maintain alignment and posture under active loading; specifically, the gravitational force directed through the upper extremities when load-bearing. In Plank and Side Plank, core engagement prevents the lumbar spine from arching excessively. When the low back collapses, the abdominal muscles stretch and lose tension, compromising stability and increasing risk of lumbar strain. This highlights the importance of engaging transversus abdominis and rectus abdominis to create a natural and supported spinal position. In Side Plank, the obliques also play a crucial role in preventing the trunk from sagging, offering lateral stability while the body is suspended on a single arm and the lateral edge of the foot.

> Stabilization is *the* major job for the abdominal muscles (in collaboration from the pelvic floor and back musculature). Core stabilization has many benefits beyond strength and tone in the abdominals:
> - It stabilizes the spine in particular and the torso as a whole.
> - It stabilizes the ribs and pelvis.
> - Stable and toned abdominal muscles hold the organs (or organ column) in place and support the vertebral column (especially at L4-L5).
> - Together, the spine, organ column, and abdominal muscles stabilize us during movement.

One key aspect of core stabilization is pelvic floor engagement. In arm-standing shapes, auspicious pelvic alignment can help prevent excessive lordosis (arching) of the lumbar spine. For example, in Plank, a slight posterior pelvic tilt helps support the lumbar curve, engaging the lower abdominals and deep spinal muscles. This tucking of the tailbone (which is generally contraindicated in upright standing shapes) assists in engaging the low ribs toward the pelvis, enhancing stability and allowing for ease of breath. In Table Top, core engagement ensures that the lumbar curve remains natural while the shoulders stabilize the weight of the torso. In practicing and teaching core and pelvic stabilization, it is helpful to attend especially to the deepest of the four layers of abdominal muscles, namely, transverse abdominis for deep inner stability. Activation of transverse abdominis and upward contraction of the pelvic floor are natural on exhalation; on inhalation the abdomen remains soft and resilient (with some gentle slow-twitch muscle action). Activation of external and internal obliques (the second and third layers of the abdominal muscles) is especially accessible when adding rotation or side-bending to standing, seated, or other shapes. If activation of the diaphragm is an additional teaching goal, *pranayama* practices such as slow-motion *kapalabhati* may be helpful. Tricks and movements for discovering core stability are presented in the following table.

In addition to pelvic alignment and pelvic floor engagement, stability in arm standing is supported by the various layers of abdominal and back muscles. For example, in Side Plank, lateral stability is maintained by the obliques and quadratus lumborum, which prevent the hips from sagging toward the floor. In Downward Facing Dog, core stability supports the elongation of the spine as the hips and navel lift and the arms press into the ground. The engagement of the deep abdominals prevents the thoracic spine from collapsing and allows for a lengthened, grounded position.

Core stabilization also facilitates movement from shape to shape. For example, transitioning from Plank to Yoga Pushup and back to Plank requires a steady engagement of all core muscles to prevent sagging or excessive arching. This dynamic stabilization maintains stability and protects the lumbar spine during transitions. Similarly, in Table Top, engaging the core prevents the low back from collapsing as the shoulders bear weight, setting up stability for movements such as Bird Dog or variations to create balance challenges, rotation, or lateral flexion.

## *Practice And Teaching Tips For Core Stabilization*

- Laugh, cough, or clear your throat – these actions engage the core and can help develop interoception of the muscles we seek to strengthen and awaken

- Place a block between the thighs or knees to awaken the adductors in the legs – they are often helpful in kick-starting transverse abdominus and pelvic floor engagement as they are fascially linked; squeeze and release quickly for several repetitions

- Practice squats – inhaling downward into the squat and exhaling upward out of the squat – focus on upward and inward movement from the pelvic floor on up when rising out of the squat

- Come to Table Top; slowly, slowly, slowly move the shoulders ahead of the hands – at some point, when you are just about to lose your balance, the deep core muscles will naturally kick in

- Come to Table Top and move into Bird Dog – one arm and the contralateral leg raise; sway forward and back and/or side-to-side, challenging your balance; yet again, the core will kick in spontaneously

- Come to Table Top and move into Bird Dog – one arm and the contralateral leg raise; tap the lifted elbow to the lifted knee under your chest

- Come to Table Top and find a natural spine with gentle core and pelvic floor engagement; with the exhalation lift the knees off the ground and hover for a few rounds of breath

- Come onto your back, fully outstretched with all limbs on the floor; lift one leg to make a 90° angle at the hip joint; then lower the leg slowly; if this is too difficult, bend the knee of the lifted leg

- Come onto your back with legs raised up in the air; slowly lower one leg toward the floor – if this is too difficult place your hands under the buttocks till the core strengthens

- Sit in Boat with both feet on the ground; straighten one knee to raise that leg upward in a diagonal; make sure to maintain the natural spinal curves, especially in the lumbar region

- Lie prone; with an inhalation, let the movement of diaphragmatic contraction lift the chest and shoulder off the ground in a hands-free low Cobra; with the exhalation return to the floor and hug the low ribs into the abdomen; suspend the breath until you feel the urge to inhale; repeat twice

- Find Bridge and Candlestick as appropriate for conditioning, using blankets under the torso for comfort and adequate props for emotional and physical support (e.g., contraindicated for osteoporosis)

For a sample of a basic core stabilization practice, check out Brems's *YogaX Core Stabilization* class at https://youtu.be/We6gIj-EWJw

Finally, when the body is horizontal to the ground, such as in Plank, Side Plank, and Table Top, core stability is enhanced by a tucked pelvis. This subtle pelvic action supports the lumbar spine by counteracting the natural tendency in these shapes to hyperextend. Drawing the ribs toward the pelvis and maintaining core integrity creates a solid, connected line of energy that supports the upper body and relieves excess pressure on the wrists and shoulders.

*Coordinating Core Stability with Easeful Breath*

In arm standing yoga shapes such as Plank, Side Plank, Downward Facing Dog, and Table Top, the relationship between stability and breath ease is a dynamic interplay that requires careful awareness. On one hand, deep core engagement (especially activation of the transversus abdominis, pelvic floor, and deep spinal stabilizers) provides the foundational support necessary for safe alignment and load-bearing through the upper body. On the other hand, such engagement can restrict diaphragmatic movement, impeding the natural flow of breath. Understanding how to balance these two aspects is crucial for sustaining arm-standing shapes with both structural integrity and respiratory freedom.

---

**Experiencing Core Engagement/Stabilization**

**Experience 1**
- Lie on your back
- Place the hands such that the thumbs are at the bottom of the low ribs and the little fingers are at the tops of the anterior superior iliac spine
- Lift the head a few inches off the ground; shoulders stay put

**Experience 2**
- Sit in a chair or in Hero, making sure your spine is in its natural position (this will not work if you are slouching)
- Place the hands such that the thumbs are at the bottom of the low ribs and the little fingers are at the tops of the ASIS
- On an exhalation, forcefully stick out your tongue

*What did you notice?*
You likely felt the engagement of the core muscles under your hands, as well as a shortening of the distance between the low ribs and top of the hips (i.e., your little fingers and thumbs move close together).

---

When the core is engaged to stabilize the pelvis and spine during arm standing, the transversus abdominis and pelvic floor create a corset-like compression around the trunk. This stabilization is vital for protecting the lumbar spine and maintaining alignment, especially when the body is horizontal to the ground, as in Plank or Side Plank. However, this same compression can limit the excursion of the diaphragm, which relies on the ability of the abdominal wall to yield slightly during inhalation, allowing the lungs to expand. Overly rigid core engagement, such as bracing or hollowing out the belly excessively, can hinder this natural movement, leading to shallow, constricted breaths.

The challenge is particularly evident in shapes like Downward Facing Dog, where spinal elongation and core stability are required simultaneously. Drawing the ribs toward the ASIS creates the necessary spinal integrity, but if done too aggressively, it can inhibit the diaphragm's descent during inhalation. This is why practitioners sometimes experience a sense of breathlessness or strain when overly engaging the core in extended holds of Downward Facing Dog. Similarly, in Plank, excessive abdominal bracing may stabilize the low back but can result in shallow chest breathing, diminishing the sense of expansiveness through the rib basket.

Effective practice in arm-standing shapes requires cultivating a dynamic stability, a form of core engagement that is supportive *and* responsive. Rather than rigidly locking the core, just enough tone is created by the transversus abdominis and pelvic floor to maintain alignment while allowing subtle movements of the abdominal wall during breath cycles. This approach enables the diaphragm to move freely and to expand the low rib basket. It can help to cue softening on the inhalation while maintaining length through the spine, and gently engaging the core on the exhalation. This rhythmic pattern supports diaphragmatic movement and maintains the natural curves of the spine, especially in shapes like Table Top and Downward Facing Dog. In Side Plank, a similar balance is found by engaging the obliques and transversus abdominis enough to prevent collapse, while allowing the waist region to expand in all directions during inhalation. Understanding how to coordinate stability with easeful breath makes it possible to stay in arm-standing shapes with spaciousness and ease, shifting away from bracing or gripping to easeful support and fluidity that allow the core to remain dynamically active and enhance endurance.

As an aside, individuals who have difficulty activating the pelvic floor (i.e., in yogic terms, who cannot seem to find root lock) or transverse abdominis often have a weaker, less efficient natural diaphragmatic breath and less intraabdominal pressure on the exhalation. Relatedly, clients who do not breathe diaphragmatically often have pelvic floor dysfunctions. Of course, all breathing involves the diaphragm to some degree. However, diaphragmatic range of motion and strength are not givens; co-contraction of core and pelvic floor is not easily accessed by all students. In particular, chest- and reverse breathing patients can have difficulty coordinating these muscles as they breathe – being habituated to (overly) use their chest muscles instead.

Balance = openness & stability
This can apply in body, breath, and mind

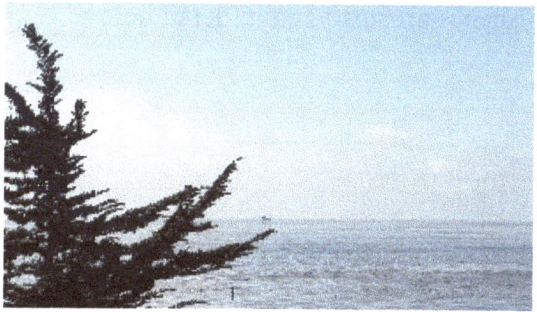

| | *Tips for Grounding, Expansion, and Stability in Arm-standing shapes* |
|---|---|
| *Grounding* | • Ground and root through the hands and arms<br>• Ground the scapulae on the back body – feel the settled energy<br>• Settle the scapulae into a grounded and rooted position on the back<br>• Connect to the earth through the parts of the body in touch with the ground<br>• Breath out to root and ground, to connect to the earth<br>• Concentrate the mind on releasing into the earth, on creating connection<br>• Settle into the shape, leaning into the direction of its energy |
| *Stability* | • Engage the core and draw in the perineum to create a stable presence<br>• Let the breath create stability in the torso – sensing into the stable presence of each inhalation<br>• Find a *drishti*, or focal point for the eyes to create steadiness in the gaze<br>• Stabilize the wrists through creating an unwavering and dynamic connection to the earth<br>• Stably align the glenoid fossa with the wrists to optimize weight-bearing in this key joint<br>• Integrate and stabilize the shoulder girdle as appropriate for the shape (e.g., scapulae retracted and depressed)<br>• Consciously locate the center of gravity and appreciate the dynamic forces of stability<br>• Draw the low ribs toward the top of the pelvis to engage the core with a stabilizing force |
| *Expansion* | • Release through the crown of the head<br>• Identify the line of energy that supports lightness in the shape<br>• Expand through the edges of the shape on the resilience of stability at the core<br>• Feel the resilience of the low rib basket with each breath in – allowing the low ribs to move outward and upward freely<br>• Expand through the back body<br>• Find length and uplift in the spine even in inverted (or half-inverted) shapes<br>• Lengthen through the spine<br>• Invite the mind to be present and explore with spacious awareness |

## Analysis and Experience of Sample Arm Standing Shapes

The following arm-standing shapes are analyzed in detail below:
- *Table Top*
- *Downward Facing Dog*
- *Plank*
- *Side Plank*

The cueing guidance offered for each shape needs to be considered in the context offered in the *general principles for arm-standing shapes*. The basics discussed above need to permeate the cueing for all these shapes. The additional cueing, shape by shape, offered here is icing on the cake. Always incorporate integrated holistic yoga cueing that addresses the following teaching principles:

- *Accessibility* – creating access through variation, adaptation, affiliation, individualization, and person-centeredness
- *Intentionality* – embedding the practice of each shape in the overall arc of the session, grounding in the theme for the class and the meaning of the practice
- *Beneficence* – honoring the wellbeing of each student and always making sure to first do no harm
- *Holism* – cueing all *koshas* or layers of experience in all shapes, never forgetting that each shape has reverberations into and is affected by all *koshas* – it is not enough to cue anatomy; also address energy and vitality, thoughts and emotions, behavioral and action choices, even community and interbeing
- *Integration* – in teaching *asana*, integrate breathwork, concentration and mindfulness, as well as the ethical principles and lifestyle practices of yoga

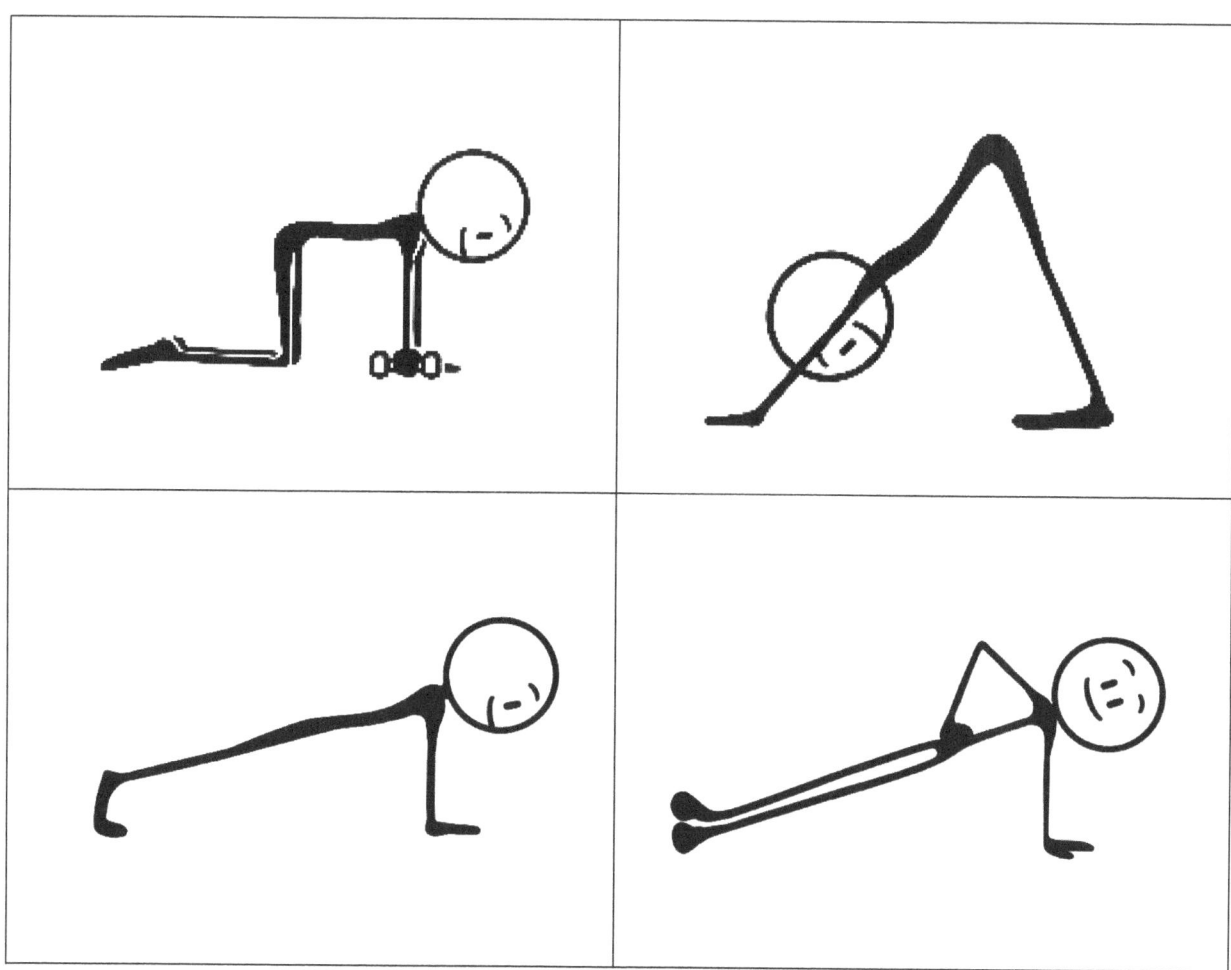

## Table Top or Bharmanasana

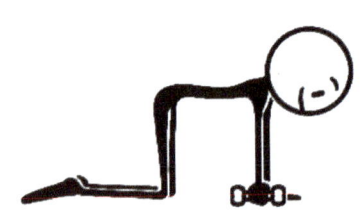

Table Top is a ubiquitous and versatile shape that serves as both a preparatory and recovery shape. With hands, knees, and feet grounded, the spine is invited into a naturally aligned position, offering a stable base for many transitions and variations. This shape cultivates a sense of balance between engagement and release while emphasizing alignment, stability, and connection between breath and movement. Though simple in appearance, Table Top invites deep engagement with physical alignment and provides an opportunity for grounding and energetic balance. It is also a wonderful shape for creative exploration, serving as an inviting base for other shapes and movements to follow. There can be much invitation for flow and creativity and many other shapes can emerge from Table Top. It is also an excellent resting shape to return to, especially when care is taken to support wrists and knees with appropriate props.

### Benefits

Table Top provides multiple benefits, physically, energetically, and mentally:
- *Grounding through hands and knees*: This shape creates a strong sense of stability, as hands and knees anchor the individual's experience to the earth, providing a stable and solid foundation physically and emotionally.
- *Experience of neutral spine*: Table Top invites awareness of spinal alignment and movement, helping practitioners find and maintain a natural position and flow, essential for healthy posture and movement in daily life.
- *Builds core and shoulder strength*: By stabilizing the spine and engaging the abdominal muscles, Table Top helps build strength and endurance in the core and shoulders.
- *Enhances body awareness*: Table Top promotes interoception and proprioception, encouraging practitioners to refine their body mechanics and connection to their moment-to-moment experience.
- *Can work with balance*: This seemingly stable shape offers an opportunity to explore subtle balance work, especially when variations involving lifted legs or arms are introduced.
- *Calms the mind*: The simplicity of Table Top encourages a gentle inward focus, promoting ease and mindfulness that can settle the nervous system.

### Cautions

When practicing Table Top, keep in mind the following considerations:
- *Wrist pressure*: For students with wrist sensitivity, encourage the use of padding under the hands or suggest walking the hands slightly forward to reduce the angle at the wrists. Wedges under the hands or transitioning to forearms can also be helpful.
- *Knee sensitivity*: Place a blanket under the knees for students experiencing discomfort, ensuring that the body is properly supported.
- *Shoulder instability or injury*: Emphasize the importance of engaging the hands to activate shoulder muscles and prevent collapse.

- *Hyperextension*: Encourage awareness of the elbow joints, preventing hyperextension by keeping a soft bend in these areas.
- *Neck tension:* Remind students to tuck the chin slightly, elongating the cervical spine while maintaining a soft, natural neck position.

*Preparations*

Table Top is an excellent base for preparing for many of the shapes and typically does not require special preparation. However, if that is a desire, to prepare for Table Top, guide students through movements from standing or seated that create awareness and alignment in shoulders, core, and hips. Such movements help warm up the spine and a more typical position in space and encourage mindful connection to breath:
- *Cat-Cow flow*: From standing or sitting, gently flowing between spinal flexion and extension helps create awareness of spinal alignment and breath synchronization.
- *Shoulder mobilization*: Shoulder shrugs, circles, and related arm movements begin to awaken the musculature of the shoulder girdle.
- *Standing pelvic tilts*: These tilts bring focus to the relationship between the pelvis and spine, helping students develop awareness of how to access a natural and healthful alignment and interaction.
- *Standing hip extensions*: Stretching one leg back while maintaining a natural spine helps engage the core and mobilize the hips, while maintaining a sense of stability.

*Key Alignment Invitations*

Table Top encourages natural spinal curves and balanced engagement throughout the torso. A few key alignment invitations promote a well-balanced and engaged Table Top while allowing for individual exploration of what feels most wholesome and supportive in each student's body.
- *Invitations related to hands and arms*:
  - *Wrists under shoulders*: Invite wrists to find a healthful spot either directly under or slightly ahead of the shoulders, with even pressure across the palms to distribute weight and reduce wrist strain. Adjust hand placement by walking them forward and or outward as needed to enhance sensations in the wrists and fingers.
  - *Activate the arms*: Keep the arms lightly engaged, avoiding collapse into the shoulder girdle by maintaining a gentle external rotational movement of the arms (without moving the hands anywhere, creating isometric engagement).
- *Invitations related to knees and legs*:
  - *Knees under hips*: Invite placing the knees directly under or perhaps slightly behind the hip joints. The tops of the feet rest comfortably on the mat. A blanket or cushion under the knees can create greater ease and access.
  - *Engage the thighs*: Lightly engage the inner thighs, as if gently drawing the knees toward each other (i.e., adduction) to stabilize the pelvis, including the sacroiliac joints. Adding internal rotation in the hip joints may create additional ease or opportunity for exploration.

- *Invitations related to core and pelvis*:
  - *Engage the core*: Gently lift the navel toward the spine, creating stability in the torso without overly tightening the core muscles. It can be helpful to explore finding the middle way by first over- then under-engaging before finding center.
  - *Natural pelvis and lumbar alignment*: Find the balance between an overly arched low back and a tucked tailbone, creating a natural position for the pelvis that promotes ease and support in the entire spine.
- *Invitations related to spine and head*:
  - *Lengthen through the spine*: Maintain the natural curves of the spine, expanding from the tailbone through the crown of the head.
  - *Elongate the neck*: Slightly tuck the chin to elongate the cervical spine, avoiding strain in the neck. Keep the gaze soft and slightly forward or down.

## Variations and Exploration

Table Top offers a range of creative variations to explore balance, strength, and flexibility These variations invite exploration within the foundation of Table Top, offering options for different needs and interests, as well as opportunities for students to move with inner-directed creativity that brings joy into the movements.
- *Table Top crunches*: From Table Top, invite students to draw one knee toward the nose or opposite elbow to engage the core.
- *Bird Dog*: Encourage lifting one hand or leg off the mat (perhaps keeping the toes on the mat, but extending the knee) to explore balance and proprioception while maintaining core engagement.
- *Integrated backbend*: Lift one leg, bend the knee, and reach back with the same-side hand to hold the foot (perhaps using a strap to connect the limbs), integrating a gentle backbend and shoulder opener.
- *Fire Hydrant*: From a natural spine, invite students to lift one knee out to the side (hip abduction and flexion), engaging the external hip rotator muscles.
- *Cat-Cow variations*: Explore lateral flexion, lengthening to one side and then the other.
- *Using props*: Blocks or small exercise balls under the hands or knees can offer additional exploration, perhaps by adding balance challenge to movement.

## Recovery

After practicing Table Top and its variations, offer these options to release tension and transition back to an easeful state. These recovery movements support the body's and psyche's transition from activation to relaxation, helping to restore balance and ease.
- *Child*: Offers a gentle release for the low back and shoulders, helping the body reset.
- *Gentle standing or seated forward folding*: Lengthens the spine and releases tension in the hamstrings and low back.
- *Gentle seated twist*: Helps release tension in the spine and may release over-efforting through gentle rotation.
- *Pelvic Tilts*: Help neutralize the spine and pelvis, bringing balance back to the body after engagement in Table Top.

*Additional Teaching Tips*

To help students explore Table Top in a more nuanced and creative (perhaps joyful) way, explore these additional teaching suggestions:

- *Invite alignment exploration*: Encourage students to explore what feels balanced and stable for their own bodies. Alignment may look different for each individual. Invite them to move from Table Top in unusual, creative, flowing, and joyful ways.
- *Invite awareness of breath*: Help students notice how breath moves through the body and supports core engagement while maintaining a sense of spaciousness. Invite exploration how breath supports opening the body on the inhalation (e.g., side rotation with one arm lifted) and drawing inward with the exhalation (perhaps reaching the arm under and through the other side).
- *Use props for comfort*: Blankets or blocks can provide additional comfort and stability for wrists, knees, or alignment exploration. Exploration of balance by using blocks or wobble boards under hands and knees can invite the 'ceptions as well as joy.
- *Imaginative cueing*: Invite students to imagine their spine as a long, balanced bridge, connecting the head to the tailbone with lightness through the limbs. Invite imagery related to opening and closing, to being a 'human stretching rack' and similar visualizations.
- *Creative exploration*: Encourage students to get creative with Table Top, using it as a base for growing into other shapes or exploring balance variations.

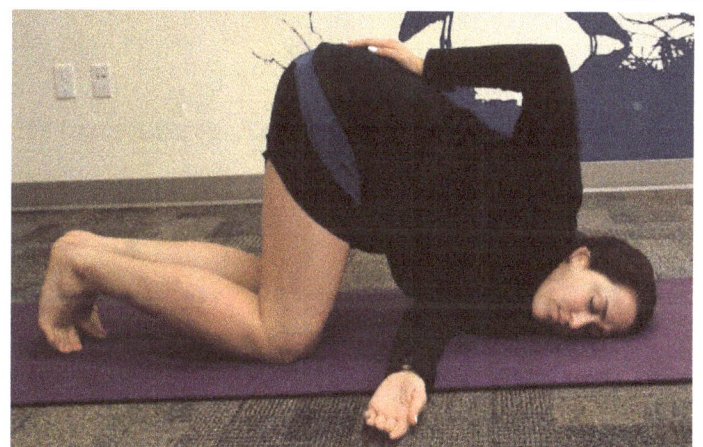
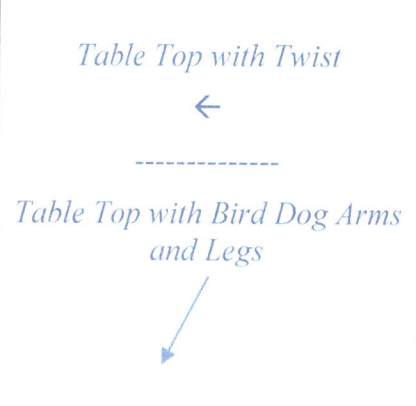

*Table Top with Twist*

←

----------------

*Table Top with Bird Dog Arms and Legs*

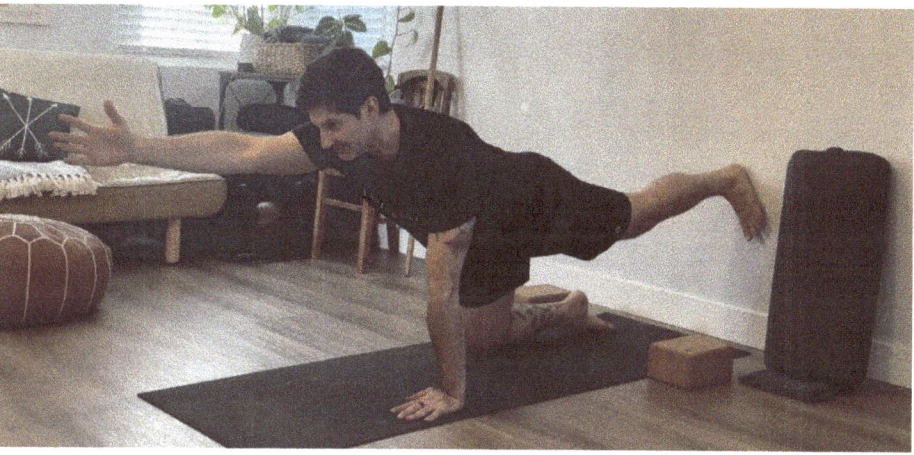

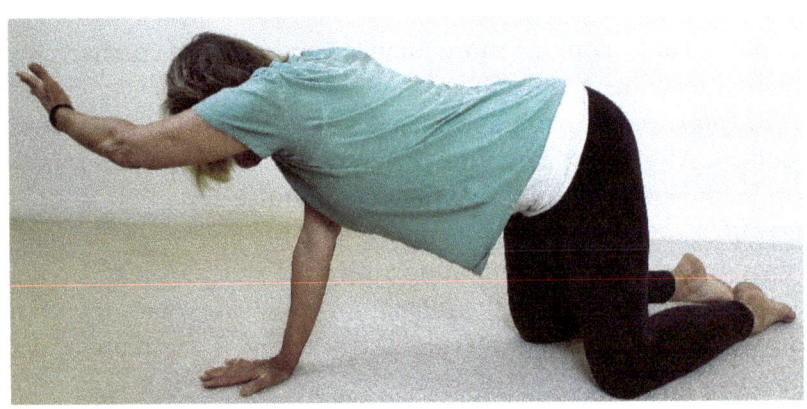

*Table Top with Lateral Flexion*

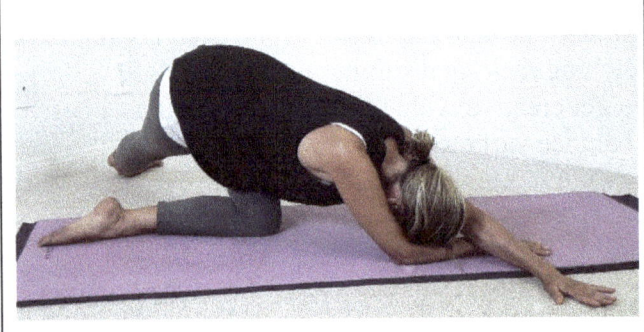 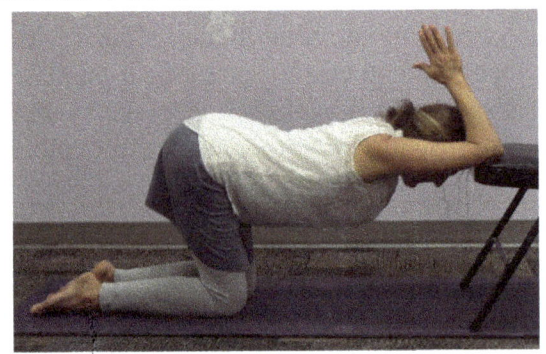

*Table Top with Creative Variations*

----------------------

*Table Top with Strength Variations*

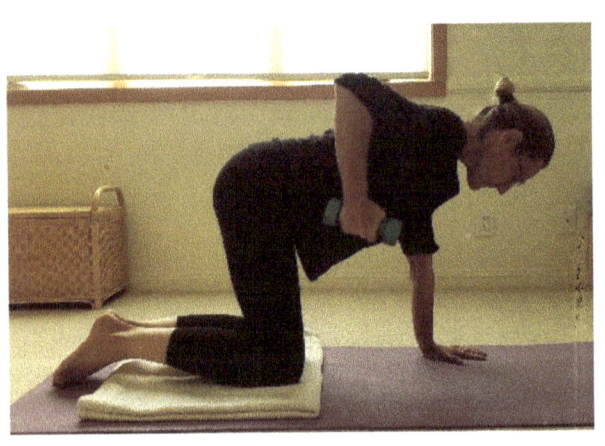 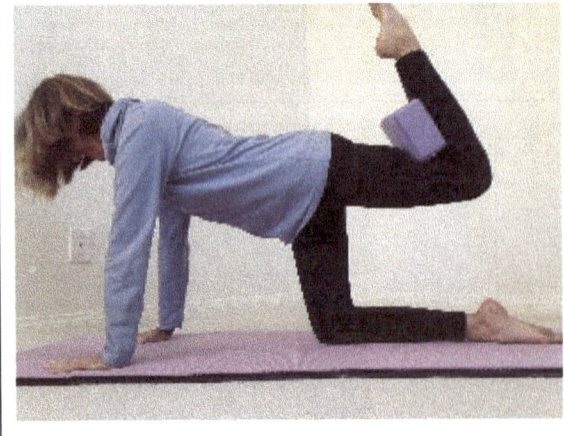

### Downward Facing Dog or Adho Mukha Svanasana

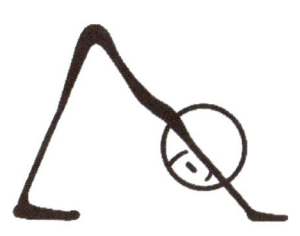

Downward Facing Dog is a powerful half-inversion that invites practitioners to connect with strength, flexibility, and alignment. Downward Facing Dog brings awareness to the full body, engaging arms, legs, spine, and core while encouraging resilience throughout the posterior chain. Though commonly practiced, Downward Dog is not a one-size-fits-all shape and every student's expression looks different based on individual anatomy, flexibility, and comfort. It is important to offer variations to ensure that this foundational shape becomes accessible and feels safe for everyone. By offering a personalized approach to Downward Facing Dog, students can explore the shape in a way that feels empowering, supportive, and safe in all layers of experience.

#### Benefits

The benefits of Downward Facing Dog extend to all layers of experience, from the physical to the mental, making it a wholesome addition to any practice as long as it is practiced with an honest balance of effort and ease:

- *Full-body stretch*: Movement into and out of Downward Facing Dog creates resilience in the shoulder girdle, hamstrings, calves, arches of the feet, and hands, promoting mobility, strength, and ease throughout the back body.
- *Strengthens arms and legs*: By engaging arms and legs, Downward Facing Dog builds strength and stability in the upper and lower body.
- *Energizing and grounding*: As a half-inversion, Downward Facing Dog can simultaneously energize the body by creating more easeful circulation of blood throughout the body, including to the brain, while grounding the practitioner tangibly through the hands and feet.
- *Enhances postural alignment*: The expansiveness invited in the spine during Downward Facing Dog helps create length and openness along the back body, encouraging healthy alignment and energetic ease.
- *Encourages breath awareness*: By creating space in the chest and rib basket, Downward Facing Dog supports mindful breathing, promoting a sense of calm and relaxation, especially if the exhalation is emphasized.

#### Cautions

While Downward Facing Dog offers many benefits, several important considerations are best kept in mind:

- *Wrist pressure*: For students with carpal tunnel syndrome or wrist discomfort, this shape can place significant pressure on this vulnerable area. Variations, such as using blocks or wedges under the hands or practicing at the wall, can reduce strain and over time increase strength and ease.
- *Leg tension*: Tightness in the hamstrings, calves, and Achilles tendons can create discomfort, especially in the back of the legs. Encourage softening or bending the knees to prevent excessive strain.

- *Hypermobility*: Hypermobile students may hyperextend the knees and the low spine. They benefit from cueing related to micro-bending the knees and creating core engagement. They do *not* benefit from cueing that increases lumbar curves (such as lifting the sitz bones). Special attention may be necessary to help hypermobile individuals develop proprioceptive awareness of hyperextension (awareness that is often missing for them).
- *Eye disorders, high blood pressure, and headaches*: As a half-inversion, Downward Facing Dog may be contraindicated for those with eye issues (such as vitreous or retinal detachment, or glaucoma), high blood pressure, or headaches. Safer alternatives such as Child or Puppy could be offered instead.
- *Shoulder sensitivity*: Shoulder injuries or tightness may require variation, such as adjusting hand placement or turning the fingers out slightly to reduce tension.

## *Preparatory Movements*

To prepare the body for Downward Facing Dog, incorporate movements that mobilize the shoulders, activate the core, and create mobility in hips and legs. Following are a few suggestions about useful preparatory movements; many more exist and always include the six movements of spine in any orientation in space. All preparations offered for practicing Table Top and explorations in Table Top itself are helpful for Downward Facing Dog.
- *Knee-down Plank*: Engages the arms, shoulders, and core, building strength and awareness needed for proper alignment in Downward Facing Dog.
- *Cat-Cow*: Helps mobilize the spine and create a connection between breath and movement, preparing the body for the spinal elongation of Downward Facing Dog.
- *Forward Folds*: Mobilizes the hamstrings and releases tension in the low back, preparing the legs for the resilience required in Downward Facing Dog.
- *Lunges*: Creating movement and energy in the hips and hamstrings prepares the body for the flexion at the hips required in Downward Facing Dog

## *Key Alignment Invitations*

Downward Facing Dog is often cued as a *resting* shape, but it requires active engagement from head to toe and restfulness is elusive for many students. The key to finding balance and ease in this shape lies in prioritizing healthful and individualized spinal alignment cues and emphasizing leg *strength* over the mobility required by straightened knees or heels touching the floor. Individually-adapted hand placement (with regard to how far apart the hands are from one another on the mat) can be equally transformational. As always, inner experience supersedes outer shape. Here are a few essential alignment invitations:
- *Invitations related to hands and arms*:
  - *Explain the nuance of arm movements*: To move the arms up and overhead (as the pelvis lifts and draws back), the shoulder joints naturally rotate exteriorly. There is no need to cue this unless you visually see a student struggling with creating a resilient alignment in the back of the shoulder girdle (i.e., incomplete flexion of the shoulder joint). Once students' arms are overhead, creating a directional movement toward internal rotation will greatly stabilize the joint.
  - *Adjust width of hand placement*: Encourage students to adjust the width of their hands, exploring what happens when they first narrow and then widen their hands apart. Often

the final and most comfortable placement of the hands is wider than they might expect. Auspicious width between the arms and hands can reduce tension in the shoulders.
- o *Find optimal hand activation and lift*: The internal rotational movement in the glenohumeral joint is greatly supported by pressing into the inner hand, the space around the thumb and index finger. Spreading the fingers and grounding through the palms helps distribute weight and protect the wrists. A sense of lift at the transition point between the palm and wrists can be useful – imagine trying to create enough space between hand and floor in this spot so that a person could slide a piece of paper between them.
- *Invitations related to legs and hips*:
  - o *Lift the pelvis up and back*: Guide students toward finding length in the spine while maintaining a soft bend in the knees. Most students are well-served by bent knees, especially if the hamstrings are tight and pulling on the low back. Care of the hamstrings and low back can be offered by inviting a bend in the knees. Once adequately warmed up or over time, some individuals may explore extending their knees. It will be helpful to become aware of possibly hyperextended knees among hypermobile students; in such cases inviting a slight bend into the knee will be stabilizing.
  - o *Engage the thighs*: Invite students to lift through the front of the thighs and engage the legs by imagining (but not actually) turning the feet outward or inward. Drawing the kneecaps up works for some, however, beware of hyperextension in the knee joint.
  - o *Ground through the feet*: Even if the heels do not touch the floor, encourage a sense of grounding through the balls of the feet and pressing through the heels. A blanket, towel, or wedge under the heels can be helpful to feel this grounding sensation very tangibly.
- *Invitations related to spine and torso*:
  - o *Lengthen the spine*: Prioritize creating length in the spine (and natural alignment in the lumbar) over straight legs or reaching the heels to the ground. Encourage students to maintain natural spinal curves, especially in the lumbar region, avoiding rounding through the back or collapsing between the shoulders.
  - o *Engage the core*: Draw the navel up and in toward the spine, creating stability in the torso and preventing the low back from collapsing. Avoid a banana shape (i.e., a sagging of the torso's midsection toward the ground) and do <u>not</u> cue moving the sternum or heart toward the floor (sometimes heard in yoga classes).
- *Invitations related to head and neck*:
  - o *Natural curve of the neck*: Keep the neck in line with the spine, allowing the head to be positioned without tension. For most students, it is helpful to imagine the head being between the upper arms with a gentle gaze toward the floor. It can be helpful to cue arm adduction until the student can feel their ears on their arms – this leads to an optimal head placement. Once achieved, re-release the arms to their most auspicious width. Another very helpful cue for the neck region is to relax the muscles at the base of neck, rather than cueing pulling the shoulders away from the ears.

### *Variations and Exploration*

Downward Facing Dog can be varied in many ways to suit a variety of physical, energetic, and emotional needs or desires. Here are some variations to explore:
- *Wall or Chair Dog*: Practicing the V-shape of the scapulae on the rib basket by standing with the hands at a wall, seat of a chair, or countertop instead of the floor reduces pressure on

wrists and shoulders. This can be especially helpful for individuals who are relatively new to the practice or are dealing with wrist or shoulder sensitivities.
- *Blocks under hands*: Placing the hands-on blocks or small barbells (holding the 'handle' between the two ends) can elevate the upper body, reduce wrist pressure, and invite more spaciousness in the shoulders. Hand width remains crucial in this variation.
- *Rolled blanket under heels*: For students with tight calves or Achilles tendons who cannot place their heels on the mat, placing a rolled blanket, wedge, or bolster under the heels can create a more grounded and supportive experience.
- *Restorative version*: Using a bolster or folded blankets under the head allows the body to rest more fully while maintaining the shape's basic structure. This makes Downward Facing Dog a more restorative, yet still actively engaged and empowering experience.
- *Puppy*: For students who prefer a more supported half-inversion, Puppy offers a gentle alternative that creates resilience in the shoulders and spine without weight on the wrists or hands. In Puppy, the extremities rest on the ground – with knees, shins, and tops of the feet on the earth; elbows on the mat, with forearms lifted and palms touching (perhaps) above the head; the forehead rests on the ground, a block, or a blanket.
- *Dolphin*: For students with wrist issues, is can be helpful to choose Dolphin, in which the forearms are placed on the ground, often with hands clasped.
- *Spa Dog*: The student steps into a strap loop and draws the strap upward to place it across the low front portion of the pelvis, across the hip creases essentially. The other end of the loop can be held by another person or can be secured to a hook or door handle. The student moves into Downward Facing Dog from standing, holding the strap in place with one hand and then allows the strap to help create the upward and backward movement of the pelvis.
- *Revolved Dog*: Unweighting one hand and reaching it through to the ankle or outer shin of the opposite leg can add a gentle and active rotation to this shape. It is a wonderful variation for cultivating balance and core strength.
- *Wild Thing*: This version is to be used with discernment as it invites heart opening, balance challenge, and core engagement. It can be offered in a playful and joyful way that invites exploration and enjoyment of the journal, rather than striving for a particular outer shape.

## *Recovery*

After practicing Downward Facing Dog, recovery movements may be offered that release tension and restore balance to body, mind, and emotions:
- *Child*: This gentle resting shape allows the spine and shoulders to release after the engagement of Downward Facing Dog.
- *Seated Forward Fold*: This option is a gentle release for the hamstrings and letting-go of low back tension.
- *Gentle Shoulder Rolls*: These gentle movements can release residual tension in the shoulders and neck.
- *Wrist Circles*: Wrists mobilization can reduce discomfort from weight-bearing.

## *Additional Teaching Tips*

To help students find ease and alignment in Downward Facing Dog, consider these additional suggestions:

- *Invite ongoing breath awareness*: Breath is a great indicator of excess effort. Guide students toward noticing how breath can support movement and how movement affects breath. Encourage them to use the feedback from the breath to find the most healthful expressions and variations of Downward Facing Dog. Focus on the exhalation may invite a greater sense of ease.
- *Emphasize individual alignment based on interoception and neuroception*: Remind students that everyone's Downward Facing Dog looks different. Encourage them to find what feels balanced and sustainable for their body, rather than focusing on an idealized or sought-after outward shape.
- *Offer a variety of props for support*: Blocks, blankets, walls, and chairs can make Facing Dog more accessible for all levels of practice. Creativity invites each student into their most healthful expression.
- *Imaginative cues*: Invite students to imagine their body creating an upside-down "V" shape, rising up dynamically and enthusiastically through the hips while grounding luxuriously through the hands and feet.
- *Avoid cueing a "resting" shape*: For many students, Downward Facing Dog is anything but a resting shape. Avoid cueing it as such and only make reference to this possibility with detailed guidance on finding adaptations and variation that create this restfulness for individual students.

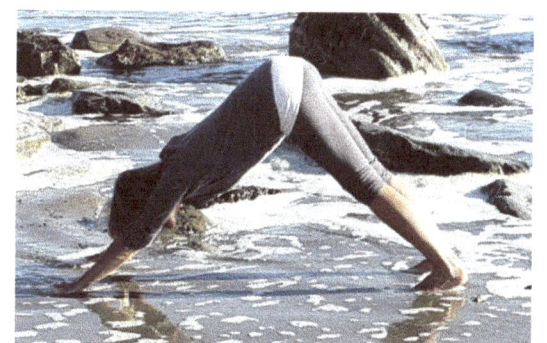

*Downward Facing Dog*

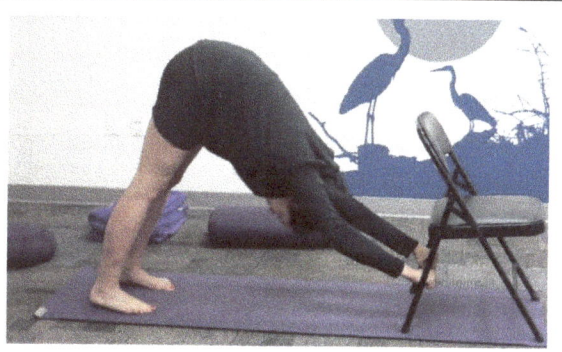

*Downward Facing Dog with lift under the hands*

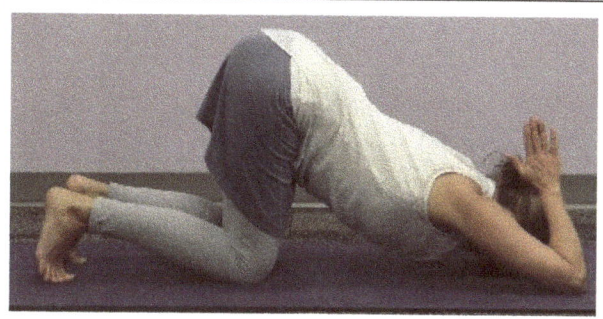

*Puppy – finding ease within effort*

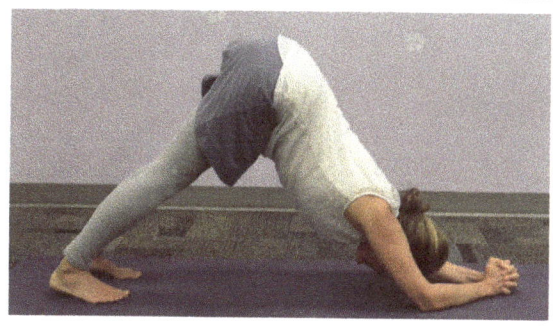

*Dolphin – creating strength with respect for the wrists*

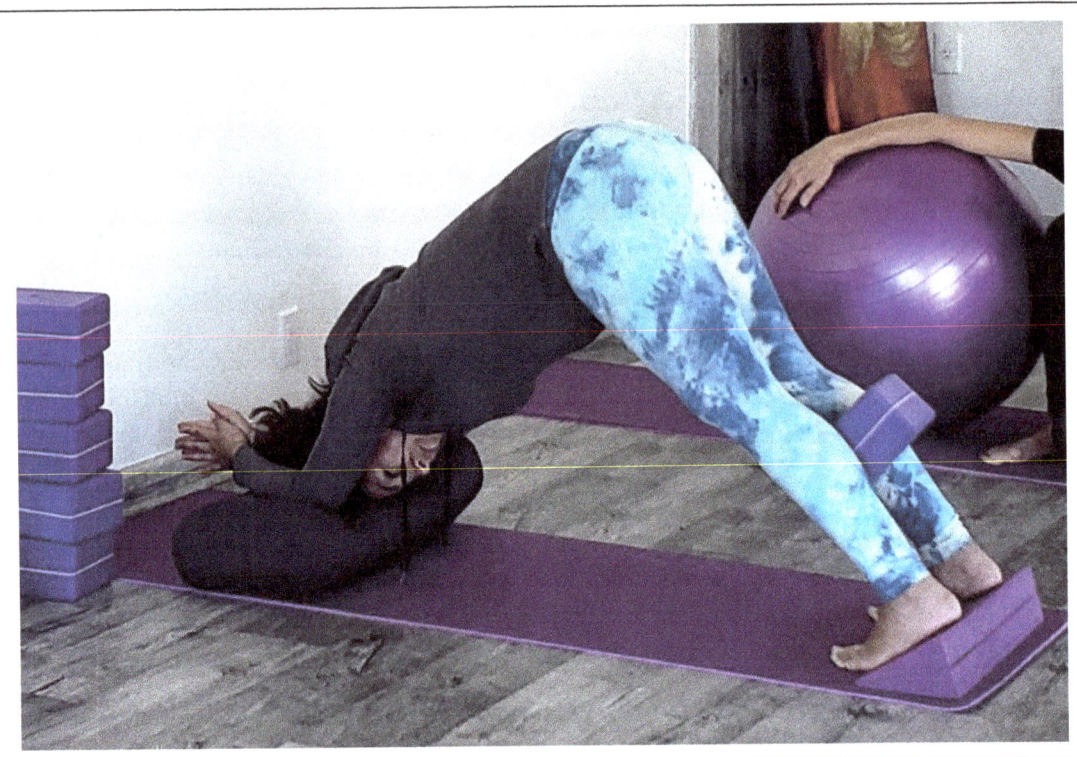

*Supported Dolphin – finding ease within effort*

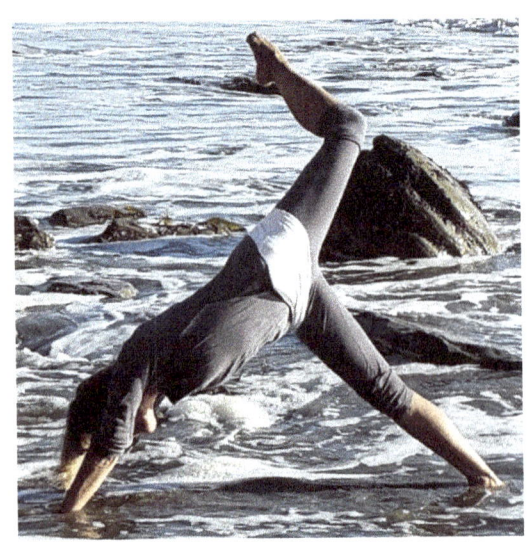

*Wild Thing – joy of playfulness with no concern for outer shape*

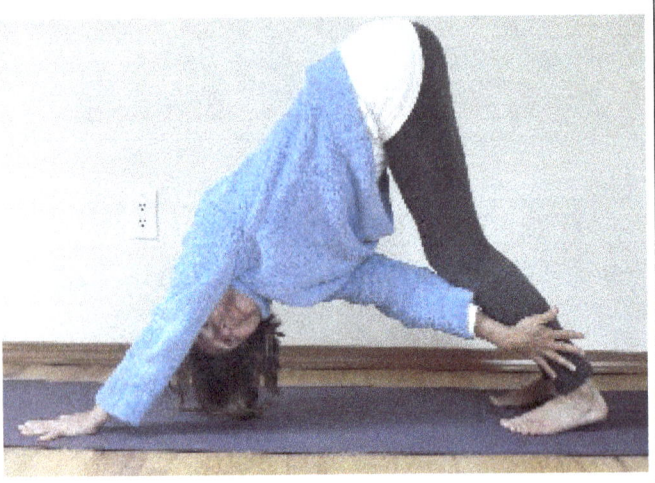

*Revolved Down Dog – the opportunity to add balance and rotation*

## Plank or Phalakasana

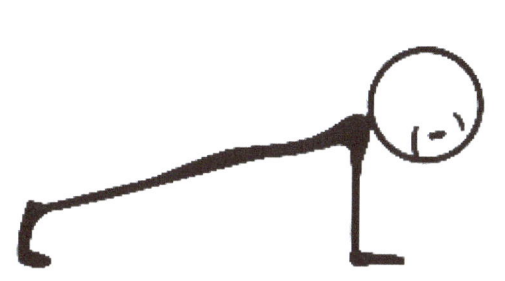

Plank is an empowering, full-body strengthener that challenges the practitioner's core, arms, and legs while fostering physical and emotional endurance and mental focus. Often considered a foundational part of many yoga practices, this shape encourages alignment, stability, and balance in all layers of experience. As is true for all shapes, Plank looks different for each individual depending on their strength, body structure, current needs, and experience. Offering variations and adaptations allows everyone to explore the shape and its associated movements safely and effectively.

### Benefits

Plank provides a wide range of physical and mental benefits:
- *Core strength and stability*: By engaging the transverse abdominis (deep core muscles), Plank strengthens the core, improves posture, and enhances balance, physically and emotionally.
- *Upper body strength*: This shape targets the arms, shoulders, and chest, building strength in the entire upper body.
- *Leg engagement*: Pressing the heels back helps activate the legs, especially the quadriceps, creating an integrated full-body experience of strength and vitality.
- *Endurance and concentration*: Holding Plank requires mental focus and concentration, promoting mindfulness, mental clarity, and perseverance.
- *Invigorating all layers of experience*: This shape energizes body, vitality or breath, and mind, with its emotions and thoughts, promoting a sense of presence and readiness.
- *Core awareness*: Plank encourages students to connect deeply with their physical and energetic core, crucial for cultivating stability and ease in other shapes and daily life.

### Cautions

Although Plank offers great benefits, it is important and helpful for wholesome expressions of the shape to be mindful of certain cautions; including all of the following as well as those listed for Downward Facing Dog.
- *Wrist discomfort*: Students with carpal tunnel syndrome or wrist issues may experience discomfort. Variations, such as using fists, forearms, or blocks, can reduce wrist strain.
- *Pregnancy*: For individuals who are pregnant, especially in the second and third trimesters, Plank may place strain on the abdominal muscles. Variations such as Wall Plank or Plank on the knees can be more supportive.
- *Low back sensitivity*: Sagging in the low back can lead to discomfort or injury. Strong core engagement may prevent this.

*Preparatory Movements*

To prepare for Plank, incorporate movements that strengthen the arms, engage the core, and promote shoulder stability. All preparations offered for Table Top and Downward Facing Dog apply to Plank as well. Table Top explorations and the six movements of the spine are excellent preparations and warm-ups.

- *Table Top variations*: These movements build arm and leg strength while encouraging awareness of shoulder alignment and core stability.
- *Downward Facing Dog*: This shape offers preparation through shoulder engagement and core activation.
- *Wall work for shoulders*: Many types of movements in this category can support the shoulder girdle, creating stability and mobility for accessing Plank with less strain; samples are discussed and shown in Chapter on 13 heart-opening shapes.
- *Core strengthening movements*: Simple core activations like Cat-Cow with focus on engaging the transverse abdominis can help build strength for maintaining Plank.
- *Work on the knees*: Practicing Plank with knees on the floor can offer valuable strengthening before attempting Plank with knees lifted.

*Key Alignment Invitations*

In Plank, alignment and engagement in all layers of experience are essential for safety and effectiveness. The following cues may help invite students into a sustainable and supportive expression of the shape:

- *Invitations related to core strengthening and spinal alignment*:
  - *Engage the core*: Invite students to draw their navel toward the spine, as if tightening a corset, to activate the transverse abdominis. This action stabilizes the spine and prevents the low back from sagging.
  - *Beware of sagging*: A banana-shaped torso may indicate lack of core engagement. Cue students to draw the navel toward the spine to help them engage the deep core muscles. Actively sticking the tongue out can help activate these important postural support muscles. Drawing the low ribs toward the iliac spine is helpful.
  - *Neck alignment*: Keep the head in line with the spine, with the gaze slightly ahead of the hands to avoid hyperextension of the neck.
- *Invitations related to hands, arms, and shoulder girdle:*
  - *Align the shoulders*: Shoulders are stacked directly over the wrists, with the shoulder blades drawing down the back. Avoid overly squeezing the shoulder blades together (scapular retraction); instead, encourage a broad support across the upper back.
  - *Press the ground away through the hands*: Grounding through the palms and feeling a slight rebound from the earth can stabilize shoulders and prevent collapse in the wrists.
  - *Watch out for shoulder misalignment*: Watch out for collapsing into the shoulders or drawing the shoulder blades too far together or too far apart. Cue a middle way alignment of the shoulder blades that invites strength in the upper body without over-engagement.
  - *Keep an isometric balance between serratus anterior and rhomboids*: Do not let the shoulder girdle drop forward or collapse. Stability in this shape relies on flexion and extension in the elbow and in the glenohumeral joint. This requires the scapulae to be stabilized on the back via that isometric action of the rhomboids and serratus anterior.

- *Invitations related to feet, legs, and pelvic girdle:*
  - *Leg engagement*: Press the heels back strongly to activate the quadriceps and fire up the legs. This engagement helps create a straight line from head to heels and prevents sagging in the hips.
  - *Beware of under-engaged legs*: Many students forget to engage their legs and then struggle with maintaining wholesome alignment. Encourage pressing through the heels and lifting through the thighs to activate and empower.
  - *Pelvic alignment*: Neutralize the pelvis by drawing the tailbone slightly toward the heels without overly tucking or arching the low back. This helps prevent hyperextension in the lumbar lower spine and stabilizes the sacroiliac joints.
  - *Look out for hips that are lifted too high*: If the hips are lifted too high, it can take away from the core work and shift more weight into the shoulders. Encourage a straight line from head to heels.

## Variations and Exploration

Plank can be varied in many ways to suit individuality related to all layers of experience, including strength, endurance, familiarity, and physical, energetic, mental, and emotional needs:
- *Wall Plank*: Practicing with the hands against a wall reduces pressure on the wrists and can be a good starting point for beginners.
- *Knees on the floor*: This variation offers more support while still engaging the core and upper body.
- *Hands in fists*: This reduces wrist pressure by placing the hands in a neutral position, often useful for those with wrist discomfort.
- *Forearm Plank:* By lowering to the forearms, students can reduce wrist strain while still engaging the core and upper body.
- *Plank with one leg raised:* Lifting one leg adds a balancing challenge and relies on even more core engagement.
- *Heels pressing into a wall:* Placing the heels against a wall can help students activate the legs more fully and find more active and empowered alignment.
- *Transition to Yoga Pushup:* Place the arms close to the torso, flex the elbows, and slowly release to the earth with control and power.

## Recovery Movements

After practicing Plank, recovery movements allow body, nervous system and vitality, and thoughts and emotions to relax and reset:
- *Gentle Downward Facing Dog*: Lifting up through the hips offers a gentle stretch for the shoulders and legs that allows the core to relax.
- *Table Top*: Finding support on the knees offers a neutralizing position to release tension in the back and shoulders; adding Cat-Cow can offer even more of a reset.
- *Child*: Full-body flexion provides a calming release for the spine and helps relax an overly activated nervous system.
- *Resting on belly:* Lying on the belly with one cheek to the ground allows the body to release any residual tension, especially in the core and low back. It also resets emotions and energy.

## Additional Teaching Tips

To help students find strength, steadiness, and wholesome alignment in Plank, consider these additional suggestions:

- *Cue breath awareness*: Remind students to focus on their breath during Plank, as holding the breath can lead to excess tension.
- *Emphasize individual alignment*: Encourage students to find what works best for their body rather than aiming for a particular external shape.
- *Offer support for wrists*: Be mindful of wrist sensitivity and offer upright alternatives or props to reduce strain.
- *Encourage core engagement*: Remind students that wholesome core activation is key to finding ease and stability in Plank.
- *Preparation in Table Top and Downward Facing Dog*: Plank is very well sequenced after keen attention to alignment and practice in these helpful preparations.

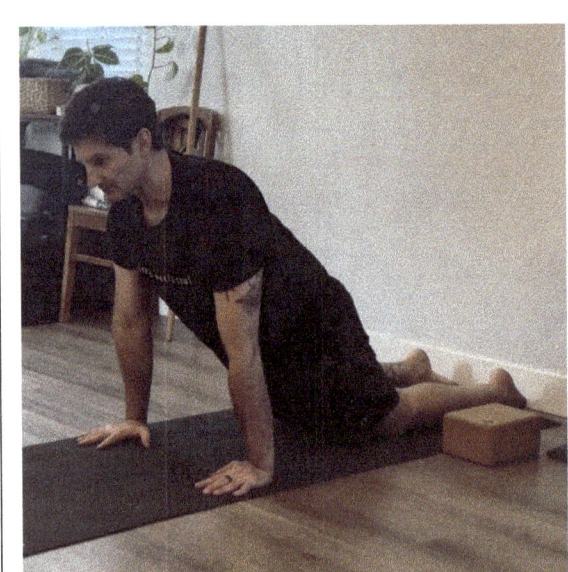

*Plank with Knees Down – moving toward strength-building*

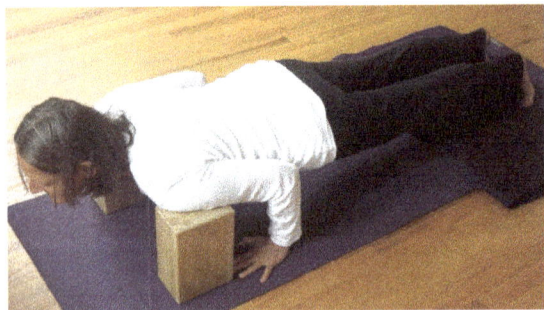

*Plank with Shoulder Props – creating proprioceptive awareness*

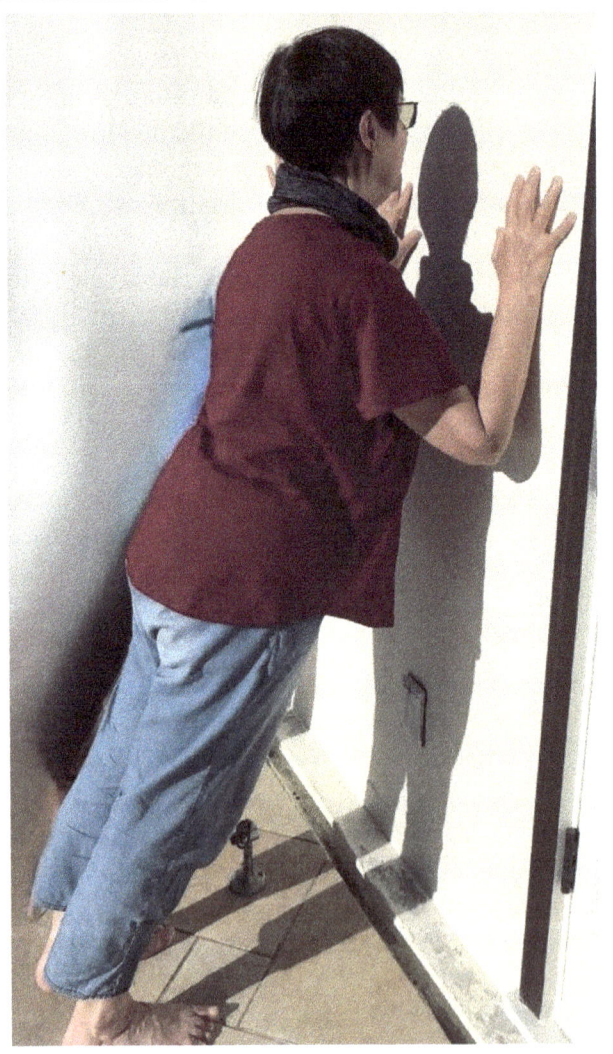

*Plank at the Wall – embracing supports*

## Side Plank or Vasisthasana

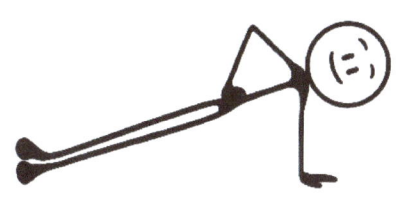

Side Plank is a dynamic, strengthening shape that cultivates balance, stability, and inner strength in all layers of experience (body, energy, and mind). It engages the core, arms, and legs, while inviting a sense of spaciousness and expansion. The shape challenges physical endurance and mental focus, encouraging practitioners to find joyful steadiness in the midst of intensity. As is true for all shapes, Side Plank looks and feels different for each individual depending on strength, body structure, mind stories and emotions, and prior experience. Offering variations and adaptations allows each student or client to explore the shape safely and with integrity, honoring their unique anatomy, energy, and current needs.

### Benefits

Side Plank offers a broad range of benefits for body, breath, and mind:
- *Core strength, stability, and endurance*: Side Plank activates the deep core muscles, including the obliques and transverse abdominis, enhancing overall core stability and support for the spine.
- *Upper body strength*: Side Plank engages the shoulders, arms, and wrists, building strength throughout the upper body, especially the shoulder gridle. It can, over time and with careful practice, counteract wrist pain, including from carpal tunnel syndrome.
- *Leg activation*: Pressing into the feet and engaging the legs helps stabilize the entire body, building strength in the thighs and improving balance.
- *Balance and concentration*: Balancing on one hand and one foot encourages deep focus and mindfulness, fostering mental clarity and presence. Balance and concentration in all layers of experience increase resilience and capacity to endure and cope.
- *Spaciousness and length*: The extended arm and lengthened side body create a sense of expansion and openness, while cultivating a feeling of lightness and freedom. This can translate into emotional wellbeing and mental resilience, even joy and a sense of accomplishment.

### Cautions

Although Side Plank offers many benefits, it is important to approach the shape with mindful attention to any areas of sensitivity:
- *Wrist discomfort*: Bearing weight on one hand can place pressure on the wrist. Variations, such as practicing on the forearm, may reduce strain on the wrists. Although the weight-bearing of Side Plank can worsen carpal tunnel syndrome in its acute phase, over time, it can help alleviate it, if taught with care and calibrated exposure to weight-bearing.
- *Shoulder or neck tension*: The weight-bearing nature of the shape may lead to tension in the shoulder girdle or neck for some individuals. Finding a healthful hand and shoulder placement can help alleviate discomfort. Using a stabilizing foot variation can also be useful.

- *Low back sensitivity*: The deep core engagement required in Side Plank helps support the low back, but without sufficient activation, this area may feel strained. Encourage mindful core and pelvic floor engagement to support spinal health.

## Preparatory Movements

To prepare for Side Plank, movements that warm up the wrists, engage the core, and stabilize the shoulders are beneficial. All preparations already noted for the preceding arm-standing shapes will be helpful for Side Plank. Side Plank is offered later in a single practice or over the course of series of practices as it is demanding in all layers of experience; physical, energetic, and emotional readiness are key to success.
- *Side body stretches*: Simple stretches that open the side body help create space and awareness in preparation for the lengthening in Side Plank.
- *Shoulder strengthening movements*: Exercises that stabilize the shoulder girdle, such as wall work (see Chapter 13), Dolphin, or Downward Facing Dog, provide a strong foundation for Side Plank.
- *Plank*: Practicing Plank first engages the core, shoulders, and arms, building strength and stability in preparation for Side Plank.

## Key Alignment Invitations

In Side Plank, alignment plays a crucial role in finding strength, balance, and openness. The following alignment invitations can help guide students into a wholesome and supportive expression of the shape. Most alignment cues offered for Downward Facing Dog and Plank will also be helpful, modified to accommodate the single-sided and open-hearted version of Plank.
- *Invitations for the core and spine*:
  - *Engage the core*: Invite students to lift through the belly and engage the deep core muscles to support the spine and prevent sagging in the side body.
  - *Lengthen the spine*: Encourage a long, natural spine, creating a straight line from the head to the heels. This elongation helps prevent unnecessary strain and supports balance.
- *Invitations for the arms and shoulders*:
  - *Align the shoulders healthfully for strength*: Invite the top shoulder to stack directly over the bottom shoulder, creating a stable foundation for the upper body. Invite the scapulae to move firmly onto the back and down.
  - *Press through the hand*: Encourage students to press the earth away with the bottom hand, feeling the earth push back (gravitational rebound) to stabilize the shoulder and prevent collapse. For some students, the bottom hand may need to move away from being directly under the shoulder joint as this increased angle may lessen some of the pressure.
  - *Extend the top arm*: Reaching the top arm toward the sky or overhead adds a sense of expansiveness and balance, helping to create openness in the chest, side body, and mind.
- *Invitations for the legs and feet*:
  - *Place the feet auspiciously*: The feet can be stacked on top of each other or staggered, depending on the student's balance and comfort level. Both options help ground the shape and support leg engagement.
  - *Activate the legs*: Invite students to press through the heels and engage the thighs of both legs, creating stability, power, agency, and support throughout the entire lower body.

o  *Use a kickstand*: One foot can be grounded ahead or behind the body to create a kickstand for greater ease and less weight-bearing in the arms.

*Variations and Exploration*

Side Plank offers a variety of adaptations and explorations, allowing students to experiment, even play, with the shape in a way that suits their needs and abilities:
- *Forearm Side Plank*: Practicing with the forearm on the ground reduces pressure on the wrist while still engaging the core and upper body.
- *Knee on the ground*: Placing the bottom knee on the floor provides more support for the lower body while allowing for exploration of balance and core engagement.
- *Kickstand*: The foot of the top leg (with knee bent) can be placed on the ground in front of the bottom leg, making a kickstand to bring more ease and balance to the shape. It is also possible to bring the top foot behind the bottom leg, which encourages more heart opening in the shape.
- *Top leg lifted*: For an added challenge, lifting the top leg off the ground deepens core engagement and challenges balance. It is also possible to lift the top leg and place foot in Tree position, resting the foot of the lifted leg on an accessible location on the bottom leg. Lifting the top leg increases weight-bearing on the bottom leg.
- *Hand on a block*: Using a block under the bottom hand can elevate the floor and provide more ease in maintaining alignment.

*Recovery Movements*

After practicing Side Plank, movements that release tension in the wrists, shoulders, and core can help the body reset and recover:
- *Child*: This grounding shape allows the shoulders and wrists to relax while calming the nervous system.
- *Downward Facing Dog or Table Top*: These shapes may relax the core and to middle back. They may not work well for students with less arm strength as they still require significant work in the shoulder girdle and arms; thus, use these with discernment and only with strong students.
- *Resting on the belly*: This relaxing shape invites ease into the nervous system, reflection, and a healthful letting go of tension in the muscles
- *Gentle twists*: Seated, supine, or reclined twists help release tightness in the side body and low back.

*Additional Teaching Tips*

To help students cultivate strength, stability, and ease in Side Plank, consider these supportive teaching suggestions:
- *Encourage breath awareness*: Remind students to stay connected to their breath, allowing it to guide them through the intensity of the shape. Expansiveness can be cued with the inhalation; drawing inward with strength can accompany the exhalation.
- *Offer individualized alignment cues*: Invite students to explore a version that feels balanced and supportive for their body and mind, rather than aiming for a specific outer shape.

- *Support wrist and shoulder health*: Be mindful of wrist and shoulder sensitivities, offering props or variations as needed to reduce strain and increase comfort. Working on the forearm for a while can create more access to the shape early on.
- *Focus on core engagement*: Emphasize the importance of core activation, as this is key to finding stability and ease in Side Plank

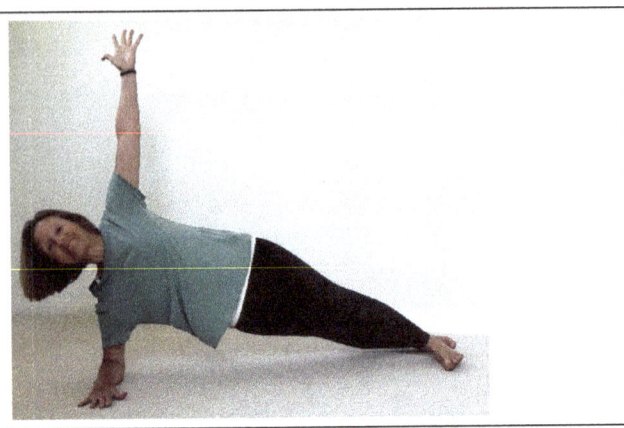

*Side Plank
– on elbow with feet staggered*

←

--------------------

*Side Plank on knee with kickstand*

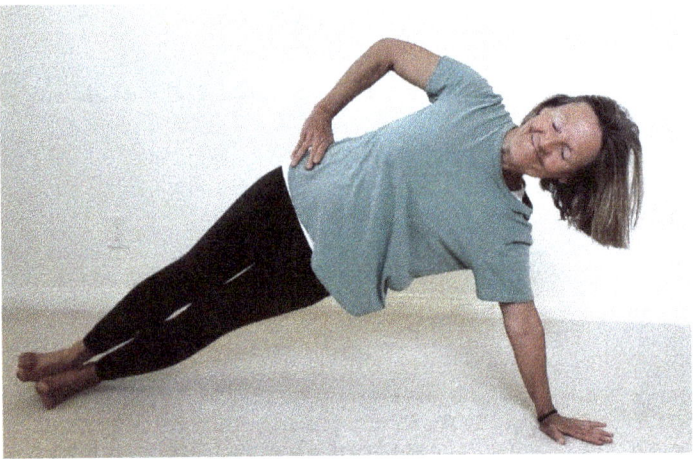

*Side Plank
– with Kickstand for balance*

→

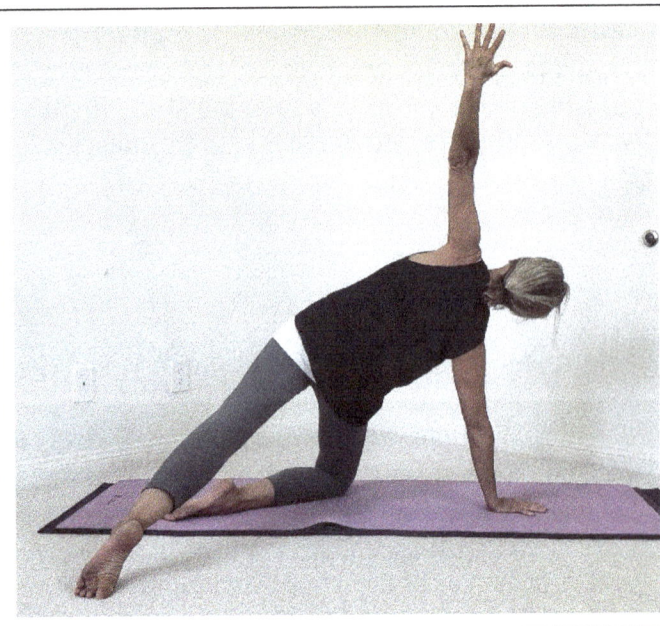

# Chapter 10: Upright Seats

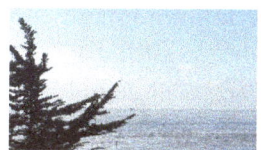

This chapter covers foundational upright seats, offering optimized teaching strategies that allow for individual tailoring and careful discernment about how and which shapes to offer, as well as about how to cue alignment informed by interoception, proprioception, exteroception, and neuroception. General principles for this category of yoga *asana* are provided and apply to most if not all seated shapes. Specific follow-up guidance is added for the chosen sample shapes.

## Anatomical Foci for Upright Seats

Upright seats create an anatomical foundation based in the pelvis and legs, relying on the lower appendicular skeleton for grounding and rooting. They depend on easeful access to the natural curves of the spine, the capacity to create core stabilization, and keen awareness to the various structures and movement characteristics of the pelvic girdle. Special attention is necessary to take good care of the knees, which in seats have to absorb any tension created between the ankle and hip joints that is the result of range of motion that is restricted in some manner. The potential for torquing the knee needs to be held in mind to make sure that knee health receives proper attention through facilitating additional range of motion above and below and through the ample use of props.

Seats clearly come in a great variety of shapes. Regardless of the chosen seat, it is key to find natural upright seated shapes that ground the body with ease and comfort by exploring the utility of props or supports (e.g., chairs, zafu, benches, blankets, bolsters, and even walls). Propitious seats allow clients to ground into the earth, expand toward the sky, and stabilize at the core. Seats for meditative or breathwork practices are enhanced by consciously choosing how to place the hands (e.g., in the lap, on thighs, palms up or down; with hands placed in the lap, a lift [e.g., pillow] can bring ease to the arms and maintain an open-heart). Contemplative upright seats can also be enhanced by conscious choices about whether to close the eyes to withdraw attention from outer sense impressions or to keep them open (e.g., at half-mast with a soft gaze point).

A variety of seats are explored in this chapter; many other options exist. Of course, for individuals who have difficulty accessing the floor, natural upright seats can be beautifully engaged on a chair or other appropriate surface (for example, on a meditation bench).

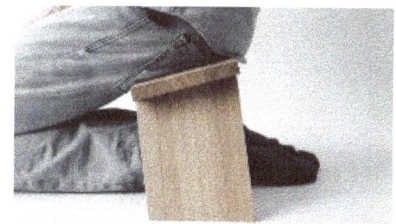

### *Natural Spine*

In seated shapes, such as Easy Seat, Hero, Diamond, and others covered in this chapter, maintaining the natural curves of the spine is essential for both structural integrity and energetic flow. Since the topic of the natural spine has been amply covered elsewhere, only a few comments about the natural spine in the context of seats are offered here. In sitting (on and off the mat), natural spinal alignment, honoring the gentle cervical and lumbar lordosis as well as the thoracic and sacral kyphosis, facilitates optimal breath capacity, reduces strain on the intervertebral discs, and supports sustainable sitting for purposes of *asana*, *pranayama*, and *meditation*. When the spine is allowed to retain its natural curves without forced straightening or exaggerated rounding, the vertebrae are stacked with integrity at all three joint points (the facet joints and the disc-vertebral body connection), promoting stability and mobility in a seat as our evolution to bipedalism intended. Props, such as blankets, bolsters, or cushions, beneath the sitz bones and the tops of femurs (more about this below) can be invaluable for supporting the natural curves of spine, allowing the pelvis to tilt forward slightly so that the spinal curves are engaged and preserved with ease. This gentle natural alignment in the spine, on a steady based created by the pelvis and legs, creates a foundation for inner stillness, easeful optimal breathing, and sustainable comfort in seated practices and daily life.

## *Core Stabilization*
(see Arm Standing above and refer back to Chapter 5 in the Anatomy Section)

Seated shapes rely on core stabilization in a similar manner as standing shapes. Stabilizing from the center outward plays a vital role in supporting the trunk, spine, pelvis, and ribs during sitting (on and off the mat), ensuring healthful alignment and ease over time. Engaging the deep core musculature (including the transversus abdominis, multifidus, pelvic floor, and diaphragm) creates a stable foundation that maintains the natural curves of the spine and preserves the integrity of the pelvic positioning. Subtle engagement of the pelvic floor invites an upward energetic lift during sitting, encouraging a sense of lightness and effortless axial extension through the spine. Simultaneously, the postural spinal muscles activate to sustain endurance and stability in the torso, reducing strain and preventing collapse during prolonged sitting. Integrated core engagement (discussed in detail previously and thus not repeated here) allows seated shapes to become anchored as well as spacious, stabile in a dynamic manner, and supportive of optimal breathing and contemplative practices.

## *Pelvic Girdle – Structures and Relationships*

The pelvic girdle serves as the central foundation for seats – in yoga *asana* and in daily life. To recap, structurally, the pelvic girdle consists of a bony ring formed by the ilia, sacrum, and the sacroiliac (SI) joints, as well as the pubic bone, pubic symphysis, ischia, and acetabula. Each of these elements contributes to the transfer of weight from above (i.e., from the axial and upper appendicular skeleton) and the maintenance of stability during sitting.

At the back of the pelvis, the SI joints connect the ilia to the sacrum, facilitating the transfer of weight from the axial and upper appendicular skeleton to the lower limbs. The SI joints are structures deserving of key consideration in sitting and in cueing seats in yoga *asana*. The SI joints are inherently designed for stability (recall their role in the construction of the junction between sacrum and ilia like a keystone arch), further supported by a powerful network of ligaments that limit excessive movement. Nevertheless, the SI joints allow for a small range of motion (approximately 2 millimeters) to accommodate activities such as sitting, standing, and walking,. Issues arise when there is too much movement between the ilia and sacrum, creating separation or compression that places excessive stress on the joints and their ligaments, potentially leading to destabilization and/or dysfunction. Hormonal changes during menstruation, pregnancy, and lactation can also increase ligamentous laxity, further challenging SI stability. The width of the pelvis plays a role in this vulnerability; women generally have acetabula that are farther apart, increasing strain on the SI joints, which can contribute to a higher incidence of SI-related discomfort.

At the front of the pelvis, the pubic symphysis connects the left and right pubic bones, completing the bony ring and providing additional stability during seated positions. In seated shapes, the ischial tuberosities (sitz bones) serve as primary contact points with the ground (along with the tops of the femurs – to be explored below). The hamstrings attach to the ischial tuberosities, which means that hamstring flexibility has a direct bearing on pelvic alignment and comfort during sitting. Tension or restriction in the hamstrings can pull on the ischium, rolling the pelvis posterior and thus limiting its ability to tilt forward gracefully, an anterior positioning that is key for maintaining the natural curves of the spine in seated shapes.

The acetabulum, formed by the convergence of the ilia, ischia, and pubic bone, is the socket that receives the head of the femur. Its slight anteversion (15°) allows the pelvis to roll over the femoral head during seated shapes, enhancing spinal alignment. For this reason, gentle internal rotation of the femur can facilitate a forward tilt of the pelvis, supporting the natural lumbar curve in seated positions. It is important to recall that depth and orientation of the acetabulum as well as shapes and angles of the femoral head and neck vary significantly across individuals, affecting comfort and range of motion in seated yoga *asana*.

Understanding these anatomical relationships in the pelvic girdle informs alignment and stability during seated shapes, optimizing comfort and minimizing strain during sustained sitting practices. This understanding needs to be translated into cueing specific movement dynamics and alignments that can be helpful to clients who are invited into seated yoga *asana*.

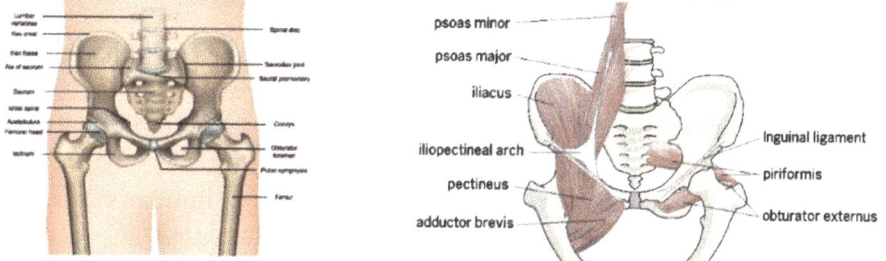

Figure 2.9 Pelvic girdle. (Data source: istock.com)   Figure 2.10 Hip flexors and rotators. (Data source: Istock)

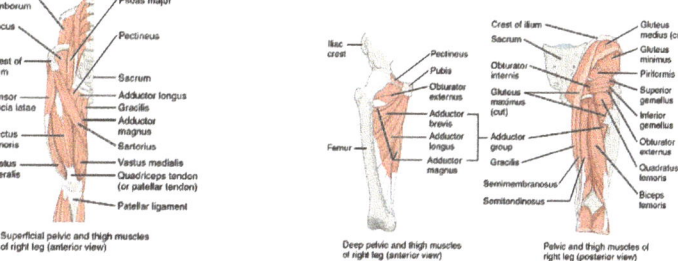

Figure 2.11 Muscles moving the femur in the acetabulum. (Data source: OpenStax; https://commons.wikimedia.org/wiki/File:1122_Gluteal_Muscles_that_Move_the_Femur.jpg; Creative Commons Attribution 4.0)

## Helpful Muscle Actions and Movement or Alignment Concepts

Understanding the unique structure and biomechanics of the pelvic girdle is essential for effective cueing and alignment. The pelvis functions as a bony ring, composed of the ilia, sacrum, ischia, pubic bone, and acetabula, and it is fundamentally designed for stability and weight transfer. Movements and adjustments in seats must respect the inherent stability of the sacroiliac (SI) joints and the interconnected nature of pelvic movement.

Because the pelvis is a rigid bony ring, both sides move together as a unit. Contrary to common yoga cueing, the pelvis cannot be 'opened like a book', fixed and stable during rotation or lateral flexion, or rotated asymmetrically side-to-side without undue risk of sacral corkscrewing. Cueing that suggests such actions is anatomically inaccurate and places undue strain on the SI joints and surrounding connective tissues. Instead, healthful pelvic movements integrate the two ilia, sacrum, and pubic symphysis as a single cohesive structure. The pelvis move as one unit – it cannot move in bits and pieces; yoga *asana* cueing and alignment must honor this structural reality.

Next, a natural pelvis is *not synonymous* with the sacrum being vertical to the ground. The pelvis, when aligned naturally, is in a slight anteriorly tilt, typically ranging between 30° and 40°. A useful image is that of the pelvis as a basin ( an understanding that arises from the German translation of pelvis as "*Becken*", translated as basin in English). When this basin is overly tilted forward, water would spill out the front; when tilted back, water would spill out the back. Natural alignment allows the imaginary water to remain level, neither spilling forward nor backward. Cueing such natural pelvic alignment in seated shapes, allows the sacrum to wedge naturally against the ilia, enhancing SI joint stability, supporting natural spinal curves from the lumbar to the cervical spine, and minimizing unnecessary strain in the low back.

To support healthful pelvic alignment in yoga practice, the *use of props* is often key to finding healthful and sustainable alignment. For example,
- A block or blanket under the seat elevates the hips, encouraging a gentle anterior tilt and preventing lumbar rounding.
- Placing a cushion or bolster between the wall and the sacrum can remind students to maintain the pelvic anterior tilt without collapsing backward.
- If leaning on something is necessary while sitting, a chair with lumbar support can help establish the proper pelvic angle in seated meditation or *pranayama*.

One of the more common misalignments in seated (and standing) shapes is the tendency to tuck the pelvis. While sometimes cued as a supposed means to protect the low back, excessive tucking actually may decrease SI joint stability and disrupt the natural lumbar curve. Over time, such action can lead to compensatory strain in the lumbar spine and SI joint discomfort. A better approach is to encourage students to find the natural tilt that allows the sacrum to wedge comfortably into the ilia, supporting the spine from its foundation.

It is crucial to understand what it means to yoga *asana* cueing that the SI joints and pubic symphysis are designed for stability, not flexibility. While a slight range of motion is natural and necessary for gait and postural adjustments, intentional or exaggerated movement in these areas during yoga seats can destabilize the joints and stress the surrounding ligaments. This is especially important to remember in seated forward folds and seated twists. To work with this understanding, yoga professionals ideally cue students to move the pelvis as a single, integrated unit rather than trying to mobilize one side independently of the other. This caution preserves the structural integrity of the SI joints and pubic symphysis reduces unnecessary ligamentous strain.

Finally, with regard to the hip joints, in seated shapes that require external rotation of the femurs (e.g., Butterfly, Half Lotus, Lotus), students may encounter limitations that are not muscular but structural, determined by the depth and orientation of their acetabula. Gentle internal rotation or micro-adjustments may support a more balanced pelvic position. However, it is helpful to remind clients that openness in the hips is not solely a matter of flexibility but often a reflection of bony limits. This acknowledgment encourages respect for individual anatomy and reduces the risk of femoral leveraging from forcing an arbitrary outer shape and excessive range of motion. By cueing with awareness of the pelvic girdle's structural realities, yoga professionals can help clients find ease, stability, and spaciousness in their seated shapes and forward folds, building the foundations for a comfortable and sustainable practice.

## *Tailored Foundations for Different Seated Shapes*

Seated shapes can be categorized by the starting orientation of the hip joint; namely, some begin in neutral or adduction, while others begin in abduction:
- *Neutral or Adduction*: Shapes such as Staff (*Dandasana*), Hero (*Virasana*), and Cow Face (*Gomukhasana*) start with the hip joints either in neutral or adduction. These shapes typically allow for easier grounding of the femur to the back plane of the body through active internal rotation.
- *Abduction*: Shapes such as Easy Seat (*Sukhasana*), Bound Angle (*Baddha Konasana*), and Lotus Variations (*Padmasana*) begin with the hip joints abducted. In these positions, grounding the femoral head and achieving the anterior tilt of the pelvis may be more challenging. However, even a modest degree of internal rotational movement can significantly enhance stability and ease.

In seated yoga *asana*, the interrelationship between the demand on the hip joints, the effect on the knees, and the reverberation into the lumbar spine play pivotal roles in achieving comfort and structural integrity. The alignment of these key areas affects the ease with which the spine can maintain its natural curves, the stability of the pelvis, and the overall grounding of the shape. Grounding the weight of the torso into the tops of the femurs, just forward of the sitz bones, provides a stable foundation for most, if not all, seated shapes. This intentional distribution of weight *across the sitz bones and femurs* supports the slightly anterior pelvic tilt, which –in turn – facilitates the natural forward angle of the sacrum and the natural lumbar lordosis.

To further stabilize seated shapes, a subtle internally rotating motion of the femurs helps seat the femoral heads solidly and securely in the acetabula, allowing the pelvis to root effectively without strain. Maintaining the relationship between internal rotation and pelvic positioning is crucial to maintaining the spine's integrity, especially during long-held seated shapes, such as to support breathing or contemplative practices.

> *A note about internally or externally rotating a bone …*
>
> *Rotation is a <u>movement</u>, not a position.* A bone may be in external rotation in the joint and yet internal rotation can be engaged here. This may be largely isometric or it may move the bone in the socket more toward neutral. Ditto for a bone that is internally rotated – we can still engage an action of external rotation.
>
> This understanding can help bring more ease into seats in and of themselves; seats as a foundation for other shapes, such as twists and forward folds; and forward folds per se (not just from seated).

*Troubleshooting Seats for Appropriate Propping*

If the lumbar spine rounds or loses its lordotic curve and the pelvis cannot adjust forward due to compressive or tensile restrictions, the practitioner may need to increase the angles at the hip joints. This can be auspiciously achieved by lifting the sitz bones and tops of the femurs on a prop to allow for a more accessible forward tilt of the pelvis and restore natural spinal alignment. Soft, loose-weave cotton yoga blankets can be particularly helpful to accomplish this, with different folding variation for different seats.

- For Easy Seat, Lotus, Staff, Butterfly, and other seats grounding into the backs of the upper legs, it helps to fold and use a needed blanket as follows: Fold the blanket three times along it narrow axis to create an eighth fold; place the blanket with the folded edge facing forward. Then take the back (lose) edge of the blanket and fold it back (toward the front) to make an extra edge about 1/3 to ½ of the way into the blanket. Settle the sitz bones on the highest setting of the blanket (toward its back) and the femurs on the lower setting in the front; the rest of the legs are draping off the blanket onto the floor.
- For Hero, Diamond, and other seats grounding into the shins (i.e., with legs folded under), consider the following blanket options: Fold a blanket twice to create quarter folds; place the shins on the blanket and let the feet drape of the back. If discomfort remains in the ankles, knees, or hips, consider the following additional blanket supports, as follows:
  - *Pelvis*: If the pelvis still rounds posteriorly, add more blankets under the hips; if blankets do not suffice, add a block or bolster on the first layer of blankets and then cover it with a second layer.
  - *Ankles*: If discomfort remains in the ankle, for some individuals it may take a stack of two or three blankets for the ankles to be comfortable; it may also be supportive to take small rolled towels or washcloths under each ankle.
  - *Knees*: If discomfort remains in the knees and/or the pelvis is not in its natural anterior tilt, lean forward out of the seat to be able to slide a quarter-folded blanket into the back of the knee joints – use the hands to hold the blanket in place inside the crook of the knee joint and sit back on the calves; the blanket will bring additional height to the pelvis and a bit of release into the knee joint. Alternatively, a bolster can be placed between thighs and calves.

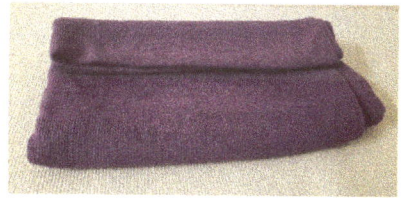 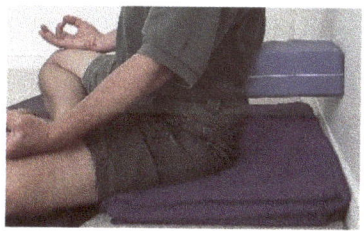 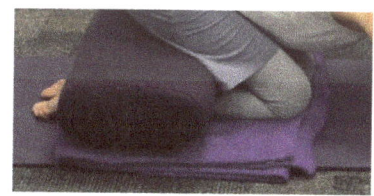

If knees are still challenged by the seat, it is important to investigate further. Healthful seated positions require a balanced link between the hip and knee joints. Limitations in hip mobility, particularly in external or internal rotation, may transfer strain to the knees in certain seated shapes. If, in Easy Seat, Butterfly, and Lotus or Half Lotus, the knees remain higher than the pelvic rim (even after propping as described above), the following added support may be helpful:
- Support the hips with yet another set of props to see if this will lower the knees any more.
- *If no*: Place props under the knees to prevent strain or injury to support them. It is fine that they are higher than the knees as long as they are fully supported. Additional folded blankets can be used for this purpose. It can also work to angle a block under the thighs – the block should not be flat on the ground as this will make the edge of the block cut into the thigh; angling the block prevents this uncomfortable pressure.

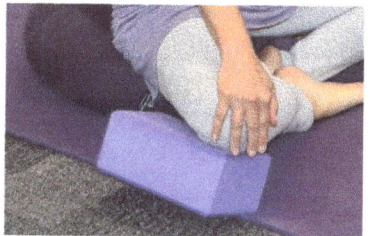 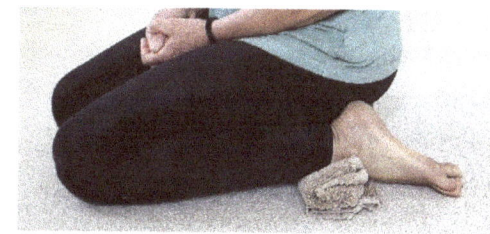

| | *Tips for Grounding, Expansion, and Stability in Upright Seats* |
|---|---|
| Grounding | • Ground through the seat, generally slightly forward of the sitz bones – notice side to side differences and ground equally; especially in asymmetrical seats (e.g., Cow Face)<br>• Ground through the heads of the femurs, feeling supported by the earth … or by the supports you are sitting on<br>• Depending on the seat, grounding may happen through the tops of the femurs (which are moving to the back plane of the body)<br>• Ground through any part of the legs touching the ground<br>• Grounding action through the hands (e.g., in staff when hands are placed on the floor behind the back)<br>• In cross-legged positions, find balanced grounding with props as needed; switch sides for equal or balanced exposure<br>• Ground into props as appropriate (e.g., under the knees; under the sitz bones)<br>• Ground through the breath<br>• Ground through the mind – dropping attention downward<br>• Ground into a settled state of mind – calming thoughts and emotions with compassion and lovingkindness |

| | |
|---|---|
| *Stability* | - Engage the core and pelvic floor muscles
- Draw the low ribs toward the top of the hips
- Engage the leg muscles, e.g., drawing knees toward chest, especially if legs are straight (e.g., Staff)
- Engage the breath
- Stabilize your attention and invite a sense of calm into the mind
- Bring the mind into the present-moment experience of the seat – as it grounds, expands, and stabilizes
- Find your inner strength
- Make intuitive adjustments to stabilize your seat
- Find joy in your inner strength and fortitude |
| *Expansion* | - Bring ease to the lumbar spine by offering a lift under the sitz bones as appropriate
- Open the angle at the hip joint to bring ease to the low back
- Lift up through the spine with each inhalation, creating spaciousness between vertebrae
- Imagine a string at the crown of the head being gently pulled/tugged toward the ceiling/sky
- Lift upward through the arms and finger tips
- Find length in the spine
- Find distance between the vertebrae
- Lift the rib basket off the pelvis
- Let the mind be expansive
- Invite lightness into your emotions |

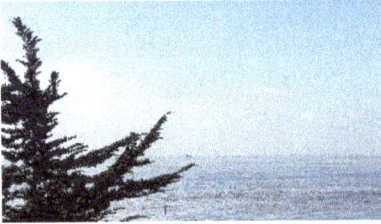

## Analysis and Experience of Sample Upright Seats

The following seats are analyzed in detail below:

- *Easy Seat*
- *Hero*
- *Staff*
- *Bound Angle*
- *Diamond*
- *Cow Face*

The cueing guidance offered for each shape needs to be considered in the context offered in the general principles for upright seats. The basics discussed above need to permeate the cueing for all these shapes. The additional cueing, shape by shape, offered here is icing on the cake. Always integrate integrated holistic yoga cueing that addresses the following teaching principles:

- *Accessibility* – creating access through variation, adaptation, affiliation, individualization, and person-centeredness
- *Intentionality* – embedding the practice of each shape in the overall arc of the session, grounding in the theme for the class and the meaning of the practice
- *Beneficence* – honoring the wellbeing of each student and always making sure to first do no harm
- *Holism* – cueing all *koshas* or layers of experience in all shapes, never forgetting that each shape has reverberations into and is affected by all *koshas* – it is not enough to cue anatomy; also address energy and vitality, thoughts and emotions, behavioral and action choices, even community and interbeing
- *Integration* – in teaching *asana*, integrate breathwork, concentration and mindfulness, as well as the ethical principles and lifestyle practices of yoga

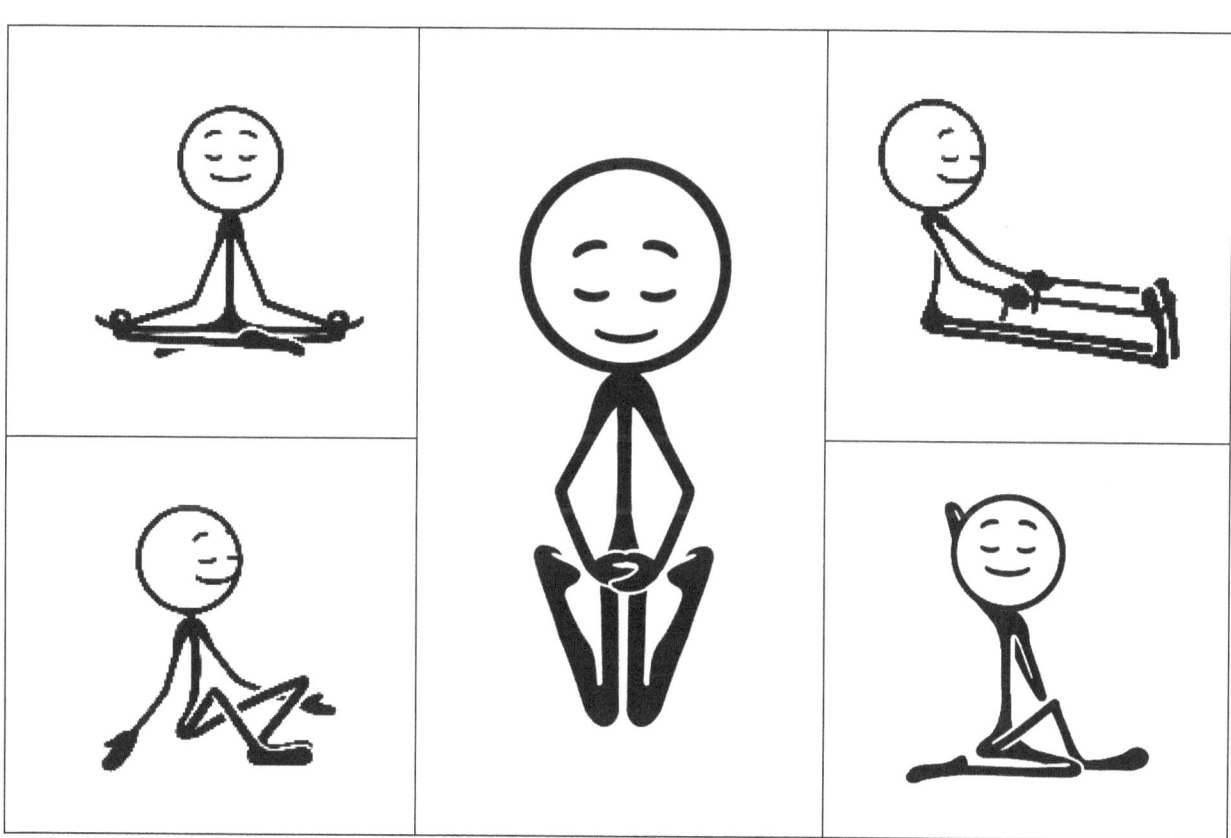

## Easy Seat or Sukhasana

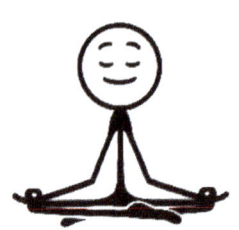

Arising from abducted, external rotated hip joints, Easy Seat is a seated shape that invites practitioners to cultivate a sense of grounding, balance, and inner awareness. This seat encourages a connection to the breath while fostering a calm and steady state of mind. Though it appears simple, this seat has much complexity and can feel demanding – which can make calling it Easy Seat ironic for some students. Each person's experience of Easy Seat may differ based on individual anatomy, mobility, and strength, especially in the slow twitch erector spinae and core muscles. Variations and adaptations may increase access to a wholesome and accessible expression of this foundational seated shape. The seat is also complex in that it demands much of the hip joints, which will move in the frontal, sagittal, and transverse planes as the shape involves hip abduction, flexion, and rotation. Through a personalized approach to Easy Seat, students can explore what feels supportive, empowering, and nurturing to them in all levels of experience – body, vitality, and mind.

### Benefits

The benefits of Easy Seat can be experienced in the physical, mental, and energetic layers of being, arising in large part from the grounded and mindful expression of this seat:
- *Creates grounding and calming*: Sitting close to the earth creates a sense of stability that can soothe the nervous system and invite a feeling of calm emotion and centered, undistracted mind.
- *Supports mindful breathing*: The open and upright shape encourages spaciousness in the abdomen and rib basket, promoting a steady, even breath and enhancing breath awareness.
- *Promotes spinal alignment and relaxation*: The shape invites the spine to find a natural lift, lengthening upward while the lower body grounds into the earth, encouraging both alignment and relaxation. Sensing into gravitational rebound creates integration between grounding, expansion, and stability.
- *Aids meditation and concentration*: The simplicity and accessibility (via props and tailored alignment) of Easy Seat make it an auspicious shape for meditation, allowing the mind to focus inward with fewer distractions from physical discomfort or efforting.

### Cautions

Although Easy Seat is generally accessible, a few considerations can help make the experience more comfortable:
- *Knee discomfort:* Sitting with the legs crossed may cause tension or discomfort in the knees, particularly for individuals with anatomy that results in less mobile hip joints. Placing a blanket or cushion under the hips and upper thighs and/or the knees themselves may alleviate discomfort (see *Variations and Exploration*).
- *Hip tightness:* Some students may feel restricted in the hips, making it challenging to sit comfortably. Sitting on a folded blanket or cushion to elevate the hips above the knees can create more ease.

- *Low back and sacroiliac strain:* If the spine collapses or rounds, it can create strain in the low back. Conversely, excessive lordosis and commensurate gripping or bracing may equally challenge posture and ease. Encourage natural pelvic and spinal alignment, and length in the spine by gently lifting through the crown of the head, and anchoring through the sitz bones and upper femurs.
- *Attention challenges:* Sitting still may be a challenge for individuals with perpetual distractibility or need for motion. Giving a focal point for attention (e.g., adding a breath observation exercise) may be helpful. Calibrated increases in length of time spent in the seat may be needed, with short 'sits' in the beginning.

## *Preparations*

Preparing the body for Easy Seat can involve movements that create mobility and ease in the hips, low back, and spine. Engaging in the six movements of the spine in a standing shape or from Table Top is a great way to start with individuals who cannot yet sit easily. These preparatory movements cultivate a sense of readiness for Easy Seat, inviting warmth and mobility before settling into stillness.
- *Hip circles:* Gentle circular movements of the legs from a standing or Table Top position to help mobilize and prepare the hip joints.
- *Gentle forward folding:* Soft forward folding while seated in a chair via a Table Top to Child flow can release tension in the low back and hips.
- *Gentle twisting:* Spinal rotations with natural movement of the pelvis, while standing or in Table Top, can create a sense of spaciousness in the torso and encourage a more upright posture.
- *Cat-Cow movements:* From standing or Table Top, flowing between spinal flexion and extension helps warm the spine and connects movement with breath.

## *Key Alignment Invitations*

Finding ease in Easy Seat often involves subtle adjustments and awareness rather than fixed alignment. The following invitations encourage a balanced and grounded shape and suggest ongoing recalibration in a mindful and present-moment manner: These alignment invitations help create a balanced, comfortable Easy Seat that emphasizes the inner experience of the shape rather than striving for a specific outward appearance. Easy Seat is most sustainable and accessible if carefully tailored to the anatomy of the student.
- *Invitations related to the legs, pelvis, and hips*:
  - *Anchor through the sitz bones and tops of the femurs:* Guide students to feel a connection to the earth through the sitz bones and tops of femurs, allowing the pelvis to rest comfortably in a natural middle-way position. If needed, suggest sitting on a folded blanket or cushion to create a slight forward tilt of the pelvis.
  - *Explore the leg position:* Invite students to experiment with how closely they bring their feet toward the body or how wide they allow the knees to fall. Comfort in the hips can often be found by adjusting the distance of the feet from the pelvis.
  - *Explore knee alignment and comfort:* The close connection between the hip and knee joints requires that attention be paid to creating comfort in the knees – avoiding torquing (the tendency for the knee joints to move beyond their natural range of motion to

accommodate restricted range of motion in the hip joints). If the knees are higher than the hips, students are encouraged to sit on a bolster, blanket, or block until the strain in the knees is gone. If the knees float off the ground, a blanket or block can be placed under them so the legs can unfold to the side without strain in the groin musculature.
- *Invitations related to the spine:*
  - *Create length in the spine:* Encourage an upward lift from the base of the spine through the crown of the head. Imagine the spine lengthening like a tree growing toward the sky while the sitz bones and tops of the femurs remain firmly rooted.
  - *Create a natural spine and pelvis:* Invite students to experiment with lumbar rounding (kyphosis) and lordosis to find the middle way adjustment of the pelvis that aligns the spine easefully in its natural curves, avoiding the extremes of collapsing vs. bracing.
  - *Softly release the shoulder girdle down:* Allow the shoulders to rest away from the ears, similar to cueing in Warrior 2 (arms resting on an imaginary shelf). This helps create space in the upper body while maintaining ease within effort. Ensure that the scapulae rest in an easeful and slightly retracted and depressed position (V-shape).
- *Invitations related to the hands and arms:*
  - *Rest the hands with intention:* Offer options for hand placement, such as resting them on the knees with palms facing up or down, or bringing the hands together in the lap or at the heart. Each placement can create a different energetic experience, which is helpful to explain.
- *Invitations related to the head and neck:*
  - *Align the head comfortably:* The head may gently lift in line with the spine, with the chin slightly tucked and drawn back, and jaws level to the ground. Encourage students to find a position wherein the neck feels spacious and free of tension. The manubrium maneuver (covered in Chapter 13, Back Bends or Heart Openers) can be helpful with neck alignment.

## *Variations and Exploration*

Easy Seat can be adapted in various ways to enhance comfort and support different physical, energetic, and emotional or mental needs. These variations provide options for exploring Easy Seat in a way that feels inviting, comfortable, and supportive.
- *Seated on a cushion, blanket, block, or chair:* Elevating the hips can reduce tension in the knees and create a more comfortable and natural position for the spine. Sitting on a chair with legs to the sides can make Easy Seat accessible to most trainees; focus is on rising up through the spine and creating comfort under the feet to make sure the knee joints are supported.
- *Using a wall for support:* For additional stability, students can sit with their back gently resting against a wall, which may help those with low back challenges. A lovely option is to sit a few inches from a wall with a yoga block between the top of the sacrum/bottom of the lumbar and the wall. The block supports the spine without eliminating core engagement and need for presence of mind.
- *Wide-legged Easy Seat:* If Easy Seat with folded legs feels restrictive or unsustainable, students may sit with their legs wider apart in a "V" shape, which can be more accessible for tight hips, especially if the pelvis is also elevated and thus supported by a blanket, bolster, or block.

*Recovery*

After practicing Easy Seat, it can be helpful to return to the same shapes offered in preparation. Additionally (and depending on overall practice arc and intention), it can be helpful to incorporate the following movements that restore balance and ease. These recovery movements help to integrate the experience of Easy Seat, providing a smooth transition from stillness to movement.

- *Seated forward folding:* A gentle forward fold from a seated position can release the hips and low back.
- *Supine twisting:* Lying down and twisting the spine can alleviate tension and stretch the back.
- *Legs-Up-the-Wall:* This restful shape promotes circulation and helps to relax the body.
- *Gentle shoulder rolls:* Releasing any remaining tension in the shoulders can help transition back to a state of relaxation.
- *Wiggles, shakes, or gentle jogging in place:* Intuitive movements that gently mobilize the entire body can be very invigorating and resetting for the nervous system after having been in Easy Seat for a while.

*Additional Teaching Tips*

To help students find ease and alignment in Easy Seat, consider these additional suggestions:

- *Invite a gentle focus on breath and breathing:* Encourage students to use the breath as a guide for finding comfort in the shape. Awareness or observation of breath and breathing can reveal areas of tension and invite presence of mind.
- *Invite exploration and play:* Remind students that there is no "perfect" Easy Seat. Encourage them to explore variations and find what feels most grounded and balanced.
- *Use props creatively:* Blankets, blocks, and cushions can create a more accessible shape for everyone, enhancing comfort and alignment. Take ample time to invite students to find prop supports that allow them to feel the ease of Easy Seat.
- *Emphasize interoception and neuroception:* Guide students to tune into the sensations in their bodies and allow these inner experiences to inform their outer shape. Cueing for a sense of safety allows students to realize the importance of physical comfort in creating emotional ease.

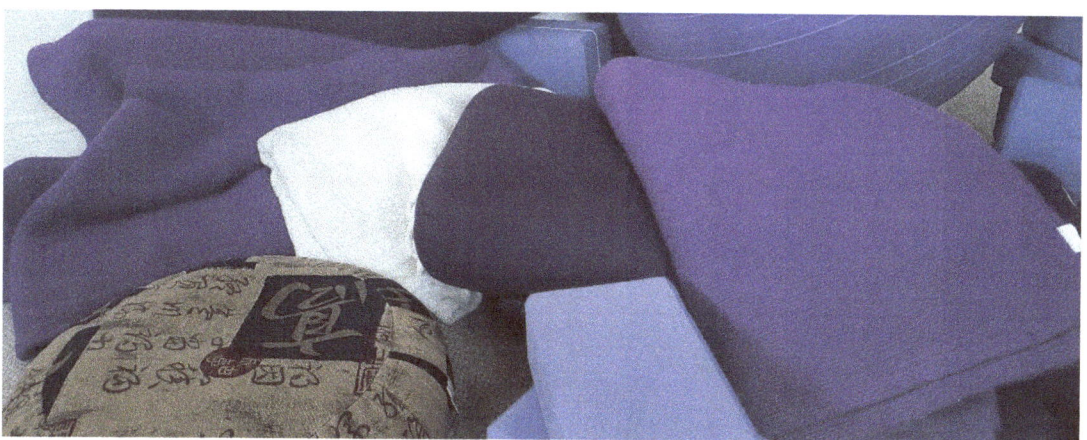

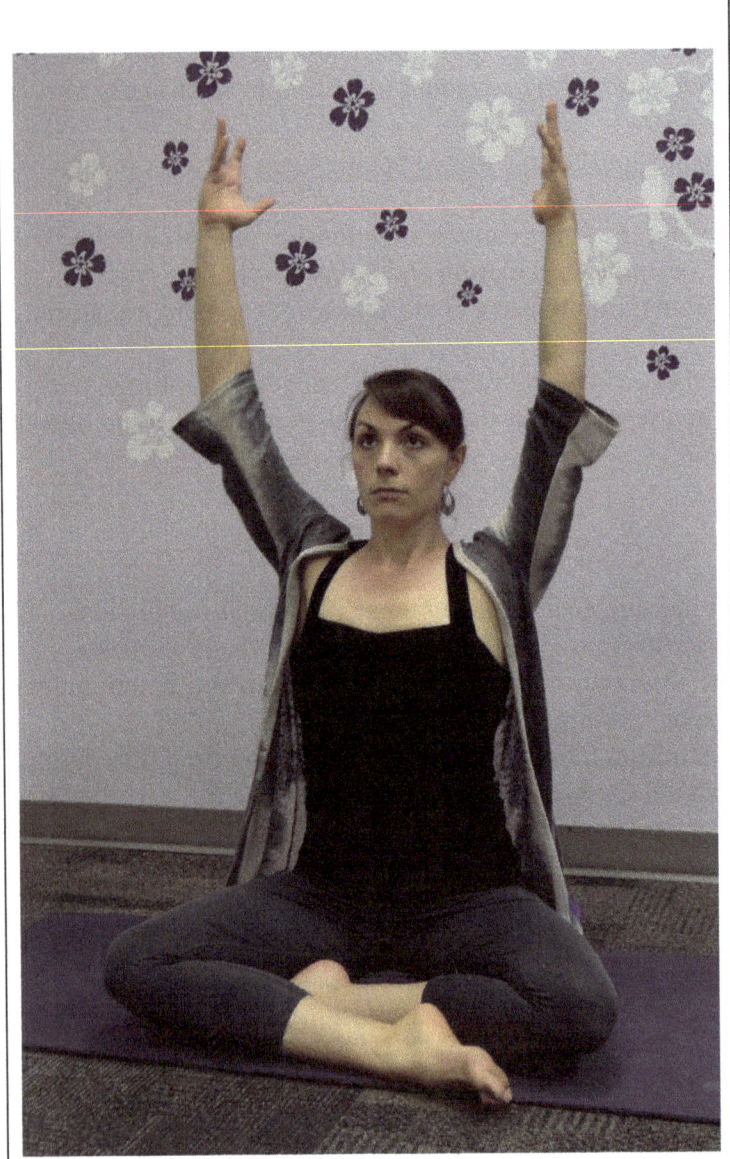

*Easy Seat with Extended Arms*
*– grounding and extending from a stable base*

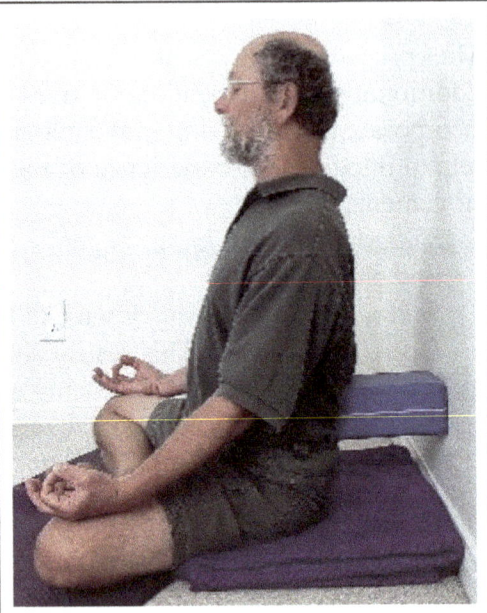

*Easy Seats*
*– embracing the support from props and walls to access presence and joy*

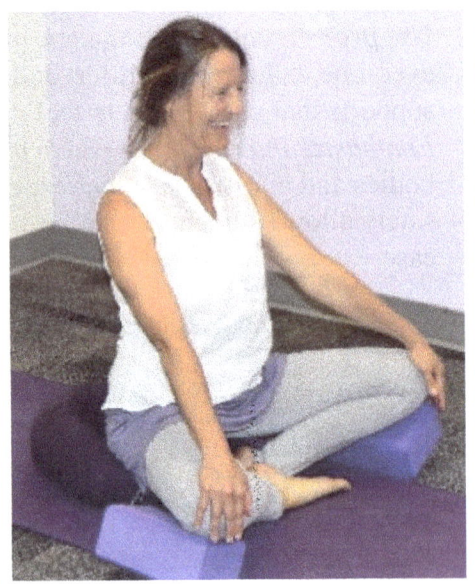

## Bound Angle Seat or Baddha Konasana

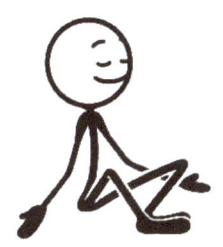

Bound Angle is a seated shape arising from hip joint abduction and external rotation that invites a sense of grounding and inward focus while creating resilience and openness in the inner thighs, groins, and hips. The experience in this shape can vary greatly depending on the unique anatomy and qualities of each body, making it important to explore different variations and approaches that support individual needs. This shape may be strongly contraindicated for individuals with a history of sexual abuse due to the open leg position. Careful use of props, such as a blanket over the entirety of the lower body, may create accessibility. However, this shape is not so essential to a yoga practice that it should become more important to access the shape than it is to help create an environment that optimizes the opportunity for the neuroception of safety.

### Benefits

The potential benefits of Bound Angle include the following, always weighed against the potential risk for individuals who have a history of sexual trauma:
- *Creating ease in inner thighs, groins, and knees*: Hip flexion and external rotation facilitate a gentle opening, which increases flexibility and comfort in these regions of the body.
- *Grounding and calming experience*: The seated shape connects the body with the earth, offering stability and a sense of rootedness.
- *Opening the inner hips*: As the knees relax outward, the inner hips have the opportunity to release tension, promoting increased mobility and ease.
- *Supporting an upright spine*: Bound Angle invites a long spine and attentive posture, encouraging mindful breath awareness and alignment.

### Cautions

Several considerations can help make Bound Angle sustainable and safe. The primary caution is psychological: sexual trauma (if known) requires consideration about the appropriateness of this shape. Additional cautions are of a physical nature and include the following:
- *Deep knee flexion and external rotation*: This shape can be challenging for knees that are not prepared for intense flexion or that are attached to hip joints with limited range of motion. If discomfort or a sense of knee torquing arises, it is imperative to use props such as blankets or blocks to support the knees and/or to access a more comfortable experience.
- *Tightness in the inner thighs or hips*: When the hips are not yet ready for significant external rotation, the sensation in this shape may feel intense. Moving the feet farther away from the pelvis may offer a gentler experience. Tight hips have limited range of motion and can create significant strain (torque) on the knees. Preparing the hips is therefore important not only as a warm-up, but also as an assessment.
- *Excessive spinal flexion*: Emphasizing a forward fold once in the seat (a common practice) is contraindicated for most students. It can create significant strain in the lumbar spine, even in the sacroiliac joints, and tends to create excess kyphosis in the spine. If a forward fold is

cued, inviting a movement of the navel toward the feet can help preserve a sense of length and openness in the torso. (also see *Cautions* for *Forward Folding* below).

## *Preparation*

Preparing the body for Bound Angle can facilitate a more comfortable and connected experience across all layers of being. Of course, an appropriate warm-up also includes the six movements of the spine. A few suggested preparations are as follows; many more exist. These preparatory movements create a sense of readiness in body, energy, and mind; they invite a more accessible experience in Bound Angle. Again, remember that great caution is necessary with individuals who have sexual trauma histories. For them, it may be physically helpful to engage in the preparations only and to leave out the complete expression of this shape altogether.

- *Hip flexion and external rotation*: Gentle movements that explore hip flexion, such as seated stretches or leg swings, can help mobilize the hips.
- *Knee flexion practice*: Moving the knees in and out of flexion, such as in a seated position, helps prepare for the deeper bend in Bound Angle.
- *Spinal movement*: Depending on the focus of the shape, preparing the spine with both extension and flexion can allow for greater ease and adaptability.
- *Easy Seat*: Sitting in a cross-legged position before Bound Angle can establish a grounded base and encourage connection to the breath. However, it can also create over-effort or strain because of the increased time period spent in abduction and internal rotation of the hip joints.

## *Key Alignment Invitations*

Subtle alignment choices can create a supportive experience in Bound Angle while fostering inward focus, in an environment of optimized opportunity for neuroception of safety for students. Bound Angle feels like a very exposed seat to some students and care needs to be taken to empower students into their own agency about how to approach the seat. Exploration and careful awareness is therefore cued in all realms: physically, energetically, and emotionally. These alignment invitations can help to create a balanced seat, focusing on inner experience rather than outer expression. Tailoring the seat to individual anatomy is key to a free flow of energy and optimizes the capacity to retain calm emotions and mental clarity.

- *Invitations related to legs and feet*:
  - *Engage from the feet up*: Bringing the soles of the feet together emphasizes a pressing into the outer edges and a releasing of the inner edges of the feet. This engagement of the feet creates stability in the legs and grounding energy in the body.
  - *Create open ease in the inner thighs*: Rolling the thighs outward (via external rotation of the hip joint) encourages a gentle release toward the floor, allowing the knees to open outward without force. Emphasize a gentle or active release of the legs rather than pressing the knees down, allowing for a natural and gradual unfolding. The goal is <u>not</u> to bring the knees to the ground; range of motion is obtained actively, not passively.
  - *Optimize ease in legs and hips*: Adjusting the distance between the feet and the pelvis allows for exploration of different depths, with the feet closer to the pelvis creating more demand and the feet farther away offering a gentler experience.
  - *Props for the knees*: Most students need a prop under the knees to find ease in this seat and to prevent straining the groin and adductor muscles.

- *Invitations related to pelvis and spine*:
  - *Honor the individual anatomy of the hip joint*: Pivoting the hips slightly toward the feet encourages movement from the pelvis, rather than focusing on the position of the knees or ankles, supporting a balanced shape. Many students do not have the range of motion in the hips to bring the knees to the ground. Thus, cueing should suggest moving within one's own joint anatomy (including using props in the most auspicious and compassionate ways).
  - *Create health in the spine and pelvis*: Maintaining a natural spine can be supported by inviting low ribs to move toward the anterior superior iliac spine and allowing the torso to extend axially, without creating hyperextension in the lumbar. Similarly, it is helpful to scan and cue interoception and proprioception for excessive rounding (flexion in the spine). Elevating the hips on a blanket or cushion may be useful to find natural spinal alignment, releasing tension in the groins, and protecting the knee joints.
- *Invitations related to upper torso, shoulders, and arms*:
  - *Rest the hands in a supportive position*: The hands may hold the feet, rest on the thighs, or support the knees in a way that feels steadying, without pressing down.
  - *Release bracing*: Letting go of gripping or efforting in the shoulder girdle allows the breath to move freely, creating a sense of ease in the upper body.

## Variations and Exploration

Bound Angle offers a wide range of variations to adapt the shape to different bodies and needs. Variations and carefully introspective explorations allow for a personalized approach, making Bound Angle adaptable for different levels of practice and comfort. The cueing of movements and explorations, rather than cueing for attaining particular outer shapes is key for Bound Angle.
- *Exploring the relationship of feet to pelvis*: Changing the foot-to-pelvis distance can adjust the intensity of the opening, with the feet closer to the pubic bone creating a stronger sensation in the hips and the feet farther away offering a gentler experience.
- *Individualizing for stability and ease*: Using a block under or between the feet can provide stability and encourage engagement in the muscles around the pelvis. Supporting the knees with blocks or blankets allows for a more comfortable experience in the hips and inner thighs, reducing discomfort in the knees. Elevating the hips on a folded blanket or bolster can help release tension in the inner groins.
- *Honoring range of motion in the hip joints*: Exploring a forward fold or reclining back on a bolster provides different sensations, with a forward fold intensifying the experience and a reclining position offering a restorative option. Forward folding is best not cued as a matter of course as it may lead to unfortunate alignment in the spine and excessively strain in the knees. It can be cued for students who have excellent interoception and proprioception and who know how to honor their body bodies' limits.
- *Restorative Bound Angle*: Using ample propping offers a calm and easeful way to continue experiencing Bound Angle, with the back supported on props so that there is an easeful leaning back into supports at optimal height to allow for extension in the hip joints without stressing the low back or sacroiliac joints.

*Recovery*

After exploring Bound Angle, deliberate movements are offered to release and restore in a manner that supports a balanced transition onward in the practice. These movements can arise from a supine position, from a seat, or even from standing. Choices of change in positioning in space depend on the arc of the class and the intention of the offering:

- *Standing shapes with movement and/or concentration:* Returning to a standing position encourages body, energy (nervous system), and mind to release and reset. This may mean standing in Mountain or engaging in wiggling, shaking, and jogging to release tension via gentle and intuitive movements.
- *Gentle twisting*: Easeful spinal rotations – supine, standing, or seated – can release tension in the low back and hip joints.
- *Lifting through the hips:* Lifting the hips from a prone position (e.g., such as in a gentle Bridge lift-and-lower) counterbalances hip flexion and rotation, as well as gently opening the front of the body.

*Additional Teaching Tips*

To help practitioners explore Bound Angle Shape with awareness and comfort:
- *Cultivate the four 'ceptions*: Invite a focus on inner sensations rather than on how far the body can move or reach, creating space for a personal experience of the shape. Invite interoception and proprioception to cultivate inner experience and agency, rather than striving for an outer shape.
- *Use props freely and with wisdom*: Offer various props and supports to encourage optimal accessibility, creative exploration, and person-centered adaptability.
- *Integrate breath awareness*: Guide the breath to bring awareness to areas of tension, release bracing, and invite the breath to create needed muscular or mental engagement.

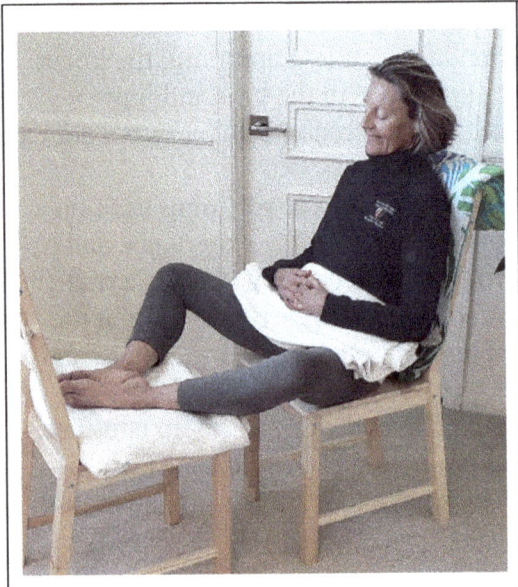 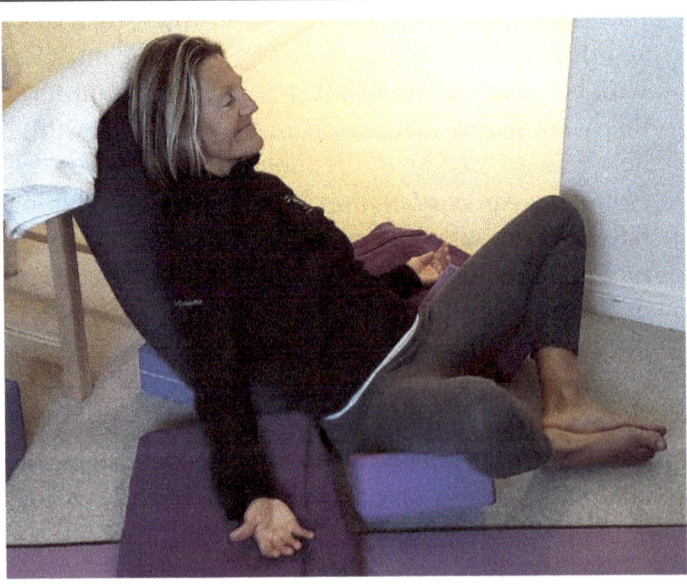

*Seated and Supported Bound Angles – embracing support and ease*

## Hero or Virasana and Diamond or Vajrasana

Hero and Diamond are grounding seated shapes that invite practitioners to connect with stability, openness, and inner strength or fortitude. Although Hero and Diamond can provide a sense of rootedness and spaciousness, they are not necessarily physically or emotionally accessible and comfortable for everyone. Creative and wholesome use of props can make these seats more person-centered, tailored to individual anatomy, energy, and mind states. The experience of Hero and Diamond varies based on individual anatomy, flexibility, and comfort, and offering variations and agency in decision-making allows students to explore these seats in a manner that feels safe, supported, and empowering. Diamond (also known as Thunderbolt) requires hip joint movement in the sagittal plane; Hero adds internal rotation (transverse plane) and slight adduction (frontal plane).

### Benefits

The benefits of Hero and Diamond extend beyond the physical, touching on mental and energetic aspects to create a balanced and wholesome experience:
- *Invite grounding and centering*: Sitting close to the earth fosters a sense of stability and rootedness, calming the mind and drawing attention inward.
- *Support resilience in the knees, ankles, and thighs*: Both seats invite mobilization and resilience, enhancing flexibility while relieving tension in these areas of the body.
- *Enhance upright posture*: With the hips settled between or on top of the feet, the spine can find a natural lift, encouraging alignment and balance in the upper body.
- *Increase breath awareness*: The open, upright shapes create space for the diaphragm and rib basket, promoting a deep connection to nasal, diaphragmatic breath.

### Cautions

Although Hero and Diamond offer many benefits, several considerations can help make their experience more accessible and comfortable:
- *Intense flexion in the knees*: Sitting in Hero or Diamond places the knees in deep flexion, which may be challenging for some. Elevating the hips on blocks or folded blankets can alleviate discomfort.
- *Tight thighs or ankles*: If the quadriceps or ankles feel tight, the stretch created in these seats may be intense. Allowing the feet to move slightly wider or placing a cushion between the calves and thighs creates more space.
- *Low back and sacroiliac strain:* If the spine collapses or rounds, it can create strain in the low back. Conversely, excessive lordosis and commensurate gripping or bracing may equally challenge posture and ease. Encourage natural spinal and pelvic alignment, gently lift through the crown of the head, and anchor through the sitz bones and upper femurs.
- *Pressure on the ankles due to plantar flexion*: If plantar flexion feels intense, a rolled blanket or washcloth underneath the front of the ankles can decrease the stretch and reduce discomfort. Sliding a folded blanket under the length of the shins, with the feet draping off the blanket can create more accessibility and ease.

*Preparations*

The six movements of the spine are always a supportive warm-up for these seats. Beyond that, preparing for Hero and Diamond can involve movements that create mobility and ease in the hips, knees, and spine. Additionally, inviting preparatory work with the feet and ankles is helpful and only limited by the teacher's or student's creativity. These preparatory movements create warmth and readiness, setting the stage for a grounded experience in both seats.

- *Flexion of the knee joint*: Gently bending and straightening the knees helps to prepare students for the knee flexion in Hero and Diamond.
- *Quad stretches*: Stretching the quadriceps from a standing or prone position helps release tension in the front of the legs.
- *Plantar flexion exercises*: Alternating the ankles through dorsi- and plantar flexion can warm up the ankles and calves, making these shapes more accessible.
- *Fancy footwork*: Any number of foot mobilizations are useful. More detailed instructions for fancy foot work can be found in https://youtu.be/eV4EHsesRIg and in Chapter Six.

*Key Alignment Invitations*

Finding ease in Hero and Diamond often requires subtle adjustments and awareness of the body's sensations. All alignment cues offered for Easy Seat will come in handy for Hero and Diamond as well. Additionally, the following alignment invitations encourage a balanced, grounded, and expansive shape that is built around each student's anatomy. These alignment invitations emphasize inner experience over outward appearance, helping students find comfort and stability in both seats. Some students will have a preference over one seat or the other; begin with the more accessible seat and slowly – over time – introduce the other.

- *Invitations related to the pelvis and legs:*
  - *Support the sitz bones in Hero*: For most students, Hero is only auspiciously accessible while sitting on folded blankets, blocks, or cushions. These supports under the sitz bones and tops of the femurs provide support for the spine and reduce strain on the knees. This adaptation elevates the hips above the knees, creating spaciousness and preserving the natural curves of the spine.
  - *Support the fronts of shins in Diamond*: For most students, Diamond is more accessible while sitting with a folded blanket under the length of the shin bones, allowing the ankles to be in less flexion and the feet to drape off the blanket. For some students, a blanket between the thighs and calves can be transformative and protective of the knee joint.
  - *Adjust the feet for comfort*: Encourage students to explore the distance between their feet, allowing them to move slightly wider apart as needed to accommodate the shape of the thighs and hips, as well as to create ample space for a prop to support the sitz bones and femurs.
  - *Release strain in the tops of the feet and ankles*: Allow the tops of the feet to rest on the mat, grounding the legs and inviting a softening in the ankles. Place a rolled-up washcloth or hand towel between the fronts of the ankles and the ground for individuals who feel excessive strain in the ankles. Bringing a folded blanket under the length of the shins and ankles, so that the feet drape off the blanket edge can be transformative for many students.

- *Invitations related to the spine:*
  - *Preserve the natural curve of the spine*: Encourage maintaining a natural spine by engaging the core and lifting through the crown of the head. A support such as a block or blanket between the feet helps maintain natural alignment.
  - *Lengthen through the spine*: Guide students to find an upward lift from the sitz bones through the crown of the head, imagining the spine reaching toward the sky and finding easeful axial extension.
  - *Gently engage the core abdominal muscles*: Subtle engagement of the deep core muscles supports the spine and prevents excessive flexion or extension in the low back.
- *Invitations related to the shoulders and arms:*
  - *Rest the hands comfortably*: Invite students to place their hands on their thighs, with palms facing up or down, or to bring hands together in their lap. This positioning influences the energetic quality of the shape, with palms facing up encouraging openness and palms facing down grounding the practice.
  - *Soften the shoulders*: Encourage the shoulders to relax away from the ears, bringing ease into the entire shoulder girdle.
- *Invitations related to the head and neck:*
  - *Place the head in line with the spine*: Allow the head to lift gently from the base of the spine, with the chin slightly tucked down and back, helping maintain a naturally aligned and tension-free neck.

## Variations and Exploration

Hero and Diamond can be widely adapted to accommodate different needs and preferences:
- *Prop between the feet:* Sitting on a block, bolster, or folded blanket elevates the hips and reduces pressure on the knees. Review prop use suggestions presented earlier in this chapter.
- *Blanket between calves and thighs:* Placing a blanket in this area creates more space in the knee joint, making it easier to sit comfortably.
- *Rolled blanket under the front of the ankles:* A rolled blanket can help decrease the intensity of plantar flexion and provide additional support.
- *Rotating the torso right and left:* Gently rotating from side to side can release tension in the spine and create a dynamic experience of the shape.

## Recovery

After practicing Hero or Diamond, consider incorporating movements that help release tension and restore balance. The following recovery movements facilitate a smooth transition from the depth of these seats to a more relaxed physical state and easeful nervous system platform.
- *Release flexion in the joints:* Moving into supine or prone positions allows the knees and ankles to relax and recover from the deep flexion, perhaps adding supine or prone windshield-wiper motion.
- *Standing with movement and/or concentration:* Returning to a standing position encourages the body to release and reset.
- *Releasing forward:* This movement, if completed with internal rotation in the hip joints, can relieve tension in the thighs and low back, allowing the body to soften.

- *Lifting through the hips:* Lifting the hips (e.g., gentle Bridge lift-and-lower) while lying on the back counterbalances the seat and gently opens the front of the body and hip joints.
- *Wiggling, shaking, and jogging:* Release tension through intuitive movements.

## Additional Teaching Tips

To help students find ease and alignment in Hero or Diamond, consider these additional suggestions:

- *Encourage breath awareness:* The breath can guide exploration in the seats, helping soften areas of tension and deepen the experience.
- *Emphasize personalization:* Remind students that these seats do not need to look the same for everyone. Invite them to find a propped shape that feels balanced and sustainable for their body and nervous system.
- *Use props creatively:* Blocks, blankets, and bolsters can support different aspects of these shapes, making them more accessible and inviting.
- *Invite interoception, proprioception, and neuroception:* Guide students to tune into their inner sensations, letting the experience inform the seats and their interactions with breath and mind rather than focusing on outward appearance and trying to meet inner expectations.

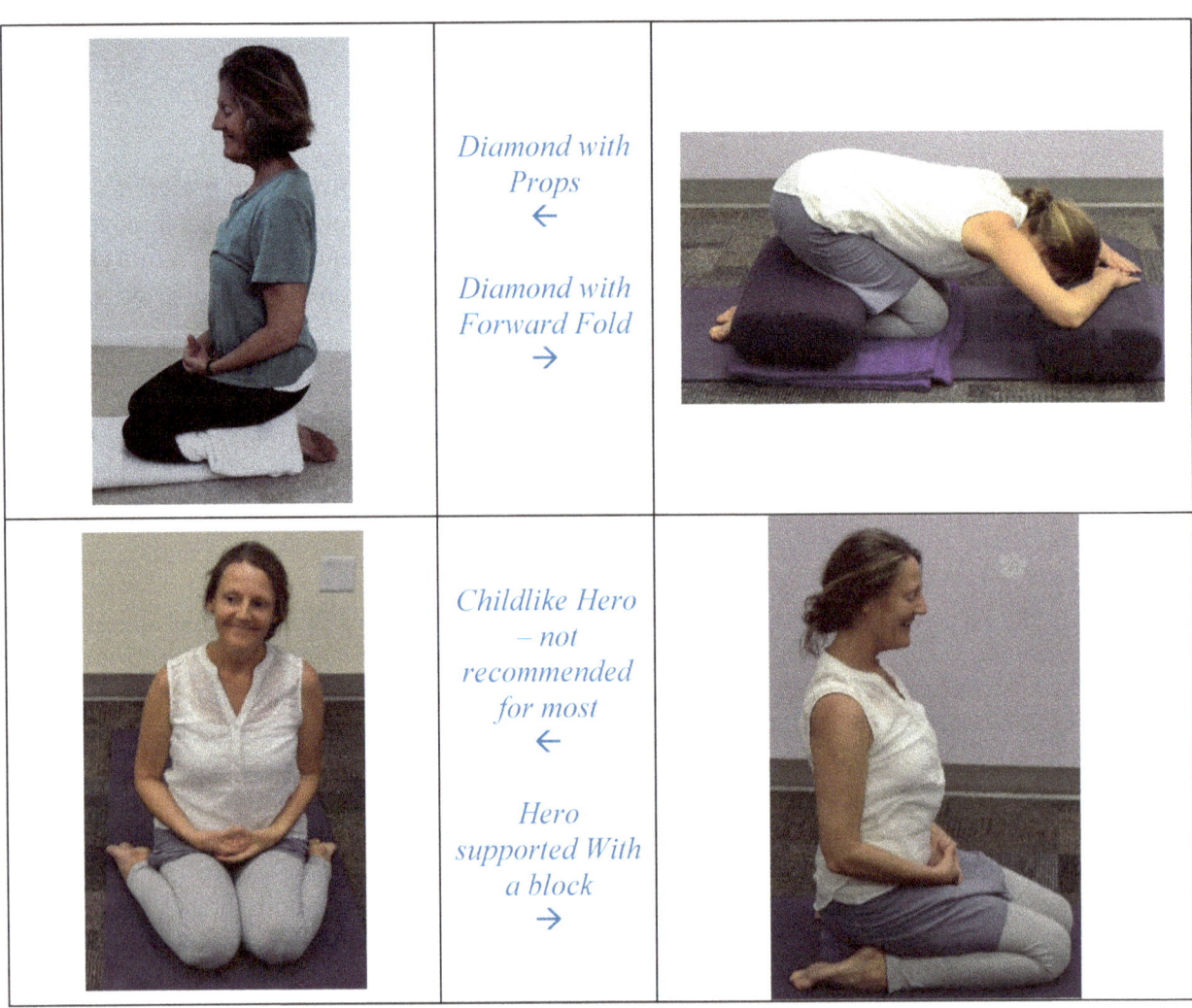

*Diamond with Props* ←

*Diamond with Forward Fold* →

*Childlike Hero – not recommended for most* ←

*Hero supported With a block* →

## Staff or Dandasana

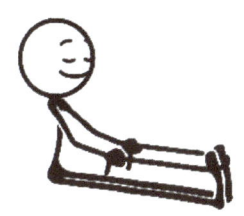

Staff is a seated shape that encourages a sense of stability and mindful alignment, fostering resilience in the legs, spine, and core. The experience within this shape can differ significantly based on individual anatomical variations, making it valuable to explore different approaches and adaptations that address individual student preferences and needs. Although it appears simple on the outside, Staff can be challenging. It is best accessed with subtle engagement and conscious awareness. Difficulties experienced in Staff often manifest in other shapes, making it a useful diagnostic tool for body mechanics and areas of tension. As is true for Diamond, Staff requires flexion in the hips (movement in the sagittal plane), without necessitating significant movements in the frontal or transverse planes.

### Benefits

Exploring Staff may offer the following benefits:
- *Establishing foundational alignment*: The engagement in the legs and core provides a stable base that can serve as a foundation for other seats, twists, and forward folds.
- *Mobilizing the hamstrings and calves*: Maintaining active legs promotes ease in these areas, encouraging resilience in the back body, especially the thighs, lower legs, and lower spine.
- *Supporting a naturally-aligned upright spine*: Staff invites awareness in the spinal column, allowing for the experience of a lengthened torso and balanced seat.
- *Enhancing core awareness*: Engaging the core muscles helps stabilize the pelvis and low back, creating a strong connection through the midline. The symmetry of the shape can contribute to sacroiliac joint strength and integrity.
- *Improving posture*: This shape strengthens back muscles and builds core strength, contributing to better posture in daily life.

### Cautions

Several considerations and cautions about common challenges help make the experience of Staff more accessible, beneficial, and sustainable. Other cautions noted in Chapter 12 about Forward Folds may also be helpful.
- *Hamstring tension*: For individuals experiencing hamstrings tightness, the pelvis tends to tilt backward, leading to excessive rounding in the lumbar spine. Elevating the hips by sitting on a folded blanket, cushion, or bolster may provide access to ease in the spine and may allow the pelvis to move into its natural slightly anteverted position.
- *Challenges in ankle mobility*: If the ankles feel tense, focusing on gently pressing through the heels of the feet may assist in lengthening the calves and creating a more comfortable seat. Working with props can be helpful (e.g., a strap around the balls of the feet – more below).

### Preparations

Preparing the body for Staff can promote a more connected experience, always preceded as appropriate by exploring the six movements of spine. Preparatory movements help create

readiness in body, breath, and mind, inviting a more accessible and stable experience in this seat. Specifically, all preparation offered for Easy Seat and Diamond and the following preparation may prove useful.
- *Hamstring mobility*: Gentle mindful movements such as leg swings, gentle standing forward bends, or seated hamstring releases can create ease in the back of the thighs. For example, practicing Downward Facing Dog against the wall may help prepare the hamstrings, inviting resilience and warmth.
- *Core activation*: Engaging in movements that bring awareness to the abdomen, such as gentle twists or small seated lifts, can prepare the core for maintaining an upright shape.
- *Spinal warm-ups*: Integrating spinal extension and rotation can allow the spine to move freely, reducing tension before sitting in Staff.

*Key Alignment Invitations*

Small shifts in alignment can create a supportive experience in Staff, allowing for individualized exploration. Working with mindfulness of inner experience, more so than outer alignment, is key to ease and wholesomeness in Staff.
- *Invitations related to the legs and feet*:
  - *Extend actively through the legs*: Invite a gentle pressing of the heels away from the body, with the toes pointing upward or flexed toward the body, to create a feeling of length along the entire leg. This can help ground the seat and bring energy up through the spine.
  - *Engage the front of the legs*: Draw the thigh muscles upward toward the hip crease while extending through the back of the legs to the heels.
  - *Ground through the sitz bones*: Feel a stable connection to the earth as the sitz bones and tops of the femurs anchor down, while extending upward through the crown of the head.
- *Invitations related to the pelvis and spine – also see cueing for Easy Seat*:
  - *Tilt the pelvis forward slightly*: Allowing the pelvis to find a slight anterior tilt may help align the spine naturally. Sitting on a blanket or cushion can be a useful way to support this alignment. Note: For hypermobile students, this cueing may not be helpful; be sure to observe and adapt invitations based on students' anatomy.
  - *Create length in the spine*: Invite a sense of reaching up from the base of the spine through the crown of the head. Rather than forcing the chest upward, imagine a gentle lifting upward of the rib basket while releasing tension in the shoulders and neck.
  - *Align the head naturally on the spine*: Tuck the chin slightly and draw back from the ears to bring the head in line with the spine (i.e., prevent forward head alignment). This subtle action can help engage the back of the neck and encourage length through the cervical spine.
- *Invitations related to the upper torso and arms*:
  - *Rest the hands mindfully*: Place the hands on either side of the hips, with the palms pressing down or the fingertips touching the floor. This connection can assist in lifting the spine and opening the heart space without excessive effort. Alternatively, if working with a strap around the feet, the hands clasp the strap and gently tug back to create engagement between the hands and feet.

- o *Release bracing in the shoulders*: Invite the shoulder girdle to relax downward. Scapulae can release naturally down and back. Releasing gripping in the shoulder girdle and torso allows the breath to move freely and promotes a sense of engaged ease in the upper body.
- *Invitations related to body proportions*:
  - o Variations in leg length, arm length, and torso length and structure can influence how Staff feels to each student. Differences in scapular positioning on the rib basket as well as tightness in legs and hips create challenges related to extending the spine fully or find ease in arm placement. Careful observation and tailored cueing can help create more easeful access to a wholesome inner experience of this seat.

## Variations and Exploration

Staff can be offered with a variety of explorations and adaptations to suit different bodies and needs. These variations provide options for exploring Staff in a manner that honors body proportions and creates alignment that feels comfortable, compassionate, and supportive.

- *Exploring support under the hips*: Sitting on a folded blanket or bolster may help individuals with tight hamstrings or low back tension to experience more comfort and stability in the shape. It can facilitate a slight anterior tilt in the pelvis, making pelvic and spinal alignment more natural and easeful.
- *Using a strap around the feet*: Holding a strap around the balls of the feet assists in creating a sense of length in the spine and legs without straining. It also encourages wholesome and mindful engagement in arms and legs as they calibrate the tension on the strap that connects them, engagement that creates easeful effort and a sense of stability.
- *Bending the knees slightly*: For individuals with significant tightness in the hamstrings, a gentle bend in the knees creates accessibility and releases strain in the low back. A prop, such as a rolled towel or soft cushion, is highly recommended to allow the knees to ground rather than float.
- *Using blocks under the hands*: Placing blocks under the hands (rather than reaching for the feet) can help elevate the upper body, supporting a natural spine. For students with long torsos, such lifts under the hands can be transformational in their experience of Staff as it will prevent slouching.
- *Lifting the arms up overhead*: To find length in the torso, the arms can lift with the inhalation and lower with the exhalation, adding a Sun Breath to the shape.

## Recovery

After exploring Staff, transitioning mindfully can restore balance and prepare the student for the next stage in the practice.

- *Seated Forward Fold with ease*: Moving into a gentle seated forward bend may help release tension in the back of the body.
- *Gentle spinal twists*: Seated or supine rotations can create ease in the spine and relieve any accumulated tension.
- *Extending the hip flexors*: Moving into shapes such as Corpse, Upward Plank, or Bridge can counterbalance the hip flexion experienced in Staff, allowing the front of the hips to release.

- *Standing movements*: Engaging in standing shapes or light movements (such as wiggling, shaking, or jogging in place) can help reset the body and bring energy back into the whole system.

## Additional Teaching Tips

To guide practitioners through Staff with awareness and care, it can be helpful to offer some of the following suggestions throughout:
- *Emphasize internal sensations*: Invite attention to how the shape feels from the inside out rather than how it looks from the outside, cultivating an experience that is unique to each individual.
- *Offer props freely*: Encourage the use of blankets, bolsters, or straps to enhance ease and accessibility in a variety of ways.
- *Integrate breath awareness*: Allow the breath to bring awareness to areas of engagement or tension, using it to create needed relaxation or focus. Opening and expanding in Staff can be connected to the inhalation; grounding and drawing inward can be cued with the exhalation.

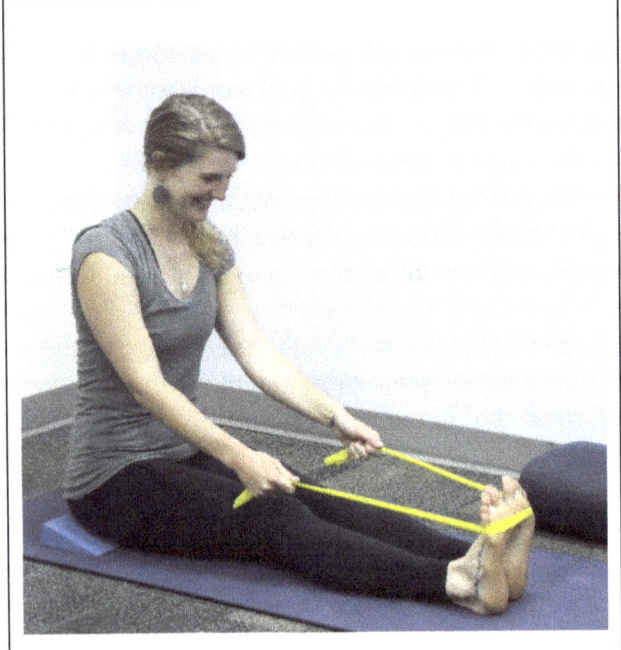
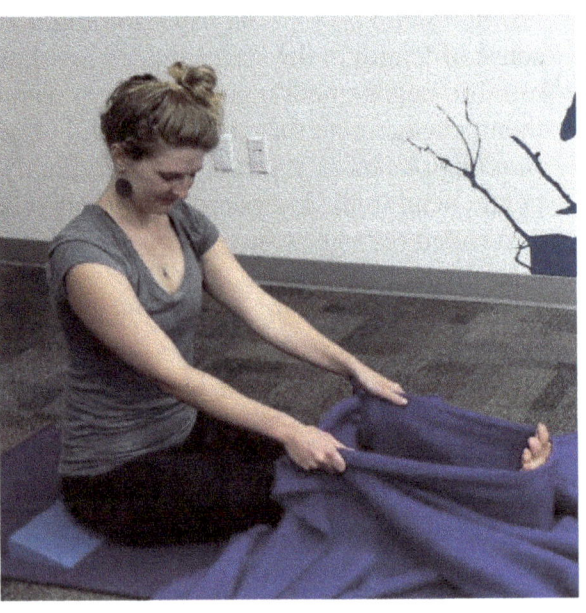

*Staff with joy and health –*
*ways of embracing the beauty of an upright seat with ease and support*

## Cow Face Seat or Gomukhasana

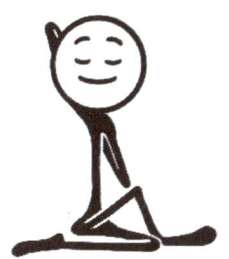

Cow Face Seat invites deep focus and connection, fostering resilience and balance in shoulders, upper back, and hips. The inner experience in this seat may vary greatly depending on each body's unique structure and needs, highlighting the importance of personal exploration via interoception and neuroception. Different variations and adaptations can help create accessibility and support a sustainable and nourishing experience. This seat requires hip joint movement in all planes with adduction (frontal plane) and internal rotation (transverse plane), as well as flexion (sagittal plane). This is a challenging seat that is to be offered with care and mindfulness.

### Benefits

Exploring Cow Face Seat offers several potential benefits, each weighed against an individual's personal needs and preferences:
- *Creating ease in the shoulders, chest, and upper back*: The shape invites gentle opening and mobilization in the shoulder girdle, promoting freedom of movement.
- *Grounding and centering*: The seated nature of the shape helps the practitioner feel rooted, encouraging a calm and steady energy while encountering challenge.
- *Supporting hip and knee mobility*: The arrangement of the legs can create ease in the outer hips, enhancing soft-tissue-related hip mobility over time.
- *Deepening resilience in various muscle groups*: The shape provides opportunity to mobilize and strengthen the hips, ankles, thighs, shoulders, armpits, chest, deltoids, and triceps.
- *Aiding chronic knee pain*: If discomfort is not acute, the leg position can help alleviate chronic knee issues by gently engaging and strengthening surrounding musculature.
- *Cultivating upright shape*: Cow Face Seat invites a naturally lengthened spine, encouraging mindful alignment supported by breath awareness.

### Cautions

Some consideration of several cautions can create an experience in Cow Face Seat that is more accessible, safer, and increasingly sustainable:
- *Shoulder sensitivity*: The positioning of the arms can create intense sensations in the shoulder joints, especially if there is existing tightness or injury. Using a strap or holding opposite elbows (as a variation) can offer a more comfortable experience. Be mindful of hyper-mobilization in the shoulder joint to prevent strain.
- *Hip and knee comfort*: Sitting in this shape may be challenging if there is discomfort in the hips or knees. Elevating the hips on a blanket or cushion can help release tension and alleviate pressure. Additionally, be cautious of torque on the knees if the hips are less mobile.

### Preparation

Preparing for Cow Face can support a more easeful and connected experience. A balanced warm-up is beneficial, incorporating the six movements of the spine. Proper preparatory

movements can establish a sense of readiness and presence, creating access to an experience in Cow Face that honors individual needs. Some suggested preparatory practices include:
- *Shoulder mobilization and strengthening*: Incorporate upward and downward mobilization of the scapula to create resilience in the shoulder girdle. Arm circles of all shapes and sizes, and in all directions offer great preparation for the glenohumeral (shoulder) joints, which have to move in complex ways in this seat.
- *Hip mobilization and strengthening*: Movements such as seated hip circles, low lunges, or dynamic hip openers can help create ease and strength in the hips. Standing shapes with a prop between the legs can help prepare the adductors and internal rotators. As tight hips can mean more strain on the knees, preparing the hips is important not only as a warm-up, but also as an assessment for how much strain may be placed on the knees in case of limited hip range of motion.
- *Spinal extension and rotation*: Gentle backbends or twisting shapes may help foster spinal mobility and prepare for an upright seat. Some of the heart-opening preparations offered in Chapter 13 can be helpful

## Key Alignment Invitations

Subtle alignment choices can support an inward focus of the mind in Cow Face, creating an environment in which practitioners can explore their unique experiences in body, energy, and psyche. Giving individualized alignment cues based on observation, exploration, and the four 'ceptions helps focus students on inner sensations, supporting a mindful approach that honors individual anatomy. As for all one-sided shapes, Cow Face is repeated on the opposite side.
- *Invitations related to the legs and hips:*
  - *Explore the positioning of the legs*: Both knees will be in flexion, one tucked under the other, with feet draping out to the sides. Ankles can be placed in the manner that feels most grounding and supportive to individual students. Mindfully exploring and adjusting the arrangement of the legs is crucial to identifying individually how to access optimal ease in the hips. The bottom leg may be extended and supported under the knee with props as appropriate for students' anatomy.
  - *Release tension in the outer hips*: Allowing the outer hips to soften toward the ground can create a sense of stability, rather than pressing the legs down forcefully.
  - *Elevate the hips for ease*: Sitting on a folded blanket can release tension in the knees and hips, promoting a balanced and supported seat.
  - *Add gentle with internal rotation of the hip joints*: Flex and adduct the legs to create resilience, engaging the adductors to stabilize the shape. Internal rotation in the hip joint supports adduction and is helpful if a forward fold were to be added to the seat (which is neither necessary nor appropriate for all students).
- *Invitations related to the shoulders and arms*:
  - *Engage the arms mindfully*: The arm on the same side as the top leg reaches up, externally rotating (thumb facing upward to the sky, like in hitchhiking) and at maximum flexion, bending at the elbow to reach toward the nape of the neck; finger tips point toward the floor. The other arm moves forward and creates internal rotation (thumb pointing down to the floor) and then bends at the elbow to bring the hand toward the back body at the middle of the thorax, in between the scapulae.

- *Adapt an arm position that supports shoulder health*: Contact may be made between the hands, or a strap can be used to bridge the gap between the hands. Using a strap between the hands or holding opposite elbows behind the back can create a more accessible experience, fostering ease in the shoulders.
- *Release bracing in the shoulder girdle*: Encourage the release of any gripping or tension in the shoulders, allowing the breath to move freely and creating a sense of spaciousness in the upper body.
* *Invitations related to the spine and torso*:
  - *Maintain a natural and energized spine*: Invite the torso to lengthen upward with axial extension, encouraging a balance between grounding and spaciousness.
  - *Support natural spinal curves*: Elevating the hips may be helpful for natural spinal alignment, preventing excessive rounding (flexion) or arching (extension).

## Variations and Exploration

Cow Face offers several explorations that can invite different bodies into the practice and encourages students to identify healthful variations. Exploring these variations allows for a tailored experience in Cow Face, emphasizing inner awareness over achieving a specific outer shape.
* *Exploring arm positions*: Using a strap between the hands or holding opposite elbows can provide support if the limbs do not comfortably reach each other behind the back. Prayer hands behind the back can offer another entirely different arm variation.
* *Adjusting the legs and hip height for comfort*: Extending the bottom leg forward, or using a bolster under the hips, can alleviate discomfort in the knees and hips.
* *Entering the shape from Table Top*: Practitioners can come into Cow Face from a Table Top position by crossing the legs at the knees and spreading the feet to sit back between the hips, which may help align the knees more easily. For some students this leads to knee torquing because of the power of gravity; thus, mindfulness is key.
* *Creating movement in the shape*: Gently shifting weight from side to side or subtly moving the arms can create resilience in the shoulders and hips.
* *Folding forward*: For students with ease in the hips, spine, and knees, a gentle Forward Fold can be explored in this seat. This is neither necessary nor appropriate for many, if not most, students. Personalized offerings are importantly based on observation by the teacher and interception by the student.
* *Side switching*: A funky way to switch sides is to plant the feet and lift the bum to circle to the side where the top foot is grounded. Make a full circle and release down. The legs have switched sides.

## Recovery

After Cow Face, gentle transitions can help restore balance and support a smooth transition to the next stage of the planned practice:
* *Releasing the shoulders and arms*: Gentle and mindful movements such as shoulder circle rolls or clasping the hands behind the back can help release residual tension in the shoulders.
* *Extending the hips and knees*: Gentle movements to extend the hips and knees can alleviate lingering tightness and creating ease after the seated position.

- *Returning to standing*: Standing shapes such as Mountain can help reset body, energy, and mind, creating grounding and closure. Wiggles, shakes, intuitive movements, and jogging in place may also be offered to invite students into a more playful recovers in all joints.
- *Lifting into Bridge*: This front body opening movement can help release tension in the hip joints and ground the shoulder blades.

Additional Teaching Tips

To encourage a mindful exploration of Cow Face:
- *Focus on inner experience*: Invite attention to the sensations within the body rather than on achieving a particular outer shape. Remind students to work from the inside out, not the outside in. Inward-focused cueing approaches create a welcoming space for each practitioner to engage with the seat in a way that feels kind and accessible.
- *Use props thoughtfully*: Offer various props to support ease and exploration. Demonstrate the seat with props to indicate that prop use is a sign of self-compassion and wisdom.
- *Guide breath awareness*: Encourage students to remain connected to the breath as a means of self-monitoring over- or under-efforting, and as a way to release tension and support engagement as needed.

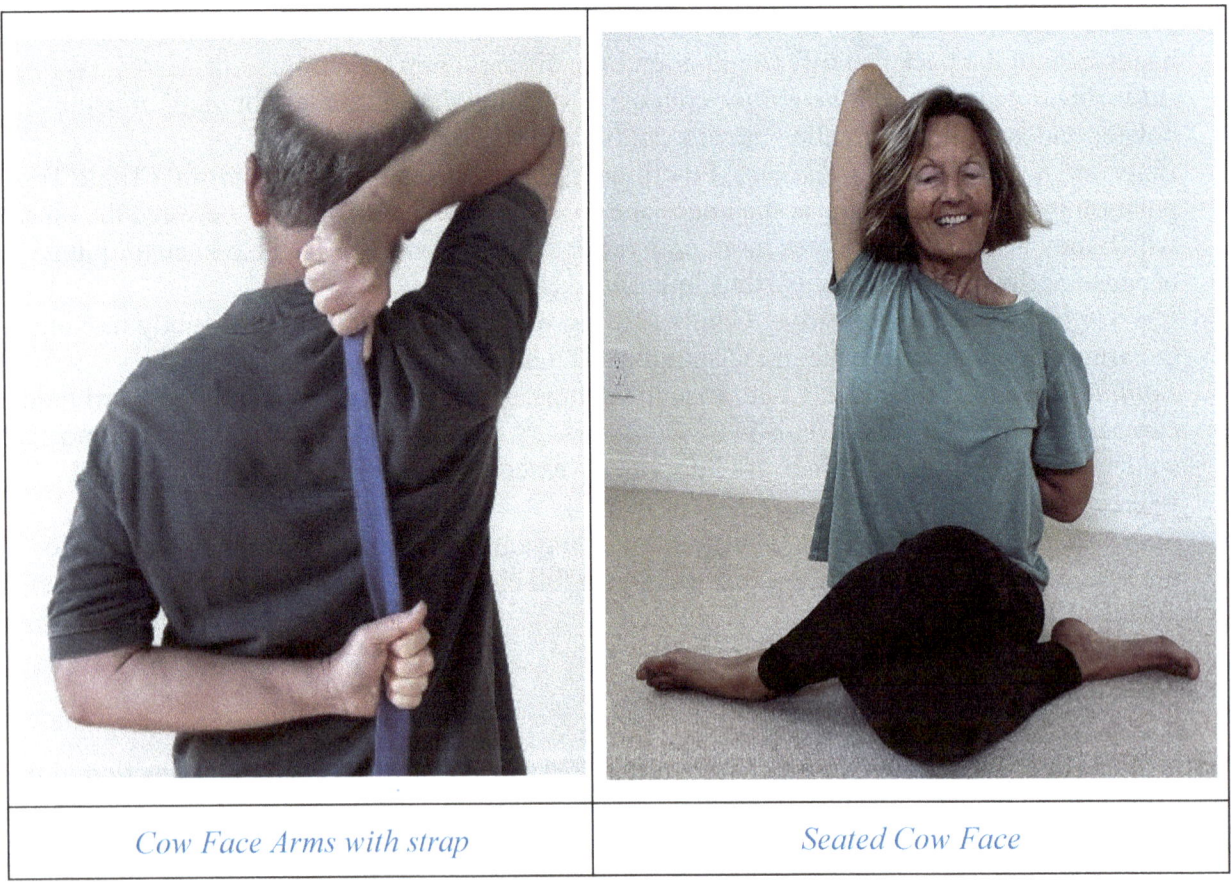

Cow Face Arms with strap | Seated Cow Face

## Chapter 11: Twists or Rotations

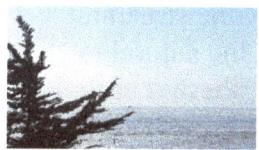

This chapter covers foundational twists and rotations, offering optimized teaching strategies that allow for individual tailoring and careful discernment about how and which shapes to offer, as well as about how to cue alignment informed by interoception, proprioception, exteroception, and neuroception. General principles for this category of yoga *asana* are provided and apply to most if not all twisting shapes. Specific follow-up guidance is added for the chosen sample shapes. Twists can unfold from standing, arm standing, and sitting. All guidance in Chapters 8 to 10 remains highly relevant and applicable – even if it is not explicitly repeated here.

Notably, this chapter begins to shift the focus from yoga *asana* as understood in terms of creating foundations – either through the feet, hands, or seat – to a focus on how shapes unfold in the various planes of movement – frontal, sagittal, and transverse. The complexity of shapes is greater and instruction is more dependent on creating attention to healthful preparation for these shapes and on understanding their specific demand characteristics.

### Anatomical Foci in Twists or Rotations

Twists or rotations move the anatomical focus beyond the natural spine and its movements in the sagittal plane. Rotations typically introduce complexity simply by adding movement in the transverse and frontal planes. They demand a sophisticated interplay of stability and mobility in the spine and pelvic region, with keen attention to creating stability in the sacroiliac region (where weight or load transfer takes place from the upper to the lower body). Simultaneously, twisting requires mobility in the upper portions of the spine with careful coordination of movement in the legs, hips, and all the joints along the path.

Twisting shapes rely on coordinated engagement of the deep spinal rotators, abdominal obliques, and muscles of the pelvic and shoulder girdles to create rotational force while maintaining spinal and pelvic integrity. Effective twisting is not solely a matter of muscular engagement; it also requires a balanced distribution of rotational force, where torque in one segment is buffered by adaptive stability in adjacent structures. Learning to initiate twists from the thoracic and cervical spines is key as these are the spinal region with the greatest access to rotation.

It is important to understand that the notion of anchoring the pelvis is not helpful. Instead, the anatomical focus in this spinal region is on movement of the pelvis as a whole unit for which mobility is supported by resilient hip joints, intuitive movements in the knees and legs, and a commitment to invite the necessary mobility into the lower appendicular skeleton that supports stability in the sacroiliac joints. Understanding this pattern and distribution of movement fosters safer, more sustainable practice, enhancing both structural stability and functional fluidity in twisting *asana*.

## Natural Spine and Pelvis

Twisting shapes are deeply informed by the structural and functional realities of the spine's segmented architecture. Understanding the natural range of motion (ROM) in each spinal region is crucial for safety and effectiveness in these shapes. It also deeply informs cueing and alignment guidance.

*Cervical Spine (C1-C7)*: The cervical spine possesses the greatest capacity for rotation among the spinal sections, with an average of 80–90 degrees of movement. Most of this rotation occurs at the atlanto-axial joint (C1-C2), commonly referred to as the '*no*' joint. This high degree of mobility allows for significant head turning, an evolutionarily adaptive capacity as it supports fast head movements in response to vigilance and identification of risk or danger. Nevertheless, in yoga *asana* practice it is generally useful to initiate twists from the thoracic spine first, allowing the neck to follow as a *secondary action*. Premature or isolated cervical rotation often results in over-reliance on neck musculature for range of motion and can disrupt the integrity of the twist. For this reason, it is generally helpful to let the neck move last, ensuring that rotational force is evenly distributed across the thoracic and cervical regions.

*Thoracic Spine (T1-T12):* The thoracic spine is structurally designed to support twisting, with an average ROM of 30–45 degrees. Its capacity for rotation is facilitated by the orientation of its facet joints, which are angled to permit rotational movement while still providing structural stability. This makes the thoracic region the primary agent of rotational movement in twisting shapes. Practitioners can helpfully focus on mobilizing this area to initiate twisting motions in the spine, promoting healthy segmental rotation that does not compromise lumbar health or sacroiliac stability.

*Lumbar Spine (L1-L5):* The lumbar spine has very limited capacity for rotation, typically between 10–15 degrees in total. This is due to the vertical orientation of its facet joints, which prioritizes flexion and extension while strongly resisting axial twisting. Notably, the lumbar region achieves its minimal rotation most effectively when it is in its natural lordotic curve; excessive lumbar extension and/or lumbar flexion further restrict its capacity to rotate (try the practice offered in the Box below). Forcing rotation in the lumbar region leads to compensatory strain, either in the intervertebral discs or in neighboring structures, especially the sacroiliac joints. Effective twisting practices encourage stabilization in the lumbar area rather than forced rotation, redirecting movement to the more rotationally capable thoracic spine.

> *Exploring twists while the spine is in lumbar extension versus flexion:*
>
> - *Test 1*: Sit in a slouch and twist to one side
> - *Test 2*: Now sit with a natural lordosis in lumbar spine and try again
>
> *What did you notice?*
> Typically, the second version will feel much easier as lumbar lordosis supports ease of rotation all the way to the cervical spine.

*Sacrum:* The sacrum is fused to the pelvis and does not independently participate in rotation, flexion, or extension. Movement at the sacroiliac (SI) joints is minimal and primarily consists of slight nutation and counternutation during flexion and extension of the pelvis, as well as gently yielding to the movements necessary for locomotion (with at most 1-2 millimeters of play in this joint). Twisting shapes *must honor* the structural reality of stability in the SI joints. This is achieved by facilitating rotational movement through the thoracic spine and allowing the pelvis to move as a whole unit, supported by resilience and natural movement in the hip joints and legs. Anchoring of the pelvis is a bad idea and is addressed in more detail below given the high risk for injury that can result over time from femoral leveraging and lumbar or sacral corkscrewing.

| Summary of Ranges of Motion by Spinal Regions | | | |
|---|---|---|---|
| Type of Motion | Cervical Spine | Thoracic Spine | Lumbar Spine |
| Rotation | 80-90° | 30-45° | 10-15° |
| Lateral Flexion | 45° | 45-50° | 20-45° |
| Flexion | 50-55° | 50° | 60-90° |
| Extension | 60° | Limited | 30° |

*Natural Pelvis*: The pelvis, composed of the ilia, sacrum, pubis, and ischial tuberosities (sitz bones), serves as the architectural foundation for the natural alignment of the spine. This basin-like structure is uniquely designed to move as a unified whole, a biomechanical reality that is mediated by its key articulations: the pubic symphysis anteriorly and the sacroiliac (SI) joints posteriorly. A naturally aligned pelvis, characterized by a slight anterior tilt, provides the optimal base for the natural curves of the spine to emerge without strain or distortion. In this position, the sacrum is angled slightly forward, supporting lumbar lordosis and evenly distributing load through the SI joints and hips.

Maintaining this subtle anterior orientation of the pelvis is important to understand, as ill-timed deviations into excessive anterior or posterior tilt disrupt the kinetic chain, leading to compensatory tension along the spinal column and altered force distribution in the hip joints. The positioning of the pelvis reverberates upward, influencing the spinal curves and the relationship between the thoracic and cervical regions. In seated twists, grounding through the *tops and backs of the femurs* rather than relying on the sitz bones preserves natural pelvic alignment, preventing posterior tilt *and* facilitating more authentic spinal rotation. Similarly, in standing twists, *internally rotating and grounding the tops of the femurs toward the back plane of the body* stabilizes the pelvis as a whole, creating the structural integrity needed for fluid, uncompromised rotation up the spine.

## Anatomical Principles for Sacroiliac Joint Health in Twists

The sacroiliac (SI) joints serve as crucial points of load transfer between the upper and lower body, functioning much like the keystone of an arch that preserves structural integrity under pressure. Positioned where the sacrum (i.e., the base of the spine) meets the ilia (i.e., the lower appendicular skeleton), these joints are designed for stability over mobility (via a robust network of strong ligaments, discussed in Chapter 5), allowing minimal movement to absorb and distribute forces while maintaining the continuity of the kinetic chain. Understanding the stabilizing role of the SI joints is crucial to healthful cueing for motion and alignment in twisting shapes. It is key to avoid undue strain at the SI joints, ensuring stability and functional alignment, as well as the *prevention of several risky movements* in the SI region that sadly are commonly invited in yoga practices.

Contrary to common misconceptions in some yoga teaching methodologies, sacroiliac pain is more often due to laxity rather than limited mobility. Encouraging excessive mobility in the SI joints as a remedy for discomfort often exacerbates the issue by further destabilizing the joints. When ligaments around the SI joints become lax, whether due to hormonal changes, repetitive strain, or inappropriate cueing during twisting shapes, the self-locking mechanism of the joints is compromised. This mechanism is what allows the sacrum to wedge securely between the ilia, transferring weight efficiently from the trunk to the lower limbs. When ligamentous integrity is lost, the sacrum is permitted to shift or rotate within the ilia, a destabilizing movement that places additional strain on already compromised ligaments. This action creates a vicious cycle of instability, inflammation, and chronic pain, often misdiagnosed as a lack of flexibility rather than the actual underlying hypermobility.

Biologically female pelvises are particularly vulnerable to SI joint dysfunction due to three key anatomical and physiological factors. First, hormonal fluctuations (particularly those associated with pregnancy and the menstrual cycle) can temporarily increase ligamentous laxity, compromising joint stability. Second, the wider distance between the acetabula (hip sockets) in female pelvises introduces greater leverage on the SI joints during weight-bearing and rotational movements. Finally, the contact surfaces between the ilia and sacrum are smaller in female pelvises, with only two segments of the sacrum articulating with the ilia, compared to three in the biologically male pelvis. This reduced surface area decreases the capacity for secure locking, making careful attention to SI stability in twisting shapes even more essential for biologically female students.

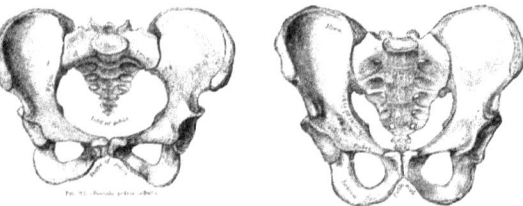

**Figure 2.12** Biologically female and male pelvises, demonstrating differences in distance between acetabula and size of SI joint. (Data source: Henry Vandyke Carter; https://commons.wikimedia.org/wiki/File:Comparison_human_male_and_female_pelvis.png;. public domain)

To support SI joint health in twisting practices, it is important to allow the pelvis and sacrum to move as a single, unified structure. Twisting forces are directed primarily through the thoracic spine rather than forced into the lumbar region, which naturally resists rotation. Additionally, spinal rotation is initiated above L1 to protect the iliolumbar ligament, which spans from L4 or L5 to the iliac crest and is particularly vulnerable to strain if twists are attempted too low in the spine. Optimal load-bearing for the sacrum and SI joints occurs when the sacrum maintains a 30–40° angle relative to the ilia. This angulation creates a wedging effect, where the weight of the trunk presses the sacrum firmly into the ilia, enhancing the self-locking stability of the joint. If this wedging action is disrupted by counternutation of the sacrum (such as through exaggerated posterior pelvic tilting or '*tucking the tailbone*'), the SI joints are effectively *unlocked*, inviting instability and increased risk of dysfunction.

Finally, awareness of the distinctions between sacroiliac dysfunction (rotational imbalances of the sacrum within the ilia) and iliosacral dysfunction (malalignment of the ilium relative to the sacrum) can inform more effective practice and safer twisting patterns. Periodically resetting the SI joints before and after twisting sequences can be a proactive measure to support long-term joint health and prevent cumulative strain (see *Box* below for a suggested practice).

> **Sample Practice for Resetting the SI Joints**
>
> *Props needed: a yoga block and strap (make a small loop)*
>
> ### Part 1
> - Settle into a comfortable supine position (as you would to prepare for Bridge)
> - Place the block sideways between the legs (to create the smallest distance between the legs; somewhat narrower than the hip joints), so it touches the thighs and calves but not the knees
> - Squeeze the whole legs (not just the knees) toward each other into the block; there may be a dragging sensation on the lateral arch of the foot – squeeze, hold, and release 7 to 10 times with the breath
> - Repeat with the block on the middle setting (i.e., legs a bit farther apart, about the distance of the hip joints); continue to make sure are not just squeezing in the knees; shift the whole legs inward (into adduction) – repeat 7 to 10 times
> - Repeat with block at the widest setting, legs a bit wider than the hips – repeat 7 to 10 times
> - Move to Part 2, staying in the same supine position
>
> ### Part 2
> - Shift the block to the narrowest setting again; take the strap loop and loop it over the knees and down the legs a few inches, cinching it so that it makes a taut hold with the legs at the narrow-block distance; remove the block
> - Press the whole legs (not just the knees) out against the strap; there may be a dragging sensation on the medial arch of the foot – press, hold, and release 7 to 10 times with the breath
> - Repeat with the strap loosened an inch or 2, so the legs are about hip distance apart; continue to press out the whole legs, not just the knees
> - Repeat with the strap loosened a bit more, legs slightly wider apart than the hip joints
>
> Neutralize, if necessary, with a few small range-of-motion Windshield Wipers (i.e., do not aim to reach the floor!) and natural-spine Bridge lifts (i.e., lift hips and torso straight up – this is not a backbend)

## *Protecting the Sacroiliac Joints in Twists*

Effective and sustainable twisting in yoga relies on understanding the anatomical realities of the sacroiliac joints and the primary risks associated with their destabilization. The SI joints are inherently designed for stability, not mobility; their primary role is to bear and transfer load between the upper body and the legs through the pelvis. In twisting, improper cueing or forced alignment can disrupt this stability, leading to strain, inflammation, and chronic discomfort. There are three main sources of risk to the SI joints in twisting *asana*: femoral leveraging, spinal leveraging, and lumbar or sacral corkscrewing. Understanding these mechanisms is essential for safeguarding the SI joints and promoting long-term spinal health.

### *Femoral Leveraging*

The first major risk to the SI joints arises from twists that involve femoral leveraging, a mechanical prying action where the femurs act as levers against the pelvis. The shape, depth, and orientation of the acetabulum (hip socket) and the angle of the femoral neck dictate the natural range of motion (ROM) in the hip joint across all planes of movement. When students or clients attempt to move beyond the natural ROM of their hip structure (e.g., as is common in wide-legged standing shapes like Warrior 2 or Triangle, where one femur is internally rotated and the other externally rotated) excess force is leveraged into the SI joints. This leverage can create excessive compression between the sacrum and the ilium on one side and excessive gapping on the other, disrupting SI stability. The twisting motion in Warrior 2 happens entirely in the thoracic and cervical spines.

To mitigate this risk, it is crucial to stabilize the SI region first and then explore the ROM of the femur within the acetabulum. Healthy cueing emphasizes that there is no universal foot or leg placement – instead deeply honoring individual variations in hip anatomy. Students are cued to move in concordance with their natural hip range of motion and *never to force* the pelvis to square off against the constraints of the femoral head in the acetabulum. In a Warrior 2, typically this means that the pelvis aligns in a diagonal, rather than ever being parallel to the edge of the mat (a *very poor cue* for alignment in Warrior 2 or Triangle).

### *Spinal Leveraging*

The second significant risk to the SI joints in twisting shapes is spinal leveraging, which occurs when the spine is forced into rotation without accommodating natural pelvic movement. This is particularly evident in shapes such as Triangle (*Trikonasana*), where the legs are positioned in multiple planes (abducted, flexed, and rotated), while the spine is simultaneously rotated and laterally flexed. The SI joints, in this scenario, are asked to stabilize contradictory forces without the ability to redistribute strain effectively. For this reason, Triangle creates biomechanical demands that exceed what SI joints can tolerate and is a direct threat to SI integrity – a risk that is completely unnecessary since Triangle taught in this way has no functional utility in daily life.

### *Lumbar Corkscrewing*

The final, and perhaps most insidious, risk to the SI joints is lumbar or sacral corkscrewing, or torquing. This phenomenon occurs when rotational forces are directed into the lumbar spine, which has very limited capacity for axial rotation (10–15 degrees across all segments). When the pelvis is rigidly fixed during seated twists or instructed to remain level during standing twists, the lumbar spine is forced to absorb the rotational demand. This not only stresses the intervertebral discs but also creates a torquing effect downward into the sacrum which is then corkscrewed inside the ilia, destabilizing the SI joints.

To avoid this, twisting shapes need to be cued in such a way as to permit the *pelvis as a whole* to rotate in the direction of the twist. This is a biomechanically natural action that is further supported by natural movements in the hips and legs, such as allowing the pelvis to lean into the twist and the knees to bend (see *Box* about natural movement in twisting below). In seated twists, the hip opposite the twist is set free to move slightly forward and up or down, and the buttock away from the twist may even lift off the ground. This ensures that the twist is initiated and sustained by the thoracic spine, where the capacity for rotation is greatest, while the pelvis and sacrum move as a single, stable unit. In standing twists, the side away from the twist is encouraged to drop down and back rather than being forced into level alignment. Knees can flex and extend naturally. These natural movements prevent rotational strain on the lumbar spine and allow the pelvis as a whole to move congruently with the twist. They are a perfect basis for healthful functional rotational movements in daily life.

*Experience natural twisting*

- Stand in Mountain and flow through a few Mountain/Extended Mountain *kriyas* to mobilize the spine a bit
- Imagine a high shelf in front of you – a bit taller than you and slightly off to one side
- Pretend you are reaching for something on that shelf, letting your body move completely naturally
- Repeat a few times with a great sense of ease and without effort; do this on both sides

*What did you notice?*

In a natural rotation, the pelvis moves as a whole. You may have noticed that quite naturally, your whole body became involved in the twist; if the twist was to the left:

- Your right arm reached up and across
- The right hip reached forward and up, while the left hip naturally moved back and down
- The right knee may have bent slightly
- The left leg may have become quite strong in the knee joint and may bear more weight than the right

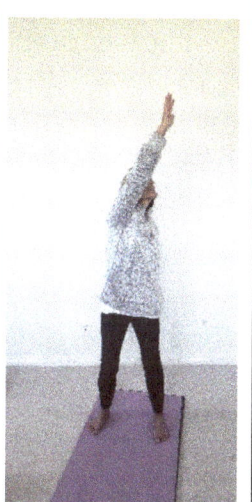
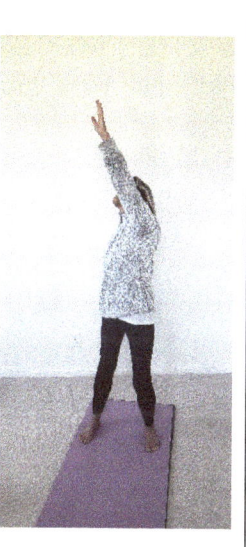

## A Few Final Asides About Twists

### Active Versus Passive Movement

In addition to the above guidance, another crucial aspect to healthy twisting lies in initiating the movement into rotations from the core muscles, the obliques, transverse abdominis, multifidus, and deep spinal rotators, even pelvic floor and back musculature, instead of relying on passive force or torque from the arms. When twists are driven by core engagement, the spine and pelvis rotate harmoniously, preserving the integrity of the lumbar and sacroiliac regions. Over-reliance on the arms to move into a twist leads to overpowering the musculature of the core and spine, resulting in destabilization and strain (often due to sacral corkscrewing). Generally speaking, active movement, during which muscles are consciously engaged to effect a movement (in this case spinal rotation), is far safer and more sustainable than passive or forced manipulation into the shape. Especially challenging and risky are twists created via binds or other outside forces, such as a passive adjustment by a teacher, especially when executed with a lot of power or force..

*Compression of Internal Organs and Fascia*

Twisting shapes often stimulate cueing about organ compression and fascial hydration – two topics that can be considered somewhat controversial in terms of the actual effects of twists on organs or fascia. Not everyone believes that twists actually serve to compress and influence the function of organs and the research about this is not deep. That said, historically and anecdotally, a general custom is to compress the right side of the abdomen first, followed by the left, as this mirrors the flow of digestion through the ascending, transverse, and descending colon, respectively. This sequencing supports natural peristalsis and optimally massages the internal organs, stimulating circulation and detoxification. For optimal organ compression and spinal length, it is typical practice to inhale to lengthen the spine before entering the twist, and to exhale while initiating the movement into the twist. Releasing out of the twist happens on the inhalation. This rhythm of breath integrates expansion and release, and may allow for structural integrity and enhanced circulation. Finally, it appears to be helpful to sequence open twists before closed twists (as the latter compress the abdomen more significantly) to prepare the body for deeper rotational work without overwhelming the visceral structures.

With regards, fascia (Myers, verbal communication in a workshop environment) indicates that immobility can lead to fascial adhesions that trap metabolic waste. Conscious, fluid movement, such as that achieved in twisting shapes, is believed to help release fascial stagnation, releasing toxins as the tissue is rehydrated and compressed. Anecdotally, it does appear to happen that students (especially those with sedentary lifestyles) can feel slightly nauseated or experience temporary detox symptoms after deep twisting practices, perhaps due to the fact that these movements stimulate organ release and fascial hydration.

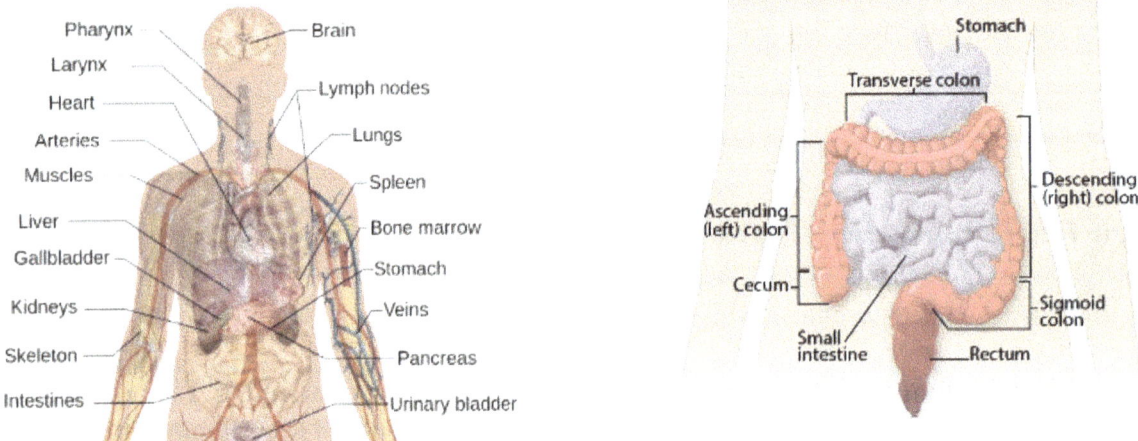

**Figure 2.13** Inner organs. (Data source: Mikael Häggström; https://commons.wikimedia.org/wiki/File:Internal_organs.svg; public domain)

**Figure 2.14** Small and large intestines. (Data source: https://www.cdc.gov/cancer/colorectal/basic_info/what-is-colorectal-cancer.htm); https://commons.wikimedia.org/wiki/File:Colon_illustration_lg.jpg; Creative Commons, 4.0.

| | Tips for Grounding, Expansion, and Stability in Twists or Rotations |
|---|---|
| *Grounding* | <ul><li>Ground through the backs of the femurs</li><li>Move the backs of the femurs toward the back plane of the body</li><li>Let the pelvis feel full and grounded as a single unit, moving as a unified whole</li><li>Use the exhalation to create a sense of rootedness as you move into the twist</li><li>Use the mind to create grounding as twists can dysregulate the nervous system and bring up emotions</li><li>Notice and calmly receive emotions or body signals – twists can bring up difficult sensation in body, energy, and mind</li></ul> |
| *Stability* | <ul><li>Keep your spine in its natural lumbar lordosis, with the sacrum nodded forward</li><li>Engage the core – yet with enough softness to allow the twist</li><li>Engage the pelvic floor, drawing inward and upward</li><li>Stabilize the shoulder girdle</li><li>Create stability in the SI joints</li><li>Allow the opposite hip to move forward to keep the pelvis stable as a whole unit</li><li>Breathe into the back body for a sense of balance and stability</li></ul> |
| *Expansion* | <ul><li>Inhale to become long and tall</li><li>Expand the spine upward and maintain length in spine with each inhalation</li><li>Find a natural spine</li><li>Resist any extra rounding (i.e., flexion, kyphosis) in the thoracic spine which is often the impulse in a twist</li><li>Imagine a slight bit of extension (slight backbend) in the thoracic spine to maintain an open heart</li><li>Move into the twist with the exhalation without losing expansiveness (open-heartedness) in the upper spine</li><li>Explore your healthful range of motion in the twist, noticing the moment natural lumbar lordosis is lost or excessive kyphosis appears in the thoracic spine</li></ul> |

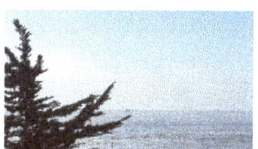

## Analysis and Experience of Sample Twists and Rotations

The following twists and rotations are analyzed in detail below:
- *Standing Twists*
- *Seated Twists*
- *Supine Revolve-Around-the Belly Twist*
- *Supported Prone Twist*

The cueing guidance offered for each shape needs to be considered in the context offered in the general principles for twists and rotations. The basics discussed above need to permeate the cueing for all of these shapes. The additional cueing, shape by shape, offered here is icing on the cake. Always incorporate integrated holistic yoga cueing that addresses the following teaching principles:

- *Accessibility* – creating access through variation, adaptation, affiliation, individualization, and person-centeredness
- *Intentionality* – embedding the practice of each shape in the overall arc of the session, grounding in the theme for the class and the meaning of the practice
- *Beneficence* – honoring the wellbeing of each student and always making sure to first do no harm
- *Holism* – cueing all *koshas* or layers of experience in all shapes, never forgetting that each shape has reverberations into and is affected by all *koshas* – it is not enough to cue anatomy; also address energy and vitality, thoughts and emotions, behavioral and action choices, even community and interbeing
- *Integration* – in teaching *asana*, integrate breathwork, concentration and mindfulness, as well as the ethical principles and lifestyle practices of yoga

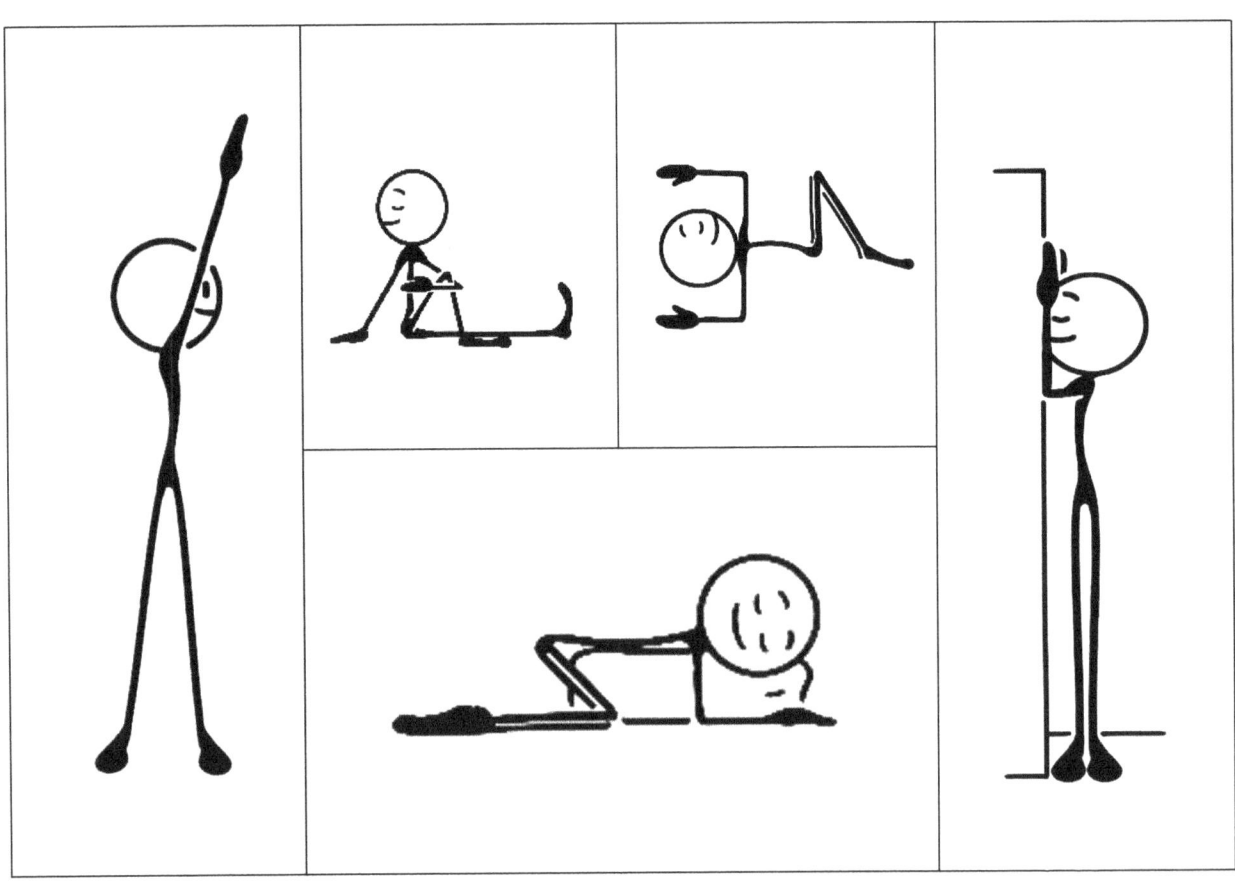

## Standing Twists from Mountain or Tadasana

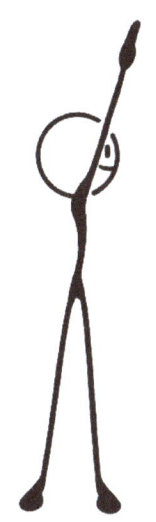

Standing Twists invite practitioners to explore the interplay between stability and ease while grounded in a stable standing shape. Standing twists can be initiated from any basic standing shape, with the instructions below focusing on twists emerging from Mountain. The *Variations and Exploration* section below expands on twists arising from Warrior 1, Warrior 3, and Triangle. Warrior 2 is a twisted shape was covered above. Regardless of starting shape, gentle spinal rotation from standing fosters balanced engagement across the torso, supporting a sense of spaciousness and resilience. Rotation is not solely a physical action; it is an opportunity to cultivate breath awareness and tune into subtle inner sensations, promoting somatic mindfulness. Although the outward shape of standing twists appears simple, the inner experience can be profound and is best varied according to individual anatomy, breath patterns, spinal mobility, and emotional state. Variations and adaptations offer personal exploration, allowing standing twists to become accessible to and beneficial for a wide range of practitioners.

### Benefits

Benefits of Standing Twists (arising from Mountain or any basic standing shape) extend across physical, vital, and mental dimensions, emerging from mindful somatic and emotional engagement with the rotation. Simple standing twists offer several positive effects:

- *Enhance rotation-based functional movement:* Learning healthful rotational biomechanics serves students well when they engage in daily living that requires twisting and turning.
- *Mobilize the spine and torso*: The rotational movement can create ease and resilience along the spine and surrounding muscles, encouraging a balance between engagement and the release of bracing.
- *Enhance breath awareness*: Twisting may promote enhanced breath awareness by gently compressing one side of the rib basket, inviting expansion and drawing inward in an asymmetrical manner.
- *Support a grounded yet mobile stance*: Establishing a stable connection with the earth through the feet while allowing for spinal rotation up high and stability down low cultivates a sense of being rooted yet free to move and explore.
- *Boost digestive health and fascial resilience*: The gentle internal compression associated with twisting can stimulate the abdominal organs and is hypothesized to support digestive function. The wringing action may help hydrate and nourish fascia.
- *Foster mental clarity*: The act of turning may symbolize a shift in perspective, inviting an experience of letting go and embracing new viewpoints, which may promote emotional release and creative thinking.

### Cautions

Although Standing Twists are generally accessible to most students, certain considerations can create a safer and more personalized experience:

- *Low back tension*: To prevent strain in the low back, guide practitioners to release the pelvis, allowing the entire pelvis to rotate into the direction of the twist to prevent undue strain on the lumbar spine and unhealthful mobilization of the sacroiliac joints.
- *Neck sensitivity*: Some students may experience tension in the neck while twisting. Allowing the head to stay in line with the chest or encouraging a gentler rotation is helpful.
- *Balance concerns*: Standing twists may present balance challenges. For those needing more stability, practicing near a wall or using a chair provides support.
- *Breathing ease*: If breath feels restricted, practitioners can ease out of the twist slightly until they find the degree of rotation at which breathing remains soft, natural, and unrestricted.

## Preparations

Preparing the body for Standing Twists can involve movements that cultivate ease in the spine, hips, and shoulders. Including these preparatory movements can help practitioners find a smoother transition into the twists. Standing twists are often a natural part of the warm-up via the six movements of the spine. These preparations can create readiness for more complex Standing Twists, warming the body, cultivating attention, and increasing emotional readiness.

- *Spinal mobilizations*: Flowing through Cat-Cow or seated spinal rolls can awaken the spine.
- *Standing lateral flexion*: Side bending can create resilience in the torso, creating opening and resilience in the muscles along the side body.
- *Hip mobilizers*: Movements such as hip circles or lunges may release tension in the hip joints, inviting greater ease in during twisting.
- *Breath-centered movements*: Deliberately and methodically connecting breath to movement fosters a deeper connection to the body, increasing awareness and length through the spine and supporting rotational movement.
- *Cueing interoception*: Preparation can focus on awareness of inner sensation to ensure that students are guided into twists with keen inner awareness.

## Key Alignment Invitations

Cultivating interoceptive and neuroceptive awareness is key to accessing ease in Standing Twists by guiding students toward subtle inner adjustments rather than striving for a particular outer shape or range of motion. Foundational alignment considerations for Mountain (or other relevant standing shapes) apply and are built upon with the addition of spinal rotation. The following alignment invitations emphasize mindful and balanced exploration, focusing on inner experience rather than outward expression. The main idea is to allow for free and functional movement, rather than overriding natural body wisdom with ill-advised cueing centered on fixing the pelvis in place (which inauspiciously results in torquing of the sacrum in the ilia).

- *Invitations related to the feet and legs:*
  - *Establish a stable foundation*: Ground evenly through the feet, feeling the connection to the earth while allowing the pelvis to rotate naturally in the direction of the twist.
  - *Release bracing in the legs*: Keep legs active without gripping or bracing; allow for a sense of fluidity in knees and ankles without promoting hypermobility.
- *Invitations related to the spine and pelvis*:
  - *Elongate upward*: Before rotating, encourage lengthening through the spine with an inhalation, imagining the crown of the head reaching toward the sky. The exhalation

invites an easeful movement into the twist, bringing the spinal rotation into the middle to upper spine (rather than the lumbar or sacroiliac regions).
    - *Let the rotation unfold naturally*: Invite the pelvis to move freely along with the spine. There is no need to try to create rotation in the lumber or pelvic region – this area is built for stability and natural functional movement allows the pelvis to move as a whole. It is best not to overcue this as most students will naturally move their pelvis into a twist.
- *Invitations related to the arms*:
    - *Encourage relaxed arm movement*: The arms can remain at the sides, gently rest on the hips, or extend outward to explore different sensations in the twist. Letting the arms swing naturally and keeping the shoulders relaxed prevents over-efforting.
    - *Add creative arm variations*: Experiment with reaching one arm forward and the other back or bending the arms at the elbows (cactus shape) to change the rotational experience. Promote ease in these movements.
- *Invitations related to the head and neck*:
    - *Choose a comfortable gaze*: The head can follow the torso's rotation, remain neutral, or turn in the opposite direction of the chest. The placement of the neck is guided by a sense of freedom from excessive strain. If the twist is offered in an ongoing rotational movement side to side (as opposed to holding a twisting shape), the head moves naturally in the direction of the twist; eye gaze follows naturally as well.

## *Variations and Exploration*

Standing Twists can arise from Mountain, Warrior 1 Lunge, Warrior 3, Triangle, and other standing shapes (they are a natural part of Warrior 2), offering numerous ways to engage individual needs and creatively explore rotational movements. Variations invite practitioners to find standing twists that resonate with their needs and interests, promoting exploration at the edge of comfort, as well as curiosity and self-awareness. Here are a few possible variations:
- *Twisting from Warrior 1 Lunge*: With the front knee bent and the back leg extended, initiate the twist from the middle to upper spine while keeping the legs stable. Stay attuned to how the shape and breath evolve as the chest opens to one side and then the other.
- *Adding a twist to Warrior 3*: A twist can be introduced by extending one arm downward (hand resting on a block or chair) and the opposite arm upward while keeping the standing leg strong. This rotational movement adds another balance challenge to the Warrior 3 shape.
- *Exploring twists from Triangle*: This is Revolved Triangle and requires specific instructions. The opposite hand moves toward the floor and the hand on the side of the rotation reaches toward the sky. For some students, Revolved Triangle is more accessible than Triangle as there is less inclination to torque the sacrum inside the ilia.
- *Practicing at a wall*: Practicing standing twists at a wall can provide additional exploration. The student stands with one side of the body at the wall, both arms at shoulder height, palms touching. The outward arm then releases from the arm at the wall and opens up into the room, ultimately reaching toward the wall on the opposite side.
- *Exploring different arm positions*: Variations such as extending the arms overhead or reaching one arm forward and the other back can change rotational dynamics and create a novel experience.
- *Twisting from Arm Standing*: see Downward Facing Dog variation with one hand at opposite knee; or Wild Thing with one hand lifted out to the side and overhead.

## Recovery

After practicing Standing Twists, incorporating movements that restore balance and ease can be helpful, and can help students transition smoothly from twisting to stillness or the next phase of their practice.
- *Shoulder releases*: Gently roll the shoulders to release any residual tension.
- *Mindful breathing*: Return to Mountain or another grounded shape and tune into the breath (perhaps with hands at heart center), allowing time for the effects of twisting to integrate.
- *Gentle spinal movements*: Incorporate Forward Folds, lateral flexion, or gentle spinal rolls to release any lingering tension.
- *Free-form movements*: Shake out the arms, sway side-to-side, or move intuitively to release tension and restore a sense of flow. Wiggling, shaking, and jogging in place can be offered.

## Additional Teaching Tips

To support ease and alignment in Standing Twists, consider these additional suggestions:
- *Guide with breath awareness*: Encourage using the breath as a guide, embracing the rotational movement on the exhalation and finding length in the spine on the inhalation.
- *Emphasize inner sensations*: Direct attention to subtle sensations within the body to deepen the experience and encourage a more mindful practice.
- *Invite self-discovery and curiosity*: Remind practitioners that the goal is not a specific range of motion but rather exploring the effect of the twist on body, breath, thoughts, and emotions.

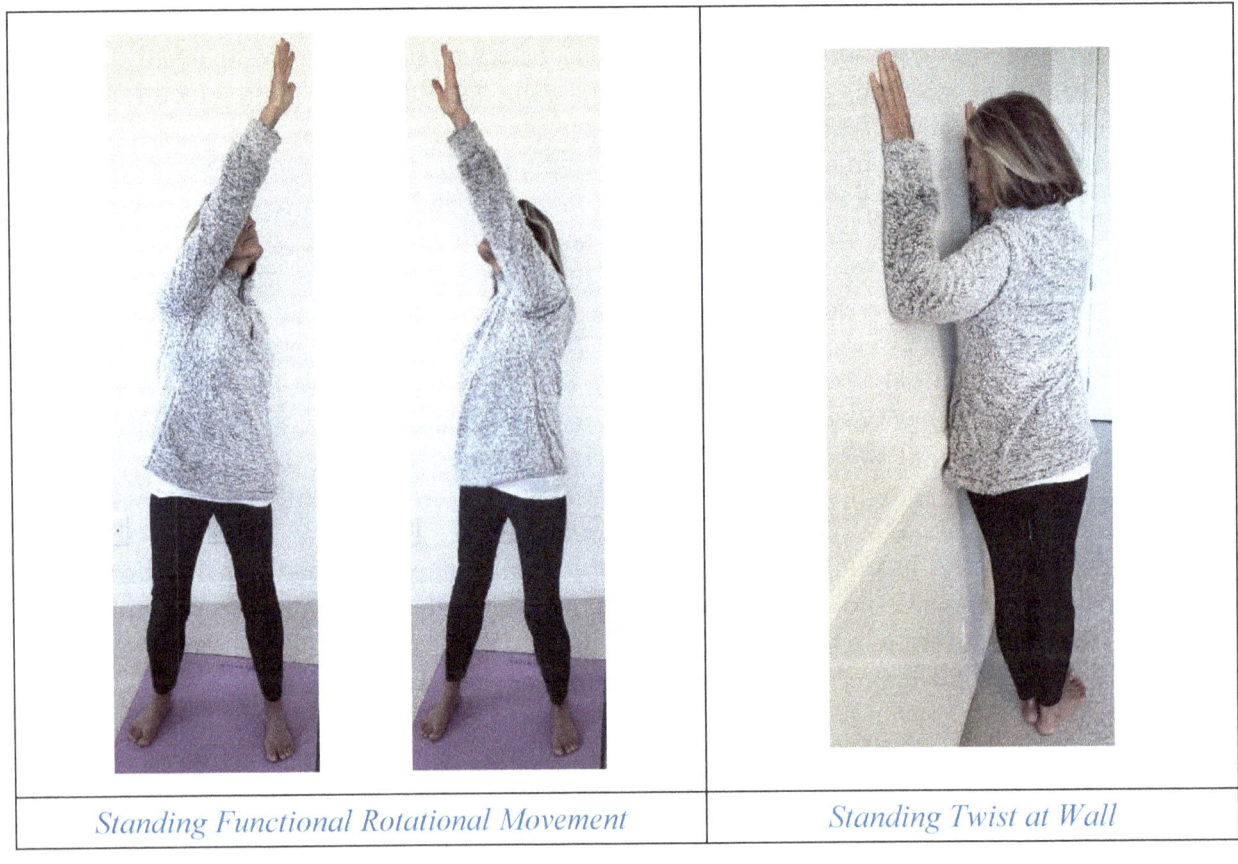

| Standing Functional Rotational Movement | Standing Twist at Wall |

## Seated Twists or Parivrtta Sukhasana

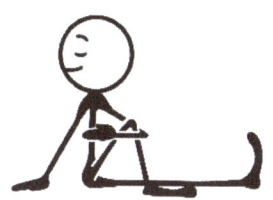

Seated Twists invite practitioners to explore the dynamic relationship between stability and ease within a grounded seated shape. Seated twists can arise from any seated shape covered above. The instructions provided here focus on a twist emerging from Easy Seat. The *Variations and Exploration* section below addresses simple seated twist that arise from Diamond, Hero, and other basic seats. For all seated twists, gentle rotation of the spine encourages a balanced engagement and release across the torso, promoting an inner sense of spaciousness and resilience. Twists are not only a physical movement, but also an invitation to cultivate awareness of the breath and subtle inner sensations, fostering a state of somatic mindfulness. Although the outward shape may appear simple, the inner experience can be deep and varied depending on each person's anatomy, breath patterns, spinal mobility, and emotional presence. Variations and adaptations can support individual exploration, making twists optimally accessible and beneficial for a wide range of practitioners, as well as creative and tailored.

### *Benefits*

The benefits of Seated Twists (arising from any of the basic seats) can be appreciated across physical, vital, and psychological dimensions, arising from mindful engagement with spinal rotations. Gentle seated twists can create the several positive effects.
- *Mobilize the spine and torso*: The rotational movement can help create ease and resilience along the spinal column and surrounding muscles and fascia, encouraging balanced engagement and release of bracing.
- *Promote mindful breathing*: Seated twists may enhance breath awareness by creating gentle compression in the abdomen and low rib basket, inviting a conscious experience of the expansion of inhalation and the drawing inward of the exhalation.
- *Encourage grounding and centering*: Establishing a stable yet dynamic and healthful base from which to create spinal rotation can cultivate a sense of connection to the earth, supporting the experience of being grounded yet mobile in a natural way as the pelvis naturally releases into the rotational movement.
- *Support digestion and fascial health*: The gentle internal compression has been hypothesized to stimulate the abdominal organs, potentially enhancing digestive function. It is also supportive of fascial health in that the gentle squeezing action creates a wringing out of the fascia, rehydrating and renourishing it.
- *Foster mental clarity*: The act of turning can symbolize a change of perspective, encouraging release and new beginnings; this shift in mental set may promote clarity and creativity.

### *Cautions*

Gentle Seated Twists are generally accessible to most students, yet some considerations can help make the experience of rotation more auspicious and person-centered:
- *Low back tension*: If there is discomfort in the low back, it is especially important to ensure that students release the pelvis into the twist. Avoid cueing the anchoring of both sitz bones –

the sitz bone on the opposite side of the direction of the twist ideally lifts and turns toward the twist to create ease in the lumbar spine and avoid corkscrewing in the sacroiliac joints. Embracing person-tailored range of motion is crucial. The hands are not used to torque (or passively rotate) the body further into rotation than spinal and abdominal muscles can create under their own power.
- *Neck tension*: Some students may experience tension in the neck during a twist. Keeping the head in a neutral position or rotating it more gently in line with the chest rather than over-rotating is helpful cueing to prevent over-efforting.
- *Hip discomfort*: Sitting in the crossed-leg position, or Easy Seat, for a twist may cause discomfort for some. Elevating the hips on a blanket or cushion can help create more ease in the pelvis. Using a symmetrical seated base (e.g., Hero) may be more auspicious.
- *Breathing difficulties*: If breathing feels restricted, the rotation is adjusted to a less intense expression, ensuring a more natural breath flow.
- *Release of toxins from tight connective tissue*: For some individuals (mostly those who tend to have some stiffness and lack of resilience in their fascia), twisting can serve to detoxify fascia and result in an increase in toxins that need to be released via blood and/or lymphatic fluid. They may experience nausea after a rotational practice. Encouraging them to drink water (perhaps with a bit of lemon juice, cayenne, and honey) after the practice may help.

## *Preparations*

Preparing the body for Seated Twists can involve movements that create ease in the spine, hips, and torso. Engaging in these warm-up movements encourages a smoother transition into the twist. Gentle seated twists are an inherent part of a warm-up via the six movements of the spine. They can be supported by the following sample preparation and no doubt many others. These preparatory movements help to establish a sense of readiness for Seated Twists, cultivating both physical warmth, increased vitality, and mental focus or attention.
- *Gentle spinal movements*: Flowing through Cat-Cow in a seated position or on hands and knees can help awaken the spine.
- *Lateral spinal flexion*: Lateral flexion from a seated or standing position can create resilience in the torso and begin to cultivate awareness of the breath.
- *Seated or standing hip circles*: Circular movements at the hip joints, inviting readiness for the twist. For some students, however, hip circles do not feel good until after they have engaged in seated twists first. Discernment is needed in cueing and sequencing.
- *Breath-centered movements*: Engaging in movements that link breath and movement can foster a deeper connection to the body, promoting awareness and lengthening through the spine before entering into the rotation.

## *Key Alignment Invitations*

Finding ease in Seated Twists depends on cultivating interoceptive awareness that guides subtle adjustments from the inside out, rather than from the outside in based on a desired range of motion. All basic alignment cues for the seat from which the twist arise apply and need to be cued before rotation is added. The following alignment invitations are focused on adding rotation to the basic seat from which the twist emerges. These alignment invitations support a mindful and balanced approach to Seated Twists, emphasizing the inner experience of the movement over an outer range of motion. The key to all alignment is freedom in the pelvis to move in a natural and functional way rather than overriding this inner wisdom of the body with unnecessary and counterproductive encouragements to anchor, fix, and hold steady through the sitz bones. Notably absent in the directions for all twisting shapes is cueing related to using the hands to find a 'deeper twist'. Instead, twists are best accessed with active engagement of the musculature in the torso – rather than striving for more range of motion via passive movement forced by the hands, strap, or another person.

- *Invitations related to the base*:
    - *Invite ease into the pelvis and stability into the SI joints*: Unlike what is often cued in yoga classes, do not anchor the sitz bones and/or tops of the femurs. Instead, the sitz bone and top of femur on the opposite side of the twist is unweighted (the opposite of anchoring) and turns toward the twist to create ease in the lumbar spine and avoid torquing in the SI joints. Embracing a person-tailored range of motion in the rotation is also crucial and means that the hands *are not used* to torque (or passively rotate or force) the body further into the twist than the spinal and abdominal muscles can create under their own power.
    - *Find ease in the leg position*: If the legs are crossed, adjust the distance between the feet and hips for comfort. Alternatively, explore a variation other than Easy Seat (e.g., Diamond).
- *Invitations related to the spine*:
    - *Create length in the spine*: Before initiating the twist, guide practitioners to elongate the spine upward with an inhalation, imagining the crown of the head reaching toward the sky. From this length, turn into the twist easefully on the exhalation.
    - *Initiate the twist from the mid to upper region of the spine*: Invite the twist to start from the middle to upper spine, allowing the movement to travel upward rather than forcing the rotation from the lumbar spine, which has very limited rotational range. Again, do not use the hands to create the rotation – let the muscles of the core do the work from the inside out for the most natural expression of the rotation.
    - *Be mindful of rib basket movement*: Gently guide the ribs to rotate without collapsing the chest, creating an even distribution of movement along the spine. Notice how the low ribs are affected by the rotation and how this experience changes with the inhalation and exhalation.
- *Invitations related to the arms and hands*:
    - *Support spinal balance with minimal to no pressure*: The hands can rest on the knees, thighs, or the ground beside the hips, providing stability without forcing or creating passive rotation or torquing. One hand may reach behind the spine and can nestle itself along the spine for support if desired – like the stick that is placed next to a newly planted tree to invite it to grow straight upward.
    - *Explore arm variations*: Extend one or both arms outward (e.g., in cactus) or overhead (e.g., at approximately 60°) to change the experience of the twist by adding additional challenge or creativity.
- *Invitations related to the head and neck*:
    - *Find a comfortable gaze*: The head can follow the rotation of the torso, can remain in a neutral position, or can rotate in the opposite direction of the rotation lower in the spine. Choice of neck placement is guided by the experience of freedom from excessive strain or tension. Invite exploration.

## Variations and Exploration

As noted, Seated Twists can emerge from any of the seats covered above in the Upright Seats section. They can be explored in a variety of ways to creatively work with individual needs and to encourage playing at the edge of comfort. The following variations are simply invitations to think of additional creative explorations.

- *Elevating the hips*: Sitting on a cushion, blanket, or block can reduce tension in the hips and low back, making a spinal rotation more accessible. It can help with freedom of movement of the pelvis into the natural twisting range of motion.
- *Using a chair*: Practicing the twist while seated in a chair can be helpful for those with limited mobility or discomfort in a floor-seated position. Encourage an upright spine and gentle rotation.
- *Twisting from other seated bases*: If the cross-legged position of Easy Seat feels restrictive, explore twists from other leg positions. Diamond or propped Hero can create more access to freedom of rotation. Bound Angle may invite more challenge. Staff offers a seat without knee flexion and may feel more easeful for some and more challenging for others. Some students thrive with one leg extended and one knee bent.
- *Standing, supine, and prone twist*: If seated rotations are not accessible, perhaps offer an alternative in other orientations in space. Standing twists are often more accessible as the pelvis automatically moves naturally and freely into the rotation.

## Recovery

After practicing Seated Twists, it can be beneficial to incorporate the following movements that restore balance and ease. These recovery movements help to smooth the transition from twisting to stillness or the next aspect of the sequence, fostering a holistic experience.

- *Gentle shoulder rolls*: Rolling the shoulders can release any residual tension.
- *Mindful breathing:* Return to the base seat and sense into the breath. Allowing time for breath awareness helps integrate the effects of the twisting motion.
- *Seated Forward Fold*: From the base seat, a gentle Forward Fold may serve to release the low back and hips.
- *Standing shape with wiggles, shakes, jogging in place or other intuitive movements*: If it makes sense from a sequencing perspective for the practice overall, rising to standing and engaging in movements can be helpful for recovery and can release tension from sitting.

## Additional Teaching Tips

To help students find ease and alignment in Seated Twists, consider integrating these additional suggestions:

- *Encourage breath awareness*: Use the breath as a guide for finding the appropriate degree of rotation.
- *Invite exploration*: Remind students that there is no goal for the range of motion in the twist. Encourage them to find a degree of rotation that feels supportive, exploratory (working the edge of comfort), and respectful of in-the-moment needs.
- *Use props creatively*: Offer blankets, blocks, or cushions to create a more accessible seat from which to rotate.

- *Emphasize inner experience*: Guide students to tune into their inner sensations, allowing these experiences to inform the shape. Closing the eyes to sense into the rotation from the inside out can be transformative as students relinquish the visual cues that may drive them into an outer goal related to degree of rotation.

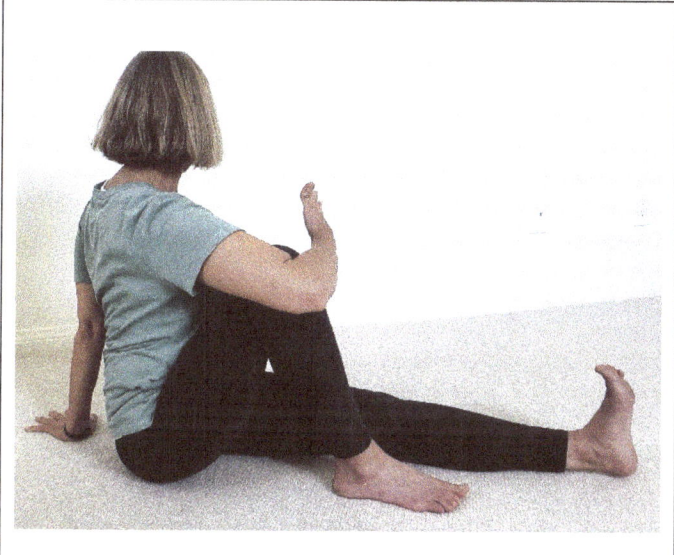

Seated Rotation – open variation

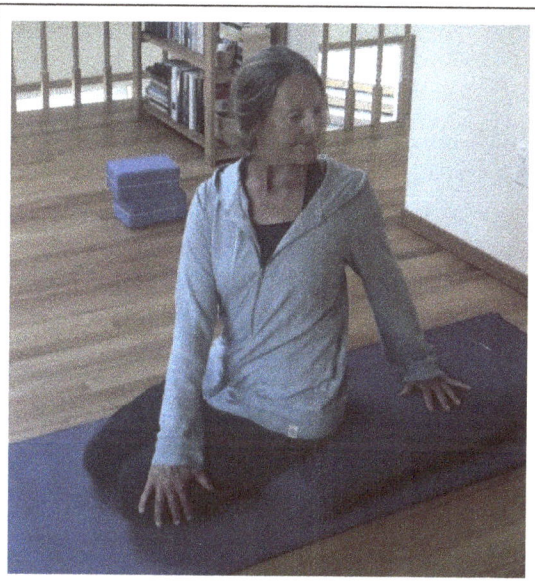

Rotated Diamond on prop under hip

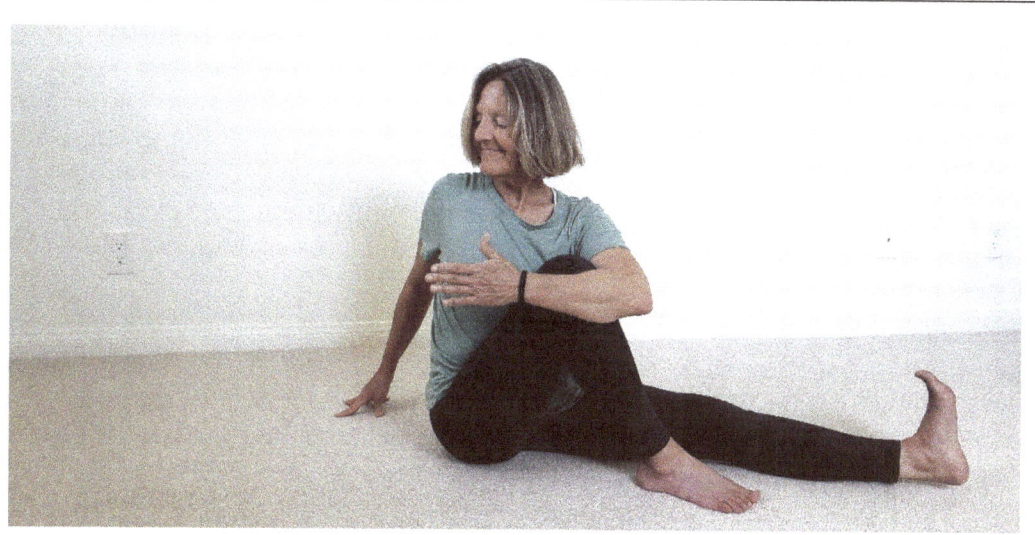

Seated Rotation – closed variation

## Revolve-Around-the-Belly Twist or Jathara Parivartanasana

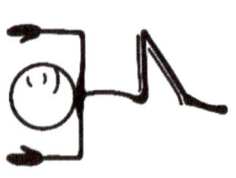

Representative of supine twists, the Revolve-Around-the-Belly Twist invites exploration of the relationship between grounded support from the back and the mobility of the spine, fostering a sense of exploration and inviting attentive curiosity. This reclined or supine shape encourages gentle rotation across the torso, originating from the middle to upper sections of the spine, exploring a wholesome range of motion and cultivating awareness of breath and inner sensations. Though the outward shape may appear straightforward, the inner experience of this supine twist brings with it some challenges that require careful calibration of instruction and expression based on students' anatomy, breath rhythm, spinal resilience, and emotional presence. Ample offerings of variations and adaptations support individual exploration, making the shape healthfully accessible and beneficial for a wide range of practitioners.

### Benefits

The benefits of the Revolve-Around-the-Belly Twist and other supine twists can be appreciated across physical, vital or energetic, and mental or emotional dimensions, emerging from mindfully embodied engagement with the spinal rotation. Supine twisting shapes may offer the following effects:

- *Mobilize the spine and hips*: The rotational movement encourages ease and resilience along the spinal column, allowing the back, pelvis, and surrounding muscles to release tension.
- *Promote mindful breathing*: The gentle rotation may enhance breath awareness by compressing one side of the abdomen while opening the other, inviting a conscious experience of inhalation's expansion and exhalation's drawing inward.
- *Support digestion and fascial health*: The internal compression may stimulate abdominal organs, potentially enhancing digestive function, and can create a wringing effect on the fascia, aiding in rehydration and nourishment.
- *Cultivate mental clarity*: The act of turning can symbolize letting go of old patterns, encouraging a shift in perspective that fosters a sense of clarity and renewal.

### Cautions

The Revolve-Around-the-Belly Twist and other supine twists are generally accessible for most practitioners, yet some considerations can help ensure a person-centered and wholesome experience:

- *Pregnancy*: As the abdomen expands, it is advisable to make the shift to reclined (rather than fully supine) twists. Twists need to be gentle with ample propping under the knees. As pregnancy advances, definitely when lying on the back is no longer healthful or comfortable, reclined and supine twists are best put on pause until postnatally. A fully supported side-lying position will be a more healthful alternative.
- *Low back discomfort, including sacroiliac instability*: If there is discomfort in the low back, decreasing the flexion in the hips and/or knees and placing a support (e.g., a cushion or bolster) under the legs create a more easeful and supported rotation.

- *Neck tension or challenges*: If tension arises in the neck, allow the head to turn in line with the chest, keep it looking in the direction of the twist, and avoid turning the head in the opposite direction from the rotation.
- *Sacrum stability*: To avoid torquing the sacrum inside the ilia, allow the pelvis to move with the rotation rather than holding it rigidly in place. Place ample props under the legs. It is may be more desirable for students, especially with sacroiliac instability, to access this supine twist from a relatively open fetal-shape side-lying position, opening the arms and heart space into the rotation (rather than from the back and moving the lower body into the twist).
- *Breathing difficulties, especially related to physiological pathologies (as opposed to psychological, such as anxiety)*: If breath feels restricted, adjust the degree of rotation of the twist to support natural breath flow.

## Preparations

Preparing for the Revolve-Around-the-Belly Twist and other supine or reclined rotational shapes can involve movements that create ease in the spine, shoulders, and hips. As always, the six movements of the spine are great preparation, and for supine twisting the six-movements warm-up can be offered in supine, standing, arm standing, or seated orientations in space. Engaging in these preparatory movements establishes a sense of readiness, cultivating physical warmth and mindful somatic and vital focus.
- *Gentle spinal movements*: Flow through spinal movements on the back that invite lateral spinal flexion, as well as flexion and extension in the hip joint to awaken the spine. Rocking the pelvis anterior and posterior is a nice option in this regard.
- *Knee-to-chest variations*: Draw one or both knees toward the chest while lying on the back to create resilience in the low back and awaken the core stabilizers.
- *Shoulder stability awareness*: Practice gentle arm presses into the floor to engage the shoulder girdle, creating a stable foundation for the twist.
- *Hip rotations*: From supine or any other orientation in space, bend the knees and explore gentle circular movements of the hip joints
- *Breath-centered awareness*: Engage in practices that connect breath with movement to enhance awareness before transitioning into the shape. Movements involving axial extension may be particularly helpful.

## Key Alignment Invitations

Finding ease in the Revolve-Around-the-Belly Twist and other supine twists involves tuning into the body's internal experiences rather than striving for an outward range of motion. These alignment invitations, focused mostly on Revolve-Around-the-Belly Twist, are also applicable to other supine twists (e.g., Windshield Wiper). They emphasize a mindful, inner-guided approach, supporting personal experience over outer shape.
- *Invitations related to the base – lying on the **back** as the starting position*:
  - *Support the spine by grounding the back*: Allow the shoulders and upper back to release tension into the floor, creating a sense of stability. Invite grounding and expansion into the back body, creating natural curves in the spine even in a supine position (i.e., there are small arches under the lumbar and cervical spines).

- *Allow the pelvis to move in the direction of the rotation*: As the knees move to one side, let the pelvis turn naturally in the same direction, finding a path for easeful movement that does not challenge sacroiliac integrity or force the twist into the lumber spine (which does not have much rotational range of motion).
- *Invitations related to the base – lying on the **side** as the starting position*:
  - *Invite the spine into its natural curves*: Find a gentle, relatively open (not fully flexed at hips and knees) side-lying, fetal position. Invite stability and expansiveness into the spine, creating natural curves in the spine even while lying on the side. Both arms reach forward and rest at shoulder height; palms may touch. Moving into the shape from side-lying rather than from being supine can be transformational for some students. Although it is unconventional, this is an anatomically sounder approach and worthwhile exploring.
  - *Open the upper body into the rotation*: Gently open the heart space by sliding the arm that is resting on top across the chest and to the other side of the body, toward the floor. It may come to rest on the floor or on a blanket or bolster, depending on spinal rotation range of motion. Alternatively, the arm and shoulder may come to rest on the floor, with the upper torso beginning to ground on the earth. The knees may natural lift away from the floor and require a bolster, blanket, or block for support.
- *Invitations related to the spine*:
  - *Guide the twist from the mid to upper spine*: Encourage the rotation to peak in the thoracic region, not in the lumbar spine and/or between the sacrum and the ilia. The lumbar spine has limited rotational range, making it crucial to allow the twist to emerge from higher up for a balanced experience. The sacroiliac joints should not be forced into an undue range of motion. Beware of sacral corkscrewing.
  - *Explore ease in the rib basket*: Notice how the ribs respond to the rotation and adjust as needed, inviting evenness in the movement without bracing.
- *Invitations related to the legs and arms*:
  - *Use leg position to guide the degree of range of motion*: Let the knees move freely, allowing them to separate as needed to find ease. If the knees do not reach the floor, place a support under and/or between them to avoid undue strain in the lumbar and sacral regions.
  - *Explore arm variations*: The arms can extend outward in a T or cactus shape or they can rest by the sides. One hand can gently rest on the opposite thigh to ground the energy toward without forcing or pressing down.
- *Invitations related to the head and neck*:
  - Allow the head to follow the direction of the rotation first. Then invite a conscious decision about whether to hold the head naturally turned in the same direction as the knees, remain in line with the spine, or turn in the opposite direction as the knees, depending on the sensation that creates a desired effect and ease in the neck.

## Variations and Exploration

There are many ways to explore the Revolve-Around-the-Belly Twist via adaptations or related supine twists to suit individual needs, align with the context of the practice, or promote creativity and exploration. These variations offer options for different levels of comfort and accessibility. They invite playfulness and individual adaptation that supports curiosity and a willingness to try something new.

- *Windshield Wiper variation*: With feet on the floor and knees bent, gently let the knees sway side to side. This dynamic movement can create resilience in the low back and hips while maintaining a natural range of motion. Alternatively, a longer hold on one side and then the other side can be invited. The goal is not for the knees to reach to floor; rather, this movement is about releasing strain in the low back and calming the nervous system.
- *Use props to create wholesome alignment*: Place a bolster, cushion, or blanket under and/or between the knees to release tension in the hips and low back. The shape may also be offered reclined with a sloping support under the back body. Supports under one or both shoulders may be helpful for some students. Similarly, supports for the head and neck can be explored.
- *Single-leg rotation*: Extend one leg on the floor while sending the opposite leg (with knee flexed or extended) across the body and the extended leg toward the floor (foot perhaps coming to rest on a block or bolster) to explore a different experience of a supine twist.

### Recovery

After practicing the Revolve-Around-the-Belly Twist or other supine twists, consider the following movements to restore balance and release any residual tension as needed. These recovery practices allow for time and space to integrate the effects of the twisting, smoothing the transition to stillness or the next aspect of the practice.
- *Knees to chest*: Draw the knees into the chest, gently rocking side to side. The level of tightness of the grip around knees will direct a massaging of the back either high into the spine (toward the thoracic spine) or all the way down to the sacrum, and anywhere in between.
- *Mindful breathing*: Lie on the back or the side and focus attention on the breath, sensing how inner somatic and vital experience may have changed with the twist.
- *Bridge shape*: Lift the hips into a gentle Bridge and roll down vertebra by vertebra to release the low back and clear the proverbial and energetic palate.
- *Standing movements*: If appropriate, rise to standing and engage in light movements to encourage ease and exploration via intuitive wiggles, shakes, or stretches.

### Additional Teaching Tips

To help practitioners find ease and alignment in the Revolve-Around-the-Belly Twist or similar supine twists a few additional considerations can serve.
- *Emphasize breath as a guide*: Encourage moving and flowing with the breath to find a healthful and compassionate degree of rotation.
- *Invite exploration*: Remind practitioners that the goal is not to reach a specific range of motion, but to explore sensation and find a supportive edge.
- *Use props creatively*: Offer blankets or cushions to create more accessible or interesting variations.
- *Focus on the inner experience*: Guide practitioners to tune into inner sensations, allowing them to shape the twist from the inside out.

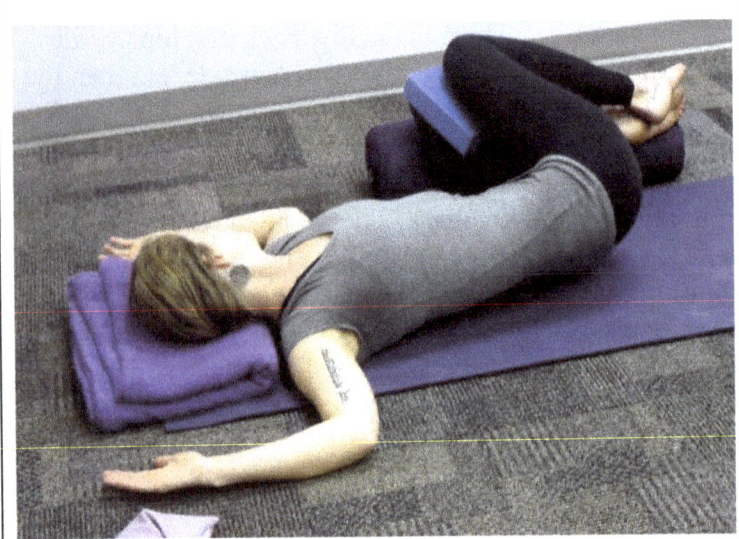

*Seated and Supine Supported Revolve-Around-the-Belly*

*- embracing ease and release*

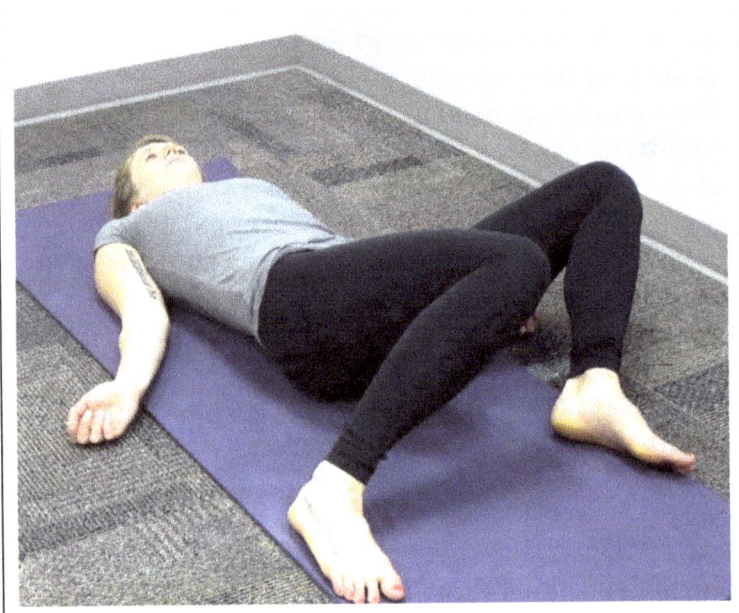

*Windshield Wiper*
*– prioritizing the health of the spine*

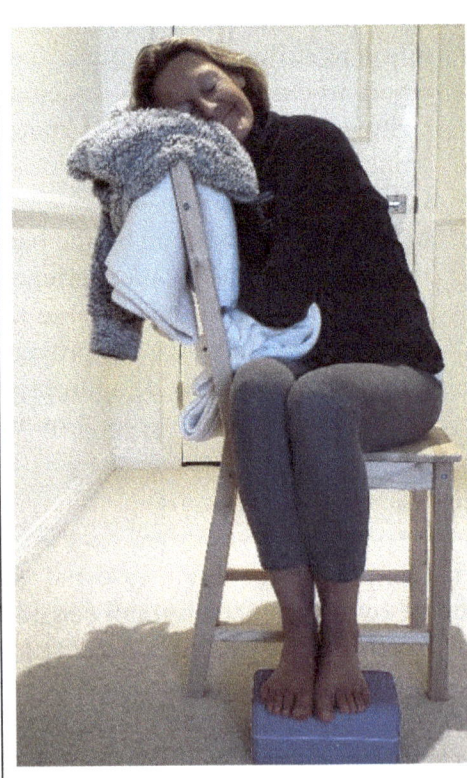

## Supported Prone Twist (with Belly on a Bolster)

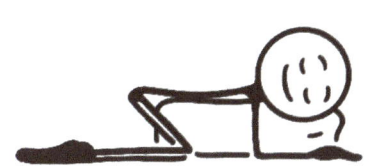

The Supported Prone Twist offers a grounding experience that invites a gentle release of tension in body, nervous system, and mind. This shape can encourage mindful attunement to breath and body, cultivating inner ease and awareness. By resting the belly on a bolster, mind and energy find support and relaxation while the body benefits from the rotation. Although the outward shape may appear restful, the inner experience is uniquely affected by each person's anatomy, breath patterns, and state of mind. Adaptations can support individual access to ease, making this twist healthful and calming for most students.

### Benefits

Engaging in a Supported Prone Twist can bring balance to body, breath, and mind via several mechanisms, including but not limited to the following:
- *Mobilizes the spine and torso*: The gentle rotation can encourage ease and resilience in the spine, creating balanced engagement across the muscles and connective tissues.
- *Enhances breath awareness*: The twist provides gentle compression in the abdomen and rib basket, inviting a conscious experience of breath expansion on inhalation and release on exhalation.
- *Encourages grounding*: With the body resting on a bolster, this supported rotation invites a sense of connection to the earth, promoting relaxation and tension release.
- *Supports digestive function and fascial health*: Gentle internal pressure from the rotation may stimulate the abdominal organs and encourage rehydration and nourishment of fascia.
- *Promote mental clarity and relaxation*: The rotational movement may create a sense of release and renewal, inviting an emotional and mental experience of calm and clarity.

### Cautions

Although a Supported Prone Twist is generally accessible, considering the following cautions can help ensure a more easeful experience:
- *Low back sensitivity*: If discomfort arises in the low back, explore adjusting the height or position of the bolster to support a comfortable range of motion.
- *Neck tension*: If there is tension in the neck, consider positioning the head in a way that minimizes strain, such as resting the forehead on a folded blanket or turning the gaze gently to the same side as the knees.
- *Hip discomfort*: If lying with the pelvis in a twisted position is uncomfortable, adding support under the opposite hip via a blanket or small cushion that turns the pelvis into the direction of the rotation can create more ease.
- *Breathing difficulties*: If breath feels restricted, allow the body to settle into a gentler (less rotated expression of the twist), ensuring a natural flow of breath.

## Preparations

Preparing for a Supported Prone Twist can involve movements that bring awareness and mobility to the spine, hips, and torso. Proper preparation can help cultivate a sense of readiness for the Supported Prone Twist, fostering physical and mental awareness. The same preparations used for seated twists are indicated. This supported twist tends to be offered at the end of a practice and therefore the entire sequence that precedes it, *is* the preparation. That said, the following prior movements are helpful:

- *Spinal flexion and extension*: Flowing through gentle Cat-Cow can awaken the spine.
- *Side-body lengthening*: Lateral spinal flexion from a seated or standing position can create a sense of space along the torso, preparing the body for the prone rotation.
- *Breath-focused movements*: Incorporating breath-centric movements creates connection to the breath and a sense of length through the spine before transitioning into the twist.

## Key Alignment Invitations

The experience of a Supported Prone Twist centers on mindful alignment that arises from inner sensation, allowing the body to find ease in a manner that is specific to each student. The following alignment invitations encourage an inwardly-directed embrace of the rotation, with an emphasis on ease and natural movement rather than on an outer shape or particular degree of rotation.

- *Invitations for the base*:
  - *Adjust bolster position for comfort*: Show how to lift the bolster onto several props to create a sloped incline. Demonstrate how to sit sideways in front of the bolster, with one hip next to the short side of the bolster, in preparation for the rotation.
  - *Find ease in the leg position*: Offer many options for placement, such as level of flexion in the hips and knees, how the legs/knees are stacked or more likely not, and how the feet drape back, perhaps with supports under the ankle.
  - *Create length before rotating*: Invite students to elongate the spine with an inhalation, feeling the space between each vertebra. As the body exhales, allow the gentle rotation to arise naturally, finding ease in the movement of turning toward the bolster.
  - *Rest the torso toward the bolster*: From the sideways seat, invite students to rotate the upper portion of the torso to turn the front part of the upper chest toward the bolster. Then release down onto the bolster. Cue tuning into sensation to find a wholesome degree of rotation and placement for the chest.
- *Invitations for the spine, including the neck*:
  - *Initiate the twist from the mid-torso*: Invite the rotation to emerge from the mid-torso, allowing the twist to travel upward. This approach helps to distribute the sensation of rotation along the upper spine rather than concentrating it in the low back.
  - *Find a relaxed gaze*: Allow the head to follow the rotation naturally, turning the gaze in the direction of the twist or keeping it neutral. Adjust the head position to ensure freedom from excess strain.
- *Invitations for the arms and hands*:
  - *Explore arm variations for comfort*: The arms can rest by the sides, extend outward in a 'T' shape, or bend at the elbows with the hands resting near the head. They can also wrap around the bolster. Each variation offers a different experience of support and balance.

*Variations and Exploration*

Supported Prone Twist can be explored in different ways to suit individual preferences and needs. The following variations can help practitioners find a version of the twist that feels inviting and beneficial.
- *Adjust bolster height*: Changing the height and angle of the incline of the bolster can greatly affect the experience of the twist. A higher bolster may create more ease, while a lower bolster may deepen the compression.
- *Use additional support*: Adding a folded blanket under the chest or pelvis can provide extra comfort and encourage a gentler expression of the shape. A prop under the head may be helpful for some to create ease in the neck.
- *Leg variations*: Experiment with different leg positions, such as bending the knees or extending one leg to the side to change the sensation in the low back and hips.

*Recovery*

The Supported Prone Twist is in and of itself a recovery shape and is most typically offered late in a sequence and followed by a transition into *Savasana*. However, it can be helpful for some students to incorporate movements that rebalance body and breath, including, but not limited to the following possibilities. These recovery movements support a smooth transition from twisting to stillness.
- *Gentle spinal movements*: Flowing through Cat-Cow or similar movements can release any residual tension in the back. Drawing the knees to chest can be helpful if any tension emerged in the lumbar spine.
- *Gentle shoulder movements*: Inviting gentle shoulder circles of various ranges of motion and guided by intuition can be helpful.
- *Mindful breathing*: Resting in a comfortable position and allowing time for breath awareness can help integrate the effects of the rotation.
- *Child or Forward Fold*: A gentle forward fold can further release the spine and hips, encouraging a sense of grounding.

*Additional Teaching Tips*

Supported Prone Twist can be a deeply restorative experience. The following teaching tips help invite ease and peaceful presence, inviting a personalized and mindful practice:
- *Emphasize the experience over the appearance*: Encourage students to focus on how the shape feels from the inside out rather than striving for an outer shape or particular range of motion. Degree of rotation is less important than sensations that arise and connection to breath.
- *Guide practitioners to settle gradually*: Allow time for the body to settle into the shape, inviting small mindful adjustments to the position of the bolster, legs, and arms to find ease. Reassure students that it is natural to take a few moments to find comfort in this complex shape.
- *Use the breath as a guide alignment*: Suggest that practitioners let the breath guide the degree of rotation. With each exhalation, invite a natural release of tension, allowing the

body to release and relax into the twist (and bolster). With each inhalation, encourage an experience of spaciousness in the torso, breath, and mind.
- *Invite practitioners to stay connected to interoception and neuroception*: Invite students to be mindful of areas of ease and areas where there may be gripping or bracing. Invite lingering tension to release with the exhalation.
- *Foster awareness of emotional responses*: Twists can evoke emotional responses as tension is released from the tissues. Encourage students to approach emotions that arise with curiosity and compassion rather than evaluation or judgment.

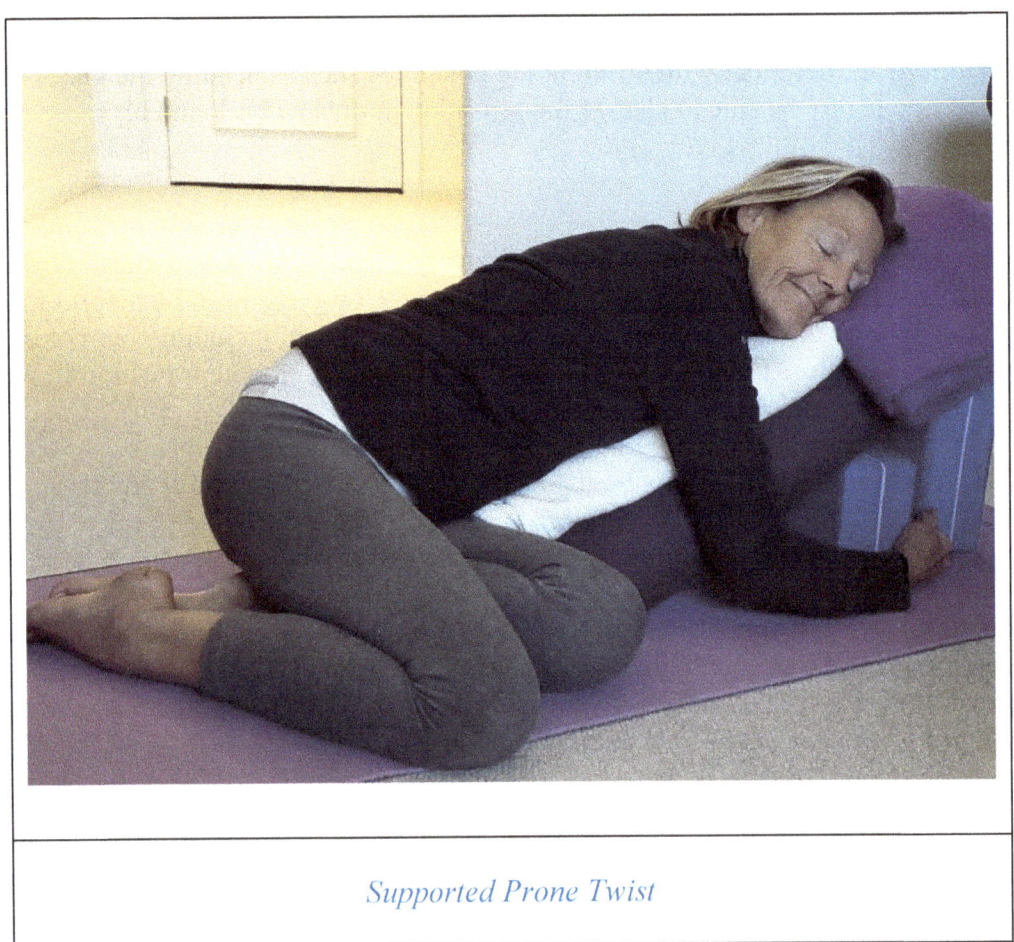

*Supported Prone Twist*

*The road of life twists and turns and no two directions are ever the same. Yet our lessons come from the journey, not the destination.*
Don Williams

## Chapter 12: Forward Folds

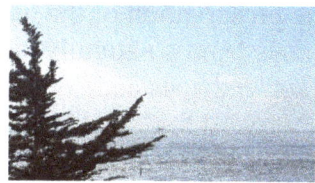

This chapter covers foundational forward folds, offering optimized teaching strategies that allow for individual tailoring and careful discernment about how and which shapes to offer, as well as about how to cue alignment informed by interoception, proprioception, exteroception, and neuroception. General principles for this category of yoga *asanas* are provided and apply to most if not all forward folds. Specific follow-up guidance is added for the chosen sample shapes. Forward Folds can unfold from standing, arm standing, and sitting. All guidance in Chapters 8 to 10 remains highly relevant and applicable – even if it is not explicitly repeated here.

## Anatomical Foci for Forward Folds

Forward folds in yoga are often misunderstood as shapes characterized by spinal rounding. While spinal flexion into our primary curve can be a part of these shapes, auspicious alignment in forward folds begins with recognizing the importance of a natural spine and a functional, healthfully positioned pelvis, with the acetabulofemoral joints – by definition – moving into flexion. Rather than focusing on the placement of the head near the legs, the intention is to fold or hinge from the hip joints with anatomical integrity and somatic awareness about what is happening in the spine during flexion in the hips. Thus, there are two possible aspects to spinal movements in forward folding: 1) the movement of the spine toward flexion (e.g., a roll-down into or out of a standing forward fold; a fully rounded, kyphotic spine in seated forward fold); and 2) the movement of the *spine with an open heart and natural spinal curve* (i.e., a shape that emerges from hinging in the hip joint with the pelvis in its most natural position). Depending on how a forward fold is accessed and expressed, there may be different preparation, risks, and contraindications.

Auspicious alignment in forward folding is not defined by range of motion (or the position of the body at end range of movement) but by the quality of action, inner awareness, and anatomical congruence. Invitations to students or clients are centered on hinging from the hips with an open heart, exploring the roles of the pelvis and femurs, and using props and tactile feedback to support bioindividual needs. Once end range of hip hinging based on natural alignment in the pelvis has been reached, a mindful decision can be made whether to deepen the forward fold via flexion of the spine. With thoughtful guidance from a yoga professional and mindful practice by the client, forward folding becomes a powerful opportunity to integrate form, function, and inner reflection. Forward folds can serve not only spinal health but also enhance nervous system balance and energetic clarity. Helpful anatomical foci include, but are not limited to the following guidance about anatomy and alignment in forward folding.

## *Natural Spine and Spinal Flexion versus Extension in Forward Folds*

Auspicious forward folding invites the preservation of the natural curves of the spine, particularly its lumbar lordosis that arises from a naturally anteriorly tilted pelvis (see below). Spinal flexion may be appropriate in some shapes and contexts, but it is not the default goal of forward folding. Generally speaking, forward folds (which always arise from flexion in the acetabulofemoral joints) may be approached in two broad ways as far as spinal alignment is concerned:

- *Spinal Flexion*: In this understanding of forward folding focus is on a rounded (i.e., flexed) back, often created by rolling down segmentally and arriving in a kyphotic fold, whether seated or standing. This approach is common but introduces compressive force to the anterior aspects of the vertebrae and discs and may challenge disc stability, particularly in the lumbar region.
- *Natural Spine or Slight Extension*: In this understanding of or approach to forward folding focus is on emphasizing hinging at the hips from a naturally aligned (slightly anterior) pelvis and keeping the spine in its natural curves or moving toward slight spinal extension. This approach emphasizes spinal lengthening, supports healthy disc spacing, and facilitates load-sharing between pelvis and spine.

Each approach has distinct anatomical and energetic effects. Some anatomists (Lasater, 2009, 2020) recommend preserving the spinal curves, especially the lumbar lordosis, to protect disk integrity given the relative weakness of the posterior longitudinal ligament in the lumbar region that provides less support to the discs during anterior compression of the vertebrae. Others (Mitchell, 2019) emphasize student choice and somatic autonomy, especially in resilient and healthy bodies. A useful teaching strategy is to begin with a natural spine and open chest, and then, if appropriate and supported, allow the spine to move into flexion with awareness. Research suggests that there may be no compelling anatomical reason to choose one version over the other, with the vertebrae and discs being able to tolerate the loads created by either approach (Clark, 2016, 2018). However, loads on the spine in seated positions have been reported to vary, with greater pressure on the disc with increasing spinal flexion.

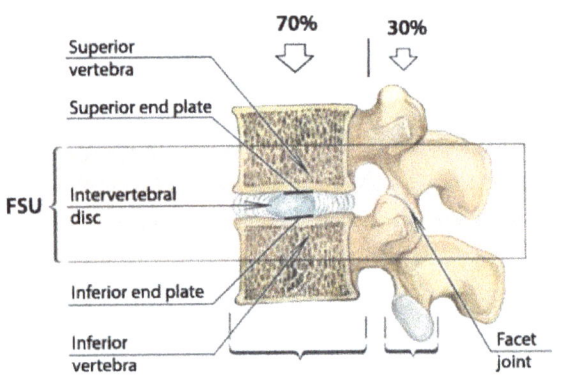

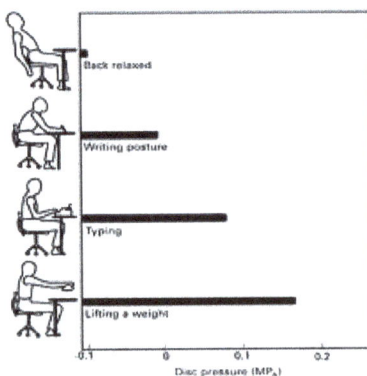

**Figure 2.15** Intervertebral disc function. (Data source: Irina Nefedova; https://commons.wikimedia.org/wiki/File:Functional_spinal_unit_(FSU).webp; Creative Commons Attribution 4.0)

**Figure 2.16** Disc pressure in various postures. (Data source: Jiqiren123; https://commons.wikimedia.org/wiki/File:Disc_Pressure.jpg; Free Art License)

A related consideration may be energetic more so than physical. Specifically, energetically, a rounded, kyphotic spine may reflect a dorsal vagal response, a self-protective, perhaps somewhat withdrawn shape. While it can be restorative in appropriate settings and within carefully created contexts, it may also evoke psychological or nervous system responses related to collapse or withdrawal. An open heart and extended sternum may help transform forward folding into a *sattvic* or ventral vagal experience, grounded and introspective without disengagement. Each yoga professional will have to decide how to cue and align forward folding. In part this may depend on the health and wellbeing of the client. Individuals with compromised health, chronic pain, or specific spinal challenges may need a different approach than young, resilient bodies with no physical or emotional difficulties or pathologies.

Each yoga professional needs to make a personal, client-centered decision about how to proceed with the greatest level of discernment and likelihood of facilitating an easeful and healthful embodiment of a given forward fold. A possible solution or compromise related to the spinal flexion versus extension debate is as follows:

- *Keep the heart open* – invite the upper chest regions to stay broad and not collapsed; offer deliberate preparations for such open-heartedness and cue it with care and skill
- *Maintain the natural curves* of the spine while moving in and out of the fold; a trick for assessing whether this is accomplished invites placing the hands on the front of the torso, with thumbs at the low rib basket and little fingers at the top of the ASIS; the same distance is maintained between the fingers on the forward fold downward and the lifting upward – the following analysis can be cued:
  - if fingers came closer together, there was likely too much spinal flexion
  - if fingers spread farther apart, there was likely too much spinal extension
  - staying with the middle way of a natural spine on the dive forward and the reverse dive upward retains the original spacing between the fingers
- *Individualize* the forward folding approach to the reality of each client or student; roll-downs and roll-ups can be used as most auspiciously fitting with student needs and resources
- Once settled into the forward fold and all feels well, individuals can be invited to *come into spinal flexion to the degree that it is auspicious for the spinal and disc health of the individual* → if flexion is desired, clients can be invited to release and let go to move inward, attending to pressure distribution on the intervertebral discs and psychological or emotional reactivities
- To exit a forward fold that involved flexion at end range of the fold with a natural pelvis, clients are invited to rise out of the shape with the same discernment, lifting the head, opening the heart, and re-accessing the natural spinal curves before rising up fully
  - remind clients to reengage attention before lifting out of the forward fold
  - encourage students to find an open heart and the natural spinal curves as they rise out of the shape

Helpful kinesthetic explorations are offered in the *Box* below. These can be integrated into a well-sequenced practice during preparation with an explanation as to their purpose. They invite interoception and proprioception as well as being a great opportunity to invite students or clients to realign themselves with the *yamas* of non-violence and truthfulness.

**Exploration of forward fold range of motion:**

- Stand with the back to the wall, feet at least 6 to 10 inches away from the wall
- Begin to fold forward slowly by rolling the entire pelvis over the heads of the femurs – take your time!
- As you slowly fold, feel your tailbone against the wall – it will begin to travel upward
- Continue to pay keen attention to the movement of the tailbone up the wall and notice when it stops moving
- When the tailbone stops moving, stop folding and note the angle of flexion at the hip joint
- This is the point at which your lumbar spine will begin to lose its lordosis if you move further into the fold
- Any further depth generally involves spinal rounding, which may be fine if unloaded, but invites consideration depending on structural and energetic goals

**Based on your experience in the kinesthetic exploration, variations of forward folding may be chosen as follows:**

- If this angle is 90° or more (i.e., the more upright you are above having the torso parallel to the ground, which is 90°), do not force deep forward folds as this will happen at the expense of the lumbar
- Work on standing forward folds with hands at the wall or seated in Staff (hips on a prop if the angle was more than 90°) with straps to increase range of motion over time

**Exploration of what is happening in the spine during forward folding:**

- Stand upright in preparation for a standing forward fold
- Place the hand on the front body with the thumbs in the region of the low rib basket and the little fingers near the anterior superior iliac spine
- Note the distance between the fingers during this standing shape with a natural pelvis and spinal curves
- Begin to engage flexion in the hip to move forward with an open heart and attend to what is happening in the hands – the goal is to maintain the same distance in the hands as this will signal whether spine and pelvis remain naturally aligned
    - If the fingers begin to come closer together, the spine is beginning to move into flexion and the pelvis may be rolling into posterior alignment
    - If the fingers are spreading further apart, the spine may have moved into excessive extension, the pelvis may be rolling further forward, and integration may be lost in the core
- The point at which spine and pelvis lose their natural curves is the end range for a forward fold with natural alignment intact. There is nothing magical about this for individuals with good spinal health. However, for clients with spinal challenges this point may signal the end-range flexion that is still auspicious for the client

## Natural Pelvis with Healthful Movement in the Hip Joints

In most bodies, a natural standing or seated shape involves a slight anterior pelvic tilt, with the sacrum slanting forward at approximately 30–40 degrees. This anterior rotation in the pelvis is maintained in forward folding as well. Forward folds originate from movement of the pelvis as a whole over the femoral heads, rather than from flexion of the lumbar spine. The articulation between the acetabulum and head of the femoral thus functions as the forward fold joint. The pelvis, including the sacrum, travels over the femur heads as a unit. This whole-unit movement, rather than isolated spinal action, generates a forward fold that is structurally sound and energetically balanced. To support this action, students can be invited to explore their natural pelvic positioning, rather than a theoretical geometric neutral. In practice, this means recognizing that 'neutral' is not a single anatomical point, but a range of positions in which the spine can remain in its most natural curves and the hip joints can articulate freely from a pelvis that still is rolled naturally forward.

Props can offer crucial support in optimizing pelvic alignment either via elevating the pelvis (e.g., on blankets, bolsters, or blocks) to allow for a natural lumbar curve and/or via propping under the knees to reduce hamstring tension that might otherwise draw the pelvis into a posteriorly tilt and the lumbar spine into flexion.

## Supportive Action via Internal Rotation of the Acetabulofemoral Joints

Once more, the hip joint is the articulation between the heads of the femurs and the acetabulum of the pelvis and is central to forward folding. Due to the anteversion of the acetabulum (~15°), internal rotation of the femurs often facilitates ease and depth in folding. Internal rotation of the femurs brings more ease to the movement (in part also because this disarms the deep six external hip rotators), helping the acetabulum roll over the femoral heads. The deep six can become overactive or tight, especially in people who do a lot of walking, hiking, or running. Internal rotation can help transcend this tension. It also helps plant the femoral head in a more balanced position in the acetabulum and facilitates grounding the femur into the back plane of the body. This positioning contributes to physical and emotional ease and rooting.

Encouraging students to explore both internal and external rotation can highlight the relationship between rotational action and freedom of movement. Internal rotation often allows the pelvis to glide more smoothly over the femoral heads and can help release any inhibiting clenching in the gluteal muscles (if present). In wide-legged folds, internal rotation often arises naturally and can be enhanced by tactile feedback or gentle engagement. Once in the fold, the gluteal muscles and quadriceps can be (re)engaged. Notably, for hypermobile students, it is typically not useful to cue internal rotation; in fact, for these individuals, gluteal activation will help invite the greater stability and control that can be of benefit. This strategy may prevent excessive passive range and contribute to long-term joint health.

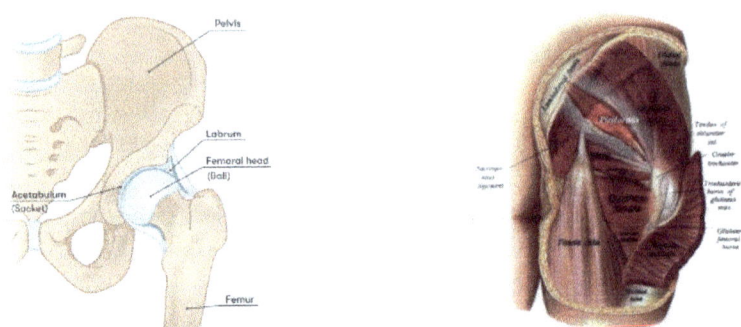

**Figure 2.17** Hip joint. (Data source: InjuryMap; https://commons.wikimedia.org/wiki/File:Hip_anatomy.svg; Creative Commons Attribution 4.0)

**Figure 2.18** Muscles affecting hip rotation and abduction. (Data source: Johannes Sobotta; https://commons.wikimedia.org/wiki/File:Piriformis.jpg; public domain)

## *Supportive Action Involving the Hip Extensors, Flexors, and Abductors*

The hamstrings (or hip extensors) are *biarticular*, which means they cross both the hip and knee joints and are placed under maximum tension when the hips are flexed and the knees extended. The hamstrings (comprised of the *biceps femoris, semitendinosus,* and *semimembranosus*) originate at the ischial tuberosity of the pelvis and insert on the tibia and fibula. Their primary actions are hip extension and knee flexion, yet their role in forward folding is distinctly one of eccentric control.

Given their biarticular nature, hamstring lengthening during forward folding can strain their origins at the ischial tuberosities if they lack resilience and capacity to accommodate deep hip flexion. Here is why: During forward folds, the hamstrings elongate as the pelvis tilts anteriorly over the femoral heads. This elongation is not passive; rather, it is mediated by a controlled eccentric contraction that modulates the descent. This tensioning action of the hamstrings manages the rate and depth of forward folding, preventing an uncontrolled collapse and guarding against excessive strain on the low back. If the hamstrings are tight or inhibited, the pelvis may be restricted from its natural anterior rotation, often resulting in compensatory flexion of the lumbar spine. This adaptation results in spinal flexion and a posterior rotation of the pelvis. Noted above, such actions may – for some individuals – place undue stress on the intervertebral discs because of the resulting compression at the anterior aspects of the vertebrae and discs. To facilitate a more effective forward fold, there must be adequate hamstring flexibility paired with intelligent engagement, allowing the pelvis to hinge forward without compromising spinal integrity.

Also affecting forward folding are the primary hip flexors, psoas major, iliacus, rectus femoris, and to a lesser extent, sartorius. They initiate flexion at the hip joint, drawing the femurs toward the pelvis or the pelvis toward the femurs. In forward folding, these muscles generally assume a state of relatively passive shortening, since the fold happens with gravity-assisted hip flexion. However, they do provide essential stabilization for the lumbar spine and anterior pelvis. Psoas major and iliacus, as deep stabilizers, create a supportive counterbalance to the posterior stretch of the hamstrings. If these muscles are excessively tight or restricted, they can inhibit the pelvis, resulting in lumbar overextension and resistance in the fold. Addressing hip flexor mobility can be helpful for facilitating the full range of hip flexion without undue lumbar strain.

Finally, the hip abductors also exert influence on forward folds. Gluteus medius, gluteus minimus, and tensor fasciae latae (TFL) function as primary hip abductors, playing a key role in stabilizing the pelvis during forward folds. While they do not directly contribute to the forward motion, their engagement helps maintain lateral stability and femoral alignment. This stability is particularly especially evident in standing forward folds, where balanced engagement prevents medial collapse of the knees and sustains optimal hip positioning. Slight activation of the abductors ensures that the femurs remain neutrally positioned, creating space in the hip joints and reducing compressive forces. This subtle engagement optimizes alignment and protects the sacroiliac joints from asymmetrical load distribution. It is particularly important for hypermobile students; it may not serve students with very tight abductor rotators.

*Helpful Muscle Actions and Preparations*

To support structurally sound and biomechanically efficient forward folding, it is essential to address the interplay of all involved muscle groups and bony structures. Cultivating hamstring flexibility through stretching and active eccentric loading helps release tension and support natural anterior pelvic rotation. As noted above, mindful approach to anterior pelvic rotation, that initiates the folding forward from the hip joints rather than the lumbar spine, ensures optimal movement and alignment. To facilitate hamstring release, teachers may emphasize reciprocal inhibition by engaging the quadriceps. Cues such as lifting the kneecaps, dorsiflexing the ankles, or flexing the toes help activate the front of the legs, allowing the back of the legs to release. In seated forward folds, using a strap between the feet and hands creates isometric engagement that reinforces length, strength, and postural integrity.

For the hip flexors, creating resilience combined with stabilization work can release tension that might otherwise limit pelvic mobility. Gentle activation of the psoas and iliacus during hip flexion may promote better access to hip hinging without lumbar strain. Abductor engagement can be subtly cued to maintain lateral stability and femoral alignment. Activating gluteus medius and minimus during the descent into a forward fold prevents the knees from collapsing inward and preserves space in the hip joints, contributing to overall pelvic health and symmetry, especially for hypermobile students. However, this action may need to be balanced with internal rotation for students with more limited range of motion.

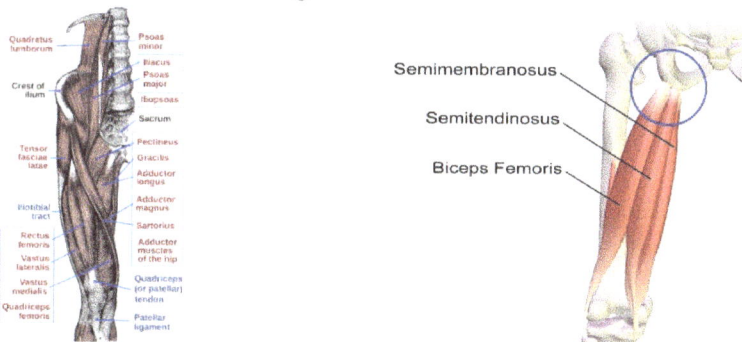

**Figure 2.19** Muscles affecting hip flexion and extension. (Data source: Jmarchn; https://commons.wikimedia.org/wiki/File:Gray430-en.svg; Creative Commons Attribution 3.0)

**Figure 2.20** Hamstring muscles – posterior views. (Data source: Paul Hermans; https://upload.wikimedia.org/wikipedia/commons/2/2b/Opgespannen_hamstrings_%28cropped%29.jpg. Creative Commons Attribution 4.0)

When students reach the end of their hip mobility but continue folding forward, the pelvis often tilts posteriorly and the spine rounds. This is not inherently problematic, but it may shift the fold from functional to compensatory. Inviting the use of props, bent knees, or reduced depth offers a safer and more integrated experience. Propping under the pelvis or knees can help reduce load if hamstrings are very tight, facilitates anterior pelvic tilt, and may prevent injury.

## Sample Practices for *Cultivating Resilience and Building Strength in the Hamstrings*

Yoga offers a large variety of ways for preparing the hamstrings for forward folding practice, attending to their need for resilience and strength. These preparations can be so powerful as to make up a significant portion of a session. They are sequenced into forward-folding practice with care, preparing the body for the resilience and fortitude required to release into healthful forward folds that work with each individual client's bioindividuality. These suggestions are an invitation for teacher creativity in working with the backs of the legs, pelvis, and low back. They invite playful yet present-minded and careful exploration with keen engagement of mind, body, and breath. They are simply a sampling of the possible preparatory work for the hamstrings.

### *Creating Resilience*

This set of sample preparatory shapes and movements for a forward folding practice emphasizes resilience via eccentric control, active flexibility, and functional adaptability across the length of the hamstrings. These preparations require mindful engagement, appropriate tailoring to individual client needs, and a natural spine where applicable. They promote neuromuscular adaptability and gently increase active range of motion.

- *Standing hip hinge with forward reach* – challenging the hamstrings eccentrically through hip flexion in a functional, upright position (essentially a preparatory version of Half-Lift [*ardha uttanasana*] or Chair-at-the-Wall [*utkatasana*], depending on hamstring resilience)

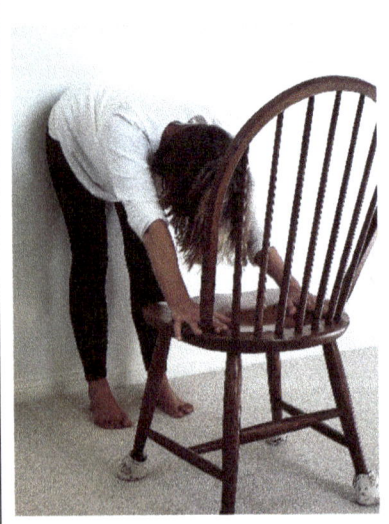

- stand with the back to a wall, facing into the room with two blocks or the seat of a chair available; place the feet hip-width apart, knees softly bent
- to begin with have the legs several inches away from the wall, while the back of the torso leans into the wall
- hinge at the hips and reach the arms forward to land the hands on the blocks or seat of chair
- keep the spine in its natural curves and the hamstrings active throughout
- slightly bend the knees; then slowly straighten them, feeling the hamstrings engage to extend the knees without locking them
- walk the feet closer and closer to the wall as the hamstrings release – the goal is not necessarily to reach the wall with the back of the heels; simply to feel the increased demand on the hamstrings as the feet move closer underneath the hip hinge
- repeat several times focusing on control and mindfulness, not speed

- *Supine active leg lowering* – Improving eccentric hamstring control while integrating hip flexor-hamstring coordination (in essence a variation of reclined Hand-to-Toe [*supta padangustasana*])

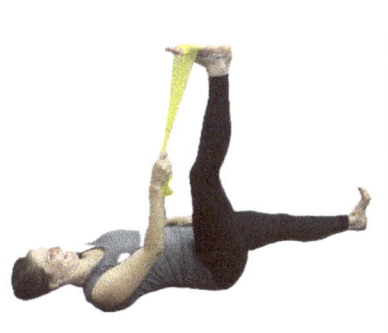

  - lie on the back with both legs extended toward the ceiling
  - engage the core and press the arms into the ground
  - slowly lower one leg toward the floor, keeping the opposite leg vertical – ideally the leg is help vertical via core strength; alternatively, the leg can be grasped with the hands behind the thigh or with a strap around the foot, ends held in both hands
  - extend the active leg's knee and avoid arching the low back as the leg moves up and down – that is, maintain the natural spinal curves and pelvic tilt
  - lower the leg as far as eccentric control is maintained and then lift the leg back up with active strength (rather than momentum)
  - repeat several times with one leg; then switch legs and repeat an equal number of times with the second leg

- *Supine hamstring slides from Bridge* (with socks or sliders) – training the hamstrings eccentrically while supporting the pelvis in its natural position

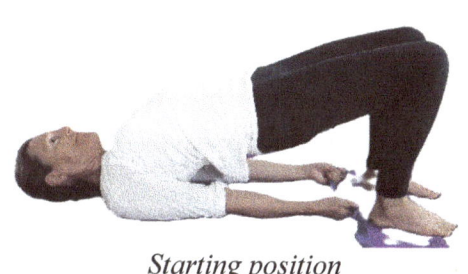

*Starting position*

  - lie on the back, knees bent, heels on sliders (or socks/towels on hardwood)
  - lift the hips into Bridge
  - exhale and slowly slide both feet forward (i.e., away from the sitz bones), inviting hamstring resilience
  - keep hips lifted and spine in its natural curves as the hamstrings respond – linger for a moment
  - then slide the heels back in under the knees, bending the knees and returning to Bridge
  - repeat several times

*Creating Strength*

This set of sample preparatory shapes and movements for a forward folding practice focuses on strength-building via concentric and isometric contractions to increase hamstring power and endurance. These preparations are offered in a context of mindful engagement, client-centered tailoring to individual needs, and attunement to maintaining the natural spine (where applicable).

- *Deadlift* – strengthening the hamstrings concentrically and eccentrically under load, using bodyweight or holding light weights in the hand

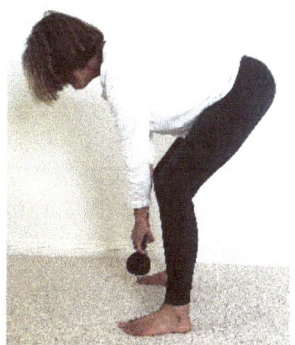

  - stand with feet wider than hip-width apart and a slight bend in the knees
  - hold a light weight (optional), and hinge at the hips, lowering the torso while keeping the spine long
  - stay mindful of the hamstrings lengthening (and strengthening) as the hips move back
  - then extend the knees, engaging the hamstrings and glutes to return to standing
  - repeat a few times – perhaps until a bit of fatigue sets in

| *Hamstring curls on a yoga ball* - strengthening the hamstrings concentrically and isometrically ||
|---|---|
| 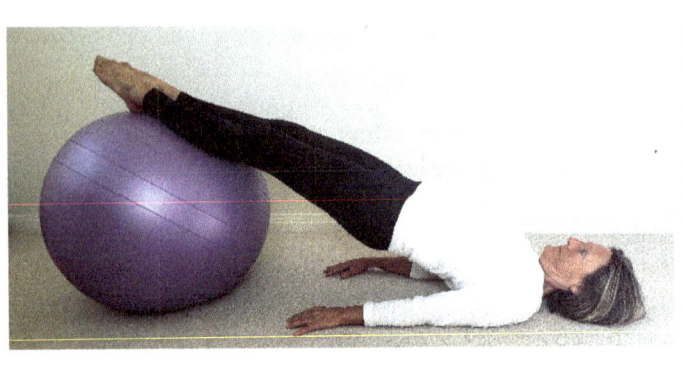 | o lie on the back with calves resting on a yoga ball<br>o lift the hips so the entire body forms a straight line (essentially moving into a Reverse Plank – with the heart facing up rather than down)<br>o bend the knees, pulling the ball toward the hips using the power of the hamstrings<br>o keep the hips lifted as the ball comes closer to the hips and avoid collapsing in the spine<br>o repeat several times |

| *Single-leg Glute Bridges* – targeting hamstrings and gluteal muscles unilaterally for strength and pelvic stability ||
|---|---|
| 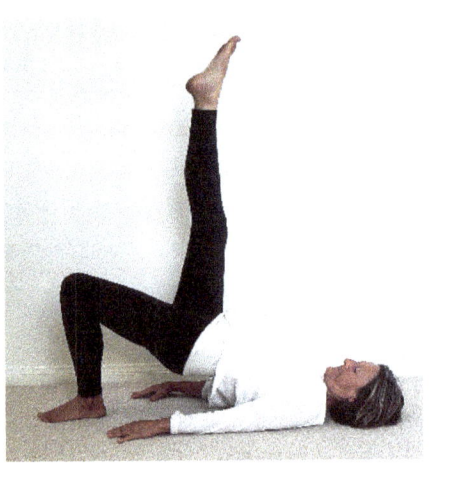 | o lie on the back with knees bent<br>o lift one leg, extending it toward the ceiling with pointed toes reaching for the ceiling; keep the other foot grounded<br>o engage the hamstrings of the grounded leg to press into the floor and lift up into Bridge<br>o stay for several breaths; then lower mindfully and with control<br>o repeat a couple of times on one leg; then switch sides and repeat on the other leg |

## *Core Stabilization*

Trunk or core stabilization has been amply covered in Chapter 4, as well as in the context of arm-standing shapes. In deeper forward folds, especially past 90° of hip flexion, balanced core stabilization supports spinal integrity. Although the abdominal wall can remain soft to allow easeful folding and breathing, a gentle engagement of the transverse abdominis and pelvic floor can support an integrated structure. Such stabilization can be accessed in a variety of ways and has been discussed in other chapters. Quick and simple hints in the moment can include an invitation to laugh or cough to feel these interdependent inner muscles. Lion's Breath on the exhalation can also be helpful. In stronger variations, such as Chair or transitions in and out of deep folds, co-activation of the core muscles provides support and coordination. Relatedly, soft and unforced exhalation can facilitate the descent or calm release into a fold.

| | *Tips for Grounding, Expansion, and Stability in Forward Folds* |
|---|---|
| Grounding | • Ground through relevant body parts on the floor<br>• Ground the femurs into the back plane of the body<br>• Engage the core as a way of anchoring<br>• Ground/anchor energetically<br>• Engage the quadriceps (draw knee caps upward; lift toes) and root down through the femurs<br>• Bring support under the knees if they are lifted off the floor<br>• Ground/anchor with the breath<br>• Invite the mind to anchor on a *drishti* (e.g., back body works well here)<br>• Deepen your awareness of sensation in the back body<br>• Ground the hands on blocks |
| Stability | • Draw in the perineum<br>• Draw the belly button toward the spine<br>• Allow softness in the belly to fold and invite stability when upright<br>• Draw the hip bones toward each other<br>• Draw the toes/kneecaps toward the hips (seated)<br>• Stabilize the shoulders first; then mobilize as needed<br>• Engage the quadriceps to invite resilience and balance into the hamstrings<br>• Engage a Lion's Breath to turn on the core muscles that support stability<br>• Laugh or cough to feel the engagement of the core and pelvic floor<br>• Find a *drishti* to stabilize attention and presence |
| Expansion | • Lengthen the spine to create space between vertebrae<br>• Maintain length in spine and end the fold when natural lumbar lordosis is lost<br>• Lengthen the back body<br>• Stabilize the shoulders first; then mobilize as needed<br>• Find softness in the abdomen as you fold more deeply<br>• Find length in the back muscles<br>• Lengthen from the soles of the feet to the crown of the head<br>• Find lightness in the torso<br>• Reach through the fingertips<br>• Reach through the crown of the head |

## Analysis and Experience of Sample Forward Folds

The following forward folds are analyzed in detail below:
- *Standing Forward Fold*
- *Seated Forward Fold*
- *Head-of-Knee Fold*
- *Wide-Legged Standing Forward Fold*
- *Wide-Legged Seated Forward Fold*
- *Child*

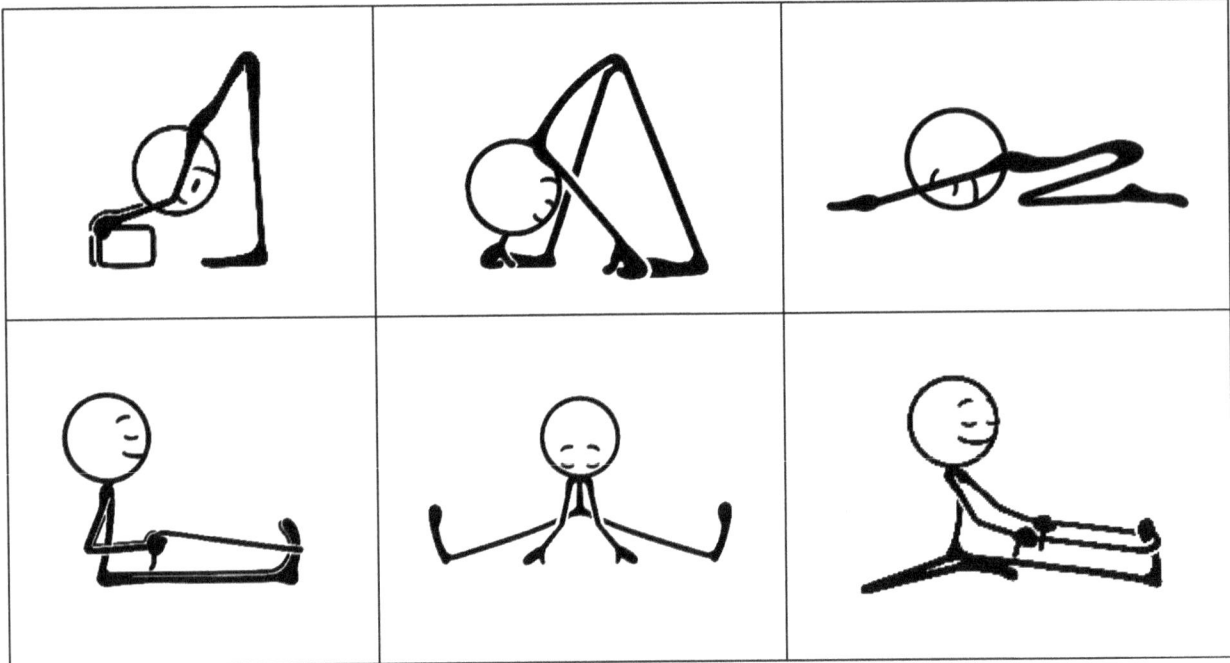

These forward folding shapes are considered foundational and if yoga professionals understand how to cue these shapes, they will be able to cue most any forward fold. They can simply apply all exemplified principles with wisdom and discernment, using their experience with practicing and teaching these shapes.

The cueing guidance offered for each shape needs to be considered in the context offered in the *general teaching and anatomical principles for forward folds*. The basics discussed above need to permeate the cueing for all these shapes. The additional cueing, shape by shape, offered here is icing on the cake. Always incorporate integrated holistic yoga cueing that addresses the following teaching principles:

- *Accessibility* – creating access through variation, adaptation, affiliation, individualization, and person-centeredness
- *Intentionality* – embedding the practice of each shape in the overall arc of the session, grounding in the theme for the class and the meaning of the practice
- *Beneficence* – honoring the wellbeing of each student and always making sure to first do no harm
- *Holism* – cueing all *koshas* or layers of experience in all shapes, never forgetting that each shape has reverberations into and is affected by all *koshas* – it is not enough to cue anatomy; also address energy and vitality, thoughts and emotions, behavioral and action choices, even community and interbeing
- *Integration* – in teaching *asana*, integrate breathwork, concentration and mindfulness, as well as the ethical principles and lifestyle practices of yoga

## *General Concepts about Forward Folding*

Many aspects of forward folds hold constant across several of the dimensions covered for individual shapes. Thus, following are general comments about benefits, cautions, preparations, recovery as applicable to all covered forward folds. After this general discussion, instructions are provided for five individual forward folding shapes, providing key alignment cues, variations, and any additional teaching tips for each.

### *Benefits*

Forward folding offers physical, mental, and energetic benefits, through enhancing the balance between effort and ease in all layers of experience (i.e., body, breath, and mind). These shapes invite introspection and self-reflection, creating a perfect environment for cultivating a yoga practice guided from within not without. Forward folds are healthful as they invite the following (and possible more) benefits:

- *Improve flexibility and mobilizes the back body*: Forward folds stretch and develop resilience in the hamstrings, calves, and low back. This promotes an opening action in these areas, facilitating energetic flow from the feet upward through the entire spine, enhancing overall flexibility and mobility.
- *Release tension in the spine and shoulders*: Forward folds help elongate the spine while activating the core to create stability. These actions promote spinal health and alignment, keeping the spine strong and supple. Additionally, allowing the head and neck to release while folding reduces tension in the neck and shoulders and creates a sense of ease.
- *Calm mind and body*: The inward, introspective nature of forward folds, when combined with mindful breathing, encourages grounding, release, and letting be. Emphasizing an extended exhalation during forward folding helps calm the nervous system and quiet the mind, making these shapes effective for stress release and emotional balance.
- *Improve circulation*: The half-inverted nature of forward folds supports improved blood flow, invigorating the body while promoting grounding. Increased circulation helps oxygenate tissues, also boosting energy and mental clarity.
- *Stimulate digestive organs*: The gentle compression of the abdomen during forward folds massages and stimulates the digestive organs, perhaps aiding in digestion and overall abdominal health.
- *Promote mindfulness*: Forward folds draw attention inward, encouraging focus on vital and somatic awareness. This introspective practice fosters mindfulness, helping practitioners connect with the present moment and cultivate a calm and centered mind.
- *Enhance posture and hip mobility*: By creating resilience in the back, hips, and lower body, forward folds can support healthful and naturally aligned posture, increased hip mobility, and better overall alignment.
- *Reduce anxiety*: The calming, grounding effect of forward folds can reduce feelings of anxiety and promote a sense of peace and relaxation.
- *Ease insomnia*: Forward folds' relaxing and calming nature makes them beneficial for unwinding body and mind, improving sleep quality, and combating insomnia.

## Cautions

Although forward folding is beneficial in many ways, it is important to be aware of the following considerations:
- *Low back sensitivity*: Individuals with low back discomfort or a history of spinal disc injuries may find forward folds challenging. Maintaining a gentle bend in the knees and engaging the core can help support the low back. Moving within a sustainable range of motion and use of props are key with such individuals.
- *Hamstring tightness*: If hamstrings are shortened from much sitting (or for other reasons), there may be a tendency to pull the low back into excessive flexion. Practicing with bent knees and focusing maintaining the natural curves of the spine (rather than deepening the fold) prevents strain.
- *Hypermobility*: Hypermobile students may hyperextend the knees and the low spine. They benefit from cueing related to micro-bending the knees and creating core engagement. They do *not* benefit from cueing that increases lumbar curves (such as lifting the sitz bones). Special attention may be necessary to help hypermobile develop proprioceptive awareness of hyperextension (something that is often missing for them).
- *High blood pressure or dizziness*: As half-inversions, standing forward folds may not be suitable for individuals with uncontrolled high blood pressure or those prone to dizziness. For such students, it may be helpful to offer variation (e.g., hands rest on a chair or blocks to elevate the torso). Additionally, it is helpful to invite moving down and up slowly, leading with the torso and allowing the neck and head to follow gently. Eyes are best kept open with a gentle connection to the outer world.
- *Possible contraindications*:
  - *Herniated discs*: People with herniated or bulging discs in the low back may need to avoid deep forward folds, as they can exacerbate these condition.
  - *Sciatica*: Those with sciatica may find that forward folds increase pain if the sciatic nerve is compressed. Students with sciatic nerve pain may need a wider stance or bent knees to maximize comfort. Mindful practice is crucial.
  - *Glaucoma or eye pressure issues*: The inverted nature of forward folds can increase pressure in the eyes. Those with eye conditions like glaucoma should consult a healthcare provider before practicing these shapes.
  - *High blood pressure*: Inversions can increase blood pressure. Those with hypertension need to be cautious with deep forward folds or avoid them if their condition is not well-controlled.

## Preparations

To prepare for forward folding, it is helpful to incorporate movements that create mobility in the legs, release tension in the spine, awaken the breath, and create a smoother transition into the fold. The six movement of the spine are used as a warm and then progress to some of the following possible preparations. These preparatory movements help build warmth and mobility.
- *Hip joints movements*: Mobilizing and becoming aware of the hip joints is helpful to engaging the hip joints as the forward fold hinge (and prevents excessive rounding in the lumbar spine).

- *Gentle lunges*: Create space in the hips and engage the legs, preparing the body for the deeper fold in a standing forward fold.
- *Half lifts*: Mobilizes the spine and the hip joints while engaging the core, providing a gentle introduction to these dynamics in forward folds.
- *Knee-to-chest standing balance*: Enhances awareness of the hamstrings and provides a gentle warm-up for the muscles of the back body. It also warms up the hip joints for flexion.
- *Cat-Cow*: Encourages a connection between breath and spinal movement, setting the stage for a more mindful journey through the movement down and back up.
- *Hamstring resilience*: See *Sample Practices for Hamstrings* above.

*Recovery*

After practicing standing forward folds, restorative movements (which happen to be very similar to the preparations) help integrate the experience and release residual tension. These recovery movements create a smooth transition from the activation of folding forward to a grounded and relaxed state. Other (or no recovery) movements may be indicated if the next step in the practice involves more forward folding or inversion into Headstand.

- *Knees-to-chest*: A gentle way to release the low back and create ease in the spine after folding forward.
- *Spinal rotations*: Gentle twists can release the spine and create ease across the back, shoulders, and neck.
- *Standing lateral flexion*: Side bends can create lateral movement that may release tightness accumulated during forward folding.
- *Intuitive movement*: Gentle wiggles, shakes, shoulder rotations, and even light jogging can feel like a supportive relief.

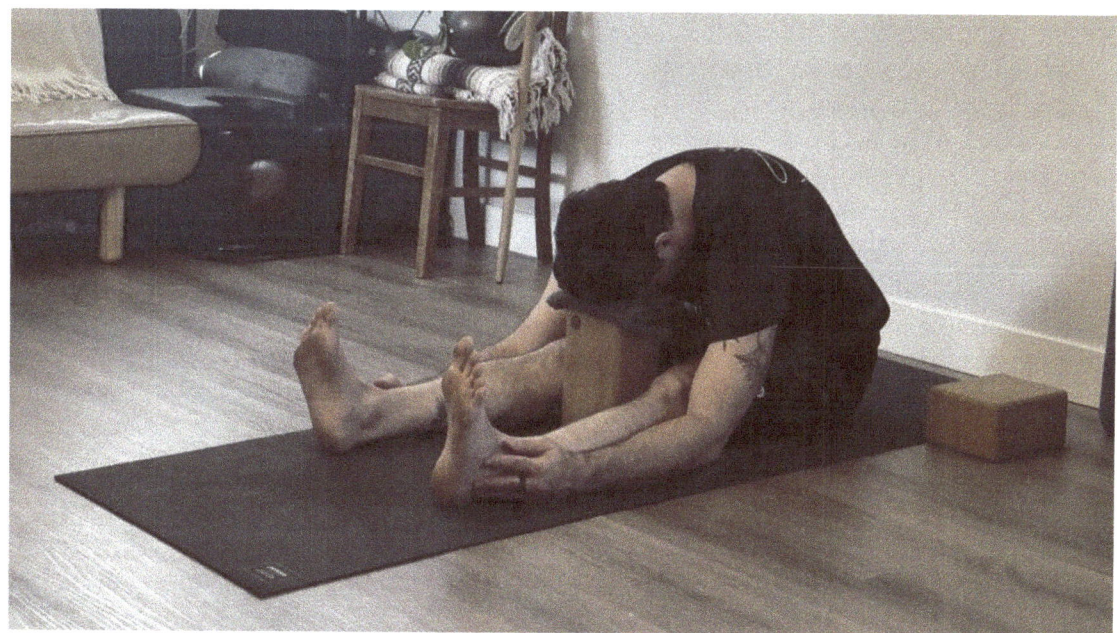

## Standing Forward Fold or Uttanasana

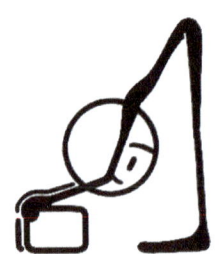

Standing Forward Folds are grounding shapes that emerges from Mountain and invites an exploration of ease within effort, strength within mobility, and resilience within mindful surrender. These folds bring awareness to the physical and vital relationship between legs, pelvis, spine, and breath. Though widely practiced as if accessible in a standard approach, Standing Forward Folds present unique opportunities for individual expression based on natural differences in anatomy, mobility, and psychological comfort levels. The experience of a standing forward fold is therefore best tailored to meet students or clients where they are, via offering variations as a matter of course to invite and prioritize a wholesome and embodied experience that arise from students' bioindividuality, not from an idealized outer shape.

### Key Alignment Invitations

Although folding forward from Mountain may appear straightforward and intuitive, finding balance and wholesome alignment in the shape involves a dynamic interplay of engagement and release, of attention and interoception. Inner experience is prioritized over achieving any specific outer appearance. These alignment invitations emphasize a complex and nuanced approach that encourages students to explore what feels most supportive and balanced for their body, while being open to feeling new sensations and changing unhealthful somatic pattern locks.

- *Invitations related to feet and legs*:
  - *Ground through the feet*: Invite practitioners to spread their toes and feel a connection with the earth. Pressing evenly through the feet can help distribute weight and create a sense of grounding. Grounding through either three or four corners of the feet can be invited (as discussed in Mountain).
  - *Moving into the fold*: Cueing from Mountain to Forward Fold emphasizes the hip joints as the origin of the fold (not the low back, which is the default of many students). Educating students about the hip joints as their forward fold hinge is key to inviting a healthful release forward. Demonstration is key to help student understand this concept.
  - *Bend the knees as needed*: A slight bend in the knees can ease tension in the low back and hamstrings, allowing for a more easeful fold. Practitioners can experiment with varying the bend to explore what creates the most comfort. It is important to remain vigilant about students who are hypermobile – they have a tendency to hyperextend the knees without awareness. They too benefit from a slight bend in the knees, but for the opposite reason of students who lack resilience in the back body.
  - *Engage the thighs*: Encourage students to lift through the front of the thighs to create stability (and strength) in the legs and around the knee joints. This subtle engagement supports the low back and deepens the sense of grounding.
  - *Internal rotation of the hip joint (legs)*: Internal rotation can greatly support more ease in a Forward Fold for students who have tightness in the back of the legs. Note: this cue may be contraindicated for hypermobile students as it will create even more flexion in the hips and extension in the knees and lumbar spine.

- *Invitations related to the spine and torso*:
  - *Maintain the natural curves of the spine*: Rather than aiming to reach the hands to the floor, prioritize creating space between the vertebrae along the length of the spine. Imagine the crown of the head releasing toward the ground while aiming to maintain natural curves, especially in the lumbar spine. For some students, this will feel like a slight backbend within the Forward Fold on the inside (because of their habit to flex excessively through the spine due to modern life causing them to lean over devices). For this reason, it can be helpful to invite awareness of outer shape in this position as students may lack accurate proprioception.
  - *Engage the core*: Gently drawing the navel in toward the spine supports the low back, and prevents moving either too far into flexion or extension in the lumbar, supporting the notion of a natural secondary curve. Core engagement, via drawing the low rib toward the hips, creates stability while moving into the fold, supports staying folded with healthful alignment, and tends to increase interoceptive awareness. It is helpful, however, to ensure that students are not braced or gripped; finding natural core engagement is key.
- *Invitations related to the head, neck, and shoulders*:
  - *Release tension*: Students can benefit from being invited to bring ease into the head, neck, and shoulders, allowing all to release toward the earth. Gentle 'yes' and 'no' motions of head and neck can invite a sense of ease.
  - *Allow the shoulder to be at ease*: There is no need to cue shoulder placement. The shoulder girdle can find its natural alignment and there is no hard and fast rule about where it should end up (no need to cue drawing the shoulders away from the ears or shoulder blades drawing together).
  - *Find a balanced gaze*: If looking downward causes discomfort, students may find it helpful to rest the gaze on a spot slightly forward on the mat. Such alignment suggests the use of a prop under the hands for more wholesome alignment along the length of the spine.

## Variations and Exploration

Standing Forward Folds can be varied creatively to honor different needs and preferences. These variations allow for exploration of the shape in a way that best suits each individual's body, creating a supportive and nourishing experience. Possible variations include but certainly are not limited to the following:

- *Hands on props*: Elevating the hands by placing them on blocks or the seat of a chair can make the fold accessible, allowing for healthful alignment in the spine and reducing strain in the back of the legs.
- *Ragdoll variation*: By crossing the arms and holding opposite elbows, the practitioner can create a sense of release in the shoulders and upper back. Slightly swaying side to side can help shed lingering tension.
- *Wide-Legged Forward Fold*: If a narrow stance feels constricting, stepping the feet wider apart can provide more room for the pelvis and low back to release.
- *Halfway lifting*: For those who prefer not to fold deeply, remaining in a halfway lift with the hands on the thighs, shins, blocks, or chair can offer a gentler alternative that still mobilizes the spine and engages the core.

- *Half-Lift* at the wall: Gaining support from the wall here is minor; the wall is for balance and the core is used to create the strength for the lift (unlike Downward Facing Dog at the wall, which looks very similar but involves strong pressure of the hands into the wall)

*Additional Teaching Tips*

To facilitate a healthful and accessible experience of moving into a Standing Forward Fold from a standing position, some of following suggestions may be helpful and create increase interoceptive and proprioceptive awareness.
- *Mindful breathing*: Invite students to notice how the breath influences their experience of the shape. Paying attention to the rhythm of inhalation and exhalation can help find a balance between effort and ease. Breathing into the back body is encouraged as forward folding (especially with the legs together) can result in labored breathing due to constriction in the front body.
- *Individual experience*: Remind students that the shape is expected to look and feel different for each person. Encourage them to explore variations and alignments that feel supportive from the inside out, rather than focusing on achieving a specific external goal. There is nothing magical about touching the hands to the floors and grounding the palms on the floor. The same grounding and introspection can arise from hands and palms on blocks, chairs, bolsters, or thighs.
- *Creative prop use*: Blocks, blankets, chairs, and straps can be used to make forward folding accessible in a grounded way and provide easeful and exploratory pathways into the fold.

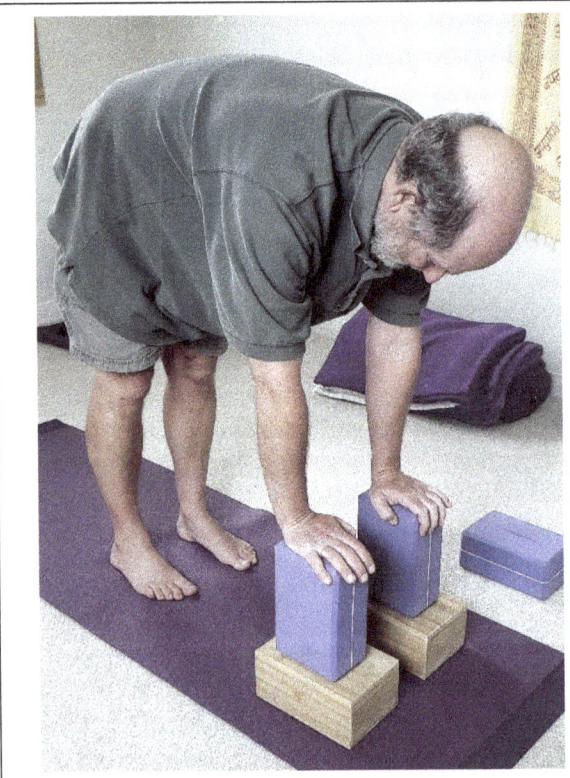
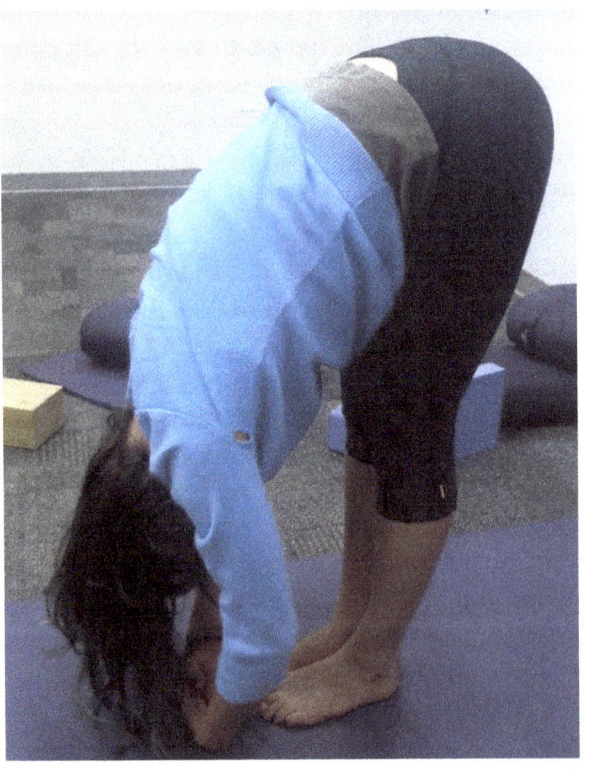

| *Standing Forward Half Lift with Support* | *Standing Forward Fold – Ragdoll* |

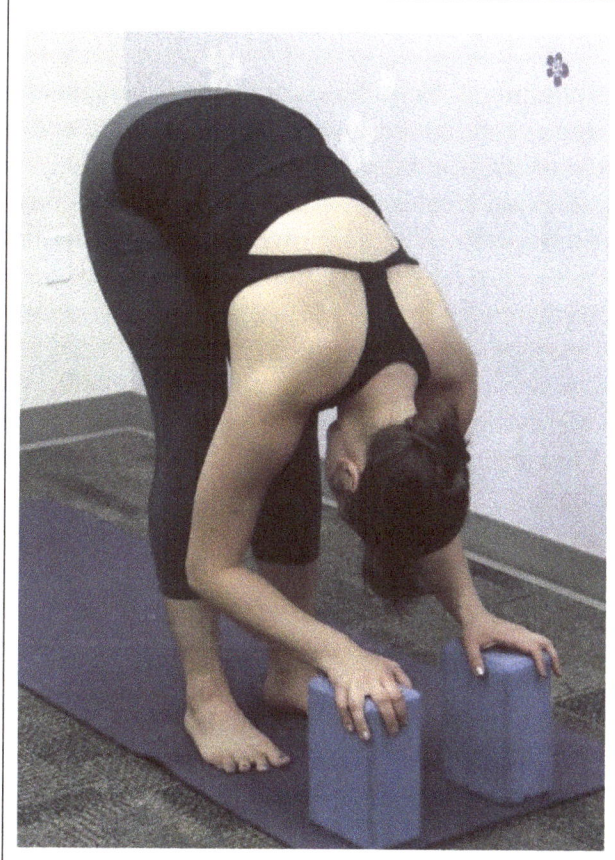

*Standing Forward Fold with Head Released*

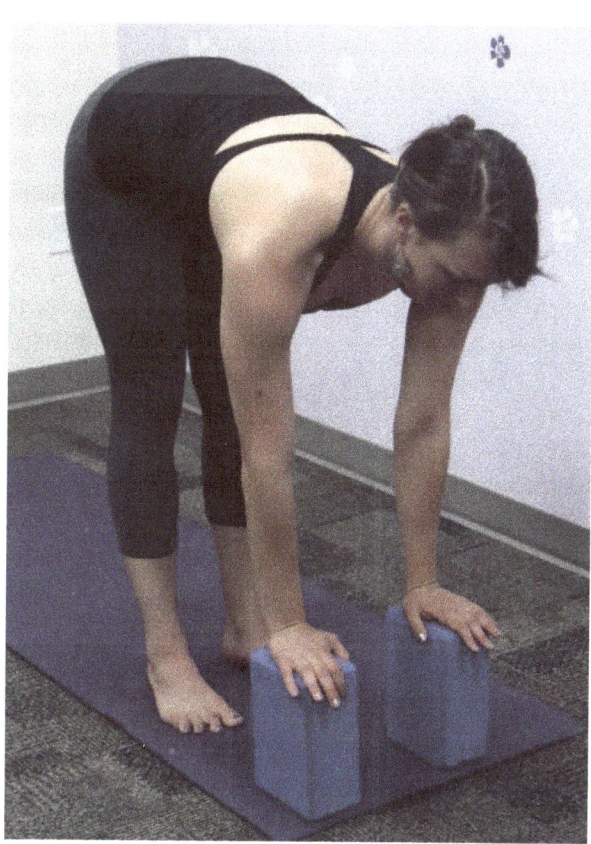

*Standing Half Lift*

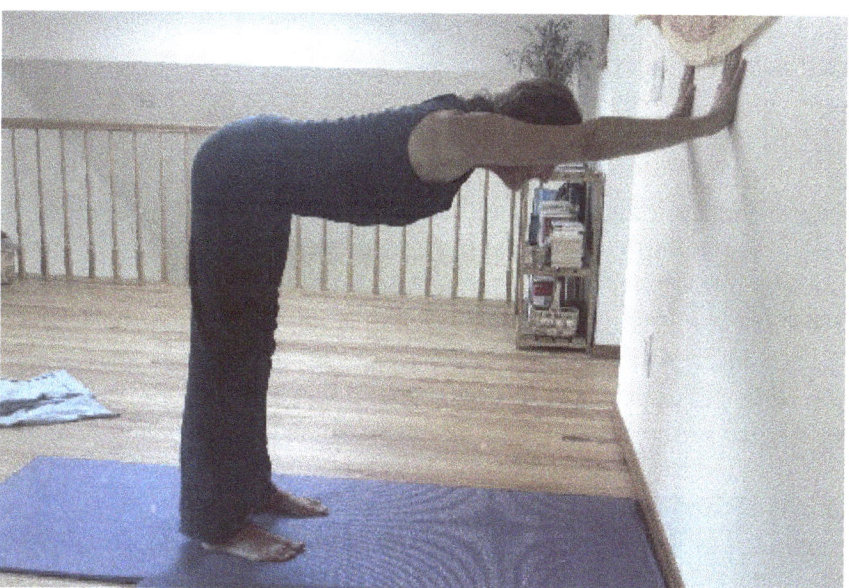

*Standing Half Lift at a Wall – no force in hands*

## *Wide-Legged Standing Forward Fold or Prasarita Padottanasana*

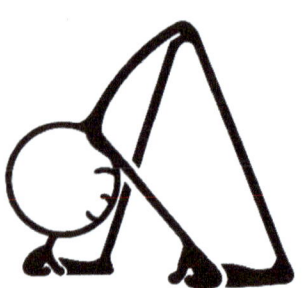

Wide-Legged Standing Forward Folds are expansive shapes that emerges from a standing base with the feet as wide apart as is comfortable for the individual's anatomy. The wide-legged starting position creates a balance between grounding and freedom of movement. This fold invites exploration of ease within stability; it releases tension in the back body and cultivates resilience and openness. By embracing individual anatomical differences and unique preferences, practitioners can experience many ways of forward folding that reflect their bioindividuality rather than a single idealized shape. Wide-Legged Forward Folds may be more accessible than folds accessed from Mountain, thanks to the wider base.

### *Key Alignment Invitations*

Wide-Legged Forward Folds combine grounding, mindful release, and supportive alignment through inviting strength and mobility. The following alignment cues aim to encourage a sense of ease and inner awareness, guiding practitioners to tune into their body's experience rather than focusing on the external appearance of the shape. They promote an interoceptive and neuroceptive experience of stability and resilience that allows sensations to arise within a context of optimized opportunity for the experience of safety and mindful presence.

- *Invitations related to feet and legs*:
  - *Ground through the feet*: Practitioners are invited to find a foot placement that supports a sense of stability and ease. The width of the feet is guided by hip anatomy and is chosen in a manner that protects the knee joints. Spreading the toes and feeling grounded through either the three or four corners of each foot can add to students' deep sense of connection to the earth.
  - *Initiate the fold from the hip joints*: Practitioners are guided to hinge at the hips as they fold, letting the hip joints – not the low back – initiate movement. This approach emphasizes natural spinal curves and helps release unnecessary bracing as well as excessive flexion or extension in the lumbar spine.
  - *Bend the knees if helpful*: A soft bend in the knees can release tension in the back of the legs and low back, allowing for a more easeful fold. This adjustment also supports practitioners with hypermobile joints by discouraging hyperextension.
  - *Engage the thighs*: A gentle lift through the thighs stabilizes the legs and supports a more stable experience of the base; it also creates resilience and prevent torquing around the knee joints. Both serve to further enhance the grounding and settling of the nervous system that is invited in this shape.
  - *Explore gentle internal rotation*: For students who experience tightness in the back of their legs, slight internal rotation of the legs may create more freedom in the fold. However, for hypermobile practitioners, this cue may be counterproductive, as it may increase create instability in joints (rather than ease).

- *Invitations related to the spine and torso*:
  - *Maintain the natural curves of the spine*: Rather than cueing a goal of reaching for the floor, invite practitioners to prioritize a natural curve in the spine with a natural sense of space between the vertebrae. As they fold, they may feel a slight backbend in the spine, depending on their natural tendencies.
  - *Engage the core*: Gently drawing the navel in toward the spine supports stability, helping maintain alignment without excessive bracing and also preventing collapse or lack of effort. Core engagement can also be cued to bring more awareness to the inner body and to get in touch with the ensuing resilient stability in the spine.
- *Invitations related to the head and neck*:
  - *Ease tension in the neck*: Encourage practitioners to let go of bracing in the neck and allow the head to release toward the earth. Gentle 'yes' and 'no' movements can help create creativity, comfort, and relaxation in this area.
  - *Consider the gaze*: If looking downward causes discomfort, practitioners can also choose to direct their gaze forward after placing their hands on a prop to support such alignment with ease.

### Variations and Exploration

Wide-Legged Standing Forward Folds offer space for exploration and adaptability to suit a range of individual needs. The following variations provide accessible entry points and opportunities for students to create a fold that feels supportive, individualized to their somatic and vital needs, as well as adapted to their emotional and mental presence in the moment. They help create folds that reflect mobility, balance, and easefulness and that are deeply authentic to in-the-moment needs and experiences.

- *Hands on props*: Placing the hands on blocks or a chair can create a more accessible fold, enabling healthful alignment through the spine and easing tension in the back of the legs. With use of these props, head and shoulders can release more freely.
- *Ragdoll variation*: Crossing the arms and holding opposite elbows can encourage a sense of release in the shoulders and upper back. Gentle swaying from side to side may help release residual tension.
- *Half lift with hands under the shoulders*: This variation involves bringing the hands on the floor, aligned directly under the shoulders, with the spine in its natural curves and parallel to the floor. This orientation in space creates length along the spine and releases compression in the low back. The crown of the head reaches forward, engaging the core and building resilience in the back body. Hands can be placed on a prop to create even more ease in the shape.
- *Halfway lifting*: For students who prefer less flexion in the hip joint and less demand on the back body, a halfway lift with hands on thighs, shins, blocks, or chair offers a gentler experience that helps develop strength and resilience in spine and core over time. The 90° angle in the hip joints is compassionate for students with tighter back bodies.
- *Downward Facing Dog torso*: Walk the hands forward (on the ground or bringing along blocks under the hands) from the fold until the torso is aligned as if in a (wide-legged) Downward Facing Dog position. This decrease in hip flexion helps practitioners create more space through the arms, spine, and back body. This variation can feel expansive and

grounding, supporting ease in the back and shoulders. Width of hand placement is adjusted as described in Downward Facing Dog as there is weight-bearing in the hands.
- *Rotations*: Rotational spinal movements (that include movement of the pelvis as a whole and integrated unit as discussed in twisting shapes) offer an additional element of challenge and playfulness in forward folds. With one hand rooted on the floor and the other reaching up, practitioners can explore rotation through the spine that invites ample movement through the length of the spine, and opening in the heart space, and mobility of the pelvis. This movement is initiated by the grounded hand pushing into the floor or prop and letting rebound support the rotation as well as the lift of the opposite arm. The upper arm does not over-effort or lead the way; it responds to the grounding strength of the hand that pushes away the floor. Rotations support openness in the shoulders and upper body; the grounded hand maintains stability.
- *Threading the needle*: From the fold, with one hand resting on the earth or a prop, reach up with the other arm to its side of the body and then reach it across the body to the other side, threading it under the grounded arm. The shoulder of the reaching arm moves toward the ground, creating significantly deeper rotation. This variation challenges the spine, back, and shoulders and needs to be offered with care. All cautions and guidance about twisting shapes apply.

## *Additional Teaching Tips*

To create an environment that promotes awareness and supports individual experiences, consider these additional teaching cues:
- *Mindful breathing*: Remind students to notice the rhythm of their breath and its influence on the fold. The inhalation can be used to invite a sense of expansiveness and opening; the exhalation can help create a sense of release as well as inviting a drawing inward with stability and strength. Sensing into the back body can be a powerful way of inviting diaphragmatic breathing.
- *Encouragement of individual experience*: As always, it is key to invite students to let the shape emerge from the inside out, not the outside in. Folds tend to bring out a desire to flex deeply and strain across the back body. It helps to remind practitioners that the focus is on a healthful inner experience rather than an idealized external shape. Creating new mental patterns of honoring needs is invited with such cueing during this more introspective approach.
- *Creative prop use*: Offer blocks, chairs, blankets, or bolsters under the hands and head as options to make the fold accessible in a beneficial and intentional manner. Practitioners can be invited to explore variations that best support their needs – *without* implying that use of props makes shapes easier or less healthful.
- *Imagery and metaphor*: Invite students to imagine their spine lengthening between earth and sky, creating a sense of dynamic length, opening, and space throughout the fold. Some students like the image of stress draining into the earth through the limbs and/or the crown of the head.

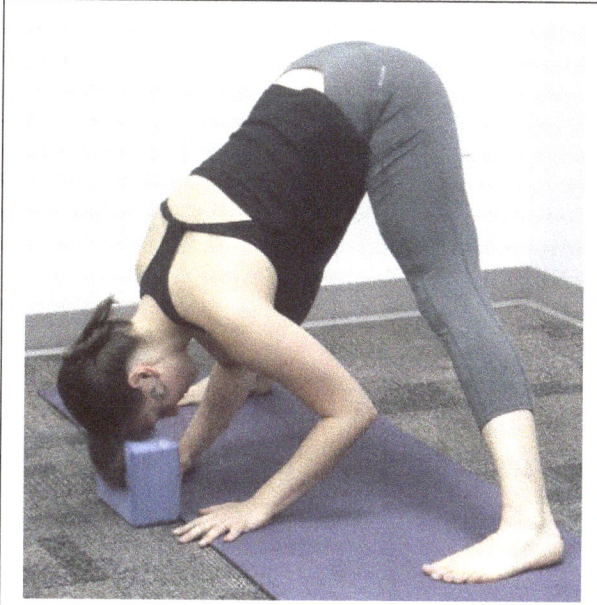 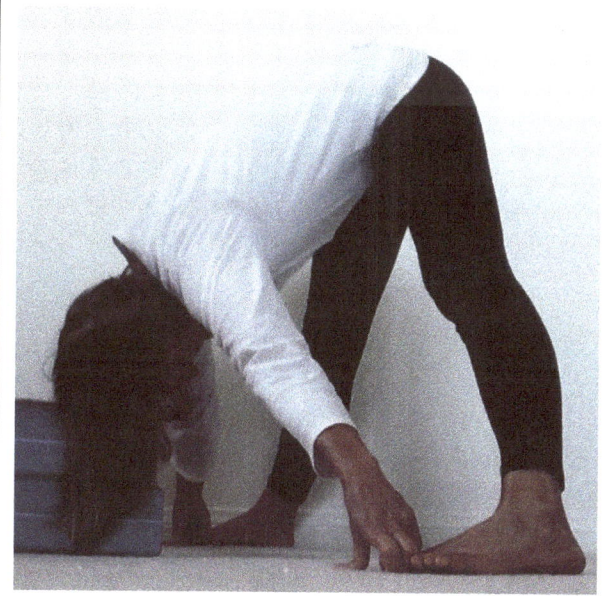

*Wide-Legged Standing Forward Fold with Supported Head*

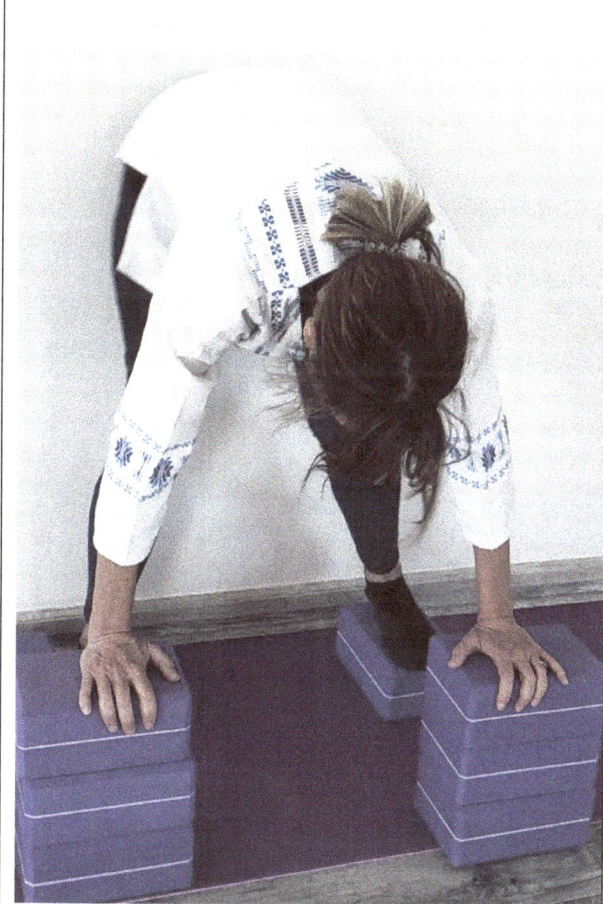

*Wide-Legged Standing Forward Fold with Heel Lift*

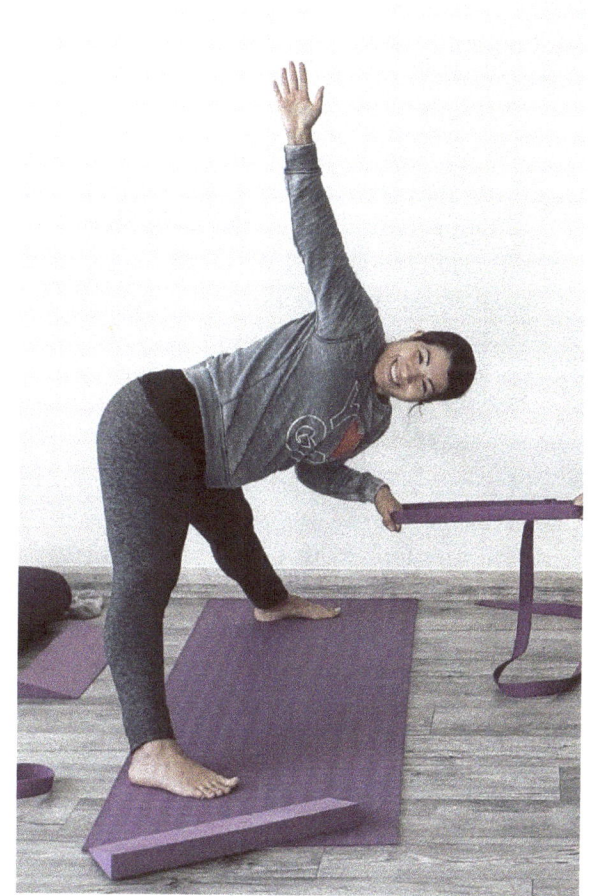

*Wide-Legged Standing Forward Fold with Rotation*

## Seated Forward Fold or Paschimottanasana

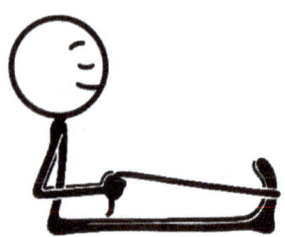

Seated Forward Folds are grounding and introspective shapes that invite practitioners to explore a balance between release and gentle engagement. From a seated position with the legs together (i.e., Staff), these folds gently mobilize the back body and encourage resilience, especially in the spine, hamstrings, and low back. By inviting each individual to honor their unique anatomy and comfort, Seated Forward Folds become a personal exploration of ease, inner awareness, and mindful movement, rather than a fixed outer shape. The goal is not to place the torso on the legs. The goal is a mindful journey forward, with optimal flexion in the hips that honors the natural curves of the spine. For many students, this means that they may not move very far past Staff.

### Key Alignment Invitations

A Seated Forward Fold emerges from a coherent and optimized seat in Staff (see Chapter 10). It encourages stability, release, and gentle activation throughout the spine, legs, and core. Alignment cues foster a deeper connection with inner experience, allowing the outer shape to unfold naturally from inside without a specific goal in mind.

- *Invitations related to the legs and feet*:
  - *Ground through the legs*: Invite practitioners to ground through the backs of the legs, bringing gentle awareness to the connection between the sitz bones and heads of the femurs. Pressing evenly through the length of the legs can create a stable foundation and support ease through the back body.
  - *Engage the thighs*: A subtle engagement of the quadriceps can provide stability and resilience in the legs, while minimizing strain in the knee joints. This engagement offers a feeling of activation in the legs and invites the fold to come from the hip joints (without rounding the back).
  - *Slight bend in the knees if needed*: A gentle bend can be beneficial for those experiencing tightness in the hamstrings or low back. It will be helpful to place a prop under the knees (rather than letting them float).
- *Invitations related to the spine and neck*:
  - *Hinge at the hips*: Guide students to fold forward by moving from the hips rather than rounding the back, inviting a release of tension in the lumbar spine. This movement pattern encourages gentle mobilization and can feel grounding and supportive as they fold. Many students are best served by remaining relatively upright in this shape rather than actually reaching the torso toward the legs.
  - *Maintain natural curves in the spine*: Encourage practitioners to start by creating length in the spine, imagining that they are maximizing the spaces between the vertebrae. Initiating the fold from this upright position supports natural spinal curves and prevents excessive bracing or straining.
  - *Engage the core*: A gentle engagement of the core may stabilize the spine and prevent collapsing forward. Drawing the navel slightly inward can encourage strength and interoceptive awareness, creating a balanced experience of ease and stability.

- o *Reach the abdomen toward the legs*: Rather than rounding forward and down, flexion comes from the hips which means the belly reaches toward the thighs. The heart space stays open.
- o *Allow the neck to remain a natural extension of the spine*: The head can stay in line with the spine and a gentle tuck of the chin and drawing back through the ears can create ease. It is not necessary to drop the head forward (tucking the chin), a common misconception that students have because it makes them feel as though they are more 'deeply' in the forward fold.
- *Invitations related to the arms and shoulders:*
  - o *Find engaged and intentional arm and hand placement*: The arms are invited to reach forward toward the shins or toes, actively engaged and awake. Depending on torso and extremity proportions of students, hands will land naturally on the legs, floor, or a prop. Engagement and connection can be invited by using a strap around the feet, held in both hands. The linking of hands to feet (which for a few students may not require a strap) creates a sense of connection between the hands and the feet and honors the natural curves the spine.
  - o *Invite shoulder blades to settle*: Remind students to allow their shoulder blades to settle naturally down the back, which supports openness across the front body, especially the heart space.. This subtle engagement can prevent rounding of the shoulders and maintains the natural curves of the spine.
  - o *Relax through the hands and fingers*: Encourage students to release any gripping in the hands and fingers, particularly if reaching toward the feet or holding a strap. Gentle, relaxed hands promote a sense of ease, inviting the whole upper body to participate in the fold without excessive bracing.

## *Variations and Exploration*

There are many variations and explorations that honor the diversity of practitioners' needs and anatomies. The following options and other creative adaptations help personalize the fold, allowing each practitioner to find a balanced and supportive entry into Seated Forward Folds.
- *Elevate the hips*: Sitting on a folded blanket or bolster can assist in tilting the pelvis forward, which supports a more aligned spine and reduces tension in the hamstrings and low back. This simple elevation encourages a fold without forcing depth.
- *Bend and support the knees*: For those experiencing tension in the back of the legs, a slight or even significant bend in the knees can release strain and support natural curves in the spine. This option supports comfort and encourages resilience in the back body.
- *Wrap the hands around the feet or use a strap*: Reaching hands to the feet, ankles, or using a strap around the soles of the feet can support a feeling of connection along the back body. Rather than pulling, this option is an invitation to relax into the fold and release any bracing while maintaining the natural curves of the spine.

## *Additional Teaching Tips*

To create a compassionate, individualized experience of Seated Forward Folds, consider these additional teaching suggestions:

- *Invite a breath-guided fold*: Encourage practitioners to coordinate the fold with the breath. The inhalation invites length through the spine; the exhalation invites the hinging forward and releasing downward. This mindful rhythm can create a balance between effort and release, bringing a calming, yet focused quality to the shape.
- *Support a gentle exploration of depth*: Rather than aiming for a final destination, invite students to pause periodically as they fold, noticing the sensations and adjustments their body makes along the way. By inviting these pauses, practitioners can cultivate patience, acceptance, and awareness of the subtle changes that arise when moving gradually.
- *Engage imagery of grounding and expansion*: Encourage students to feel as though their sitz bones and upper femurs are rooted into the earth, providing stability, while their spine lengthens upward from the hips to the crown of the head, creating a sense of spaciousness.
- *Encourage ease in the upper body*: In Seated Forward Folds, there is often a tendency to create tension in the shoulders, neck, and jaw. It can help to bring awareness to these areas and let go of unnecessary bracing.
- *Offer time for reflection in the shape*: Seated Forward Folds invite introspection; introspection requires patience and attention. It is helpful to invite students to linger for several breaths so that their experience can deepen gradually.
- *Stay with diaphragmatic breathing*: As students fold forward, invite them to visualize the expansion into the back body (middle to lower) with each inhalation and a softening with each exhalation. This focus maintains diaphragmatic breathing, a sense of openness, and freedom in the spine.
- *Encourage non-judgmental observation*: Forward folds can bring up emotions or internal resistance. Gently remind students to observe whatever arises in the shape without judgment, using the fold as an opportunity to practice self-acceptance and compassion. This approach can foster a reflective and nourishing experience.

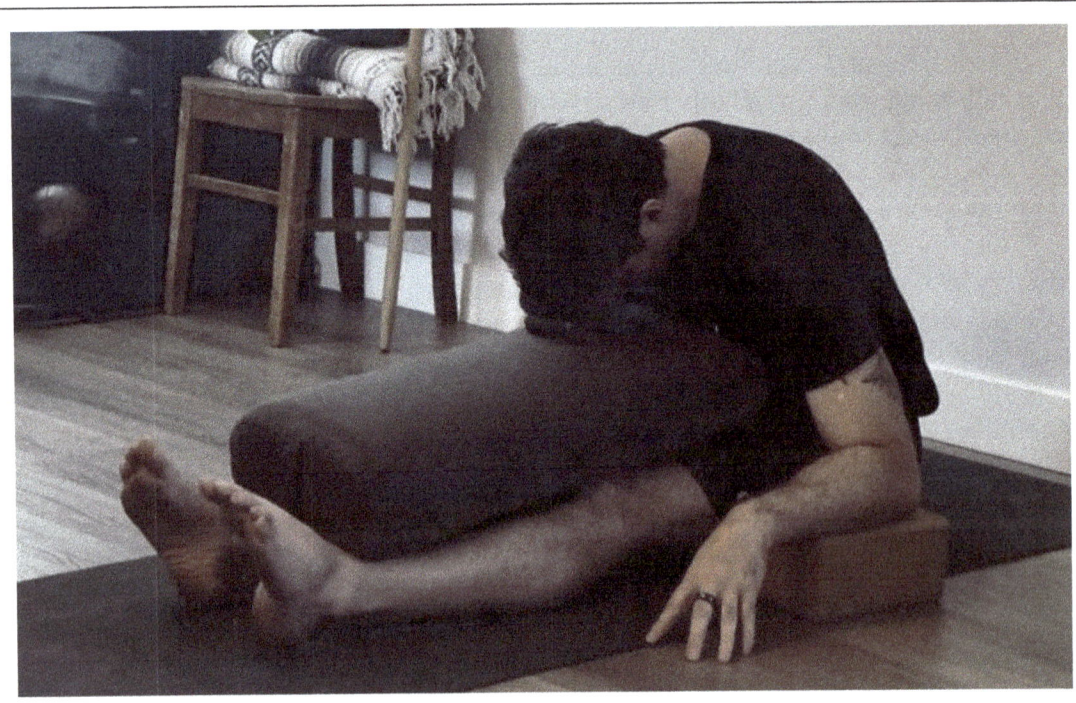

Seated Forward Fold with supports

## Wide-Legged Seated Forward Fold or Upavistha Konasana

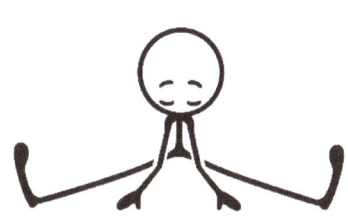

Wide-Legged Seated Forward Folds invite openness and introspection; they offer a balance of grounding, gentle activation, and ease. With legs wide and spine elongated, these folds encourage a gentle exploration of resilience in hips, thighs, and spine. Rather than reaching toward a specific destination, practitioners are invited to explore their unique expression of the shape through mindful movement and personalized adjustments. The wide legs create more anatomical ease; however, it is useful to recall cautions about wide-legged positions in the context of students who have histories of sexual trauma. For them, the anatomical ease may be offset by emotional challenge present in this more vulnerable shape. As was true about Seated Forward Folds, the goal is not to bring the body to the floor; the goal is to explore natural range motion and to embrace one's own anatomy and vitality.

### Key Alignment Invitations

In Wide-Legged Seated Forward Folds, alignment becomes an exploration of stability and inner awareness that encourages practitioners to connect with their own unique embodiment of the shape. Rather than aiming for an idealized outer shape, alignment cues focus on cultivating ease and resilience, so that each individual can find their own unique rhythm, expression, and range. The guidance below supports mindful engagement and a deep relationship with sensations, emotions, and breath, encouraging an experience that unfolds naturally from within rather than being imposed from without. Again, it is important to stay mindful of possible emotional challenges that may arise from the wide-open legs. A standard Seated Forward Fold may be a good alternative as may be an option to work with a blanket covering the legs and lower body.

- *Invitations related to the legs and feet*:
  - *Root through the legs*: Encourage students to ground through the backs of the legs, sensing their connection from the sitz bones and upper femurs down through the heels. This rooting helps build a stable base and invites greater ease in the fold.
  - *Draw up through the thighs*: Grounding the femurs to the earth can engage and stabilize the legs, inviting resilience while feeling supported. This activation helps guide the fold from the hips and maintains length along the spine.
  - *Bend the knees if helpful*: Clients experiencing tightness in the inner thighs or low back may benefit from a gentle bend in the knees. Adding support, such as a rolled blanket or mat, beneath the knees invites ease and groundedness without the need to force the shape.
- *Invitations related to the spine and neck*:
  - *Fold from the hips*: Invite students to move from the hip joints rather than the low back, allowing the spine to stay in its natural curves and maintaining ease in the lumbar and sacral regions. This movement pattern grounds the fold in the hips, honoring students' natural range of motion.
  - *Maintain spaciousness through the spine*: Encourage students to begin with a sense of length from tailbone to crown, as though expanding the spaces between the vertebrae. This axial extension cue can support natural spinal curves, minimizing strain and encouraging ease.

- ○ *Engage the core*: Subtle (not braced) core activation, drawing the navel slightly inward and upward and drawing the low ribs toward the hips, can stabilize the fold and prevent collapsed disengagement. This gentle drawing in helps promote resilience and self-awareness during the fold.
- ○ *Reach the abdomen toward the floor*: Rather than rounding forward and down, flexion comes from the hips which means the belly reaches toward the floor. The heart space stays open.
- *Invitations related to the arms and shoulders:*
  - ○ *Explore different hand placements*: Students can reach forward with hands resting on the legs, floor, or a prop, depending on their comfort anatomically, energetically, and emotionally. Engaging a strap around the feet (if accessible and appropriate, especially in the context of sexual trauma) offers a grounded, connected feeling that facilitates ease in the upper body. Note: this requires a longer strap due to the distance between the feet.
  - ○ *Invite the shoulders to settle*: Encourage students to allow the shoulder blades to settle naturally on the back, opening the heart space without forcing the shoulder blades back. This subtle invitation prevents tension and supports relaxed presence in the fold.
  - ○ *Let go of gripping in the hands*: Remind students to release tension or bracing in the fingers and hands. Gentle relaxation fosters ease in the hands, arms, and shoulders reverberates throughout the upper body and helps the fold feel spacious and balanced.

## Variations and Exploration

Wide-Legged Seated Forward Folds invite students to explore unique adaptations that honor their body's needs and add a layer of creativity. Creative variations kindle curiosity and bring newness into the fold, allowing participants to be playful and exploratory. These variations offer a supportive, individualized experience and tailor the shape to each individual's unique needs.

- *Resting on the forearms*: For a grounded experience, students rest their forearms on a tower of blocks, bolsters, or a large yoga ball between the legs. This option invites connection to the earth, settles the students into the shape, and yet maintains ease in the back body.
- *Supported twist variation*: To invite a gentle twist into the fold, students can bring one hand to the opposite leg and let the other arm move upward or rest on the floor behind. This gentle rotation can create a dynamic experience in the fold.
- *Lateral flexion/rotation exploration*: Instead of folding directly forward, students can explore rotating and then leaning the torso over one leg (and then the other), reaching both arms in that direction or placing the opposite hand on the thigh. This variation invites resilience and opening into the side body and encourages a different experience into the spine and hips.
- *Explore a connection between hands and feet*: If students have access to a long strap or scarf, they may wrap it around the feet, holding one end in each hand to connect hands to feet. This connection offers a sense of containment and engagement for some students, helping them feel more grounded and centered in the fold. Caution is necessary with students who have trauma experiences as bound shapes can become triggering.
- *Reclined variation*: For a different approach to the shape, students can explore a reclined version by lying on their back and opening the legs wide, perhaps with a yoga ball between the knees. This restful adaptation creates a similar sense of openness and grounding, inviting relaxation while allowing the hips to release. Again, caution is necessary with students who have trauma histories.

*Additional Teaching Tips*

The following tips aim to encourage mindful and introspective experiences in Wide-Legged Seated Forward Folds. They reiterate the beauty of bringing the other limbs of yoga into the experience of *asana*.

- *Create a rhythmic collaboration between breath and movement*: Invite practitioners to connect movement to their breath by finding length on the inhalation and releasing forward on the exhalation. A breath-guided approach fosters somatic mindfulness and grounds the mind in present moment awareness.
- *Pause to explore inner awareness and/or concentration*: Encourage students to take small pauses as they fold, noticing how their body feels in each stage of forward movement. Pauses invite patience, curiosity, and a sense of discovery; they connect students more deeply to their inner experience.
- *Encourage grounded and expansive imagery*: Invite students to feel their legs rooting into the earth, while imagining length through the spine as they fold. This imagery can foster feelings of stability, grounding, and heart opening.
- *Support ease in the upper body*: Invite students to release unnecessary tension in shoulders, neck, and jaw, particularly if they are reaching forward. Such awareness encourages a relaxed and open experience.
- *Stay with diaphragmatic breathing*: Guide students to breathe into the middle and low back, expanding with the inhalation and gently releasing with the exhalation. This focus on diaphragmatic breath invites spaciousness, vitality, and natural spinal alignment.
- *Invite compassionate contemplation*: Forward folds, especially with the legs wide apart, can bring forth internal resistance and vulnerable emotionality. Gently remind students to observe these feelings without judgment, using the shape as a space for self-acceptance and kindness. Give permission to abandon the shape if it does not serve their psychological wellbeing in the moment.

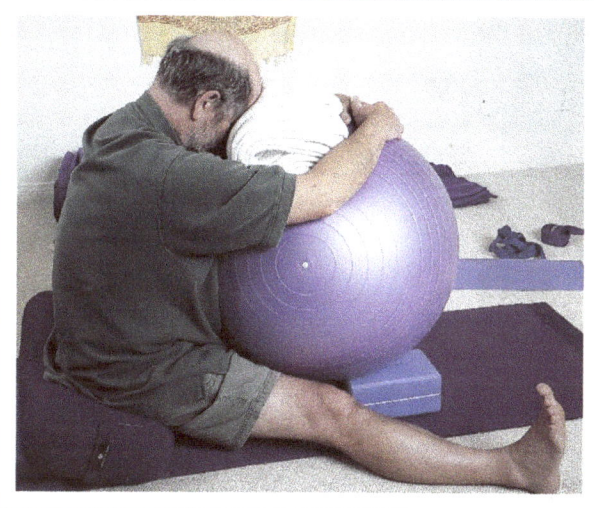
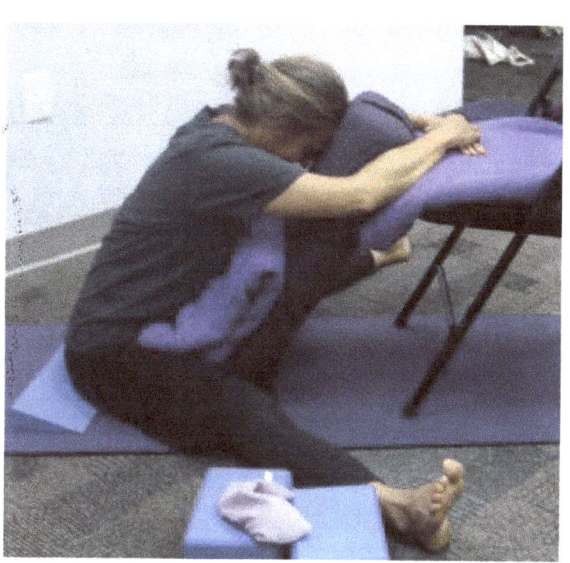

*Wide-Legged Seated Forward Folds*

*– super-supported →*

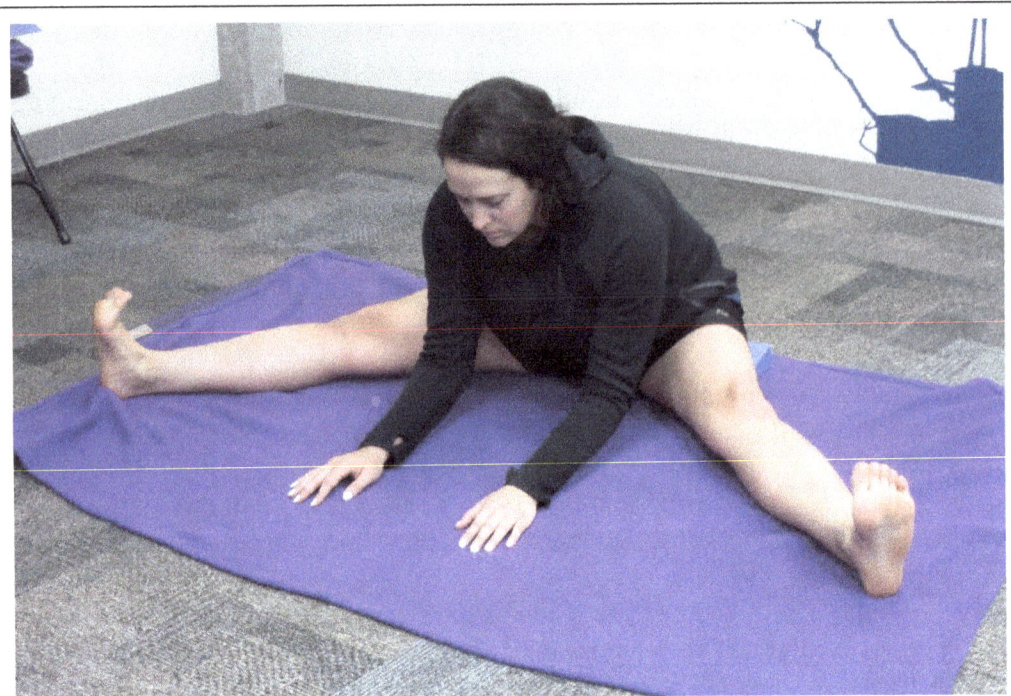

*Wide-Legged Seated Forward Folds with discerning engagement*

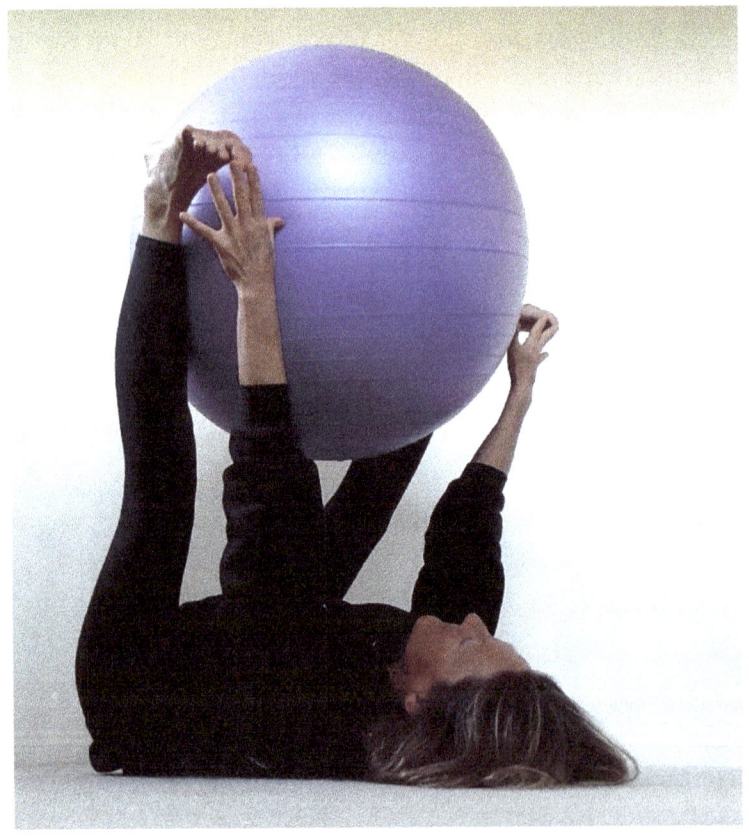

*Supine Wide-Legged Seated Forward Folds*

## Head-of-Knee Shape or Janu Sirsasana

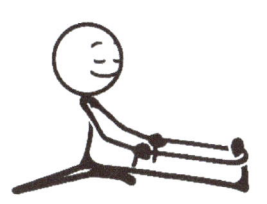

Head-of-Knee invites quiet introspection, allowing for a grounded connection by nestling the base of one foot against the inner thigh of the opposite leg. With one leg extended and the other drawn inward, the shape encourages an emotionally safer inner focus. It invites resilience along the back, hamstrings, and side body, adding a subtle rotation in the torso and opportunity to explore inner experience rather than reaching an outer goal. A gentle approach invites clients to embrace a personal embodiment that reflects all layers of experience. Head-of-Knee creates space for contemplation, opens pathways for emotional experience and regulation, and invites reflection and wisdom. To clients with trauma experiences, this shape may feel more grounding and protected than Wide-Legged Folds.

### Key Alignment Invitations

In Head-of-Knee, alignment cues focus on stability, grounding, settling, and embodiment. They encourage movements informed by inner sensation, vital experience, and emotional unfolding. The fold promotes resilience by guiding awareness from the pelvis upward along the spine, helping establish a unique experience of stability coupled with mobility, and effort within ease. The fold arises from Staff and alignment cues for Staff are equally important to Head-of-Knee.

- *Invitations related to the legs and feet:*
  - *Gently move into the leg positions*: From Staff, bend one knee and draw the bent leg toward the chest. A gentle hug of the leg to the body can create compassion and proprioception. From this position, gently root through the extended leg while laterally rotating the hip joint of the bent leg to let the knee move outward and toward the floor. The knee does not need to land on the floor – instead honor the range of motion in the hip joint (see guidance for Warrior 2 based shapes) and use a prop under the knee to support it, rather than forcing it to the floor and torquing this precious joint. The sole of the foot of the bent leg nestles itself to the inner thigh of the extended leg.
  - *Root through the extended leg*: Gently press through the back of the extended leg, feeling a grounded connection through the heel, sitz bone and top of the femur. This rooting can cultivate ease and support while gradually folding. A prop under the knee to prevent floating and/or hyperextension of this joint is helpful for some students.
  - *Create ease in the knee of the bent leg*: Stay attuned to the bent knee, continuously monitoring sensation and adding a blanket, bolster, or block underneath to optimize wholesome alignment. A gentle release of the knee into a support encourages comfort in the hips and helps maintain stability in the shape.
  - *Create engagement in the meeting of the legs*: Press the foot of the bent leg into the inner thigh of the extended leg and the thigh into the foot, creating an isometric action of stability. For some students, this may require a prop – either between the sole of the foot and the thigh (e.g., a small block on its side) or between the outer ankle and the ground (e.g., a small folded towel).
- *Invitations related to the spine and neck:*
  - *Move into the fold with patience*: Prioritize the base (all body parts touching the earth and each other) and only invite a forward folding movement once the base is stable and

easeful. Before folding, it can be very helpful to lift upward through the arms (e.g., Sun Breath) and rotate slightly to the opposite side of the extended leg. Linger in this axially-extended rotation and wait for an exhalation to rotate forward over the extended leg.
    - *Move forward from the hip hinge*: To fold over the extended leg, move from the hip joints to maintain length along the spine, letting the shape open from the hips rather than rounding the low back. This gentle hinge from the pelvis honors its natural range and encourages comfort. It is fine if the opposite side of the pelvis lifts slightly. This can be very protective for the sacroiliac joints and reflects somatic wisdom.
    - *Do not grasp for reaching the torso to the leg*: Create a fold that honors individual range of motion. For many students, a strap between the foot of the extended leg and the hands can be very helpful (see guidance for Seated Forward Fold).
    - *Elongate through the spine*: Imagine creating length from the tailbone to the crown, sensing each vertebra in gentle alignment. This expansive energy invites natural spinal and pelvic alignment, supporting spaciousness in the low back and side bodies.
    - *Center through the navel*: A light drawing inward of the navel engages the core subtly, supporting a stable and energetically releasing fold. Gentleness in this engagement is key to foster awareness and resilience. Cueing the drawing of the low ribs to the anterior superior iliac spine (ASIS) is an alternative.
- *Invitations related to the arms and shoulders:*
    - *Explore hand placements*: Place the hands either on the extended leg, beside the hips, or with a gentle reach forward. Each placement offers a distinct experience, allowing for balanced engagement and ease. A strap between foot and hands can be grounding.
    - *Allow the shoulders to settle naturally*: Feel the shoulders release, letting the shoulder blades rest softly on the back. This gentle release supports openness through the chest, encouraging an expansive heart space and ease in the upper back.
    - *Find ease in the hands and fingers*: Allow the hands to relax without gripping, especially if they are holding a strap. Releasing the fingers and palms helps the whole upper body and neck unwind, fostering a calm sense of presence.

## Variations and Exploration

Head-of-Knee invites personalized adaptations to create uniquely supportive experiences that align with each practitioner's needs. Explorations of this shape invite students to find a deep sense of connection and letting be in all layers of experience. They guide practitioners into becoming their own teacher as they identify their natural range of motion and how to meet their needs for comfort and self-discovery.
- *Rest the forehead on a support*: Use a bolster, large yoga ball, or folded blanket beneath the forehead (i.e., with the prop gentle resting near the extended leg) to encourage grounded presence. This support under the forehead allows for a calm, nurturing experience while maintaining length in the back without over-stretching.
- *Invite a gentle twist*: Experiment with placing one hand on the bent leg and the other behind, gently twisting to one side. This subtle rotation reveals sensations in the spine and can invite a more dynamic expression of the shape.
- *Add lateral flexion*: With both arms reaching toward the extended leg, experiment with gentle side body stretching. This variation creates space along the side body.

- *Connect the hands to the extended foot*: Use a strap around the extended foot, holding each end to create a contained connection. This engagement supports a grounded feeling, particularly helpful for students seeking a tangible, stable focus in the fold.
- *Prone adaptation*: For a more relaxed experience, release the torso onto a large yoga ball or onto a bolster leaning against a chair.

## Additional Teaching Tips

The following tips create an opportunity to deepen the introspective experience within Head-of-Knee in a manner that connects students deeply to their inner sensations and breath. It continues to cultivate the interoceptive and introspective quality of other forward folds, in a shape that invites a bit more of a sense of rooting and grounding.

- *Synchronize movement with breath*: Encourage students to find length on the inhalation, and to invite a sense of easing into the fold with the exhalation. Connecting breath with movement grounds the mind into easeful concentration.
- *Pause to explore inner sensation*: Invite students to take gentle pauses, sensing how the body feels in each small adjustment. Pauses create a spacious, mindful approach, opening a pathway to self-awareness and compassion.
- *Embrace imagery for grounding and openness*: Invite students to visualize their sitz bones and femoral head of the extend leg grounding into the earth while feeling length along the spine. This imagery encourages stability and an open-hearted feeling in the shape.
- *Ease in the upper body*: Encourage students to release unnecessary tension in the shoulders, neck, and jaw. Awareness in these areas invites a relaxed experience that unfolds naturally.
- *Commit to nasal and diaphragmatic breathing*: Guide students to breathe gently into the belly, side waist, and low back, sensing the inhalation as a gentle expansion and the exhalation as a gentle letting be. Diaphragmatic and nasal breathing invites calm resilience and a supportive rhythm throughout the shape.
- *Invite compassion and lovingkindness*: Acknowledge that Head-of-Knee, with its subtle asymmetry, can evoke physical and emotional challenges. Encourage students to observe any internal sensations without judgment, allowing the shape to create an opportunity to practice compassion and loving self-acceptance.

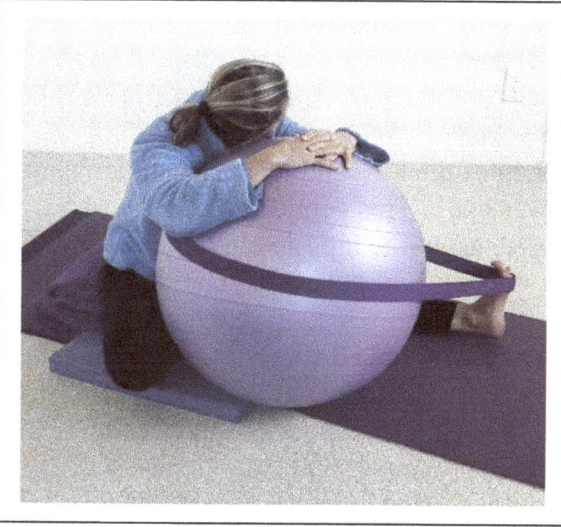

*Supported Head-of-Knee Shape* ←

*Head-of-Knee Shape* →

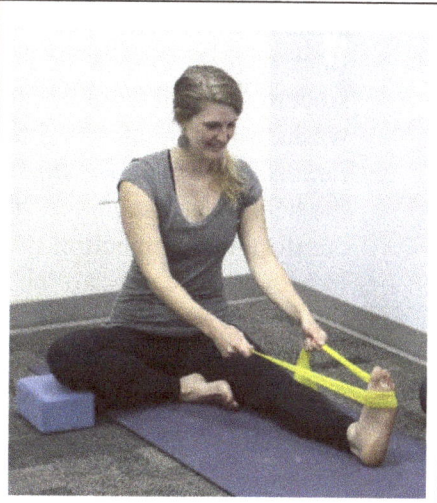

## Child or Balasana

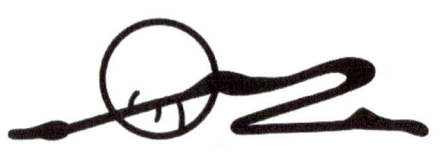

Child seeks to create an opportunity to experience safety, rest, and inward focus. It offers a grounding experience as the body folds in on itself. However, for some students Child can have the opposite effect as it is very similar to the physical posture of collapse and self-protection in the face of extreme danger or life threat. It is key to understand how Child affects students emotionally and to invite them to find an open-hearted resting shape if Child is triggering. For some students, the tight fold of Child is not anatomically restful or respectful. They can be better supported with more space between the legs and torso through ample use of supportive props.

For students who experience Child in a positive manner, the rested torso and forehead creates a shape for connection, nurturance, and relaxation. It encourages a journey inward, quieting the mind while allowing the body to let go. Child can be a space for deep introspection, giving students permission to connect to their breathing, to let go of a distracted mind state, and to reconnect with natural vital rhythms.

### Key Alignment Invitations

In Child, alignment guidance emphasizes ease and security, inviting students to connect with natural diaphragmatic and nasal breathing and to a grounded and supported present-centeredness. Cues focus on inviting personal comfort and a carefully tailored personal experience, promoting inner ease over outer shape. Again, for some students, Child must be cued very carefully based on their nervous system adjustment to the shape and their anatomical structures' interaction with it. Child arises from Diamond and all cueing guidance and cautions for that seat are helpful in creating a solid base from which to move forward.

- *Invitations related to creating a base from which to fold:*
  - *Ground softly through the lower legs and tops of the feet*: Allow the shins and tops of the feet to settle into the mat, feeling the connection from toes to ankles to knees. Grounding helps create stability, allowing the lower body to settle into ease. Sitting on a single or a stack of folded blankets, with the feet trailing off can help create a softer base. Many students benefit from a blanket between the thighs and the calves, as well as from a rolled washcloth or small towel under the front of the ankles.
  - *Release tension in the hips and thighs*: The weight of the hips and torso can sink toward the heels, releasing excessive bracing in the lower body. This gentle invitation fosters comfort and connection in the fold, creating resilience in the hips and low back. However, ease may not be accessible for some students without a soft support between thighs and calves, such as a folded blanket.
  - *Consider knees slightly apart or together*: Find a comfortable distance between the knees; a slight opening of the knees can create more space for the torso, while closer knees increase a sense of containment. Adjusting knee placement offers each student the freedom to choose a variation that feels supportive, physically and emotionally.

- *Invitations related to moving forward into the fold:*
  - *Fold forward from a stable and comfortable base*: The forward fold needed for Child proceeds as do all other forward folds - from the hip hinge. It is key to have props at the ready to receive the torso. For many students, the connection between torso and thigh requires an intermediary such as a bolster, blankets, or cushions. Props to receive the head are also important, such as a block softened with a folded towel or blanket.
  - *Move slowly without expectation*: Let the forward fold happen slowly and gently with ample time to gather appropriate props and supports and to allow the breath to adjust. Attend to spine, neck, arms, and shoulders along the way, based on observation of how students settle forward.
- *Invitations related to the spine, neck, and head:*
  - *Lengthen from tailbone to crown*: Imagine creating space along the spine, from the base of the tailbone to the top of the head. Gentle elongation (or axial extension) supports natural alignment.
  - *Allow head and neck to release*: Rest the forehead on the mat or, much more likely, on a prop, so that the neck and head can relax fully. This sense of support can relieve tension along the neck and upper back, promoting gentle relaxation through the head and shoulders.
  - *Center through the core*: Slight engagement through the core can support a feeling of containment in the lower abdomen and grounding in the torso. This subtle stabilization fosters resilience and allows the spine to come to rest naturally.
- *Invitations related to the arms and shoulders:*
  - *Encourage shoulders to ease downward*: Invite the shoulder girdle, including the shoulder blades, to come to rest naturally. Cueing may suggest a release of gripping or tensing in the shoulders to encourage a restful experience.
  - *Experiment with arm placement*: Place the arms either extended forward, relaxed at the sides, or reaching slightly backward with palms facing up or down. Each option offers a distinct experience, allowing for a unique expression of comfort and ease in the shape.
  - *Let go of gripping in the hands and fingers*: Fingers and hands are invited into a sense of ease, releasing tension or gripping. The fingers may naturally curl slightly inward. Gentle relaxation in the extremities promotes ease in the upper body.

## Variations and Exploration

Child invites unique variations that honor individual needs, creating a restful, introspective experience. These adaptations provides an opportunity for self-expression and discovery, and make the experience of Child more anatomically personalized and emotionally accessible.

- *Rest with a prop under the torso*: Place a bolster, blanket, or large cushion under the chest and belly for support, which allows a deeper release along the back. Propping fosters comfort and may be especially grounding for those who seek extra containment. The prop can be placed between the legs if the knees are apart, or on the thighs if the legs are closed.
- *Side-stretch variation*: Experiment by reaching one arm to the opposite side, inviting a gentle stretch along the side body. This subtle shift brings a dynamic experience to Child, invites resilience into the spine and rib basket, and creates a more active shape.
- *Bring a blanket between the thighs and calves*: For a more lifted and spacious feeling, students can place a folded blanket or cushion between their calves and thighs. This option

fosters a sense of safety and support, helpful for students who may feel vulnerable in the fold. The lift can be even higher (e.g., a bolster) if the base of Child is created from Hero rather than Diamond.
- *Forehead on a block or bolster*: Elevate the forehead with a block (softened with a towel or blanket) or bolster to maintain ease in the neck and upper body. This option creates a slight lift and for some students may relieve strain in neck or shoulders. For some it also makes the shape feel less confining emotionally and physically.
- *Supported supine Child*: To experience a similar grounding in a different orientation in space, students can enter a Child-like shape from lying on their back. From a supine position, they clasp the backs of the legs with knees bent, drawing the legs in gently toward the chest. This restful alternative provides ease and avoids some of the emotional or anatomical challenges of prone Child. The back body can relax and there is no or little compression of the front body.

## Additional Teaching Tips

Additional teaching tips support a mindful, introspective experience within Child, as students are encouraged to connect with their breathing and inner sensations and invited to create a calm and grounding experience on the inside, regardless of the shape they create on the outside.
- *Connect breath with gentle movement*: With the front body compressed, Child provides a perfect opportunity to invite students to feel the breath in their side ribs, waist, and back bodies. They can attune to the rhythm of breath opening up these regions on the inhalation and gently drawing inward on the exhalation. Staying attuned to this rhythm supports somatic and vital awareness and a natural sense of presence.
- *Invite diaphragmatic and nasal breathing*: Encourage students to sense expansion as they inhale and a gentle drawing inward as they exhale. Invite them to breathe nasally even in this prone shape. Child is an excellent opportunity to cultivate breathing into the back body to create more rib basket resilience.
- *Pause to cultivate inner awareness*: Suggest that students pause to sense into their body, noticing areas of ease or tension. Pauses foster introspection, curiosity, and deeper connection to experience in a gentle and exploratory way.
- *Support ease in the upper body*: Remind students to release any holding or gripping in the shoulders, neck, and jaw. This awareness encourages a soft experience that supports relaxation. Inviting a gentle smile can be helpful in creating a natural sense of ease.
- *Emphasize compassionate observation*: Recall and share that Child can bring forth vulnerability or emotion. Invite students to observe inner sensations, emotions, mental narratives, and vitality with non-judgmental open-heartedness and open-mindedness. Self-compassion in this shape can be helpful in finding a loving, kind, and nurturing expression of Child.

# Integrated Holistic Yoga Movement | 435

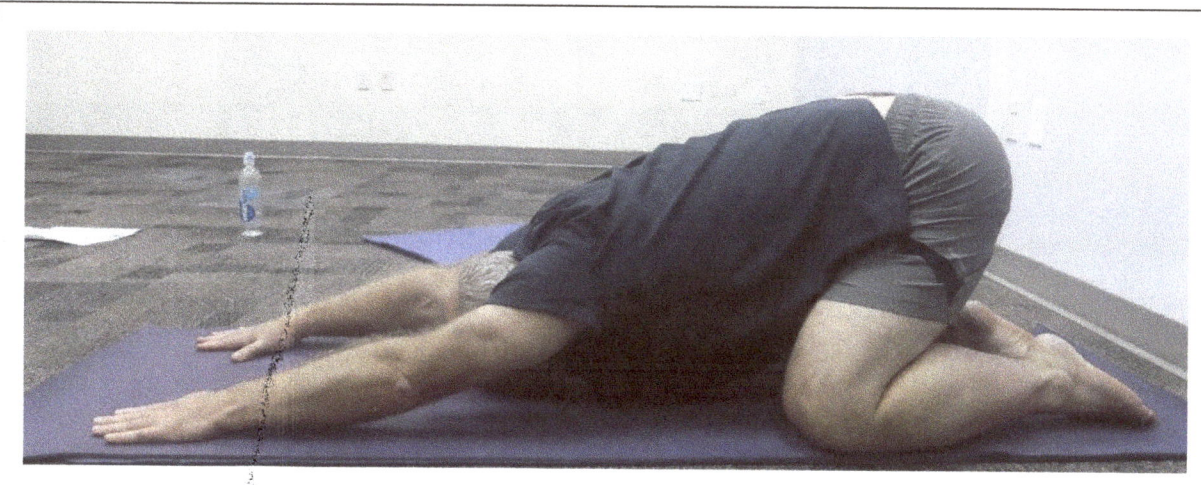
*Wide-Legged Child with arms extended*

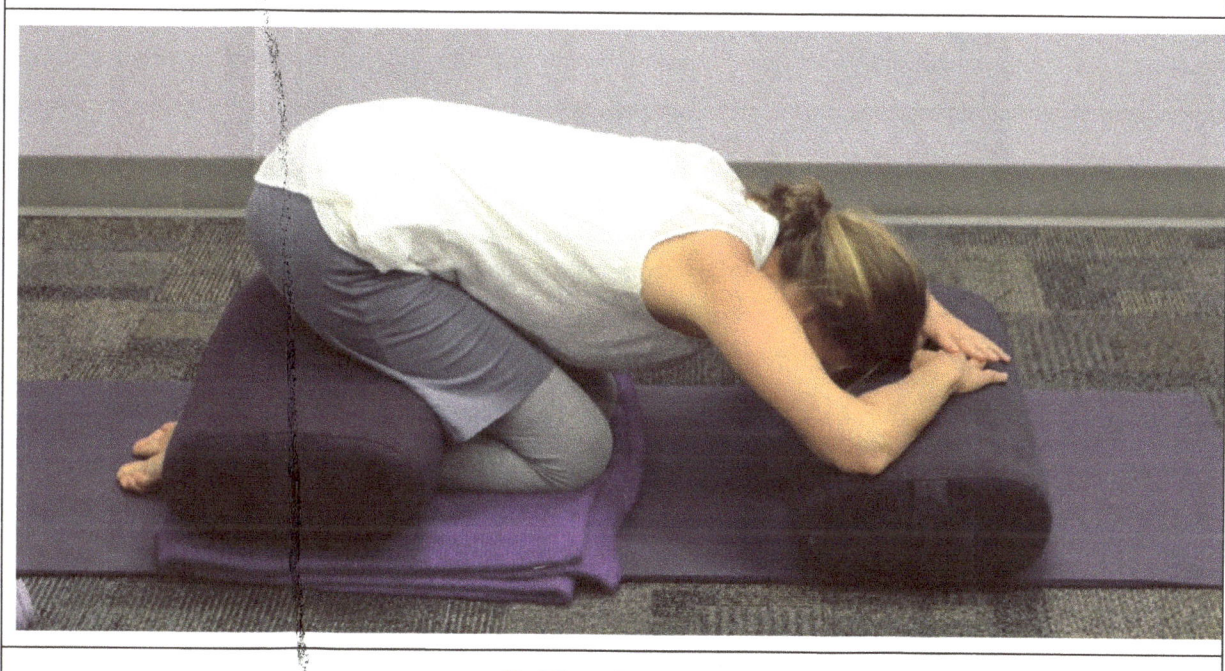
*Child with supports*

*True yoga is not about the shape of your body, but the shape of your life. Yoga is not to be performed; yoga is to be lived. Yoga doesn't care about what you have been; yoga cares about the person you are becoming. Yoga is designed for a vast and profound purpose, and for it to be truly called yoga, its essence must be embodied.*

Aadil Palkhivala

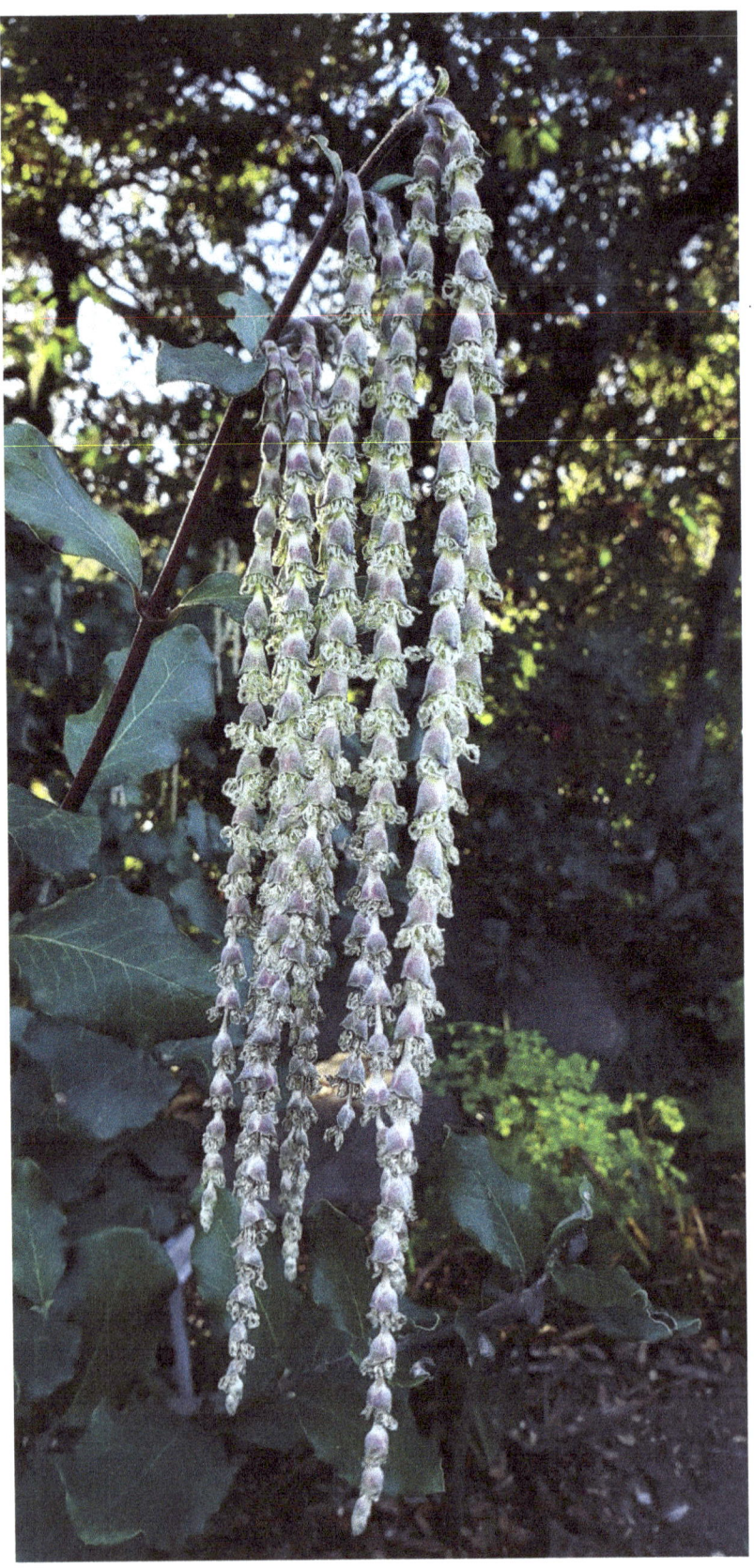

## Chapter 13: Backbends or Heart Openers

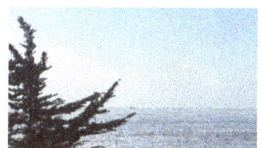

This chapter covers foundational backbends, offering optimized teaching strategies that allow for individual tailoring and careful discernment about how and which shapes to offer, as well as about how to cue alignment informed by interoception, proprioception, exteroception, and neuroception. General principles for this category of yoga *asana* are provided and apply to most if not all heart-opening shapes. Specific follow-up guidance is added for chosen sample shapes. Heart Openers can unfold from standing, arm standing, and sitting. All guidance in Chapters 8 to 10 remains highly relevant and applicable – even if it is not explicitly repeated here.

### Anatomical Foci for Backbends or Heart Openers

In teaching backbends or heart openers, it is important to note that some individuals have strong emotional or mental reactivity to these shapes. The heart-opening nature is counter to the more protective forward-folding shapes that tend to generate more of a sense of safety. Working with polyvagal states can therefore be particularly helpful in teaching backbends and in preparing students for a strong yet compassionate heart-opening practice. Because of the spinal flexion bias in modern life, it is helpful to realize that for some students even simply bringing the spine into its natural curves may feel like a backbend (e.g., this can even hold true for resting in *Savasana*). Therefore, it is helpful to think *less of backbending*, and *more of heart opening* as the frame for these shapes. This approach is also less demanding and less risky for the lower spine, as it reduces practitioners' likelihood of creating a backbending hinge in the lumbar spine.

Helpful anatomical foci include, but are not limited to the following guidance about anatomy and alignment actions in the head and neck region, thoracic region, and lumbar and sacral regions of the spine. They integrate attention to opening the front body while strengthening the back body – a physical movement integration with strong emotional implications as well.

#### *Overview of Relevant Body Regions*

Heart opening (or backbending) involves a coordinated interplay between the front of the body, shoulder girdle, back body, head, and neck. These shapes can be understood as deep extensions of the spine that stretch the entire anterior chain of the body – from the face and throat, through the chest and belly, extending into the hip flexors, quadriceps, and even the anterior legs. Simultaneously, heart opening calls for substantial engagement and stabilization in the posterior chain, particularly in the erector spinae, gluteal muscles, and hamstrings, which act to support spinal integrity and control extension.

On a myofascial level, heart-opening stretches and builds resilience in the superficial and deep front lines (as described in Myers' anatomy trains), elongating connective tissues and muscle fibers along the entire anterior surface of the body. This lengthening facilitates expansiveness through the chest and hip regions while demanding strength and neuromuscular coordination along the superficial and deep back lines to stabilize the arc of the body.

### Attending to the Whole Front Body

To achieve effective and healthful heart opening, it is essential to address each segment of the body, with attention to the anterior and posterior aspects:
- *Neck and head region*: Create openness in the throat and ensure proper alignment of the head to avoid compression in the cervical spine.
- *Thoracic region*: Mobilize the clavipectoral fascia and surrounding musculature to expand the chest and encourage upper spinal extension. Strengthen the back region for balance across the front and back body.
- *Shoulder girdle*: Cultivate both stability and mobility, allowing for a broad, spacious chest while maintaining scapular integrity.
- *Hip region*: Release tension in the quadriceps and hip flexors while simultaneously engaging the hamstrings and glutes to protect the low back and guide pelvic positioning.
- *Abdominal region*: Invite a balanced stretch and subtle engagement, ensuring the extension is evenly distributed along the spine rather than hinging at vulnerable segments.

### Attending to the Mind

The expansive nature of backbends not only challenges the physical body but also influences the nervous system and mental or emotional state of the practitioner. Intentional heart opening encourages individuals to cultivate a *sattvic* (calm, balanced) state, activating the ventral vagal pathway to maintain emotional steadiness and clarity, as well as a clear connection to all layers of human experience, including to vitality as expressed by the breath, and to the mind as expressed in emotional reactivity, mind states, and mental contents that may emerge during the practice. Full physical, vital, and mental presence and conscious awareness are crucial to navigate the possible intensity and reverberations of heart-opening shapes through the *koshas*. Psychologically, heart opening invites vulnerability – it is a shape of openness of heart that invites in the outer world and with this invitation becomes more dependent on the compassion and kindness of the response of others. Heart openers invite clients to expose their vulnerability and to become open to exploration. This energy is the very opposite to that of forward folding, which tends to be introspective, self-protective, and drawn inward.

### Preliminary Notes and Cautions

Important structural and physiological considerations are best kept in mind when guiding students or clients into heart-opening practices. Guidance includes, but may not be limited to the following consideration:
- *Anterior longitudinal ligament considerations*: The anterior longitudinal ligament (ALL) must have sufficient resilience to accommodate backbending. Any sensation of pinching in the low back (particularly at L5-S1) often stems from this ligament or the deep front line resisting extension. Working with backbends can require months of mindful practice to prevent hinging at the lumbar spine that seeks to circumvent the tension in the ALL. The goal is not to stretch the ALL – it is a ligament and needs to maintain its role as a stabilizer. The

work seeks to create a backbend that distributes across the length of the spine rather than being centered in its lumbar region.
- *Abdominal vulnerability considerations*: As the abdominal muscles are stretched during heart opening, their ability to contract forcefully is reduced. Awareness of this can help practitioners avoid over-relying on lumbar compression for range of motion. Creating softness in the abdomen without losing integration and stability is key to optimizing backbending.
- *Pregnancy considerations*: During pregnancy, deep backbends increase the stress on the *linea alba* that is already inherent in the increased size of the abdomen. This additional demand on the *linea alba* necessitates cautious engagement of backbends, and avoidance of end range of motion, to reduce the risk of undue strain and *diastasis recti* (separation of the left and right sides of the rectus abdominis along the linea alba).
- *Stimulation of the nervous system*: Heart opening is inherently stimulating, invoking strong responses in breath, mind, and body. Practitioners are well served to be made aware of the potential heightening of energy and sympathetic arousal being invited to balance them with grounding practices as necessary.

## Neck and Head Regions

In heart-opening practices, the neck and head play a pivotal role in achieving both structural alignment and energetic expansiveness. Heart-opening shapes invite the entire front line of the body to stretch, including the vulnerable and often compressed structures of the anterior neck. To fully express the backbend while maintaining spinal integrity, the front of the neck must open, and the back of the neck must strengthen to support the weight of the head in extension.

The anatomical structures primarily involved in the positioning of the neck and head during heart opening are the sternocleidomastoid (SCM) and the trapezius muscles. These muscles form the outer ring of musculature that influences head rotation and alignment. Both are innervated by the 11th cranial nerve (accessory nerve), enabling them to influence head carriage and spinal alignment in backbends. When the upper trapezius is underactive and the SCM is tight, a pattern of anterior head carriage often emerges. This forward positioning restricts cervical extension and compromises thoracic mobility, limiting the full expression of heart opening.

### Helpful Preparations and Actions

To counteract this, activation of the upper trapezius and release of the SCM allows for a more integrated lift of the head and neck, reducing strain and optimizing spinal alignment. To effectively open the front of the neck in heart opening, the head needs to shift back, paralleling the jawline with the ground. This positioning elongates the anterior cervical fascia and invites a gentle extension through the thoracic spine, contributing to the feeling of expansiveness characteristic of heart-opening shapes. It can be accessed by dropping the chin slightly forward toward the chest (not too far!) and then drawing the head backward to align it in its natural position along the spine. Engaging the trapezius while softening the SCM allows for gentle tuck of the chin and prevents excessive compression at the cervical vertebrae. It can help students to use a fingertip to guide the movement of the head (via the chin) and to visualize the cervical curve lengthening and decompressing as the back body engages to support its natural extension.

This enhanced cervical alignment also prevents collapse in the vulnerable regions of C5–C7 and compression above and below the atlas. The chin tuck can be augmented by neck strengthening practices. Both preparations are detailed in the Box that follows.

*Chin Tucks*
- Stand or sit with the natural curves of the spine, grounding through the tops of the femurs if seated
- Rise up through the crown of the head
- Use the fingers of the dominant hand and bring them to the bottom of the chin
- Use the fingers to urge the chin downward (without exerting pressure – this is a nudge, not a command) as the head slightly nods forward (nodding 'yes')
- Then, use the fingers to urge or nudge the chin back so that the head moves toward the back plane of the body until the openings of the ears align more closely with the tops of the shoulders (they may not reach the destination, but the importance rests in the fostering of the *movement direction*)
- Hold the chin tuck for a few moments
- Repeat this process often throughout the day, especially while standing or sitting for a long time
- Use this chin tuck movement every time before doing neck stretches or heart openers, including all of the following movements

*Neck Strengthening*
- Come to standing or a comfortable seat with natural spinal curves
- Tuck the chin and draw the head back as described in *chin tucks*
- Place a flexible band around the back of the head so that it spans across the region of the occiput
- Hold one end of the flexible band in each hand and use the hands to draw forward on the band while actively and strongly resisting the forward movement of the band with the head (remaining in the chin tuck position throughout)

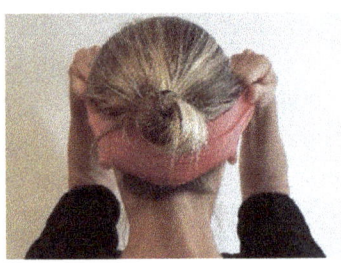

To facilitate optimal neck positioning, cranial nerve resets and trapezius releases can be used prior to entering backbends. These neuromuscular techniques stimulate the vagus nerve, inviting a parasympathetic response that enhances a sense of calm and presence during practice. This vagal engagement optimizes polyvagal regulation and invites calm presences into the uplifting energetic quality of heart-opening shapes. Incorporating these resets before backbends allows students to approach the practice from a ventral vagal nervous system platform (i.e., from a place of *sattva*), enhancing the structural integrity of the neck as well as the physiological and psychological benefits of heart opening.

*Helpful Polyvagal Practices*

**Pre-test:** Check range of motion of neck rotation

**Basic polyvagal reset exercise**
- Come to a comfortable supine position
- Interlace the hands and place them behind the head with thumbs at occiput
- Without moving the head at all (!), turn both eyes to the right and look to the right for at least 30 to 60 seconds (or until a deep sigh or yawn escapes)
- Then return eyes to center and take a moment to notice
- Repeat with eyes turned to gaze to the left
- Then return eyes to center and take a moment to notice

| |
|---|
| **Helpful Polyvagal Practices** |
| **Salamander exercise**<br>• Come to standing or to a comfortable upright seat; make sure head is in line with spine (e.g., tuck the chin and draw the head back)<br>• Sidebend neck only to the right; gaze left with the eyes; hold 30 seconds or so<br>• Bring head upright; release the eyes; notice your sensations and reactions<br>• Now sidebend neck to the left; gaze turns to the right; hold 30 seconds or so<br>• Bring head upright; release the eyes; notice your sensations and reactions<br><br>**Posttest:** Recheck range of motion of neck – note if there is a difference; typically, there is a lot more range of motion |
| **Trap release exercise**<br>• Come to standing and make ragdoll arms (hands to opposite elbows)<br>• Let the arms hang naturally in front of the low abdomen; rotate right and left about 3 to 5 times<br>• Lift ragdoll arms to shoulder height; rotate right and left about 3 to 5 times<br>• Lift ragdoll arms to above the head; rotate right and left about 3 to 5 times<br><br>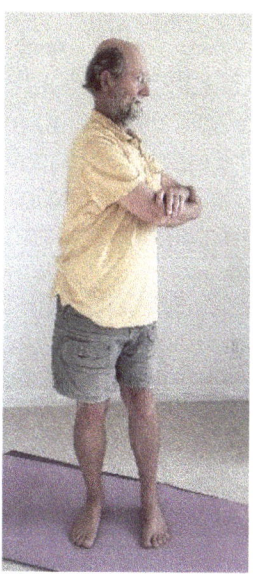 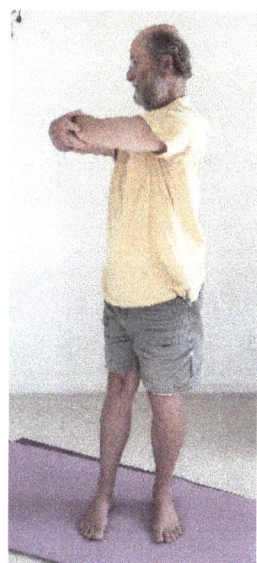 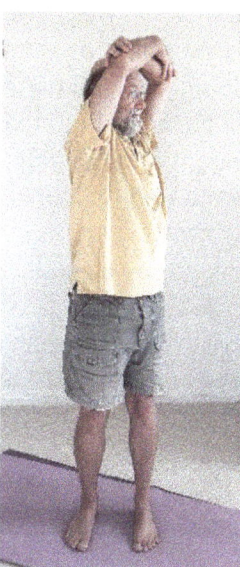<br><br>Credit for these practices goes to:<br>Rosenberg, S. (2017). *Accessing the healing power of the vagus nerve*. North Atlantic Books. |

## Thoracic Region

The thoracic region plays a central role in achieving heart opening and spinal extension. The thoracic spine, which comprises 12 vertebrae (T1–T12), is naturally kyphotic, or curved posteriorly. In backbends, the goal is to encourage extension through the thoracic spine while maintaining the integrity of the spine and avoiding excessive hinging at the lumbar segments. This requires opening in the chest and strengthening in the back.

*Creating Resilience in the Pectoral Muscles and Clavipectoral Fascia*

To create auspicious heart opening, the pectoral muscles and clavipectoral fascia (the connective tissue network surrounding the clavicles and upper chest) must be resilient. Pectoralis major and pectoralis minor are particularly influential, as their lack of resilience restricts the ability to broaden across the chest and lift the sternum. Chronic tightness in these muscles, often resulting from habitual forward rounding, pulls the shoulders into protraction, limiting thoracic mobility and inhibits range of motion in heart-opening shapes, such as Upward Facing Dog, Cobra, or Camel. Relatedly, the clavipectoral fascia serves as a structural conduit, transmitting tension across the anterior shoulder and chest. If this fascia is restricted, it binds the pectoral muscles, preventing the scapulae from retracting and the sternum from lifting. This restriction not only diminishes heart opening but also places unnecessary strain on the cervical spine as the head attempts to lift without adequate support from below.

*Creating Strength in the Back Body and Shoulder Region*

For optimal heart opening, the anterior release is ideally balanced by activation of the posterior chain. Trapezius, rhomboid, and erector spinae muscles are crucial to drawing the shoulder blades together and stabilizing thoracic extension. When the upper trapezius and rhomboids are actively engaged, the scapulae retract and depress, creating the foundation for chest elevation and ideally balancing the load on the cervical spine. Such balanced engagement allows for even distribution of the backbend along the thoracic curve, reducing the tendency to hinge excessively in the lumbar spine. It may be helpful to cue a broadening of the collarbones and gentle lifting of the sternum from the mid- to upper thoracic region, rather than relying on arching the low back.

Seated and quadruped rows (on hands and knees) are a great choice for the creation of strength and resilience in the thoracic spine. Rows create strength in the back body while opening the front body. They are a great practice that can be done daily and as a warm-up for breathwork, yoga, or other physical activity. These preparatory practices were covered in Chapter 9.

The shoulder region serves as both a mobilizer and stabilizer, depending on the heart-opening shape being practiced. Effective heart opening requires a delicate balance of scapular stability and glenohumeral mobility, ensuring the arms and upper spine can extend safely without compromising joint integrity. This means that to achieve expansive heart opening, it is crucial to prepare the shoulders for both mobility and stability. The scapulae are essential for maintaining structural integrity, especially since the shoulder girdle's only skeletal attachment is at the sternoclavicular joint. Several preparations that are applicable to heart opening were already covered in Chapter 9 in the context of arm standing and are best reviewed in preparation for guiding students into heart-opening shapes.

*Helpful Preparations and Actions*

Following are several helpful preparatory exercises that ready this region of the body for the physical, vital, and emotional impacts of heart opening. First, instructions are offered and then a few pictures are provided for additional clarity. The offered tricks and exercises create resilience in the pectoral muscles through intentional stretching and myofascial release, mobilize the clavipectoral fascia with gentle chest openers, activate the trapezius and rhomboid muscles to stabilize the scapulae and support spinal extension, and encourage thoracic mobility through segmental articulation (which serves to prevent hinging at the lumbar spine). These movements involve spinal extension, and it is helpful to ensure that the low ribs do not flare during their practice. Drawing the low ribs in adds to rib basket resilience and contributes to strengthening the intercostal muscles.

Opening of the heart (while strengthening the back) can be greatly facilitated with two prompts that can be used anywhere, anytime. Once clients have learned the two tricks that follow, they can be helpfully used for postural alignment in all contexts, and especially during breathwork.

Trick #1: *Manubrium maneuver*
Place the middle and ring fingers on the manubrium and give a gentle directional prompt for the manubrium to move slightly upward and backward without creating flare in the low ribs. This movement does not entail a strong push – it is a very gentle guidance for the heart region to open. Rather than reaching the whole sternum up to open the heart, the opening comes from the manubrium and prevents the low ribs from splaying out too much, maintaining just the right amount of core stability.

Trick #2: *Suspender move*
Place the thumbs into the axilla and point/move the fingertips upward toward the ceiling – this will invite the heart to open by rolling the shoulder girdle very slightly up and back. It helps to be sure to contract rectus abdominis to draw the low ribs toward the hips to prevent flaring. If the thumbs cannot wrap into the axilla, the palms of the hands can be placed to the side ribs, as high up the chest as possible to prompt the same opening motion. This gentle and small movement is a subtle yet effective reminder to roll the shoulders up and back to open the heart. It also invites the scapulae to move down and back and does so without creating rib flare or excessive opening.

The following exercises are wonderful back-bending preparations. They can come in handy in preparing for arm standing.
- *W with back at the wall or seated* – stand very close to or at a wall with the back body and bring the arms into a modified cactus shape to look more like a W, pressing the backs of the arms into the wall (or do this freely in the midst of a room from seated or standing – see photo below); this movement opens the clavipectoral fascia, helps with forward head (see next bullet), and strengthens the trapezius and rhomboid muscles
- *Hands-on-Block or Hands-on-Elbows Overhead Lift* – stand with the back to a wall; bring the hands to the opposite elbows (like in the trap release) or on either side of a block; lift the arms up and back to reach the wall above the head; repeat several times; switch up the grip of the elbows to break habitual patterns in how the arms interlace; this can strongly alter the experience of the movement
- *Plank/Cobra at the wall* – stand with the front body facing the wall about an arm's length distance away; place the hands to the wall at shoulder height and lean into the wall bringing the lower sternum and axillae toward the wall and sliding the arms up and down (this will essentially look and feel like a reverse W movement)

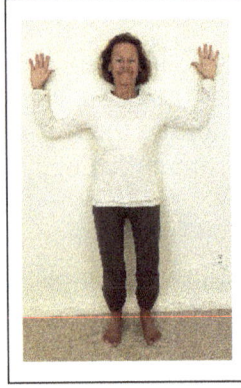 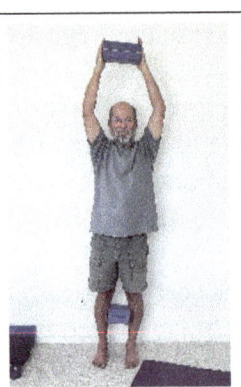 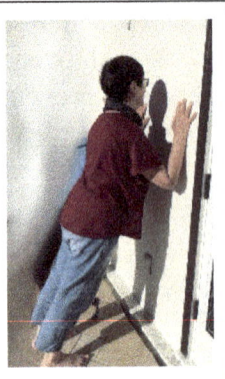 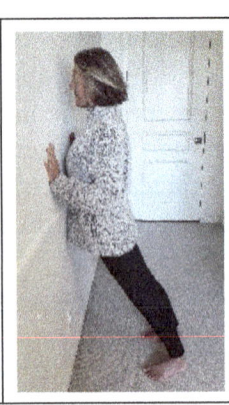

W at wall ← 
Overhead lift →
Cobra at wall →
Plank at wall ←

- *Doorway Heart Opener* (beware: this is a passive stretch and needs to be used with discernment) – come to standing, directly behind a doorway; bring the arms into goalpost or cactus position; please one forearm (elbow, length of the ulna, wrist, and hand) on each side of the doorway; lean the chest forward to open the heart through the center while keeping the low ribs tucked; release after a short hold – stay mindful throughout and do not over-effort in this passive stretch
- *Angel Wings* – lie on your back with your hands by your side with palms up; with the inhalation, slide the arms along the floor until the arms are reaching overhead on the floor, making an imaginary angel wing; with the exhalation, draw the arms back down to your side – be sure to keep the scapulae drawing toward each other and down the back; repeat
- *Snow Angel At The Wall* – stand with your back flush at the wall – if there are significant postural challenges, it is possible that the feet may need to be away from the wall a bit for the buttocks, upper back, and back of the head to touch the wall; make these adjustments with care and tuck the chin; then draw angel wings at the wall, lifting the arms along the wall up and overhead with the inhalation and lowering the arms back down to your sides with the exhalation; you can also use angel wings at the wall from a wall squat position for a little extra effort
- *Yoga Mudra* – Yoga *mudra* is a combination of several healthful spinal movements that support strength and resilience in the thoracic spine and rib basket. It can be a somewhat demanding movement for some patients and is offered once shoulder Vs and heart openers have become easeful and pleasant. Yoga *mudra* combines shoulder V, heart opening, and spinal flexion. It is complex yet very powerful as a spinal health practice. Instructions for yoga *mudra* are complex, thus a little more detail is offered.
    - Come to standing or sitting with natural curves in the spine and proper pelvic rotation
    - Interlace the fingers behind your low back
    - Draw the scapulae toward each other and down the back, lift the arms away from the region of the sacrum as high as possible without rounding the shoulders in front
    - Keep the low ribs tucked gently
    - Stay here or begin to bend at the hip joint to come toward a half lift with the interlaced hands resting on the sacrum to begin with
    - From half lift, raise the arms toward the ceiling and, if appropriate for your body in the moment, lower deeper into a forward fold; it tends to be most helpful to bend the knees
    - In a variation, come into yoga *mudra* while in Hero; then move toward Child with the top of the head placed on the floor and arms reaching up

## Pelvic Region

In heart-opening practices, the pelvic region is a crucial area of stabilization and extension; it involves releasing the front of the hips while strengthening the posterior chain to maintain integrity and protect the lumbar spine. The hamstrings, gluteal muscles, and quadratus lumborum (QL) must be strong and resilient as they help stabilize the pelvis to maintain extension through the hip joint without excessive compression in the low back.

At the same time, heart opening requires significant resilience in the psoas, iliacus, and quadriceps, as these muscles constitute much of the lower front line of the body and need to be able to lengthen so as not to draw the lumbar spine into hyperlordosis, creating an undesirable lumbar hinge (see image and more detail below). Preparatory movements such as hip flexion and extension help release tension and cultivate resilience. Additionally, stretching the adductors helps balance the inner thigh line, encouraging a neutral pelvic orientation.

To maintain structural integrity during heart opening, it is vital to:
- Ground the femurs to the back plane of the body while extending the hip joints; this action prevents the femoral heads from jutting forward, which could otherwise strain the anterior hip capsule and lumbar spine
- Introduce a micro-bend at the hip joint, allowing space for proper alignment, especially in very deep backbends such as Wheel or Pigeon (which are not covered in this Volume).
- Utilize internal rotation and/or adduction of the thighs to encourage proper femoral positioning; this can be accomplished via placing a block between the thighs to create adduction, stabilizing the pelvis

One of the most important protective mechanisms for the spine in backbends is the concept of lengthening through the entire spinal column rather than hinging from a singular point, often the lumbar-sacral junction (L5-S1). This is accomplished by:
- Cultivating a sense of lift and elongation from the base of the spine through the crown of the head
- Distributing extension evenly through the thoracic and lumbar regions instead of overloading one segment
- Maintaining the natural spinal curves rather than flattening or hyperextending specific areas

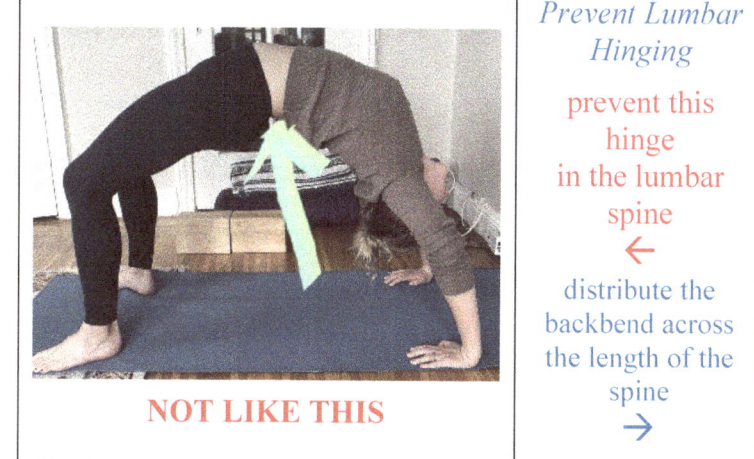

**NOT LIKE THIS**

*Prevent Lumbar Hinging*

prevent this hinge in the lumbar spine ←

distribute the backbend across the length of the spine →

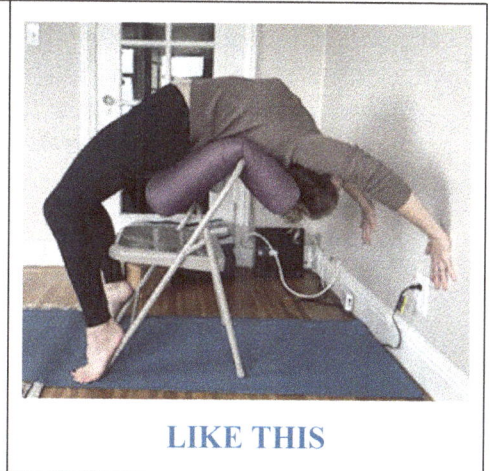

**LIKE THIS**

Another aspect of backbending is related to the biomechanics of the sacrum. In lumbar extension, the sacrum nutates – a forward nodding motion that allows the tailbone to move upward. This natural movement supports spacious and sustainable backbends. It is truly a natural movement and cueing can get in the way of easeful alignment in this region. For example, cueing related to the tailbone can become counterproductive. Specifically, contrary to some alignment cues, tucking of the tailbone in backbends may actually disrupt the natural nutation of the sacrum and compress the lumbar spine. It may be best simply to trust students' natural body rhythm: When the pelvis is allowed to move freely, the sacrum pivots gracefully, contributing to the overall arc of the backbend without creating strain.

Relatedly, to create ease and space in the sacral region in prone backbends, it can be very helpful invite the legs to widen slightly as feels natural. This gentle abduction of the hip joints, accompanied by experiment with gentle external and internal rotation, facilitates natural sacral nutation and can serve to reduce tension in the low back. That said, because of the significant bioindividuality of this body region, it can be helpful for students to experiment with different ways of landing the pelvis on the ground in prone backbends – this is truly *experimentation*, not advice to engage in one action over another. The experimentation invites successively pressing different parts of the lower front body toward the floor (from the pubis down to the femurs to the tops of feet – essentially achieving different degrees of pelvic contact with the earth) to notice when the greatest ease is accessed in the prone backbends in the lumbar and sacral regions, as well as the hip joints.

### *Helpful Preparations and Actions*

To cultivate readiness in the hip region for heart opening integrating the following preparatory techniques can help create the necessary resilience and spaciousness in the hip region, supporting heart opening while maintaining structural integrity and lumbar protection.

- *Hip circles*: from standing, arm standing, or seated draw circles with one leg at a time to mobilize the joint and releases tension in the surrounding fascia
- *Prone or lunging hip extension and flexion*: activate the psoas and iliacus for optimal lengthening and resilience from prone or lunge
- *Kneeling Frog Kriya and prone Half Frog*: prone, standing, or lunging Half Frog: targets the psoas, quadriceps, and iliacus; deepens awareness of the hip joint and opens the adductors
- *Extended Bridge with prop under the sacrum*: allow passive opening of the hip flexors while the posterior chain stabilizes – as always, use discernment with passive stretching or create an isometric action instead if there is discomfort or the goal is strength
- *Upward-facing Plank or Table Top*: strengthens the glutes and hamstrings while expanding the anterior hip line

> *"If love were a yoga pose, it would be a backbend,*
> *offering your heart to the world."*
> (Rebecca Pacheco, Do Your OM Thing, 2015, p. 106)

### Hip Extension and Flexion With Props and for Strength

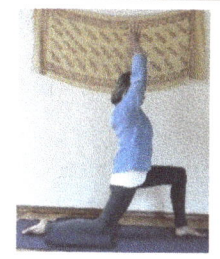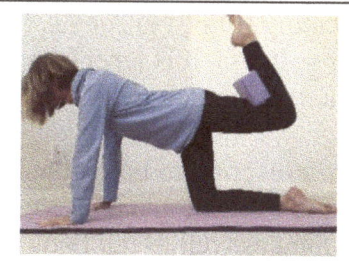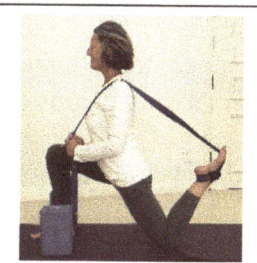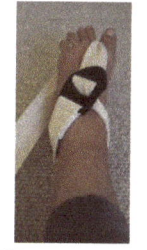

### Kneeling Frog Kriya and Prone Half Frog

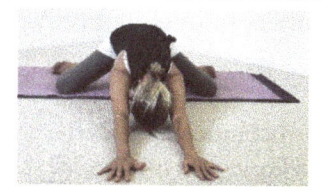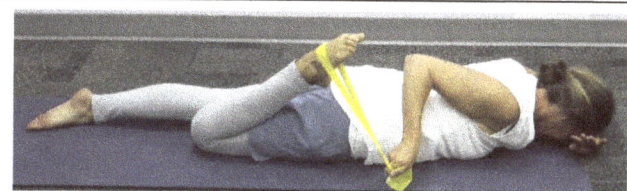

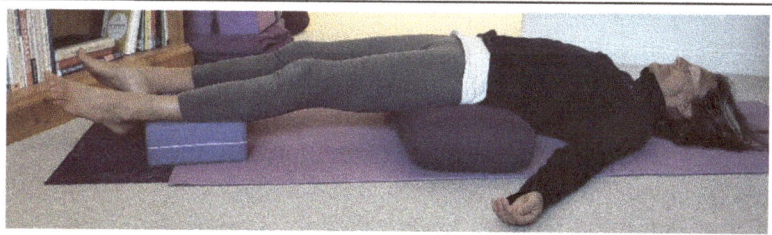

*Extended Bridge (with support under feet)*

## Abdominals and More

In heart-opening practices, the core region plays a subtle yet pivotal role in stabilizing the spine while permitting sufficient expansive extension. Unlike forward folds or twists, where core engagement primarily serves to protect and support the lumbar spine, backbends require a more nuanced relationship with the core musculature, prioritizing length and release over contraction.

To fully express a backbend, the anterior core muscles (including rectus abdominis, transversus abdominis, and obliques) are best prepared for resilience and suppleness. Over-contraction of the abdominal muscles during heart opening restricts thoracic extension and can compress the lumbar spine, counteracting the necessary expansiveness of the front body. Instead of bracing or drawing the abdomen in, it is more effective to invite the abdomen to soften, allowing anterior myofascial tissue to lengthen organically. Such softening permits the diaphragm to move freely, enhancing breath capacity and promoting a natural opening through the entire front body.

## Mind

While backbends open the heart, and thus may feel vulnerable to some or create fear for others, backbending practice in and of itself is neither risky physically nor psychologically, as long as teachers carefully guide students into empowerment and agency. With empowerment, the open heart is invited against the backdrop of intense personal engagement, responsibility, and presence; it arises from the deep inner strength of the individual who is opening the heart. The back body along the entire length of the back body is strong and engaged; thus, although the abdominals have to be soft and malleable, the shape in and of itself is full of strength, power, and beauty. Heart opening is *sattvic*, neither creating *rajas*, nor *tamas*. Heart opening is empowering in its cultivation of inner strength and outer softness. It is a perfect practice for exploring powerful psychological dimensions of yoga *asana* practice.

Heart-opening backbends are profoundly empowering to body, breath, and mind. Their expansive nature tends to bring emotional and psychological sensations and challenges to the surface, making it essential to prepare the mind as well as the body for these practices. Regardless of the strong emotional reactivity they may create, backbends can be transformative when approached with structural awareness *and* emotional attunement. Carefully designed sequencing and cueing can be therapeutic emotionally, enabling practitioners to open not only their physical heart region but also their emotional and energetic heart.

To create access to *sattvic* empowerment and inner strength, it is helpful throughout a heart-opening practice (from the opening centering to the closing meditation) to provide guidance about how to achieve emotional presence and mental engagement, encouraging open-hearted self-compassion, unwavering awareness, insightful presence, and personal responsibility for choices that signal balanced effort and ease. The following ideas can be supportive:
- Help cultivate a *sattvic*, ventral vagal state to maintain calmness and resilience throughout the practice; this can come from self-regulation as well as co-regulation with the yoga professional and/or other clients in the session
- Encourage concentration and full mental and emotional presence to support deep and sustainable opening; support emotional awareness through cueing attention to how emotions may ebb and flow during the practice, offering supports and ways to access equanimity and self-compassion as indicated by what emerges for clients
- Stay attuned to clients' responses to the practice, offering variations that honor their current state of mind and emotional readiness
- Acknowledge the possible vulnerability of the body's positioning in heart-opening shapes, especially in shapes during which the forward body is fully exposed; perhaps start with shapes that protect the body while opening the heart – such as prone backbends (e.g., Cobra, Locust) and backbends with the front body facing a wall (e.g., Camel variation at the wall)

> *"Whatever is open and elevated is stimulated*
> *and whatever is closed and lowered is quieted."*
> Hansen Lasater, 2020, p. 173

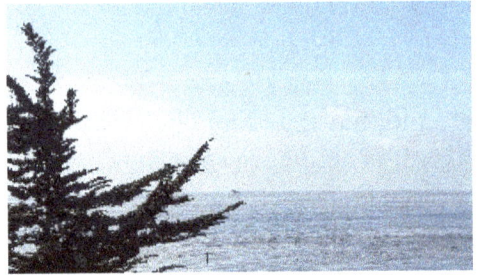

| | Tips for Grounding, Expansion, and Stability in Heart Opening |
|---|---|
| *Grounding* | <ul><li>Ground through the body parts in contact with the floor</li><li>Ground through the shoulder blades</li><li>Do not turn the neck side to side in supine shapes such as Bridge, Upward-Facing Plank, or Table Top (can compress the vertebral artery)</li><li>Ground through the breath – inhale lightly and subtly and ground into the backbend with a deliberate and long exhalation</li><li>To release the backbends, reground through a relevant body part (e.g., bring hands to hips/sacrum before lifting up/forward)</li></ul> |
| *Stability* | <ul><li>Integrate the shoulder girdle using the reverse suspender move, manubrium maneuver, or similar strategies to ground the shoulder blades (down [depression] and back [retraction]) while lifting the heart</li><li>Create a V with the scapulae – retract and depress on back</li><li>Practice a W with the arms while the back is at the wall</li><li>Attend to glenohumeral joint stability – do not create vulnerability for the joint (which can dislocate the humerus) (e.g., in Camel, bring the arms behind you via extension, internal rotation, and adduction as opposed to making a big shoulder circle that invites flexion, external rotation, and abduction)</li><li>Mindfully and softly engage the core muscles, including the perineum; allowing for stable breathing</li><li>To release out of the backband restabilize into the core; as the glutes release, core stability will be easier to re-access than in the backbend itself</li></ul> |
| *Expansion* | <ul><li>Find length in the front body – from psoas to sternocleidomastoid</li><li>Find openness in the chest (pectorals and related fascia)</li><li>Inhale to move into the backbend with spaciousness and openness</li><li>Maintain length in the spine, using the inhalation to create space between vertebrae</li><li>Face the top of head forward in prone backbends to bring the bend into the thoracic, not simply the cervical spine</li></ul> |

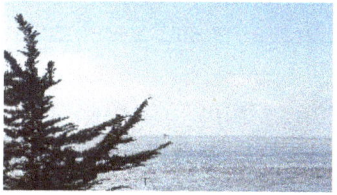

## Analysis and Experience of Sample Backbends or Heart Openers

The following heart openers are analyzed in detail below:
- *Camel*
- *Cobra*
- *Locust*
- *Bridge*

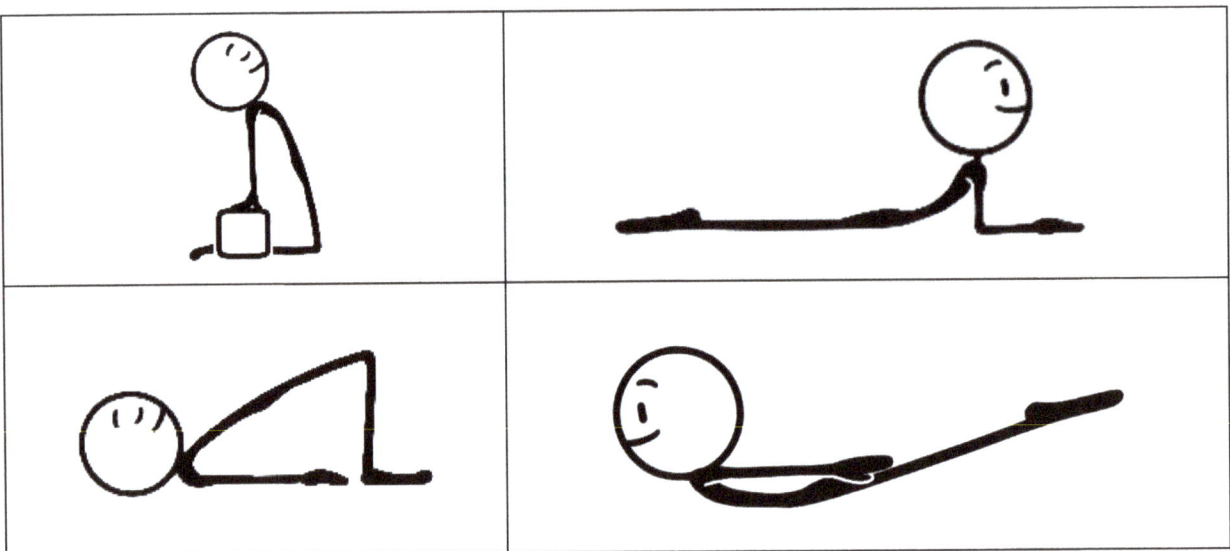

The cueing guidance offered for each heart-opening shape needs to be considered in the context offered in the general anatomy and teaching principles for backbends. The basics discussed above need to permeate the cueing for all these shapes. The general concepts below can provide further guidance for beneficial and tailored cueing. The additional cueing, shape by shape, offered here is icing on the cake. Always incorporate integrated holistic yoga cueing that addresses the following teaching principles:

- *Accessibility* – creating access through variation, adaptation, affiliation, individualization, and person-centeredness
- *Intentionality* – embedding the practice of each shape in the overall arc of the session, grounding in the theme for the class and the meaning of the practice
- *Beneficence* – honoring the wellbeing of each student and always making sure to first do no harm
- *Holism* – cueing all *koshas* or layers of experience in all shapes, never forgetting that each shape has reverberations into and is affected by all *koshas* – it is not enough to cue anatomy; also address energy and vitality, thoughts and emotions, behavioral and action choices, even community and interbeing
- *Integration* – even in teaching *asana*, integrate breathwork, concentration and mindfulness, as well as the ethical principles and lifestyle practices of yoga

## General Concepts about Backbends or Heart Openers

Many aspects of heart openers or backbends hold constant across several of the dimensions covered for individual *asanas*. Thus, following are general comments about benefits, cautions, preparations, and recovery as applicable to all covered heart-opening shapes. After this general discussion, instructions are provided for four individual heart-opening shapes, providing key alignment cues, variations, and any additional teaching tips for each.

*Benefits*

Heart Openers offer a wide array of physical, mental, and energetic benefits by promoting an opening of the heart and expansion of body, breath, and mind. Through cultivating resilience, strength, and stability, backbends balance effort and ease across all layers of experience. These shapes encourage outward expressiveness and a sense of spaciousness, making them ideal for promoting vitality and energy. Heart opening invites the following (and more) benefits, embedded into a practice of integrating effort and ease.

- *Create resilience in the front body and open the chest*: Heart openers mobilize the chest, shoulders, and hip flexors. This opening action invites a sense of spaciousness and freedom across the front superficial and deep body, encouraging a feeling of expansiveness and opening.
- *Enhance spinal mobility and release tension*: As the spine elongates and arches backwards, heart openers create space between the anterior portions of the vertebrae, promoting spinal health and resilience. By releasing tension in the low back and mobilizing the upper spine, these shapes keep the back strong and adaptable.
- *Activate and strengthen the core*: Backbends gently engage the core muscles to provide stability and yet softness as the spine extends. Gentle core stabilization activation serves to protect the low back while building balance, essential for sustaining backbends with increasing ranges of motion.
- *Invigorate body and mind*: The expansive nature of Heart Openers, combined with the necessity to invite conscious and subtle breathing, helps stimulate vitality and alertness. Heart opening can lift mood, combat fatigue, and encourage mental clarity; they are highly energizing.
- *Cultivate courage and openness*: Backbends can evoke emotional release as they challenge the body to open and expand in vulnerable ways. Heart opening can promote a sense of courage and emotional resilience, helping practitioners release fear or anxiety and embrace openness in body and mind. This shift in emotional state may promote the amelioration of depression and low energy.
- *Promote mindfulness and presence*: By inviting attention to physical and vital sensations as well as emotional and mental reactivity, Heart Openers encourage practitioners to stay anchored in the present moment. The focus required for safe and mindful heart-opening movement deepens the connection between mind, breath, and body, fostering concentration, attentiveness, and compassionate wisdom.

*Cautions*

Although Backbends offer numerous benefits, it is important to be mindful of several considerations to practice safely and with awareness. For some individuals, the open-hearted nature of backbends can be challenging emotionally; for others, it takes them to the limit of their anatomy, especially if they have postural patterns that favor spinal flexion and anterior head carriage.

- *Low back sensitivity*: Those with lumbar or sacral pain, discomfort, or history of injury may find Backbends challenging, both physically and emotionally. Creating resilience in the front body and length in the spine before arching helps support their lumbar and sacral region.

Offering variations that reduce intensity (such as practicing smaller bends or using props for support) tend to be helpful anatomically and emotionally.
- *Neck tension*: In large ranges of motion within spinal extension, many students let the head fall back; this is not a particularly helpful movement. Maintaining length in the neck and creating conscious engagement in the cervical spine helps prevent strain. Beware of unnecessary bracing in the neck and shoulders to maintain a sense of freedom of movement in the thoracic regions – front and back.
- *Hip tightness*: The hip flexors (e.g., psoas, iliacus, even quadriceps) play a key role in Backbends. Tightness across the hip joints can limit mobility and cause the lumbar region of the spine to overcompensate. Creating resilience in musculature that crosses the hip joints before and during heart opening helpfully teaches students to distribute the backbend more evenly across the length of the front and back body.
- *Breath restriction*: Heart opening can restrict the breath if there is tightness in the chest musculature and/or rib basket. Staying connected to the breath and allowing for continuous and freely-unfolding breathing enhances the experience of openness and relaxation. It is important not to sacrifice the breath for range of motion. Stress apnea (i.e., spontaneous holding of the breath) is a sign to back out of the heart opening until the breath recovers its natural rhythm.

- *Possible contraindications*:
  - *Herniated discs*: Individuals with herniated discs need to approach heart openers with care, avoiding excessive range of motion or unsupported shapes that place strain on the spine. Interoceptive and proprioceptive cueing is key to helping these students identify healthful ranges of motion and wise propping choices.
  - *Heart conditions*: Students with cardiovascular disorder or challenges (e.g., high blood pressure) best seek medical clearance before practicing extensive heart openers, as these shapes stimulate the cardiovascular system.
  - *Shoulder or neck injuries*: Participants with shoulders or neck injuries are invited to practice with mindful attention and interoception to minimize protective bracing or excessive range of motion in these regions of the body. Variations with appropriate intensity or supportive props invite safe ranges of motion and mindful movement into and out of heart-opening shapes.

## Preparations

To prepare for backbending, it is helpful to incorporate movements that mobilize the spine, open the front body, and engage the core. Some useful preparations include the following listed ideas and, of course, the six movements of spine as a warm-up. Most of these strategies have already been elucidated the anatomical foci section above; this listing represents a summary that is best understood in the context of the anatomy and psychology discussed above.
- *Spinal mobilization*: six movements of spine (e.g., standing Cat-Cow; rotations with arms in cactus), synchronized with breath to prepare the nervous system and clear an emotional pathway into backbends
- *Cranial nerve reset and trap release*: eye movements, neck movements, and shoulder movements

- *Preliminary gentle opening of the heart*: suspender move, manubrium maneuver, Cobra at the wall and similar actions
- *Mobilization of the shoulder joint*: e.g., arm and shoulder circles, Eagle arms, wall stretches (e.g., Ws, wall rotations/twists)
- *Strengthening of the shoulder joint*: e.g., dolphin swimming, movements from Table Top (e.g., Bird Dog, Fire Hydrant)
- *Opening the psoas*: e.g., Lunges, Half Frog – any shape that opens the hip flexors and creates space across the front body
- *Core engagement*: any shapes and movements that create resilience in the core (see core stabilization guidance in Chapter 9)

## Recovery

After practicing backbends, restorative movements can help release tension and bring balance back to the body. Consider these recovery shapes at the end of the complete backbending practice. It is generally *not helpful* to intersperse recovery shapes in a sequence of backbends as this may counter the careful preparation for spinal mobility (i.e., extension) and core stability. Recovery in a backbending sequence is offered toward the end of the session overall, as a physical and emotion reset and preparation for *Savasana*. These recovery movements create a smooth transition from the expansive experience of backbending to a more grounded and relaxed state that invites the restfulness and silence of an inner practice at the end of a session. They allow body, breath, and mind to release residual tension to become open to integrating the benefits of this expansive and open-hearted practice.

- *Child*: This shape offers a gentle way to release tension in the spine, especially the low back, after backbending. It also creates ease in the shoulders and hips.
- *Knees-to-Chest*: Lying on the back with the knees drawn toward the chest helps to create ease in the low back and reset the spine after deeper extensions.
- *Supine Twist*: Gentle spinal rotations release tension in the back, shoulders, and neck. Twists can help neutralize the effects of deep backbends and create ease across the body.
- *Seated Forward Fold*: Moving into a gentle, supported forward fold can help release the spine and calm the nervous system, providing a counterbalance to the energetic effects of backbends.

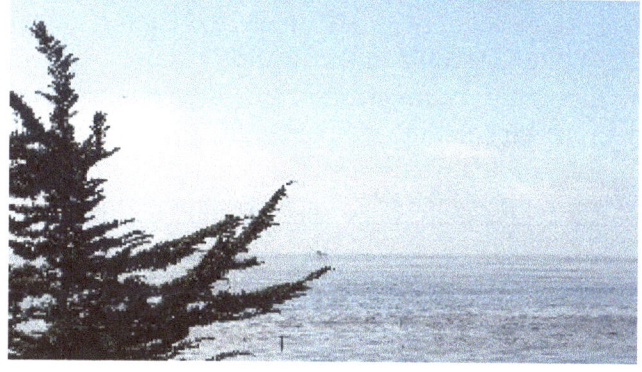

## Camel or Ustrasana

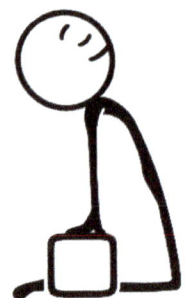

Finding ease in Camel requires a connection to interoception, neuroception, and proprioception, focusing on the experience of opening the heart, without striving for a big backbend on the outside. The following invitations offer gentle guidance for moving into Camel from a place of stability and with a mind that is concentrated on the movement into, within, and out of the shape. Heart opening has a strong psychological component and requires present-moment-centeredness in mind, breath, and body.

### Key Alignment Invitations

Alignment in Camel begins in a kneeling position that is grounded through the lower legs and feet, and relies on the entire body to create stability and ease in the spine as the heart space is opened and the back is strengthened. From a kneeling base, a gentle lift through the heart and expansion across the chest can be invited, helping practitioners experience openness without strain. Guidance further encourages engagement through the thighs and back body, allowing each part of the body to support the shape, without creating excessive tension. By cueing alignment with mindful attention and careful intention, practitioners can experience Camel as an expression of balanced resilience, in which interoception, proprioception, and neuroception guide all movement and deepen a compassionate, inner-guided expression of heart opening that is person-tailored and accessible.

- *Invitations related to the base – <u>kneeling as the starting position</u>*:
    - *Anchor through the legs and feet*: Ground through the shins and tops of the feet, allowing these areas to serve as the foundation for the rising upward that is involved in the shape. Bring vitality and mindful presence into the legs, creating a stable base from which the spine can gently lift. Kneeling on a blanket with the feet draping off the blanket (see guidance for Hero and Diamond) can be very helpful to creating easeful grounding.
    - *Ease the hips into a natural position*: Let the pelvis move naturally as a gentle curve is invited into the lower spine. Overcueing of the pelvis (e.g., cueing tucking or tilting) tends to be counterproductive as most students have a natural inclination for letting the sacrum move in coordination with the lumbar spine. Cue only if students are observed to tilt or tuck excessively (perhaps due to habits they have developed in other contexts). Notice areas of bracing, especially in the glutes, and encourage release of excessive contraction to allow for engaged openness without strain.
    - *Engage the thighs for person-centered stability*: Subtle engagement of the thighs can help maintain stability in the hips, giving support to the spine's lift and creating a sense of groundedness throughout the lower body. This engagement can be invited via use of a prop. For students whose legs tend to splay apart (abducting and externally rotating), offer a block between the legs to invite adduction and internal rotation. For students whose legs tend to migrate too far medially or rotate too far internally, offer a strap around the legs for them to press into, engaging abduction.
- *Invitations related to the spine and chest*:
    - *Lift through the front body*: Invite the heart space to gently rise, leading the upper spine into a natural arc. The manubrium maneuver can help facilitate this beautifully and not

excessively. The suspender move is a great way to find opening, either using the thumbs in the axilla or the hands high and laterally on the rib basket. The thoracic spine takes on the primary role in extension, allowing the lumbar spine to remain stable and resilient.
- *Create space in the rib basket*: Invite expansiveness in the rib basket while breathing into the front and side body. Allow breath to guide movement into heart opening, bringing ease rather than pushing or forcing excessive range of motion in the spinal extension. Attend to not excessively splaying the low ribs to maintain core stability.
- *Find ease across the shoulders and collarbones*: Release bracing in the shoulder girdle, encouraging a gentle drawing back and down of the shoulder blades (creating a gentle V movement). This light engagement supports openness in the chest and strength in the back without compressing the back of the neck or shoulders.
- *Invitations related to the arms and hands*:
  - *Explore hand placement for support*: Hands can rest on the low back, palms pressing lightly to guide the lift of the heart; alternatively, hands can reach for the heels if that feels accessible. Blocks or the seat of a chair by the heels can serve as a supportive option for the hands to land, inviting the arms into a relaxed reach without straining.
  - *Align the elbows with the torso*: Gently draw the elbows toward each other behind the back to support a healthful shoulder position. This medial engagement helps maintain integration and connection throughout the upper body.

*Invitations related to the head and neck*:
- *Allow the neck to follow the spine's curve*: Keep the neck in line with the spine, encouraging natural extension rather than hyperextending the cervical spine (a common misalignment in backbends). This position promotes ease through the entire spine, particularly in the cervical region that is often overly extended by students as they strive for a 'deeper' bend, misunderstanding the goal to be the attainment of some idealized outer shape rather than inner experience.
- *Find steadiness through a gaze point*: Gaze may gently lift upward or stay neutral, depending on comfort. Letting go of tension in the throat area supports a sense of openness without strain, creating a balanced experience for the head and neck. If students tend to hyperextend through the neck, invite the gaze to focus straight forward or downward. Often, degree of neck extension follows the direction of the gaze.

## Variations and Explorations

Camel offers many individual exploration and creativity that can align with personal needs and intentions. Demonstrating Camel in these variations invites students not to strive for an outer shape, understanding instead that they are inviting an open-hearted experience that is open yet easeful, engaged yet peaceful. Each of these variations offers an opportunity for individualized exploration, allowing practitioners to discover a personal connection to Camel and honoring their most auspicious anatomical and psychological access to heart opening.
- **Supported Camel with props under the hands**: Placing props by the heels provides a person-centered placement for the hands and promotes a grounded experience of heart opening that does not create excess strain in the low back. This variation is useful for students who tend to create a strong hip hinge (see above) in backbends and who need to retrain their proprioception to find more healthful extension across the full length of the spine.

- *Seated Camel*: Practicing a seated variation of Camel by sitting on the heels with hands resting on the low back offers a similar heart-opening experience. This gentle shape invites mobilization through the upper spine and shoulders without creating excessive strain anywhere along the length of the spine. The wall can also feel psychologically protective.
- *Wall Camel*: Students can be invited to practice Camel facing a wall, with the knees grounded against the wall and the hips moving toward the wall before inviting the spine into extension. The support of the wall for the lower region of the body tends to decrease range of motion to invite a more genuine expression of spinal extension. It also creates strong engagement in the quadriceps and psoas, inviting resilience and enhanced mobility over time.
- *Arm and foot positions in Camel*: Invite creativity in the arms by offering possibilities such as full shoulder flexion (reaching arms upward) or cactus arms. Feet can be in dorsiflexion with toes tucked under rather than planting the tops of the feet on the ground. Letting the feet drape off a support (such as kneeling on blankets or bolsters) can bring ease or novelty.

*Additional Teaching Tips*

To help practitioners find ease and alignment in Camel, a few additional considerations can serve students to find optimized and personalized experiences of the shape.
- *Use breath as a guide*: Encourage practitioners to allow each inhalation to lift the heart gently, and each exhalation to ground and release into the lower body, creating a supportive rhythm or pulsation in the shape.
- *Focus on the inner experience in body, breath, and emotion*: Guide practitioners to connect with inner somatic and vital sensations, allowing them to evolve and unfold their Camel from the inside out rather than focusing on a specific outer shape. Attunement to emotional reactivity can help create insight and acceptance.
- *Encourage curiosity and exploration*: Remind students to explore sensation with curiosity and compassion to find a sustainable and highly personal expression of Camel. Variations enhance the heart-opening experience, increase agency, and invite students into personal empowerment, agency, and responsibility for making discerning choices.

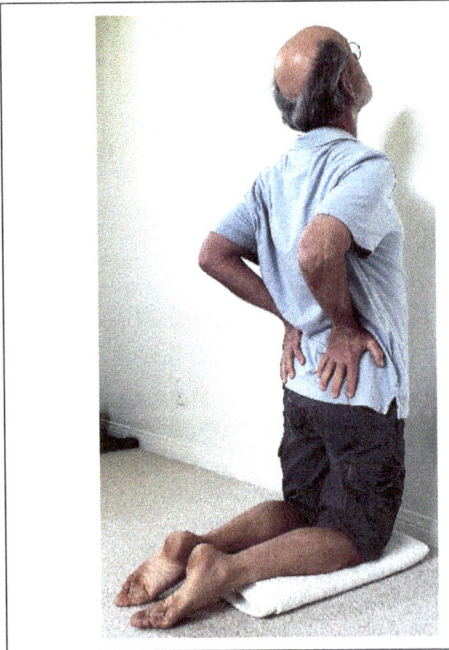

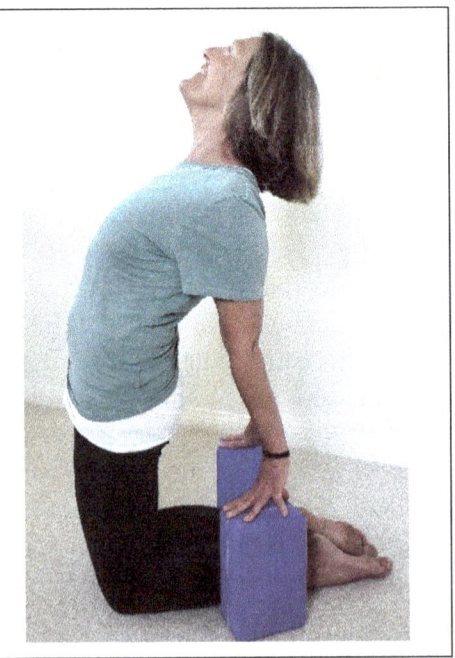

*Camel with Wall Support – creating safety with props and carefully placed hands* ←

*Camel with Floor Supports* →

## Cobra or Bhujangasana

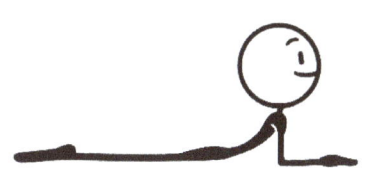

Exploring Cobra as an embodiment of resilience and openness that arises from a base of strength and vitality invites practitioners to connect deeply with inner sensations of body, breath, and mind, including emotional states and reactivities. Cobra arises from lying prone on the floor and, by its very nature, challenges students to rise up from a very grounded foundation in a gentle arc that exudes self-compassion and interoceptive and proprioceptive awareness. Cobra can be a shape in which to emphasize the development of back body engagement and strength that facilitate gentle heart opening. It is offered in a manner that _does not_ pursue an exaggerated, straining, or excessive arch, or extension, in the spine. The heart-opening, rather than backbending, properties of the shape are emphasized and cued. The guidance that follows stresses intentional cueing that invites discovery of a very stable experience in Cobra; an experience that grounds attention in present-moment awareness of all layers of experience and keeps the heart open and the back body strong.

### Key Alignment Invitations

An even and steady rise through the spine, from a prone position, is important and can be cultivated in Cobra (and related prone heart openers) by anchoring through the lower body and lifting from the heart space (rather than hinging in the lumbar spine). Intentional alignment cues help practitioners experience Cobra as a connected and compassionate whole-person experience, in which engagement and ease in one area support movement and persistence in another. Practitioners are invited to find natural openness in the front body – from pelvic girdle to pectoral girdle; a gentle lift and extension through the spine; and the experience of strength and stability throughout. Students are guided toward a mindful and sustainable experience of Cobra, emphasizing exploration, presence, compassion, interoception, neuroception, and proprioception over striving for a particular outer expression of or range of motion in the shape.

- *Invitations related to creating a strong foundation from which to lift:*
  - *Anchor through the pelvis, fronts of the legs, and tops of the feet*: Press gently through the tops of the feet and allow the legs to remain active. Feel the grounding from the feet all the way up through the pelvis, providing stability *and* lightness as the chest begins to open and lift forward. Keeping the feet in keen contact with the floor without gripping promotes a solid foundation. Invite exploration of optimal pelvic alignment – for some students, a gentle tucking facilitates engagement; for other, a gentle tilt is more healthful. One-for-all cueing (i.e.,, either always cueing anterior or always cueing posterior rotation of the pelvis) does not work as it is important to understand the starting position of the pelvis. Inviting interoception, proprioception, and student self-exploration is key.
  - *Creating the lift of the spinal extension and the openness of the heart space*: Let the lifting of the upper body arise from intentional hand placement (see more below) and attention that is directed to the back body for strength and extension in the thoracic spine as well as to the front body for openness and resilience. The resilience of the front body and the strength of the erector spinae muscles will contribute to decisions about how high to lift in Cobra. Many options exist – from a very low lift with hands floating above the earth to a high lift that can essentially transition into Seal or Upward Facing Dog.

- *Find optimal engagement in the gluteal muscles*: Although excessive contraction (i.e., bracing or gripping) in the glutes is not helpful, intentional engagement in this region is likely necessary as many students these days have some degree of gluteal amnesia (i.e., under-engage the glutes or have weak glutes that fail to participate in movement when it would be helpful for them to do so). The engagement invited into the gluteal muscles is supportive, not restrictive, of forward and upward movement in the heart space. Engagement in the glutes facilitates a natural flow of energy throughout the back body, and allows the thoracic spine to extend with evenness. Gluteal engagement can also be cued as a way to prevent a lumbar hinge.
- *Move the femurs toward the back body to enhance stability*: Subtly drawing the inner thighs towards one another (without pressing the legs together) and finding slight internal rotation help create resilience in the lower body, offering support for the spine as it arcs and the chest as it opens. Leg engagement can help practitioners maintain alignment and avoid unwholesome hinging in the lumbar spine. Notably, the opposite pattern may be needed for the rare students who start the shape overly internally rotated and adducted.

- *Invitations related to alignment in spine and chest:*
  - *Cultivate gentle spinal extension from the thorax*: Allow the heart space to open gently, rising upward and forward from the front body without overemphasizing the low back. Manubrium and suspender moves can invite this way of opening. They help students focus on a gradual lifting of the chest and upper spine rather than pushing the spinal extension into the lumbar region. This approach balances the curve through the entire spine, particularly engaging the thoracic area to promote resilience and ease.
  - *Expand across the front ribs*: Invite space and mobility in the rib basket with each breath, feeling a subtle opening across the chest with the inhalation and a sense of anchoring and grounding with the exhalation. As the inhalation invites the low rib basket to move outward and upward, a natural lift follows in the front body. The back body will respond with engagement in the erector spinae muscles, keeping the movement stable and free of strain. As the exhalation invites the ribs to draw inward and downward, along with gentle core stabilization, unnecessary arching in the lower spine is prevented.

- *Invitations related to shoulders, arms, and hands:*
  - *Establish an intentional arm and hand position*: Position the hands slightly wider than shoulder-width as optimal (refer to recommendations made about hand placement in the Arm Standing and Inversion chapters, especially in the guidance for Downward Facing Dog and Handstand), with fingers spread and palms pressing lightly into the mat. The hands are grounding points, aiding the lift from the chest without taking on the upper body's weight. This hand positioning encourages a gentle lift while keeping the lower body connected to the mat.
  - *Choose a wholesome degree of flexion/extension in the elbows*: Even in a very high lift or large range of motion in the spinal extension, it is helpful to maintain a micro-bend in the elbows to prevent overextension in these joints and create a more sustainable shape. This subtle bend helps practitioners find balance and keep the lift of the spine light and continuous, supporting an open chest without forcing the low back. For many students, there will be significant flexion in the elbows and a lower and more sustainable lift into Cobra. It is considerably better to access Cobra from the power of the core and back than the more passive spinal extension created by vigorous elbow extension or pressing of the hands into the ground. In fact, a handless Cobra is one of the best variations to offer.

- *Ease the scapulae down and back*: Encourage the shoulder blades to gently move away from the ears and toward the back, feeling a light engagement that draws energy down the back and opens the heart. Scapular movement comes from a sense of spaciousness balanced with healthful muscular effort, creating openness in the collarbones and allowing the neck to stay free from tension. The manubrium maneuver is helpful.
- *Invitations related to neck and head placements:*
  - *Keep the head in line with the spine*: Let the head follow the natural curve of the spine, avoiding forced or hyper-extension in the neck. Natural alignment fosters ease through the cervical spine, helping to prevent strain or tension in the throat. Encourage students to feel the continuity from the base of the spine to the crown of the head, moving with a sense of lightness.
  - *Find a soft gaze forward or slightly downward*: A steady gaze point, directed forward or downward (rather than upward) helps prevent hyperextension in the neck. It counteracts a tendency in many students to throw the head back in Cobra to have a (false) sense of greater opening in the front body and more range of motion in the spine.

### Variations and Explorations

Cobra offers a variety of ways for practitioners to explore their own preferences and needs for heart opening and back strengthening. Each variation can help build strength in the back body as well as mobility in the front body, while encouraging a unique and personalized experience of Cobra that neither over- nor under-efforts.
- *No-Hands Cobra*: Lifting into Cobra with the hands hovering a few centimeters above the ground is a great way to engage the core and facilitate a lift that is based on active range of motion (rather than passive range of motion that is created by the arms). It is a great way to cultivate strength in the back body, stability in the core, and opening in the heart space. This version of Cobra is a favorite and perhaps ought to become the default version of Cobra.
- *Low Cobra*: By keeping arms bent and the chest closer to the ground, Low Cobra provides a shape that emphasizes stability in the lower body and reduces compressive load on the lumbar spine. This variation allows practitioners to explore the movement through the upper back and shoulders with less intensity, focusing on gentle spinal extension and emotional regulation..
- *Wide-Handed Cobra*: Positioning hands slightly wider than shoulder width can allow for a spacious feeling in shoulders and chest. This hand placement may feel particularly beneficial for those with restrictions in shoulder range of motion and invites ease across the chest.
- *Sphinx*: Practicing Sphinx (i.e., a supine backbend on the forearms) is often described as preparatory to Cobra. This is not usually the case. For many students, Sphinx forces a passive lift as the arms contribute power to move into spinal extension. Use it and cue it with care.
- *Seal and Upward Facing Dog*: These variations invite more forceful pressure through the hands to create greater spinal and axial extension for a more lifted variation of Cobra. These progressions of Cobra serve only students who have easeful alignment in Cobra and do not hyperextend, or worse yet, hinge in the lumbar spine. It is recommended to allow the pelvis to lift up off the ground in these shapes, rather than cueing for the pelvis to remain anchored to the earth. Even the tops of the thighs will naturally lift for most individuals.
- *Wiggling Cobra*: Many movements can be added to Cobra, including slight lateral flexion and rotation. These variations can bring flexibility and fun into a more exploratory way of

being in prone spinal extension. No-Hands Cobra needs to be a familiar and accessible practice before wiggles are added to Cobra.

*Additional Teaching Tips*

To enhance the experience in Cobra, several approaches can be used that encourage movements that connect to breath, concentration, awareness, and mindful somatic and vital investigation and emotional experience.

- *Move with the breath*: Practitioners are encouraged to use the breath rhythm to support the rise (with the inhalation) and release downward (with the exhalation) in Cobra. Encourage students to inhale as they gently lift the chest, and to exhale to ground and find ease. A breath-centered rhythm promotes staying connected to the flow of *prana* within the shape and may prevent either bracing or collapsing.
- *Cultivate inner focus*: Remind students to maintain interoception, proprioception, and neuroception, noticing sensations across body, breath, and mind. Such attunement and compassionate concentration fosters a practice that emphasizes the healthful experience of strength in the back body, resilience in the front body, and stability at the core over achieving an outer shape. By focusing on subtle sensations, practitioners engage in mindfully attuned movement, rather than rigidly braced or collapsed presence.
- *Encourage self-exploration and acceptance*: Invite students to explore different variations without a goal of achieving a particular range of motion or position. Each practitioner's experience is unique, and curiosity can reveal insights about how to move the body in an authentic way. Remind students to honor their experience as the primary guide toward creating a practice that is gentle and empowering.

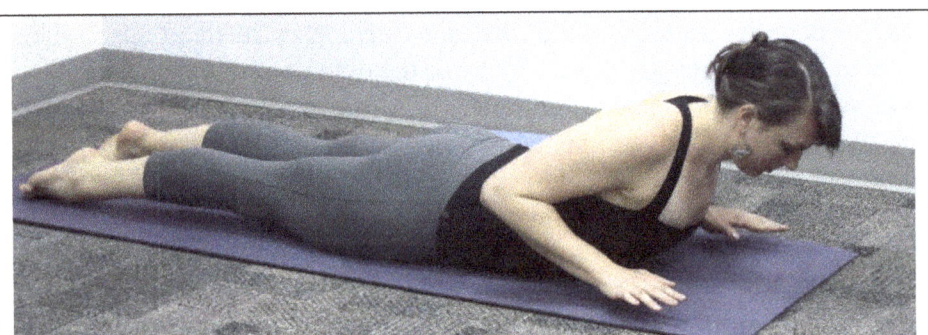

*Handless Cobra – committing to a shape created through back muscle engagement, not passive force*

*Upward Facing Dog – committing to a shape that builds inner strength rather than an outer shape allows the pelvis and upper thighs to lift dynamically*

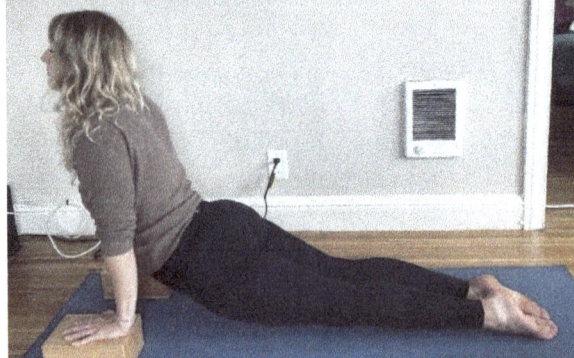

## Locust or Salabhasana

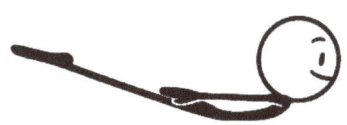

Locust offers practitioners a chance to explore grounded resilience and empowerment through the activation of the back body, linking intentional engagement with a sense of steady ease. By lifting from a supported and strong prone base, Locust invites practitioners to cultivate a steady connection to inner sensations and mental clarity, allowing them to rise with stability and calm awareness in all layers of human experience. Locust invites integrated holistic strengthening of the back body, release of tension across the chest, and openness in the front body without striving for exaggerated lift or tension. Practitioners are invited to experience Locust as a grounding shape that awakens vitality, mental focus, and emotional balance from the core outward, keeping attention on inner experience rather than on achieving a particular outer shape.

### Key Alignment Invitations

Locust invites resilient extension through the back line of the body that is a combination of front-body opening and back-body engagement. Locust combines grounding, expansion, and stability in a shape that invites resilience across the length of the torso – front (mobilization) and back (strengthening). Practitioners are encouraged to create stability, building a shape that feels dynamic and sustainable, with strong attunement to interoception, proprioception, and neuroception to find appropriate range of motion and outer expression that aligns with inner needs, anatomically, energetically, and emotionally.

- *Invitations related to building a strong foundation from which to lift:*
  - *Ground through pelvis, legs, and tops of the feet*: Connect the length of the front body to the earth with mindful awareness of finding a sense of grounding. An easeful (rather than braced) prone position is a great foundation for the strong lift from the back body that is to come. Starting from a place of relaxed ease invites a non-grasping attitude about lifting into the shape, inviting a healthful range of motion in the body and emotion in the mind.
  - *Engage the back body and the core*: The lift in Locust arises from engagement throughout the back body, strongly supported by all core stabilizers. This engagement can begin with a feeling of drawing gently inward at the navel, extending through the spine, and allowing the chest to open via strategies such as the manubrium maneuver or suspender move. Inviting core strength creates a sense of stability, supporting the lift in the upper body in harmony with the back muscles without excess efforting.
  - *Find balanced gluteal engagement to lift the legs*: To lift the legs away from the earth, a healthful activation in the glutes, without bracing, stabilizes the hips and facilitates ease in the spine, preventing lumbar hinging. Many clients benefit from cues about this gluteal engagement, given the common occurrence these days of some degree of gluteal amnesia related to excessive hours of sitting. Lifting the legs in Locust is entirely optional.
- *Invitations related to lifting with ease and an open heart:*
  - *Cultivate length through the spine*: Invite elongation of the spine, lifting through the back body in a way that feels grounded and free from strain. Encourage spinal extension to arise from the thoracic region of the spine, rather than hinging in the lumbar region. This intentional engagement of spinal extensor muscles invites spaciousness across the chest without overextending or forcing.

- *Expand through the chest and shoulders*: Invite a feeling of openness across the clavicles, allowing the heart space to open naturally. As the shoulder girdle releases away from the ears, practitioners are invited to create spaciousness that avoids forced extension in the lumbar and cervical spines. Let the heart-opening movement promote a sense of lightness and expansiveness across the front body, fostering resilience without bracing or gripping.
- *Invitations related to supporting stability through arms and hands:*
  - *Let the arms hover forward or reach back with ease*: Arms may be stretched long, forward of the head, to hover a few centimeters above the ground, with palms facing each other, or back toward the feet, with palms facing the floor or the sides of the body. Either positioning helps engage the muscles of the upper back to create steady, active, and empowered movement. Reaching the hands back without forcing can encourage a feeling of ease within effort and often feels more open and lighter than arms reaching forward. Arms reaching forward can offer more strength-building opportunities in body and mind
  - *Adjust the width and position of the arms for ease in the shoulders*: For practitioners who experience tightness or discomfort in the shoulders, adjustments in arm position, such as moving the arms outward (abduction) or slightly down (perhaps via internal rotation) toward the ground, may enhance comfort. Optimizing arm position can create easeful stability in the shoulders to allow for an unimpaired lift into spinal extension.
- *Invitations related to aligning the head and neck:*
  - *Maintain wholesome alignment in the neck*: The head follows the natural curve of the spine, aligning with the body without hyperextending or releasing too far forward (into flexion). By focusing on alignment from the base of the spine to the crown of the head, practitioners can experience continuity in spinal extension, which promotes a distribution of the backbend across the length of the spinal column and prevents lumbar hinging.
  - *Direct the gaze slightly downward or forward*: A soft gaze forward or toward the floor can help the neck remain in a neutral position, avoiding strain and injury. Creating a gaze point invites relaxation and a resilient lift through the back body. It also anchors the mind into soft focus and emotional regulation.

## Variations and Explorations

Locust provides a variety of ways for practitioners to explore strength, resilience, and alignment in a way that is grounding and empowering. Each variation allows practitioners to sense into the movement and engage the back body without overemphasizing range of motion or force.

- *Low Locust*: This variation involves a slight lift of the chest and legs, creating a more accessible entry into the shape. Low Locust emphasizes stability across the pelvis and core, allowing practitioners to tune into subtle engagement in the low back without focusing on degree of lift.
- *Arms-Engaged Locust*: Engaging the arms forward or to the sides and back can provide a different degree of effort through the upper back and offers a sense of spaciousness and openness across the chest. Playing with this variation can feel liberating for students as they get to explore which arm position and expression of Locust best accommodates their anatomy, energy, and emotional state.
- *Hands at the Low Back*: Clasping the hands behind the low back can support heart opening; the key is to use this arm and hand placement with gentleness and without force. This position encourages balance between strength in the back line of the body and ease across

heart space, allowing for grounded yet expansive stability. If the heart space collapses when the hands are clasped behind the back, widen the distance between the two hands by connecting them via a strap.
- *Leg-Only Locust*: For an experience focused on lower-body engagement, clients may lift just the legs, keeping the torso grounded. This helps build strength in the glutes and low back without involving the upper body, offering a grounded and stabilizing variation.

*Additional Teaching Tips*

To explore a variety of experiences in Locust, several approaches can facilitate playfulness. Such exploration of variations relies on mindful attunement to sensation, deep connection to the breath, and the inner emotional experience of the shapes that are being explored.
- *Use the breath as a guide*: Invite clients to coordinate movement with breath, lifting gently on the inhalation and releasing any bracing on the exhalation. A rhythmic flow or pulsation with the breath invites exploration, dynamic movements (rather than rigidity or gripping), and stable resilience.
- *Foster inner awareness and sensation*: Encourage clients to tune into subtle sensations, observing how different areas of the body engage and release with each breath and each variation in movement. By inviting awareness to the connection between breath and movement, practitioners can experience grounded presence, promoting deeper inner focus and physical and emotional stability that is resilient, adaptive, and dynamic.
- *Invite exploration and self-compassion*: Remind clients that each experience of Locust is unique, allowing room for variations that feel empowering and supportive of present-moment-experience. Self-inquiry, compassion, and acceptance are guiding principles for students who want to honor all layers of experience, from body, to energy, to mind and emotions.

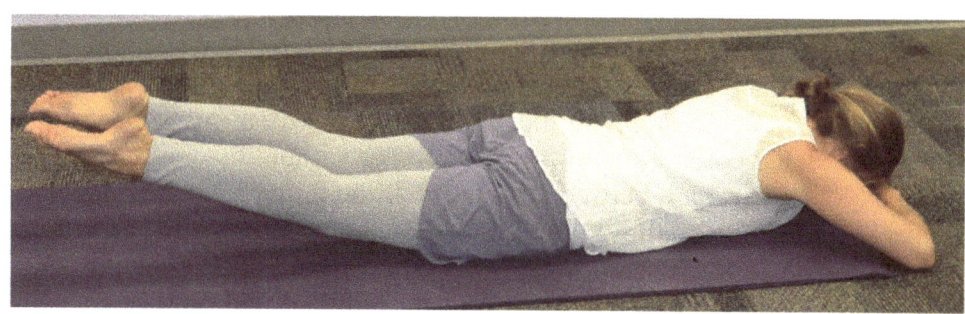

*Locust with Arms Resting – committing to a strong lift from the back body*

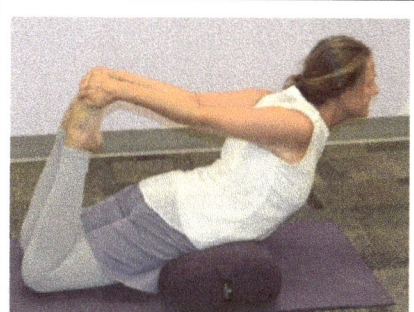

*Locust Variation – moving toward Wheel*

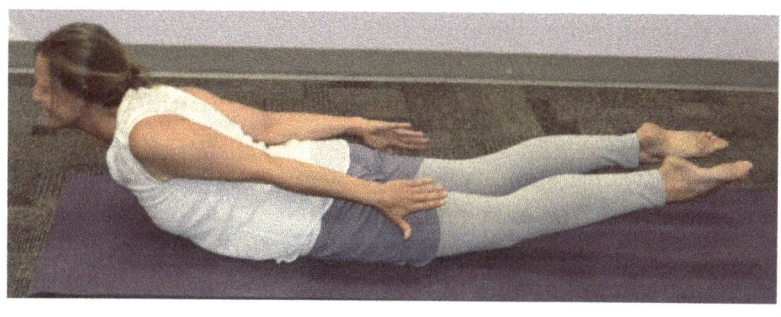

*Locust with All Limbs Lifted – keeping a natural curve in the cervical spine*

## Bridge or Setu Bandha Sarvangasana

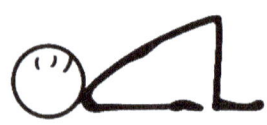

Bridge is an invitation to connect with stability and a sense of expansion, to experience inner power and strength that rises from the ground up. Bridge engages the whole back body while creating ease and opening through the front body, inviting practitioners to feel grounded yet open-hearted. Bridge offers a unique opportunity to experience a balance of resilience and calm by lifting from a strong foundation, without reaching for a particular goal (or range of motion). The following guidance focuses on cultivating interoception, proprioception, and neuroception, to help practitioners find alignment through inner experience, including attentiveness to breath and energy, as well as compassion for emerging emotions or narratives in the mind.

### Key Alignment Invitations

Bridge begins with the body lying supine, grounded through the back with knees bent and heels drawn close toward the sitz bones. It invites an even rising upward through the spine, guided by attunement to sensation in legs, hips, core, and beyond. The following alignment invitations encourage practitioners to explore a balanced lift with openness through the heart space while sustaining a profound and grounding connection to the earth.

- *Invitations related to creating a foundation:*
    - *Grounding from the feet*: Begin by rooting down through the soles of the feet, feeling the contact with the mat through all three or four corners of each foot. This grounding serves as one of two bases from which the lift occurs, creating a sense of stability through the legs that supports gentle spinal extension, especially in the mid to upper back. The feet collaborate with the shoulder girdle as a base of support.
    - *Ground through the shoulder blades*: The second base of stability arises from a deeply grounded shoulder girdle. Allow the scapulae to draw toward each other, wiggling one side inward and then the other, engaging the shoulder V in a supine position.
    - *Inviting gentle engagement in the thighs*: If the thighs tend to move away from one another, encourage them to gently draw toward one another without bracing, perhaps by gently squeezing a block or cushion between the knees. If the thighs tend to collapse toward each other, explore the possibility of tying a yoga strap (or resistance band) around the legs, just above or below the knees, and invite gentle abduction by pressing into the strap. These individually-tailored actions create resilience and stability, particularly in the hips, which allows for an even rise in the pelvis and helps maintain alignment as the chest lifts.
- *Invitations related to hips and pelvic stability:*
    - *Ease the hips into a natural position*: As the pelvis begins to rise upward away from the earth, notice excessive arching or bracing. Invite a sense of ease, finding alignment that allows for stability without strain. Such ease may require subtle engagement in the glutes that lifts the back body smoothly, without a lumbar hinge.
    - *Create spaciousness in the lumbar spine*: Encourage students to feel the lumbar spine lengthening, rather than compressing, as they rise. A grounded and engaged lower body supports the back, creating a gentle arc rather than an exaggerated lift.

- *Invitations related to lifting with ease:*
    - *Lengthen from the base of the spine*: Guide practitioners to feel a gradual lengthening from the tailbone up through the thoracic spine. Lift is achieved in a wholesome way by paying attention to the relationships between the vertebrae (preventing compression, hinging, or torquing), by not having a goal of achieving a particular height. Instead, focus is on a resilient arc that creates ease and balance along the spine and the front body.
    - *Expand the rib basket with breath*: As the chest lifts, invite each inhalation to bring a sense of spaciousness across the low ribs, allowing them to move outward and upward even in this position. This breath-centered lift in the low rib basket helps open the heart area without forcing the shape too high into the torso. With the exhalation, the low ribs gently draw downward and inward, inviting a sweet and wholesome pulsation of energy in this open-hearted alignment.
- *Invitations related to the upper appendicular skeleton:*
    - *Ground the arms for stability*: Allow the arms to rest on the mat, palms facing downward or upward, depending on individual shoulder anatomy. By pressing the hands gently into the mat, the arms support the lift of the torso while maintaining a sense of groundedness. For students who need a deeper connection to their back bodies, interlacing the fingers beneath the body, bringing the shoulder blades closer together, may bring a sense of stability during this expansive expression of a heart opening.
    - *Ease the shoulder blades downward*: Invite the shoulder girdle to release toward the mat, allowing the neck and throat area to stay unencumbered, unconstricted, and unbraced. Gentle grounding action of the scapulae helps maintain a feeling of spaciousness across the chest, while allowing the upper spine to rise up evenly.

## Variations and Explorations

Bridge offers various options for practitioners to explore different expressions of grounding, stability, and expansiveness. Each variation invites a unique experience and allows for personal exploration, enhancing the strength, dynamism, and stability in body, breath, and mind. Honoring personal anatomy, energy, and emotional reactivity remains crucial and is always emphasized when variations and explorations are offered.

- *Supported Bridge with props*: Placing a block or bolster(s) beneath the sacrum offers a restorative approach to Bridge, allowing practitioners to experience lift without excessive effort. This option promotes relaxation and creates space for breath awareness and exploration of inner sensations. (see Chapter 15 – Restorative Practices)
- *Dynamic Bridge with breath and rhythm*: Many dynamic variations exist that link movement with breath. One possibility is a pulsation with breath wherein hips lift on an inhalation and lower on an exhalation. This dynamic variation invites a rhythmic, wave-like motion that enhances awareness of breath and brings fluidity to the spine. Other dynamic variations – typically with the sacrum on a bolster or foam roller – invite the legs to be stretched up into the air and to make a variety of movements, such as scissoring side to side, moving downward toward the floor and back up (either with knees bent or extended), legs in Tree shape, and many other options that can be playfully explored.
- *One-Legged Bridge*: For those seeking a variation that increases strength, lifting one leg toward the sky while maintaining stability in the grounded leg can intensify the engagement through the back body and core. In this variation, there is no prop under the sacrum. The lift

is maintained by core and back strength. Thus, this lifted variation requires engaged attentiveness to wholesome alignment through the pelvis and spine.
- *Extended Bridge or Drawbridge*: In this variation, the knees are extended and the entire back of the pelvis is supported by a prop (ideally a yoga bolster) to create a long open-hearted arch from the toes to the crown of the head.
- *Strengthening Bridge with Extended Knees*: In this variation, the hips are suspended in the air as the feet rest on a yoga ball or the seat of a chair. Strong core, hamstring, and gluteal engagements lift the spine up in its natural curves to create a Plank-like shape with the body. This Bridge variation is focused on spinal strength more so than spinal extension; nevertheless it is a strong heart opener.

## Additional Teaching Tips

Several additional cueing tips and helpful hints can individualize and tailor the experience of Bridge. Additional cueing is about inviting introspective exploration of all layers of experience, and allowing Bridge to create access to feelings of strength, stability, and ease in body, breath, and mind.
- *Move with the breath*: Guide practitioners to find a steady rhythm with the breath, rising with the inhalation and grounding with the exhalation. This breath-centered approach brings an energetic pulsation to the shape, concentrating the mind into the present moment and cultivating a sense of resilience.
- *Encourage inner awareness*: Remind students to tune into sensations in the body, observing where they feel stability, ease, strength, or subtle engagement. Fostering a proprioceptive, neuroceptive, and interoceptive focus enhances self-attunement and emphasizes inner experience to create compassion and wisdom.
- *Invite curiosity and exploration*: Allow practitioners the freedom to explore the shape with a spirit of curiosity. Emphasize that each expression of Bridge can be unique; encourage clients to honor what feels stable and aligned for their body, energy, and mind state in each moment. Exploration builds a deeper connection to the inner teacher, fostering confidence and adaptability as well as empowerment and agency.

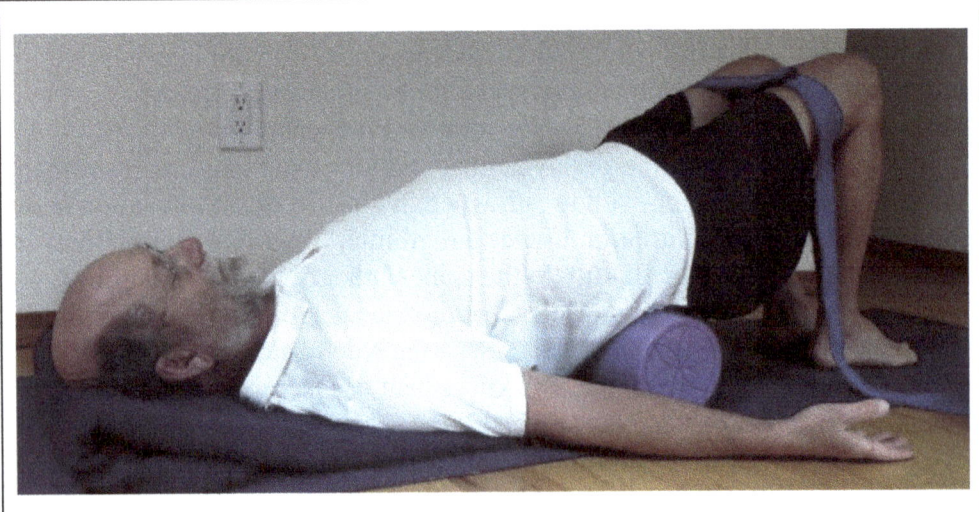

*Bridge with multiple supports*

Integrated Holistic Yoga Movement | **467**

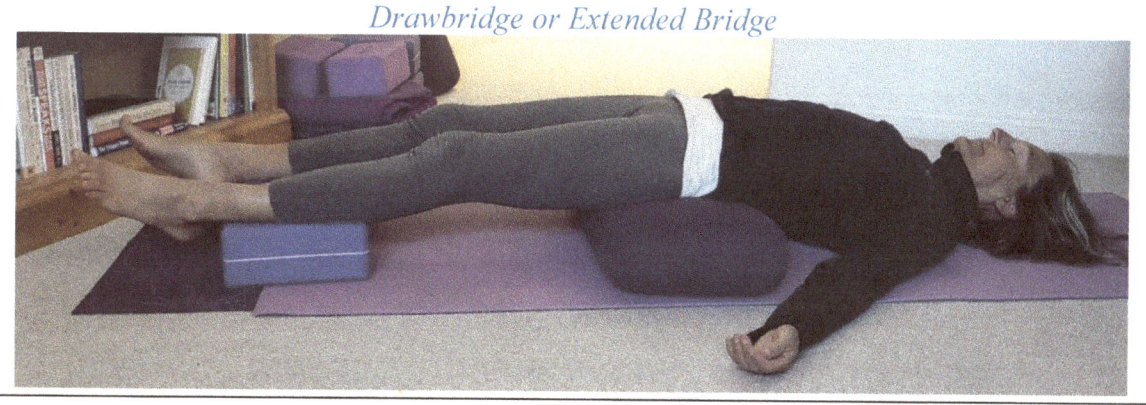
*Drawbridge or Extended Bridge*

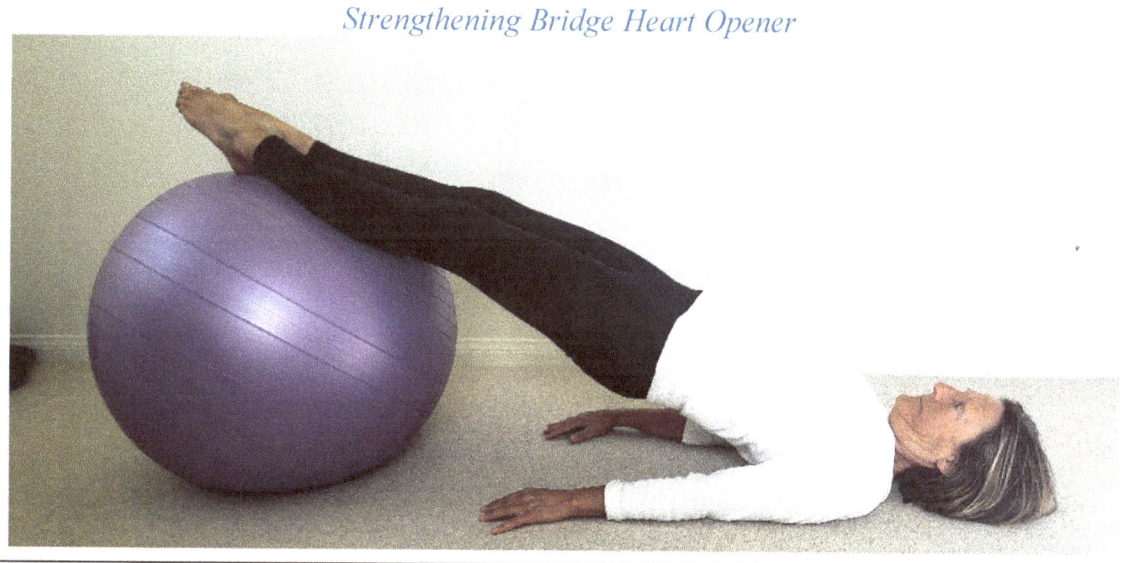
*Strengthening Bridge Heart Opener*

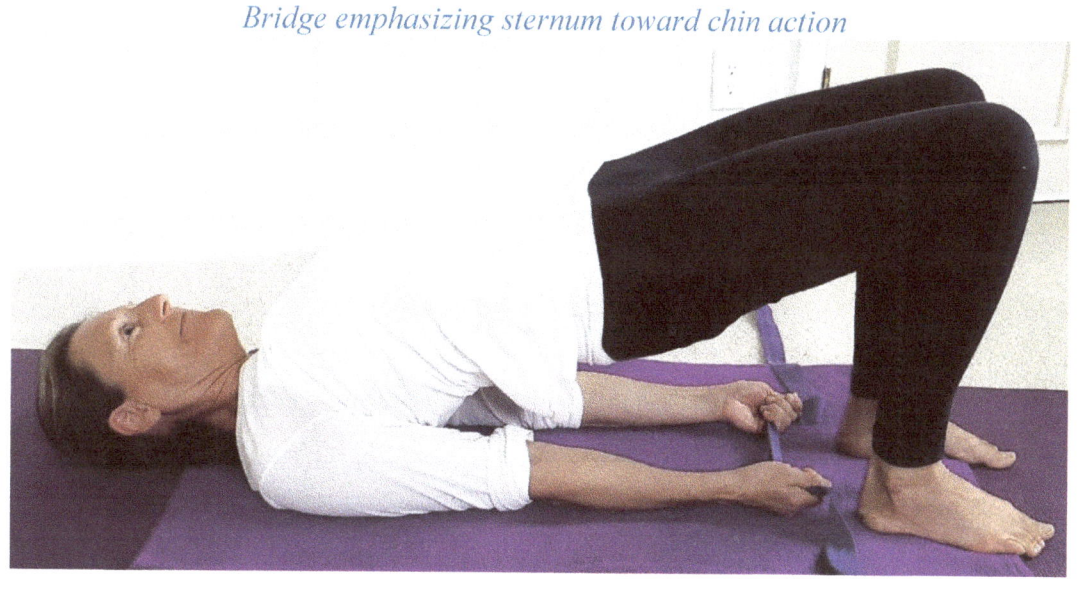
*Bridge emphasizing sternum toward chin action*

***Yama** and **niyama** (the ethical code) assist us in this reasoned restraint, acting as a firebreak for our behavior.*
***Asana** is a cleansing agent and **pranayama** begins to tug out consciousness (citta) away from desires and toward judicious awareness (prajna).*
***Pratyahara** is the stage at which we learn to reverse the current that flows from mind to senses, so that mind can bend its energies inward.*
***Dharana** (concentration) brings purity to intelligence (buddhi), and **dhyana** (meditation) expunges the stains of ego.*
B.K.S. Iyengar, 2005, Light on Life, p. 176

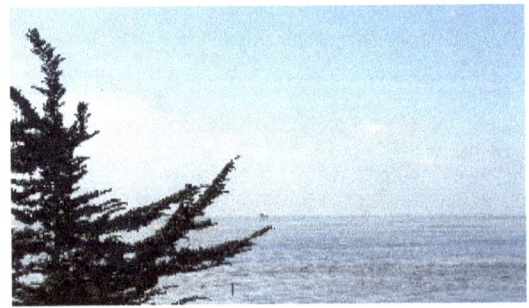

## Chapter 14: Inversions and Partial Inversions

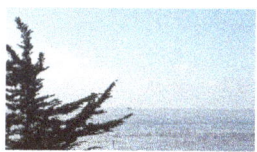

This chapter covers foundational inversions and partial inversions, offering optimized teaching strategies that allow for individual tailoring and careful discernment about how and which shapes to offer, as well as how to cue alignment informed by interoception, proprioception, exteroception, and neuroception. General principles for this category of yoga *asana* are provided and apply to most if not all upside-down shapes. Specific follow-up guidance is added for the chosen sample shapes.

### Helpful Anatomical Foci by Type of Inversion

Anatomically, inversions tend to arise out of other categories of shapes (i.e., heart openers, forward folds, arm standing). Thus, preparations for the respective anatomical practice of origin (so to speak) can guide sequencing that leads to an inversion. This sequencing rule for anatomical preparations is also true for vital and mental preparation to some degree. However, movement into an inversion requires additional careful preparation of the psyche, addressing common fears, emotions, and mental associations with going upside down.

Somewhat simplistically put, origins for various inversions can be conceptualized and understood as follows:
- Handstand can be sequenced successfully to arise from arm standing or core stability practices and also involves some of the principles that support forward folding.
- Headstand tends to arise auspiciously from a forward folding practice (informed by proper preparation with attention to core engagement, balance, and concentrated focus).
- Candlestick Shoulderstand can helpfully evolve from heart-opening practices and can become an integral part of a restorative practice. Core engagement preparation is also ideally integrated to support steadiness and ease in the shape.
- Regular Shoulderstand tends to arise from a combination of forward folding and heart opening and is a very demanding shape. Only highly propped versions of Shoulderstand are recommended for most students and in any setting that brings more vulnerable individuals to the yoga practice (e.g., in healthcare). It is not recommended as a standard practice as it has a poor risk-benefit ratio.

In other words, for each chosen inversion, sequencing, preparation, and cool-down (recovery) is dependent on how the shape is perceived biomechanically, how it blends into the overall class sequence, how psychological and anatomical intentions are framed, and how the shape is allowed to unfold. Inversions need to be taught with clarity about the demands on and reverberations into all layers of experience. However, while they require discernment and care in teaching, they are highly useful practices, especially from a psychological perspective. They increase self-efficacy and can be very empowering. To teach them, it is important to heed the following advice:

- Have a clear intention for the practice and inversion that serves as the peak; then sequence accordingly
- Develop tailored and relevant anatomical and psychological foci within the relevant shape category(ies) that apply to the correlated specific inversions

> **Special Anatomical Note about Inversions**
>
> Inversions are great for the organs and spine. Because the organs are attached to the spine, when you turn upside down, they tug on the spine, and blood and lymph move differently through the organs, with increased cardiac return. This allows the heart to slow and rest.
>
> What does not happen in inversions is greater (i.e., more voluminous) blood flow to the brain. Blood volume that flows to the brain is carefully controlled: there is always about 750 ml of blood in the brain. Being upside down does not change this absolute volume of blood in the brain at a single moment. While the face might get red, the brain will have the same amount of blood as always:
> - If the brain had more blood in it, you would have a horrible headache.
> - If it the brain had less blood in it, you would faint.

| | *Tips for Grounding, Expansion, and Stability in Inversions and Half Inversions* |
|---|---|
| Grounding | <ul><li>Ground through the hands, protecting the wrists</li><li>Ground into integrated shoulder blades</li><li>Ground into the back body if supine</li><li>Ground via the exhalation</li><li>Find a focal point or *drishti*</li></ul> |
| Stability | <ul><li>Engage the core and the perineum</li><li>Draw the low ribs to the anterior superior iliac spine</li><li>Draw navel in and up</li><li>Use *mula bandha*</li><li>Use *uddiyana bandha*</li><li>Use *jalandahara bandha* – first flex cervical spine (lowering chin); then draw chin back; or use manubrium maneuver, drawing chest to chin</li><li>Stabilize breath and mind</li><li>Find a focal point or *drishti*</li></ul> |
| Expansion | <ul><li>Once upside down, regain and maintain the natural curves in the spine</li><li>Lengthen through the spine</li><li>Expand via the inhalation</li><li>Expand energetically</li><li>Create a sense of lightness and upward movement with the breath</li><li>Expand your perspective in the full inversion – the symbolism of looking at the world upside down</li></ul> |

## Analysis and Experience of Sample Inversions

The following inversions are analyzed in detail below:
- *Handstand and Half Handstand*
- *Headless Handstands*
- *Candlestick and Supported Lifted Bridge*

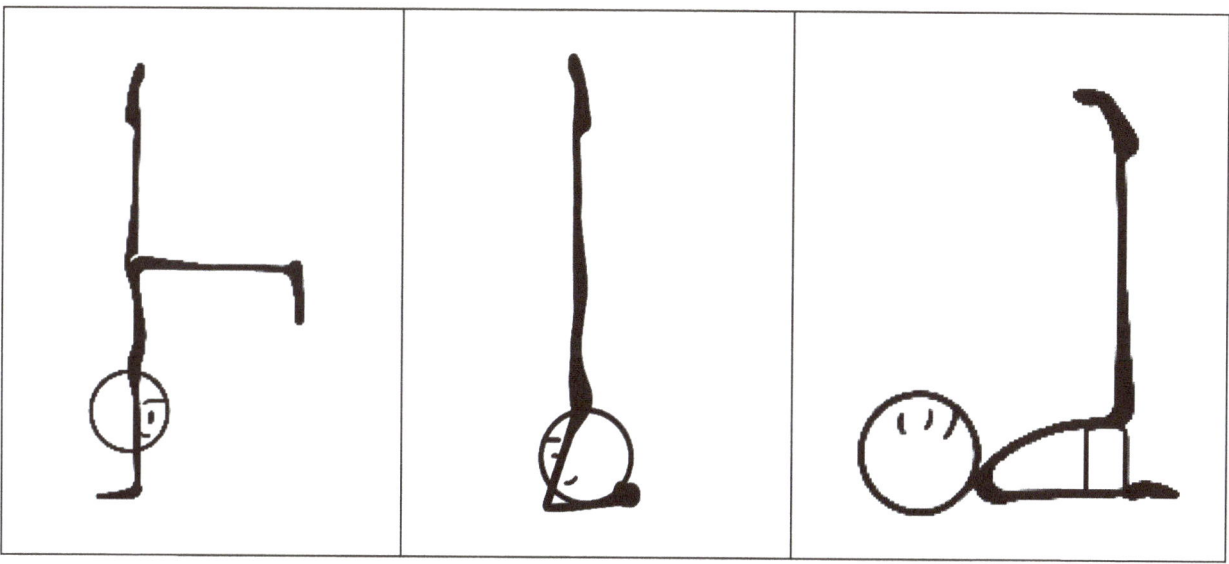

Cueing guidance offered for each covered inversion needs to be considered in the context offered in the general concepts of sequencing offered above and in Volume 1 of the Series. The basics discussed related to the emergence of inversions from specific categories of *asana* need to permeate the cueing for all inverted shapes as relevant. Additional cueing, shape by shape, offered below is icing on the cake. Always integrate integrated holistic yoga cueing that addresses the following teaching principles:
- *Accessibility* – creating access through variation, adaptation, affiliation, individualization, and person-centeredness
- *Intentionality* – embedding the practice of each inversion in the overall arc of the session, with grounding in the theme for the class and the meaning of the practice
- *Beneficence* – honoring the wellbeing of each student and always making sure to first do no harm
- *Holism* – cueing all *koshas* or layers of experience in all shapes, never forgetting that each shape has reverberations into and is affected by all *koshas* – it is not enough to cue anatomy; also address energy and vitality, thoughts and emotions, behavioral and action choices, even community and interbeing
- *Integration* – even in teaching *asana*, integrate breathwork, concentration and mindfulness, as well as the ethical principles and lifestyle practices of yoga

## General Concepts about Inversions

Many aspects of inversions hold constant across several of the dimensions covered for individual *asanas* in this category. Thus, following are general comments about benefits, cautions, preparations, and recovery as applicable to all covered inverted or upside-down shapes. After this general discussion, instructions are provided for five individual inversions (in three categories), providing key alignment cues, variations, and additional teaching tips for each.

### Benefits

Inversions invite a harmonious balance between effort and ease, building physical strength, energetic vitality, mental clarity, and emotional resilience. Through inversions, practitioners can experience a shift in perspective and nervous system regulation, enhancing vitality and emotional responsivity. By shifting the body's orientation and reversing blood and lymphatic flow, inversions such as Headstand, Candlestick Shoulderstand, and Handstand offer unique opportunities for creating balance, strength, and focus. Inversions integrate stability, grounding, and expansiveness, inviting students to cultivate confidence, engagement, agency, and equanimity. Following is a listing of specific benefits that may arise from incorporating inversions into a yoga practice.

- *Boost circulation and revitalize blood flow*: Inversions encourage increased circulation by reversing the effects of gravity, helping blood flow to the heart and brain more efficiently. This can promote oxygenation of the cells, reduce fluid buildup in the lower extremities, and stimulate the lymphatic system, supporting overall detoxification and revitalization.
- *Strengthen the core and upper body*: Shapes like Headstand and Handstand require substantial core engagement and shoulder stability. This activation builds essential strength in the core, arms, shoulders, and back, providing stability and control needed to safely balance upside down. Regular practice of inversions enhances muscular endurance and balance, as well as power across the upper body.
- *Improve balance and focus*: Balancing in an inverted position requires focus and steady awareness. Inversions cultivate concentration, body awareness, and patience, and can enhance mental clarity and focus on and off the mat. Sustained attention promotes a meditative state, inviting mindfulness into the practice.
- *Stimulate the nervous system and relieve stress*: Inversions have a calming effect on the nervous system, particularly Shoulderstand, which gently stimulates the parasympathetic nervous system. Inversions support relaxation and can help reduce stress, anxiety, and mental fatigue. By inviting students to access emotional and nervous system regulation, inversions support a sense of calm and balance.
- *Enhance spine health and decompress joints*: With proper alignment, inversions elongate the spine, relieving pressure on the vertebrae, and building structural support for spinal health by strengthening the surrounding musculature and connective tissue.
- *Build confidence and courage*: Attempting inversions challenges practitioners to overcome fear and develop trust in their own strength and agency. Inversions foster resilience and courage, encouraging practitioners to approach challenges with curiosity and openness, as they push beyond their comfort zones anatomically, energetically, and psychologically. Inversions create self-efficacy and boost self-confidence.

- *Cultivate mindfulness and presence:* The focus and alignment required for inversions naturally invite students to remain grounded in the present moment. By attuning to breath, balance, and sensations, students access mindfulness, attentiveness, and the four 'ceptions.

## Cautions and Contraindications

Inversions are either to be used with great caution or not recommended if any of the below-listed conditions are present. Proceeding with care is essential; medical clearance may be required. Involve students in the decision-making process about whether to proceed but exert your responsibility for their health and safety if you have reservations about their choices. Voice your concern if you have it – in the end, not only do you need to consider the wellbeing of your students, but you also need to protect your own safety as a teacher, physically and legally. Exercise caution and care if students present with the following issues:

- Pregnancy, especially if new to inversions – highly experienced pregnant yogis may continue for a while into pregnancy
- Closer than 12 weeks post-partum
- Glaucoma, retinal detachment, vitreous detachment (with great caution only on the latter, if the individual is an experienced yogi); medical clearance is encouraged
- Hypertension (if successfully treated, inversions may be offered with caution to an experienced yogi) and other heart conditions; students need to have medical clearance
- Arthritis, osteoporosis, or other challenges in all regions of the spine
- Asthma or respiratory issues that may be aggravated by the change in gravitational pull or by the psychological demand of going upside down
- Gastroesophageal reflux
- Recent surgery, injury, or significant accident (especially if involving whiplash)
- Lack of yoga experience, especially if self-taught and/or if combined with weak core stabilization and/or limited range of motion, limited stability, and lack of strength
- Anxiety, fear of falling, and similar psychological issues can present challenges but are not in and of themselves contraindications – work with caution and in a stepwise fashion
- Neck and spinal issues can be strong contraindications if inversions are taught with weight-bearing on the head or neck (this is not promoted here); see special notes about how to teach Headless Headstand and adapted versions of Shoulderstand

## Preparations and Recovery

As noted above, inversions are embedded in a larger, carefully sequenced practice that integrates the inversion in an intentional and meaningful way, anatomically and psychologically. Preparations and recovery are sequenced as described in the category of shapes that are most relevant to the particular inversion that is chosen. For example, if Headless Headstand is to be taught within a sequence, preparations and recovery sequences would be determined by the forward folding and core stabilization of the practice overall. Inversions are not taught in isolation of other types of shapes – they are always embedded in a greater physical, energetic, and psychological preparation and recovery.

General guidelines about how to prepare for inversions attend to anatomy, breath, and emotional or mental state. They include, but are not limited to, the following teaching principles:
- Offer proper anatomical, energetic, mental, and psychological warm-up
- Use gradual progressions into inversions, offering successive approximations
- Cultivate core strength, shoulder stability, and balance
- Make ample use of props and adaptations, including walls, partners, headstanders, and psychological support
- Integrate wholesome breathing practices that support nervous system regulation and emotional equanimity
- Invite a growth mindset that helps with allaying fears and anxieties related to going upside down; also invite a mindset of curiosity and playfulness that is less focused on a particular outcome and more so on a joyful journey
- Integrate mindfulness, interoception, proprioception, and neuroception to prepare the student's nervous system in a manner that maximizes activation of the parasympathetic branch of the nervous system and keen attention
- Remind clients to be patient about accessing a particular outer shape, focusing instead on inner preparation and willingness to explore steps toward inversions without necessarily going all the way upside down – working with imagination can be very beneficial

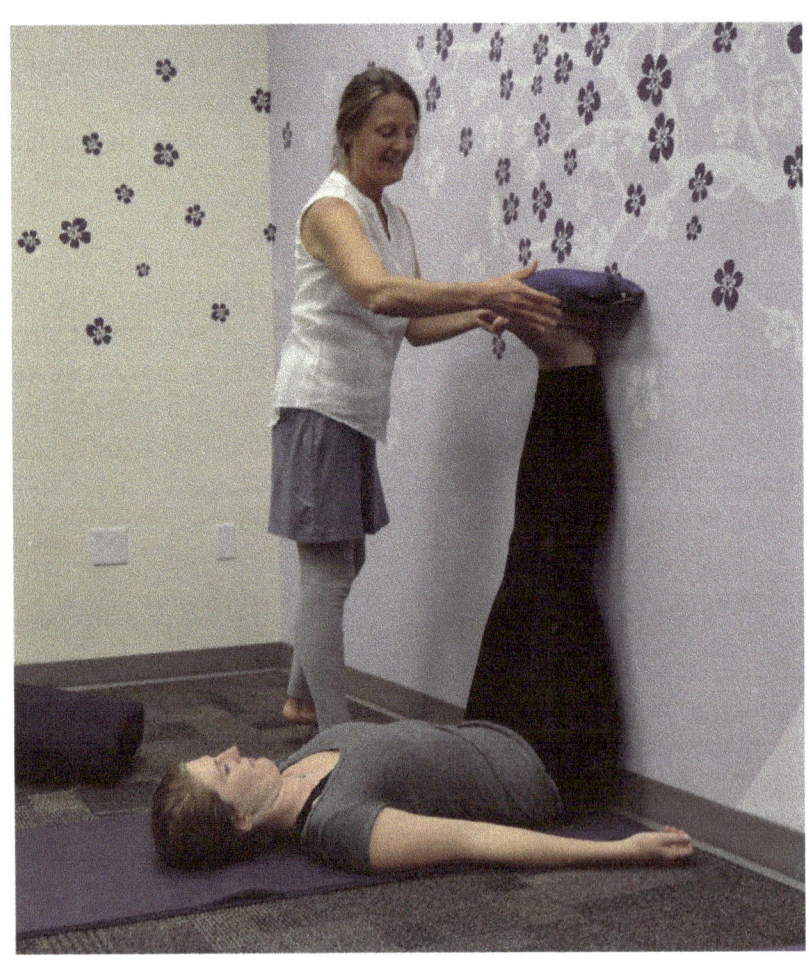

## *Handstand and Half Handstand*

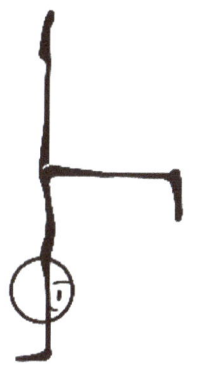

Handstand, ¾ Handstand, and Half Handstand are inversions that arise from arm standing, with forward folding alignment and engagement principles sprinkled in, as well as core stabilization and engagement. Thus, it is important to review and apply the teaching principles and guidance for all of these shapes and related preparations, alignment principles, cueing suggestions, and directional movements. Once adequate strength and interoceptive, proprioceptive, and neuroceptive awareness have been developed, it is often the emotional aspect of inversions that hold clients back from going upside down. Attending to the psychology of clients and students is as important as attending to the physical and vital layers of experience.

### *General Alignment Guidance for All Handstands*

Teaching and practicing Handstand safely requires more than strength and courage in all phases of the shape – from entering into the shape, holding stable in the shape, and exiting. It depends on cultivating wise and compassionate movement, integrated alignment, and refined proprioceptive awareness. While pathways into the shape vary with bioindividual and psychological factors of each student, certain anatomical principles form a crucial foundation for healthy alignment, in the approach to all variations of Handstand and in their maintenance.

#### *Optimizing Scapular Stabilization*

A functional and stable Handstand relies, of course, on many variables from the tips of the fingers to the tips of the toes. However, a key beginning in understanding this shape begins at the scapulae. The scapulothoracic junction, the functional articulation between the scapulae and rib basket, provides the dynamic yet stable platform from which the arms extend overhead and stabilize. The central work here involves balancing scapular depression and retraction, with strength arising from coordinated activity between the lower trapezius, rhomboids, and serratus anterior. Review of the following two anatomical principles in Section 1 may be helpful:
- Pectoralis minor (with its origins on ribs 3–5 and insertion on the coracoid process) acts in scapular protraction and depression, in balance with the trapezius muscles on the back. If balance between pectoralis minor and trapezius muscles is not available, access to scapular stability can be limited. This may occur, for example, if pectoralis minor is tight or shortened (i.e., less than resilient), as may be the case with individuals with tight anterior bodies (e.g., due to habitual forward hunching). Strength and resilience are needed in both sets of muscles for healthful scapular integration.
- Additionally, the rhomboids on the back and serratus anterior wrapping around the side body to the front, collaborate to help glide the scapulae downward and medially, an essential movement for controlled elevation of the arms without winging in the scapulae or collapsing at the base of the neck.

The scapulae must be *firmly anchored* without *rigidity*, allowing for the uplift and breathability necessary to invert without strain. This is facilitated by maintaining an open heart space, namely, unrestricted clavipectoral fascia and chest wall muscles that are resilient enough to allow the scapulae to move and stabilize appropriately. Pectoralis major and minor, when supple, allow the humeri to adduct, bringing power and grounding into the glenohumeral joint, as well as yielding to the back muscles so the scapulae can retract and depress.

### *Facilitating Mobility and Stability in the Glenohumeral Joint*

Once scapular stability is established, the glenohumeral joint (the ball-and-socket articulation between the humerus and the scapula) must allow for full shoulder flexion (i.e., moving the arms overhead). This mobility, however, requires active stabilization of the shoulder girdle as a whole, scapular placement on the back body, and grounding of the humeri in the glenoid fossae. The glenohumeral joint is most inherently stable in extension, internal rotation, and adduction (e.g., as occurs naturally in closed-chain alignments of the arms such as in *Chaturanga*). However, in Handstand, the arms are in end-range flexion and perhaps slightly abducted, which decreases joint congruence. To counter instability, internal rotation and isometric adduction of the upper arms are encouraged at end range of shoulder joint flexion to protect the joint capsule and surrounding tissues.

- Cueing internal rotation (without overdoing it) creates a muscular "hug" around the joint, activating stabilizers like the subscapularis and engaging latissimus dorsi, teres major, and pectoralis major.
- Arm standing principles, like those used in Plank and Downward Facing Dog, prepare the shoulder complex by training co-contraction between deltoids, rotator cuff muscles, and triceps.

### *Creating Integration in the Arms and Hands*

A healthful and strong Handstand relies on fully integrated arms. This integration begins at the hands and wrists, travels through elbows, and completes at the shoulder girdle. Strong and reliable elbow extension is essential for structural integrity and load transmission through the hands, wrists, and arms into the shoulder gridle and its precarious connection to the axial skeleton and clavicles. Fully extended elbows engage all three heads of the triceps brachii, especially when the wrists are pronated (palms flat, thumbs pointing inward). Supination, by contrast, limits full triceps recruitment and can compromise balance. Neck extension (moderate) can greatly support access to elbow extension through the primitive extensor reflex that is so key to human development toward upright, bipedal walking and movement. This extensor reflex is the mechanism that supports infants to move upright when they are learning to lift their heads in a prone position. Specifically, when an infant lies on the belly and wants to look up to another human being or at the world, neck extension has to be learned. When the neck extends in this way, the arms reflexively straighten (via elbow extension). This reflex can be used to significant advantage by cueing students to *extend the neck slightly* – which, given the starting position for Handstand (in a half inversion – more about this below), means looking at the ground, rather than dropping the head and looking into the room. This deliberate neck extension to trigger the extensor reflex is natural and not forced; in other words, it is not an overextension of the cervical spine and does not cause any cervical compression. Once balance is achieved in the full inversion, a gentle softening at the base of the neck can relieve unnecessary effort.

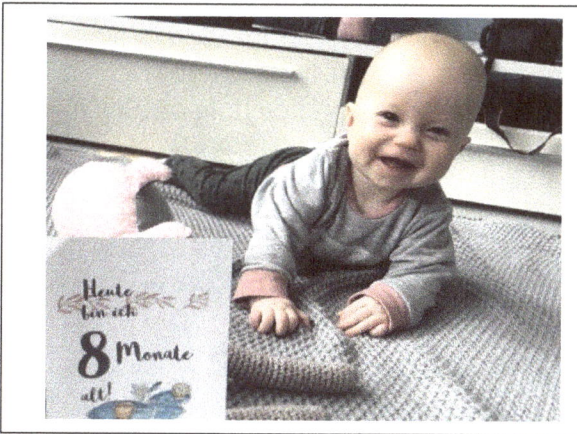

Pronate the wrist →
Extend the elbow →
Extend the neck

Use this developmental trick for handstand ☺

The final aspect that can support the extensor reflex is wrist pronation, which means stability can be further enhanced through attention to distribution of load through the hands. Pressing down through the thumb and index finger mounds (inner edge of the palm or *hasta bandha*) pronates the wrists and further contributes to the extensor reflex. This action also distributes load away from being concentrated at the wrist creases, and enhances proprioception through mechanoreceptors in the hand. Creating a hand arch (similar to the medial arch of the foot) by gently drawing the finger pads toward the palm's center, further balances muscular tone in hands, wrists, and arms and thus contributes steadiness to the base for Handstand.

### *Optimizing Hand Placement and Chest Freedom*

The width of hand placement can greatly influence openness and strength of the chest wall. If the hands are too narrow, the clavicles crowd and restrict the breath and may limit upper back mobility; if the hands are too wide apart, adduction strength may be lost. A functional method for determining ideal width is to reach both arms forward to ground them strongly into the earth (e.g., from Table Top); then engage in a few movements of shoulder flossing (dropping the sternum toward the floor and back up to mobilize the glenohumeral joint). In this motion, observe clavicular alignment and inner sensation connected to the movement:
- If the clavicles or chest feel tight or restricted, widen the hands slightly (more width in the stance)
- If these regions feel slack or unintegrated, bring the hands closer toward each other (less width in the stance)

The goal is a position in which the chest feels *open <u>and</u> capable of engagement*. This supports pectoral activation for humeral adduction, which in turn enhances shoulder girdle integrity in the inverted position.

### *Utilizing Props, Progressions, and Practical Tools*

There is tremendous value to using props intelligently to support Handstand. A blanket or wedge under the hands can reduce wrist strain, especially for beginners or individuals with limited wrist dorsiflexion or shoulder joints with restricted range of motion (see measurement for hand placement in Half Handstand below). Practicing Handstand by a wall, with a bolster, or with partner support can help reinforce neuromuscular pathways without overloading the nervous system. Such external supports are particularly useful for clients who have subtle (even strong) psychological fears of going upside down; they will not, however, make up for lacking strength and integration. Additionally, for clients with hesitations about Handstand, teaching Half Handstand (with hips over shoulders and feet on wall) or ¾ Handstand (stretching one leg up toward the ceiling from Half Handstand) can build familiarity and safety.

### Summarizing the Key Anatomical Principles at Hand

- Heart opening is literal: fascial freedom and structural balance across the anterior chest enables shoulder function and healthful breathing in Handstand
- Scapular intelligence is primary: create stability through muscular coordination, not rigidity
- Glenohumeral support comes from internal rotation and adduction at end-range flexion
- Hands and arms must function as an integrated chain, leveraging reflexive and developmental patterns that integrate elbow extension, neck extension, and wrist pronation
- Props and progressive stages help support psychological competence and confidence

## Alignments and Movements for the Base and Moving Upside Down

As noted, it can be psychologically and emotionally supportive to progress toward a full Handstand in stages and with props. Offering a wall for Handstands is extremely helpful and necessary for most students, especially in healthcare settings. Starting with the feet at the wall, Half or ¾ Handstand, for more weight distribution and nervous system regulation is a great way to introduce Handstand.

### Half and ¾ Handstand: Creating a Base and Lifting Up

These two Handstand variations require all of the foundational principles noted above as well as the most auspicious distance of the hands from the wall, where the feet will rest and that will be used to support the process of moving upside down while remaining stable in the inversion. Thus, the first step in the process is to measure the optimal distance for the hands to be away from the wall by sitting in Staff with the back at the wall:
- Lift both arms overhead (externally rotating the glenohumeral joint on the way up)
- Pronate the wrist (while extended) and notice if the backs of the hands can reach the wall while the wrist is straight (extended)
- If not, scoot the pelvis away from the wall until the whole back of both hands can comfortably rest on the wall; mark this spot on the mat
- Your hands will go to where your heel prints are at the moment when the whole back of both hands can comfortably rest the wall
- Using this method for hand placement in Half Handstand optimizes the distance for the range of motion in the glenohumeral joint. A less movable joint will result in a slightly longer distance to the wall – this personalized adjustment will create greater ease and stability
- Many students have a hard time trusting this measurement and end up too far away from the wall; excess distance from the wall compromises core stability in the shape – measure

carefully and support students in the optimal distance determination – encourage them to trust this measurement
- Place the hands where the heelprint was; move into Downward Facing Dog with the heels against the wall
- Walk one foot up the wall to land at approximately hip height once upside down; then step the second foot to join the first once both feet are planted at the auspicious height (see photo), find stability in the shoulders using all principles that were already explained above for arm standing
- If desired reach one foot toward the ceiling to move into ¾ Handstand

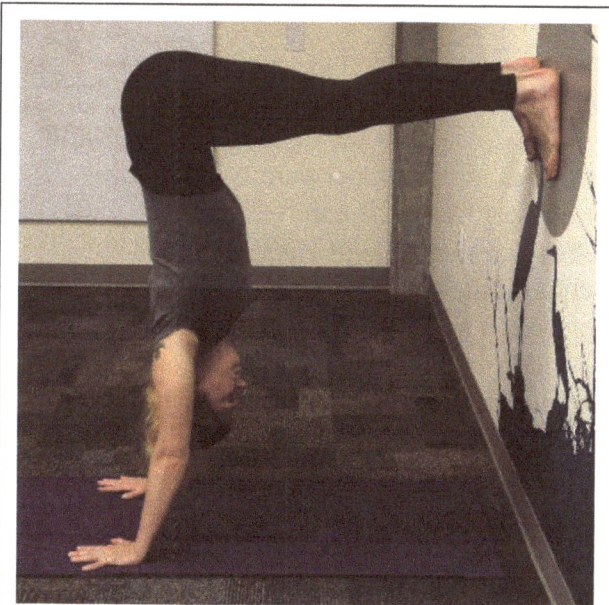

↑ *Half Handstand*

-------------------------------

*3/4 Handstand →*
*with one leg extended*

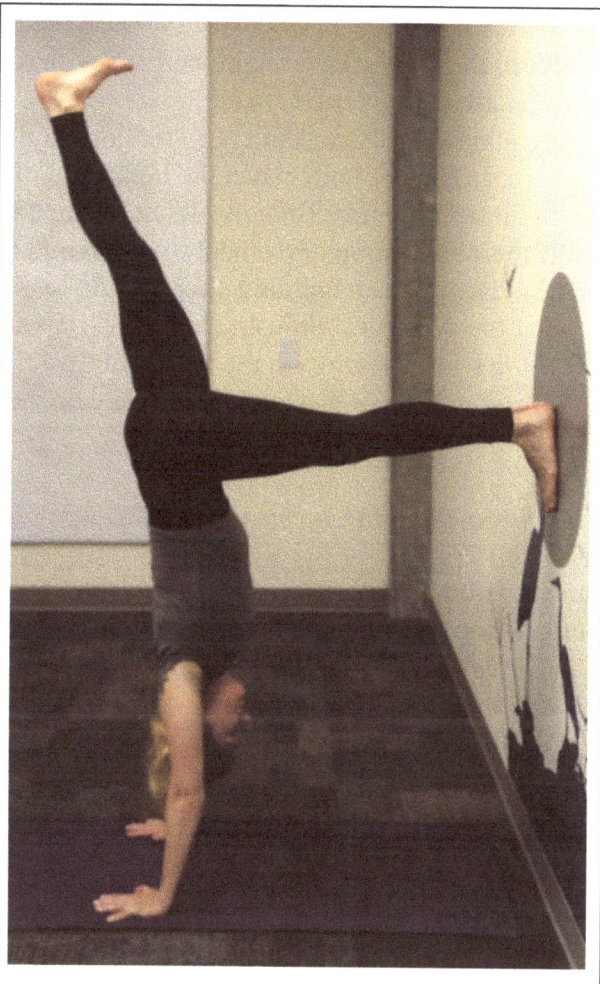

*Handstand: Creating a Base and Kicking Up*

For Handstand, when using the wall as a backdrop for psychological support, the distance from the wall is important but slightly more difficult to determine. As a general rule of thumbs, place the hands about 6 to 12 inches from the wall (with the back facing the wall; feet into the room). Often it is not clear whether the chosen distance was auspicious until the client starts kicking up; it is important to stay observant and adjust the distance from the wall with a curious spirit. From

the initial hand placement, move into Downward Facing Dog and find stability and presence in this preparatory shape and starting position. Then proceed as follows:
- Walk the feet toward the hands to move the shoulders closer to being aligned above the wrists; try to align hips toward being stacked above the shoulder – the closer and higher you can bring the hips, the higher your center of gravity and the easier the kick-up
- Step one foot forward (whichever one automatically wants to take the first step); feel the core engage naturally as you move toward the water pump shape that will allow the back leg to swing up
- Use several water pump preps to determine which leg is dominant and start the work with the naturally forward moving leg as the push leg (once Handstand come easily, it is fine to switch it up) – remember that the push leg does the work
- Keep the swing leg straight, perhaps with toes pointed and allow it to gain momentum upward and toward the wall
- Readiness for Handstand (i.e., for going fully upside down, past the water pump motion) is signaled by the body when the hips feel light while kicking in water pump; finding this lightness may necessitate walking the hips ever closer toward the hands
- If the water pump movement feels labored and heavy, practice Half Handstand and ¾ Handstand; keep building strength and resilience until the water pump movement feel light and the swing leg almost naturally swings up toward the wall and the push leg follows
- If the legs or feet reach the wall, stabilize the shoulders and core and try to remove the feet from the wall so that you stand freely on your hands; the wall is a security measure, not a resting place

*Alignments and Movements for Stabilization Once Upside Down*

Stabilization has been described elsewhere, but a few brief instructions are repeated here. This guidance applies to all versions of Handstand.
- *Core engagement/stabilization*: the core is stabilized, with pelvic floor and umbilicus drawing in but not clamping down (balance between effort and ease to allow for a sweet breath); envision low ribs drawing toward the tops of the hips (i.e., toward the anterior superior iliac spine, or ASIS)
- *Natural spine with open heart*: once upside down, beware of a banana-shaped (unstable) spine and avoid collapsed/rounded shoulders; a bolster as a prop at the wall to support the shoulders and upper back may help until strength and proprioception in the shoulders has been built sufficiently; however, do not sacrifice core engagement and shoulder stabilization if using a bolster
- *Vertical and adducted humerus with extended elbows and pronated wrists*: do not let the elbows jut out to the side – keep them extended (extend the neck); keep the humeri vertical under the glenoid – continue to create a motion that triggers adductors and internal rotators; strong pectoralis muscles are key to this adduction; keep the heart space open and stable; keep pronating the forearms and wrists and pressing into *hasta bandha*; engage slight neck extension if stability wavers

Once ready to come down, descend gently, trying to touch down the feet without sound. This requires core strength and control. Rest in Child for a few moments to prevent orthostatic hypotension. Rise when ready. Repeat if desired.

## Headless Headstands

There are two versions of Headstand – 'regular' Headstand (*Sirsasana 1*) and Tripod Headstand (*Sirsasana 2*). Regular Headstand (traditionally) is based on a triangular base of the arms, resting the load of the shapes on the two forearms and the head. Tripod Headstand arises (traditionally) from a 3-point base: the two hands and the head. However, the versions of Headstand offered here are a bit different in that *neither version brings any weight-bearing onto the head or neck*. Both are offered in variations that do not load the head or neck, in adaptations that lift the head off the ground and place the load on a base that is entirely grounded in the arms and shoulder girdle. Somewhat confusingly, the versions offered here create a *triangular* base for regular Headstand and a *rectangular* base of Tripod Headstand. Many alignment principles and much cueing overlaps both versions of Headstand; however, several key distinctions are made in hand placement, movement into the shape, and stabilization of load bearing. The overlapping principles are covered first; then distinctive features related to the respective bases are discussed separately for each version of Headless Headstand.

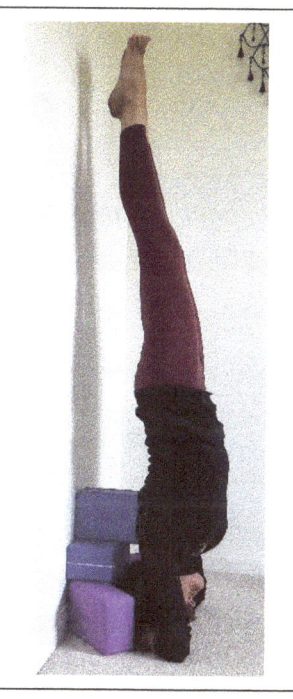

### What is Headless Headstand?

**The head is free floating in all upside-down Headstand shapes** that are recommended to be taught to the vast majority of students. That is, there is no weight-bearing on the neck and head.

### Why Teach Only Headless Headstand?
This alignment takes the risk to the neck out of the shape. The neck is not weight-bearing; the shoulder girdle is.

### How Is Headless Headstand Taught?
For ground-based Headstands, the head is lifted ever so slightly off the ground – enough that someone would be able to slide a piece of paper underneath the head.

Even more auspiciously, choose Tripod Headstand on a headstander or on two chairs. In these Headstands, head and neck hang freely; the weight is born by the shoulders.

### Key Alignment Invitations Shared by Headstand and Tripod Headstands

Headstands arise from arm-standing shapes, forward folding shapes, heart-opening and back-strengthening movements, with lots of core stability principles sprinkled in. It is therefore key to review teaching principles for these types of shapes and core stabilization practices before teaching Headstands.

Review and have clarity about all of the following central themes; refer back to prior chapters and relevant anatomy section as necessary. Most, if not all, of the anatomical and kinesiological guidance for Handstand above also applies to all versions of Headstand.

- *Mobilization and activation of the back body with resilience in the front body*: refer back to heart-opening (i.e., backbending) shapes for creating resilience in the front body and strength in the back body
    - hamstrings, calf muscles, quadratus lumborum, and all layers of spinal muscles are invited to become active and engaged – strengthening preparations in these regions are helpful
    - chest muscles are invited into resilience and an openness of heart is cultivated physically and emotionally
- *Resilience in the hamstrings*: refer back to practice principles for forward-folding shapes
    - invite resilience into the hamstrings with preparations that invite strength and suppleness – a variety of options is offered in Chapter 12
- *Core stabilization and the natural curve of the spine*: refer back to relevant sections in the chapters about upright standing and arm-standing shapes
    - offer preparations and cueing that invite engagement of the core with care to maintain healthful breathing as well as adequate engagement without bracing; bringing ease into the effort to create strength at the core (from the inside out) is key and happens not only physically but also psychologically
    - integrate attention to maintaining the natural curves of the spine even as core strength is cultivated; natural curves are maintained from the anterior rotation of the pelvis to the gentle tuck of the chin to help the head draw back, creating a natural lordosis in the cervical spine
- *Shoulder stabilization and activation – focus on the scapulae*: refer back to the pedagogy and practice principles related to arm-standing shapes and Handstand to stabilize the shoulder blades on the back with strong activation of the back muscles and resilience in the front muscles
    - scapular depression and retraction are key to balance and health in Headstand; instability in the scapulae puts neck, head, and upper back at risk
    - rhomboids and serratus anterior need to be strong and in balance with one another to be able to help stabilize the scapula on the back
    - pectoralis minor opposes the action of the lower trapezii to stabilize the shoulders; balance between the lower traps and pectoralis minor is essential to scapular stability
    - mobilized, *yet strong*, pectoralis muscles and resilient clavipectoral fascia (an open heart space) are key to this type of inversion to stabilize the scapulae and have sufficient strength for the necessary adduction of humeri
- *Shoulder mobility and stability – focus on glenohumeral joint*: refer back to arm-standing shapes and Handstand
    - the glenohumeral rhythm supports the necessary full arm flexion and abduction to reach the arms overhead
    - glenohumeral joints are most stable in extension, adduction, and internal rotation; since extension cannot be achieved in Headstand (i.e., in full flexion), it helps at least to invite adduction and internally rotation into the glenohumeral joints (i.e., humeri)
    - once mobilized and at full range (i.e., with arms overhead), stability has to be created in the glenohumeral joint via activation of internal rotation and adduction movements in that joint – isometrically engaging the arms bones toward each other and rotating them internally

*Alignments and Movements for the Base and Moving Upside Down*

Two different bases are used for the two offered variations of Headstand: one arising from the forearms; the other from the hands and shoulders. Preparatory shapes and the best shapes from which to enter the types of Headstand differ significantly.

## *Base and Lift-Up for Headstand*

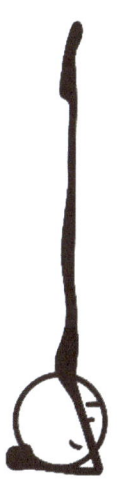

The most auspicious starting shape for regular Headstand is Dolphin, which shares the same base of the forearms. To create this base:
- Interlace the fingers and close the hands; press the bases of the thumbs and index fingers of the right hand to those of the left hand, creating strong isometric engagement to create a movement toward pronation the wrist – this helps fire up the triceps even in elbow flexion and invites internal rotation into the glenohumeral joints (for greater stability here)
- Check the location of the elbows – they are best aligned under the glenoid fossa to keep the upper arm (humerus and all soft tissue) vertical, internally rotated, and adducted; find the optimal placement of the elbows via placing them on the earth slightly narrower than usual; then let them 'scrub out 'on their loose skin; this action will reset the foundation to find elbow alignment under the glenohumeral joints – play with this until optimal placement is achieved
- Press into the ulnae, not the wrists – it is key to press the thumbs together and to lift the pinky finger side of the hands off the ground; this lift of the hands anchors the arms into the ulnae a few inches up the forearm; there is a sweet spot for ulnar grounding that is optimal to weigh-bearing on the forearms and it may take some interoceptive exploration to find it
- The downward pressure of the pronated forearms and wrists activates the triceps, the major elbow extensors – it is essentially an attempt at elbow extension within elbow flexion and creates strong isometric engagement; forearm pronation also stabilizes the glenohumeral joint and the humerus stay vertical, adducted, and internally rotated

In preparation for lifting or kicking up into Headstand, follow the sequence described below. This sequence can be broken down into steps and it is perfectly fine to stop short of going fully upside down. All preparatory steps are just as strengthening and beneficial as the fully inverted shape. It is a good idea to enjoy the process and not get attached to the outcome or the goal. Over time, body, breath, and mind will become ready to embrace the full inversion. It does not have to happen right away.
- Start in Dolphin and engage in a few rounds of Dolphin swimming, that is, begin moving from Dolphin arms in a Downward Facing Dog position to Dolphin arms in a Plank position, repeating this strength-building flow a few times; it is a great preparation for the entire body, especially the shoulder girdle and backs of the legs
- In the next step toward Headstand, move the shoulders closer toward Plank position to align them above the wrists and walk the feet ever closer hands, through and beyond a Downward Facing Dog position of the body

- As the feet come close to the hands, the back of the head presses vigorously into the thumbs; the pushing action of the head against the thumbs creates strong isometric engagement and creates the movement in the neck that activates the extensor reflex (see Handstand above)
- <u>*Let the head float – the head does not touch the ground*</u>; it should be possible to slide a thick piece of cardboard between the head and floor; the weight of the shape is ultimately borne entirely by the arms and shoulder girdle
- Try to walk the legs in close enough toward the hands to align the hips toward being stacked above the shoulders; the closer and higher the hips, the higher the center of gravity and the easier the kick-up or lift-up
- Step one foot forward (whichever one automatically wants to take the first step); feel the core engage naturally
- If you plan to push up both legs at the same time – also step the second foot forward; from here, with hips above shoulders and head floating, lift up (if possible) entirely based on the strength of the core
- Alternatively, keep the swing leg a little farther away from the hand and kick up with the push leg; kick up gently, *but only if the head is floating*: if there is any weight on head and neck, kicking up is not indicated – it is not safe
- Once one or both legs are in the air, stabilize; if both legs are in the air and leaning against the wall, draw them away from the wall – neither the legs nor feet nor any portion of the back body should be resting against the wall (unless using blocks, as discussed below)
- It is key to cultivate enough core stability to access and hold the shape from the inside out, without external support from the wall
- It is perfectly fine to move into ¾ Headstand in which only one leg is lifted up at a time – this variation has all the benefits of bringing both legs into the air (though one at a time) and may present a lovely starting point for anyone who does not yet have the self-efficacy physically or psychologically to lift all the way into the full inverted variation of Headstand

A possible set of wall props that can support a natural spine (preventing kyphosis in the thoracic spine) is shown in the images below. In this set-up, the body and legs are held upright by the strength of the core and proper alignment. The top block of the set-up simply serves to prevent collapse at the more vulnerable junction between the cervical and thoracic spine. It is positioned at such a height (via adjustment of the lower blocks) as to press gently into the upper thoracic (not the cervical) spine. This support is a help for individuals who are able to move upside down and remain stable, but need a safety prompt to prevent collapse in the upper regions of the spine.

| *Proper propping ↭ is crucial: Let Your Head Float. There is no weight on the neck or head. This requires great care in the assembly of the arms, wrists, and hands, as well as skillful use of props that is tailored to individual needs.* | *Set up support at the wall for the thoracic spine for 'regular' Headstand* 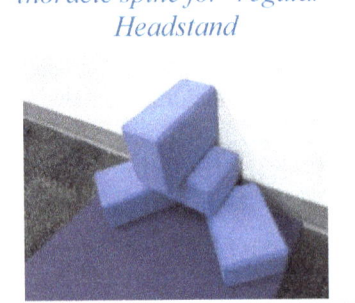 | *Create a foundation for 'regular' Headstand via discerning arm and hand positioning* 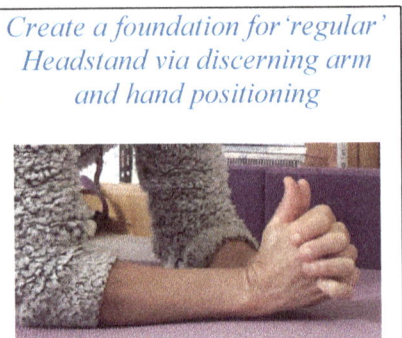 |

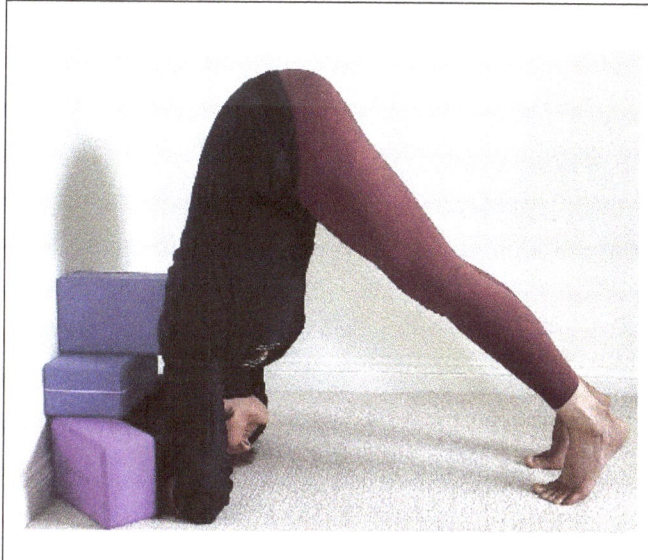
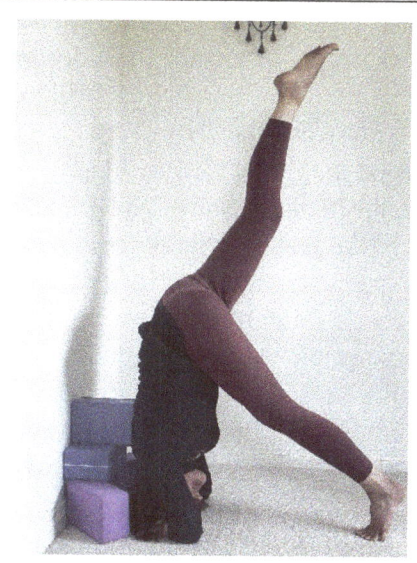

Core engagement and shoulder or base stabilization remain crucial once upside down. Several important principles are helpful:

- Ensure that the head floats and there is no sensation in the neck; the neck should be able to move freely side to side since it is not touching the ground; if this is not the case, come down as gently as possible
- Maintain core engagement/stabilization – the core is stabilized, with pelvic floor and umbilicus drawing in but not clamping down (find balance between effort and ease to allow for a sweet breath); envision the low ribs drawing toward hips
- Maintain a natural spine and open heart – beware of a banana-shaped (unstable) spine and avoid collapsed or rounded shoulders; keep the heart space open and stable; strong pectoralis muscles are key to adduction in the shoulder joints; stabilize the scapulae on the back
- Maintain vertical, internally rotated, and adducted humeri within the glenoid fossa with flexed elbows; do not let the elbows jut out to the side but keep them actively drawing inward toward each other
- Pronate the forearms and wrists and strongly press the floor away to activate the triceps; press the back of the head into the thumbs to further support the extensor reflex
- Rotate the femurs internally such that the balls of the feet might touch; the heels might turn out slightly
- To release, aim to exit in reverse from entry; strive for a soft (inaudible) landing via an engaged core

### *Base and Lift-Up for Tripod Headstand*

The most auspicious starting shape for Tripod Headstand is from a movement from Plank toward *Chaturanga*, which shares the same base of the arms and creates a movement toward a propped foundation for the shoulders. Have adequate props at hand to create a base of support under the shoulders – typically at least two to three blocks (of various heights) under each shoulder. Create the base for the Tripod Headstand as follows:

- Start in Plank and then take a slow approach to move downward into *Chaturanga* with the elbows drawn in toward the sides of the body (strong adduction in the shoulder joints); walk the feet in toward the hands, bringing the hips above the shoulders; from here, measure the height between the shoulders and ground; walk back out and set up the shoulder props to the assessed height needed to support the shoulders to float the head
- Once the props are arranged, once again start in Plank, *Chaturanga*, and then walk the feet toward the hands to stack the hips above the shoulders; place the tops of the shoulders onto their respective stack of blocks (as shown in the images below)
- The hands remain on the grounds with fingers pointing toward the blocks; press into the spaces around the base of the thumbs and index fingers, supporting internal rotation in the glenohumeral joints and a strong foundation on the earth
- The elbows are flexed and arms adducted – moving strongly and actively toward one another
- Release the crown of the head toward the floor and allow the shoulders to roll along – the tops of the shoulders will be on the blocks and the head needs to float; if the head does not float, come down and increase the height of supports until it does
- Feel the square foundation of this base: the load is distributed in the tops of the two shoulders and the palms of the two hands
- To lift up into Tripod Headstand from this aligned position, several options exist, all initiating the movement from the strength of a stable core, engaged hip rotators, and powerful legs with shoulders and arms creating a strong square base:
    - lift the knees onto the backs of the upper arms for a ½ Tripod Headstand (see image below); experiment with floating the knees, eventually perhaps extending the knees fully and coming into the full inversion
    - alternatively, lift into ¾ Tripod Headstand by lifting only one leg toward the sky

If this set-up does not work because the head cannot float, try using a headstander or two chair as shown in the images below. For any of these versions of Tripod Headstand, core stabilization is key once upside down.

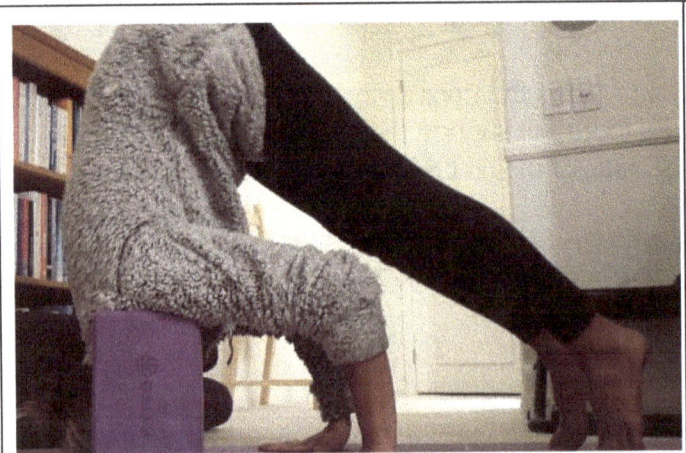 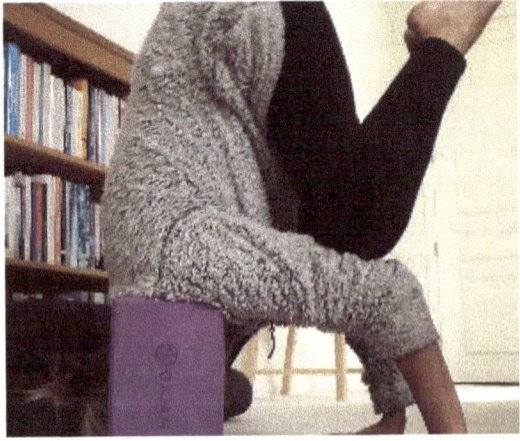

Height of the props under the shoulders is key and needs to be measured and refined with great care. The supports need to be stable and high enough to assure that the head floats, but not so high as to create imbalance or instability

Core, shoulder girdle, and base stabilization remains crucial once upside down. Several important principles are helpful:
- Ensure that the head floats and there is no sensation in the neck; the neck should be able to move freely side to side since it is not touching the ground; if this is not the case, come down as gently as possible
- Maintain core engagement/stabilization – the core is stabilized, with pelvic floor and umbilicus drawing in but not clamping down (find balance between effort and ease to allow for a sweet breath); envision the low ribs drawing toward hips
- Maintain a natural spine and open heart – beware of a banana-shaped (unstable) spine and avoid collapsed or rounded shoulders; keep the heart space open and stable; strong pecs are key to adduction in the shoulder joints
- Maintain vertical, internally rotated, and adducted humeri within the glenoid fossa with flexed elbows; do not let the elbows jut out to the side but keep them actively drawing inward toward each other
- Ground the hands strongly into the earth; stabilize the scapulae on the back
- To release downward, aim to exit in reverse order from how you entered; strive for a soft (inaudible) landing via an engaged core

Another excellent and low-risk options is to take Tripod Headstand off the ground with a headstander or two chairs on a sticky mat and with proper supports under the shoulders.

> *Using a Headstander for Tripod Headstand*
>
> A headstander (aka inversion stool, feet-up trainer, or Headstand bench) is a prop designed to help students practice Tripod Headstand without placing undue pressure on the head or neck. It typically consists of a U-shaped or rectangular wooden or metal frame with a padded support surface for the shoulders and an open space for the head to hang freely. Some versions have a sturdy base with nonslip feet; many come with handles to assist with mounting and dismounting. Use of a Headstander:
> - *Protects the cervical spine*: By removing direct load from the head and neck, it significantly reduces the risk of compression injuries.
> - *Builds strength gradually*: Helps build shoulder and core strength needed for unassisted inversions.
> - *Increases confidence*: Offers a safe way to practice upside-down without fear of falling.
> - *Improves proprioception*: Trains the body to orient itself in inverted space.
>
> To Enter Tripod Headstand
> - Kneel in front of the headstander, placing your hands on the floor or on the prop's sides.
> - Place your shoulders on the padded platform and gently lower your head into the open center so that it hangs freely without touching the floor.
> - Lift your knees onto the platform (or hop lightly from a squat), then slowly straighten the legs upward into a vertical line, using core control.
> - Once balanced, engage the shoulders and core, and breathe slowly.
>
> To Exit Tripod Headstand
> - Slowly lower one leg at a time or both together (if experienced).
> - Bring the knees to the chest and then to the platform.
> - Carefully step or slide down and rest in Child to allow the nervous system to regulate.

### Using a Headstander or Two Chairs for Tripod Headstand

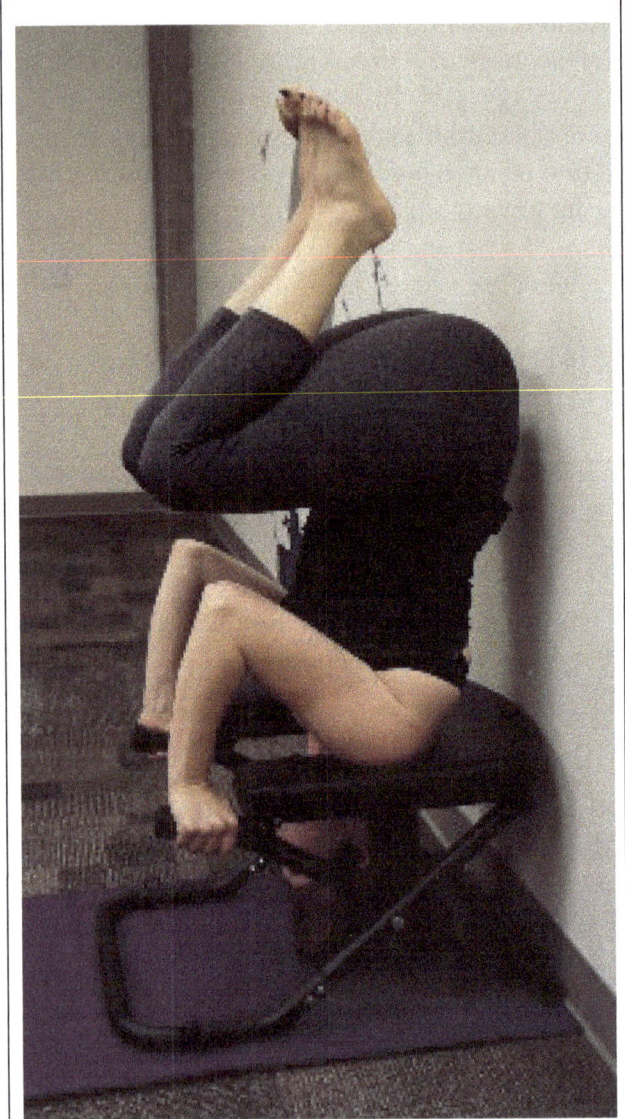 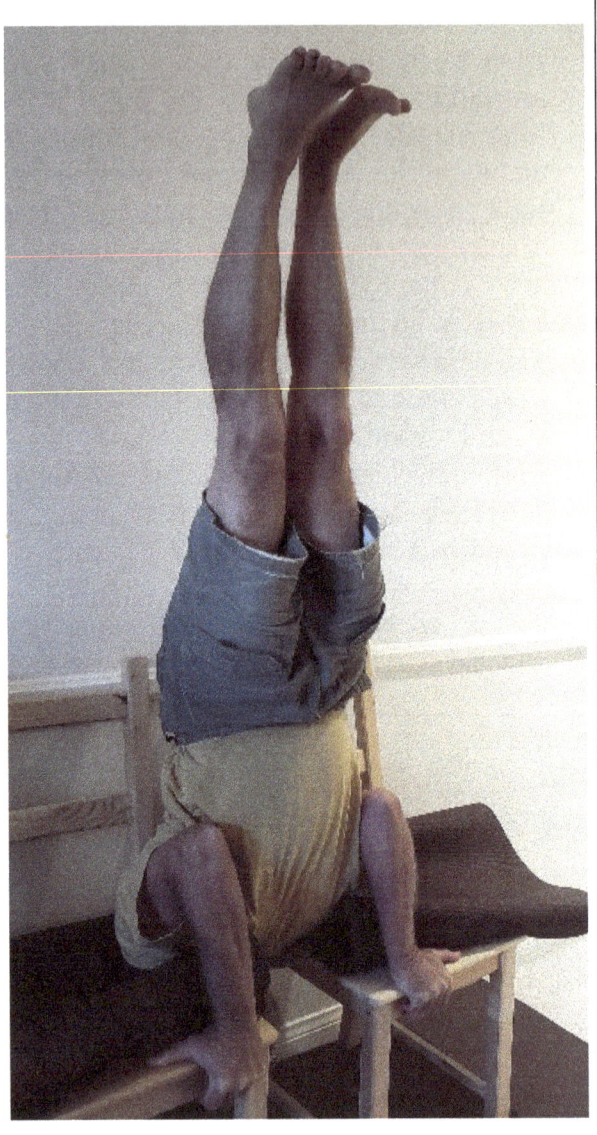

In using a two-chair set-up, make sure to move the head relatively closer to the wall than the front of the chairs. The weight of the body comes to rest at the front of the chairs, there is a danger of the chairs tipping over into the room! This is not a risk worth taking! The distance between the two chairs is such that the head can just move in between them. There needs to be ample space on either side to fully support the shoulders. All the rest is the same as pressing up from the ground or a headstander.

Clients who are new to the practice are typically best served to go up only once or twice. The second entry is helpful if it is judged to be a good reinforcement of the success of the first attempt. A second entry may be avoided if the student is tired and is less likely to encounter success again. Decompress in Child to allow the nervous system to reregulate and to prevent orthostatic hypotension. Stay upside down no more than 3-5 minutes.

## Candlestick Shoulderstand and Supported Lifted Bridge

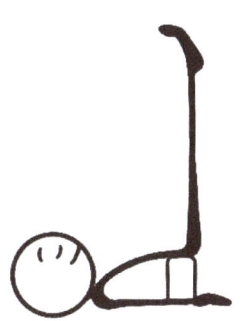

Supported Lifted Bridge and Candlestick Shoulderstand are inversions that arise from or result in a mix of backbends and forward folds. Supported Lifted Bridge (half inversion) and Candlestick (full inversion) are combinations of Forward Folds and Backbends. Thus, it is important to review and understand how to apply the underlying alignment principles, pedagogy, and practice principles for both types of shapes. Core engagement and stability remain key and resilience in the back body is very helpful. The preparation practices offered for arm standing, backbending, and forward folding are helpful in this category of inversions as well.

Other full inversions in this category include Elbow Balance and Shoulderstand. These shapes are not covered in this manual because they are not safely accessible to many individuals. Novice teachers are not ready to teach these shapes until they have a keen understanding of anatomy, physiology, and nervous system (co-)regulation as well as a keen eye for student observation that intelligently support cueing and assistance. Shoulderstand requires meticulous alignment for neck safety and bears great risk. This risk is generally not justified as this shape has little functional movement value in daily life. Further, most benefits that arise from Shoulderstand can be gleaned from excellent alternatives, including Supported Bridge and Candlestick.

Supported Bridge and Candlestick are inverted backbends and shoulder-supported inversions, respectively. Both require careful integration of spinal alignment, shoulder and cervical stability, and pelvic engagement. While Bridge can emphasize either heart opening or back-body activation (or both), Candlestick demands controlled flexion through the thoracic and cervical spine, alongside sophisticated shoulder girdle mechanics. As compared to Shoulderstand, Candlestick removes weight from the cervical spine while still offering many of the circulatory, lymphatic, and nervous system benefits of Shoulderstand. It is an accessible inversion that teaches foundational principles of spinal decompression, core integration, and shoulder girdle awareness. It provides an ideal opportunity to explore the relationship between grounded support and vertical lift, inviting the practitioner to find alignment not through force, but through intelligent engagement. The guidance that follows emphasizes joint positioning, muscular engagement, and fascial continuity, along with suggestions for healthful alignment and movement strategies. Transitioning from Supported Bridge to Candlestick creates a natural progression from extension into supported inversion, making them complementary shapes. This progression offers psychological and physiological readiness.

### Key Alignment Invitations for Bridge and Candlestick

It helps to have clarity about several central themes, hints, and tricks in preparing students or clients for Bridge and Candlestick. Bridge was covered in some detail in the context of heart-opening shapes in Chapter 13. Focus here is on building a stable foundation, promoting spinal mobility, and understanding the intricate balance of strength and flexibility required for Candlestick. The shape arises from a supine position, lying on the back, much as in the traditional shape taken for *Savasana*.

### Managing Load via Sacral Support and Pelvic Lift

In Candlestick, the sacrum rests on a prop, elevating the pelvis above the heart and head. This elevation shifts gravitational load and facilitates drainage from the lower extremities. Anatomically, the lift of the pelvis is engaged as described for Bridge (see Chapter 13) and encourages length and ease through the lumbar spine. Elevating the sacrum reduces the need for lumbar hyperextension to lift the legs toward the ceiling or sky. Additionally, the iliopsoas complex must release to allow the thighs to move into vertical alignment without excessive anterior pelvic tilt. These anatomical nuances can be greatly supported by placing a bolster or foam roller under the sacrum, not the lumbar spine. To create a stable platform, the prop needs to span the entire width of the pelvis, without a sense of arching or teetering. The small edge of a block is never appropriate as a support as it is too small for many individuals to scan across the entire pelvis and tends to land only on the sacrum. This placement can create movement of the sacrum inside the ilia – not a good idea. The width of a block can work for some individuals; however, as a matter of course, a wide prop (like a bolster) is superior – also for its softness, yet stability and strength.

### Supporting the Shoulder Girdle and Cervical Safety

Because the upper spine remains on the ground in Candlestick, the scapulae must be drawn onto the back to lengthen the neck and protect the cervical vertebrae. In full Shoulderstand, weight often shifts onto the neck, but in Candlestick, this risk is reduced if the thoracic spine is slightly lifted and the head remains neutral. Scapular depression and retraction help to lift the thoracic spine off the mat, creating space at C7–T1. The upper trapezius and levator scapulae must be resilient, while the serratus anterior and rhomboids engage to stabilize the shoulder blades. It is important to avoid pushing down into the head; there should be no pressure in the cervical spine.

From an alignment perspective, it is healthful to slide and wiggle the shoulders – typically one side at a time – toward one another in this supine position. Once the scapulae are nestled onto the back body, the upper arms and elbows can press into the mat to help lift the chest without excess arching in the lumbar spine. The back of the head rests passively (i.e., head and neck are relaxed), and the gaze stays upward so as to avoid any turning of the neck.

### Creating Core Control and Myofascial Continuity

Once the pelvis is supported and stable, the legs extend vertically toward the ceiling. The goal is not simple a passive lifting (i.e., not hanging in the joints; see Chapter 9) but active engagement of the core, hip flexors, and leg muscles to create strong and stable vertical alignment that feels active, balanced, and *sattvic*. Abdominal activation via transverse abdominis and lower fibers of the rectus abdominis supports spinal stabilization from the center. Co-engagement of the pelvic support creates additional lift and stability. The hip flexors (especially iliacus and rectus femoris) must be balanced by hamstring strength and resilience (see Chapter 12) to maintain vertical legs without tucking. The fascial lines of the Superficial Front Line and Deep Front Line are engaged but not strained, inviting a sense of lift and supported suspension.

From an alignment perspective it is helpful to encourage students to draw the pubic bone and low ribs toward one another to support lower abdominal and pelvic engagement. The legs are invited to be grounded neutrally in the hip sockets, neither internally or externally rotating (excessively). A sense of adduction can be invited by drawing the inner thighs lightly toward midline via isometric adduction to support pelvic steadiness. Reaching through the balls of the feet maintains a sense of upward lift and energy.

### Considering Neck, Breath, and Nervous System

Due to the elevation of the legs and pelvis above the heart, Candlestick stimulates baroreceptors and the parasympathetic nervous system. To take full advantage of this health-promoting alignment, care needs to be taken to ensure that the cervical spine is not under pressure and the breath remains smooth. It is important to preserve natural cervical lordosis, avoiding either flattening or pressing the back of the neck into the floor. The neck hyperextension is also avoided, especially at the transition to the base of the skull.

Inversions naturally decrease heart rate and calm the nervous system, but straining the breath or bearing down can counteract this. The diaphragm's role is therefore pivotal, as is nasal breathing (as is supports diaphragmatic breath, whereas mouth breathing inhibits it). Soft, subtle, and gentle nasal breathing will invite ease in the nervous systems and health in the diaphragm's range of motion, even as it presses up against the lifted contents of the abdomen. It is helpful to keep an eye out for breath dysregulation, by noticing any presence of chest or even clavicular breathing.

It is useful to calibrate the lift under the pelvis to achieve enough height so that the chest is open and the head and neck rest comfortable and in natural curves but not so high that the breath becomes labored or restricted. If students report or are observed to become breathless or to have pressure in the throat or eyes, invite them to come out of the shape and rest in a shape that allows for reregulation. If Candlestick is attempted again, a lower lift under the hips may be more auspicious.

### Transitioning Into and Out of Candlestick

Moving into Candlestick happens gradually and with control. Jerky or rapid movement into inversions can place strain on the spine and especially the neck. Mindful engagement of the hip flexors and core helps with a natural lift of the pelvis; straining or bracing in the arms or neck are not helpful but are often observed, especially in clients who are new to lifting into Candlestick. Support such individuals with cues of gentle movements upward. To lower down from Candlestick, clients will first need to place the feet back to the ground, lowering the legs with control and support from the full spectrum of core muscles, including pelvic floor and back muscles. Once the feet are on the ground, the pelvis is lifted a bit higher so that the teacher can remove the pelvic support (i.e., the bolster or foam roller). The descent from the ensuing Bridge is supported by eccentric hamstring control and abdominal strength to lower out of the shape gracefully and healthfully. It can be cued as a strength-building descent with the spine in its natural curves descending as a whole; or it can be offered as a spinal exploration via rolling down, slowly articulating vertebra after vertebra. This motion can be helpfully likened to the laying down a string of *mala* beads, bead by bead.

Once students have exited Candlestick, recovery can be invited that transitions the spine to its natural curves and settles any dysregulation in the nervous system or emotions. Windshield Wiper action in the legs can be helpful; the goal is not to bring the legs to the ground but simply to reset the low back. SI joint releases can be supportive (see Chapter 11). A very gentle forward fold may be helpful. As typical, choices of follow-up or recovery shapes are also guided by what comes next in the sequence.

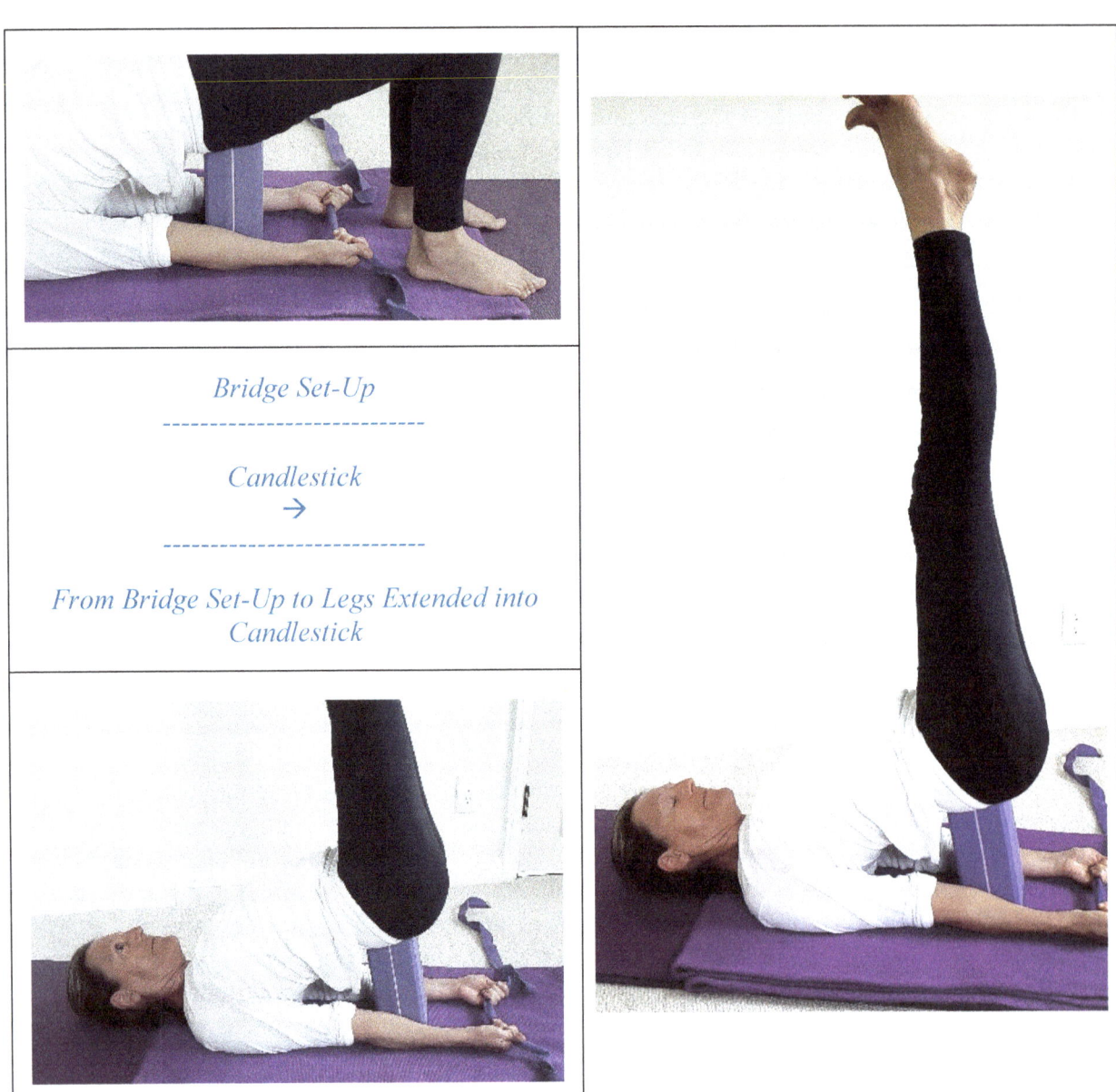

*Bridge Set-Up*

*Candlestick*
→

*From Bridge Set-Up to Legs Extended into Candlestick*

# Chapter 15: Resting and Restorative Shapes

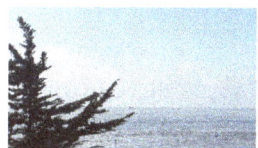

This chapter covers key resting and restorative shapes, offering optimized teaching strategies that allow for individual tailoring and careful discernment about how and which shapes to offer, as well as about how to cue alignment informed by interoception, proprioception, exteroception, and neuroception. General principles for this category of yoga *asana* are provided and apply to most if not all restorative approaches to yoga *asana*.

Restorative yoga *asana* arises out of the respective general categories of shapes (e.g., a restorative forward fold follows all the principles of forward folding in all layers of experience and then blends in the special considerations relevant to making the fold restorative and regenerative). Anatomical foci that are primary in those shapes and associated alignment principles apply directly to the related specific restorative and resting shapes but care needs to be taken to support all joints in these more passive or related embodiments of the given shapes. Primary nervous system foci are related to grounding, letting go (without buckling or collapsing), resting (without falling asleep), rejuvenating, and resetting. Restorative yoga *asana* practice is dedicated to nourishing vitality and resilience. It is generally taught in a manner that is balancing to the nervous system and applicable to all types of polyvagal states or *gunas*, integrating the exploration of affective tones, arousal, and the emergence of the *kleshas*. Restorative *asana* is typically taught in such a way that it also becomes an interior practice of yoga (most commonly either *pratyahara* or *dharana*). In tends to be more focused on creating self-compassion and awareness than on gaining insight. In other words, the work is more energetic and emotional than mental or cognitive.

## Benefits of Restorative Practices

Restorative yoga practices offer an entryway into stillness, rest, renewal, ease, and inner work, allowing students to restore their body, energy, and mind, easing emotional reactivity and cultivating compassion, lovingkindness, and peacefulness toward themselves and others. Through gentle, supported shapes, restorative yoga invites relaxation, nervous system regulation, energetic recalibration, and emotional wellbeing. Restorative practices foster a holistic sense of balance and resilience, creating a foundation for harmony, self-compassion, and self-awareness.

Not surprisingly, most if not all students or clients can benefit from restoratives. Some individuals have an easier time with restorative *asana* than others, often with *rajasic* clients turning away from such practices and *tamasic* clients seeking them out. The challenge is to help more *rajasic* students – who often stand to gain the greatest benefit from restorative work – to allow themselves to move into this very different way of being with their body, vitality, and emotionality. Clients with greater propensity toward *tamas* have an easier time with embracing these practices. With these individuals, the challenge is to make sure that they do not withdraw, disconnect, space out, or even fully dissociate during this downregulating practice. The manner of teaching is crucial to supporting individual needs most auspiciously.

Teaching clients about the benefits of restorative yoga practices may be a helpful way to create accessibility. The following benefits of restoratives can be highlighted:
- *Encourage deep relaxation and reduce stress*: Restorative yoga helps activate the parasympathetic nervous system, guiding the body into a state of relaxation. By calming the fight-or-flight response, they help stress levels diminish, alleviating tension and promoting mental clarity and calm.
- *Support nervous system regulation*: Through extended, gentle holds, restorative shapes promote a regulated nervous system, balancing overstimulation with quiet introspection. This recalibration soothes the body's stress response and fosters tranquility, provides opportunity for access to the experience of safety, and encourages resilience.
- *Enhance tissue resilience and joint mobility*: Restorative shapes gently challenge muscles and connective tissues, promoting gentle resilience that may serve to release chronic tension, increase joint mobility, and encourage ease in physical movement.
- *Promote mental clarity and focus*: The stillness of restorative yoga shapes invites practitioners to cultivate mindfulness, enhancing present-moment awareness and concentration. Quietude supports mental clarity, encouraging uncoupling from distractions and fostering a meditative state.
- *Boost immune function*: By shifting the body into a parasympathetic state, restorative yoga can enhance immune function. Calming effects help reduce stress-related inflammation and may improve the recovery and responsiveness to immune challenges.
- *Support in emotional release and self-awareness*: Restorative yoga provides space for emotional release, encouraging practitioners to process and release stored emotions in a safe environment. Resting in restorative shapes can increase self-awareness, empathy, and compassion, as students connect to their inner emotional landscape.
- *Support pain relief and healing*: Resting in gently supported shapes may alleviate chronic pain by relieving tension in muscles and joints. Restorative yoga nurtures the body's natural healing processes, supporting pain management and offering a pathway to enhanced physical comfort and ease.
- *Cultivate the mature emotions*: Restorative yoga emphasizes surrender and acceptance, inviting students to let go of *kleshas* and *vrittis* as they embrace the present moment. They are invited into accessing peace, gratitude, and connection, while cultivating compassion and lovingkindness toward self and others.

## *Cautions and Contraindications*

Although restorative yoga is generally gentle and accessible, certain conditions call for care and caution to ensure a safe and beneficial experience. A few key considerations and contraindications are best considered when teaching restorative yoga.
- Avoid prolonged holds in a single shape if there are acute injuries or acute inflammation. Be sure to offer sufficient props so that injured areas are supported and not exposed to risk.
- Be sure to prop all joints to avoid passive range of motion, where gravity pulls on limbs and creates strain on joints. Restorative shapes are not meant to increase range of motion; they are invited to for reasons of creating ease and replenishing energy.

- Use caution with props (e.g., straps), especially if there are sensitivities related to sensory processing, attention, or trauma history. It is helpful to demonstrate props before the session begins to notice reactivities among clients. It may serve to offer alternative props or setups and encourage clients to modify their restorative prop arrangements to create the greatest opportunity for the experience of a safe, comfortable environment that meets individual needs and resources.
- Be mindful with specific conditions, such as glaucoma, vitreous detachment, or high blood pressure. For example, it may be necessary with some clients **to** avoid positions in which the head is placed significantly below the level of the heart, especially for long periods of time.
- Exercise caution with hip and knee sensitivities that may be triggered by prolonged holds. It is good practice to offer ample supports under the knees or hips to prevent and alleviate discomfort. A gentle bend in the hip creases (via a prop under the knees) is very supportive to nervous system regulation as well as to physical ease.
- Be aware of anxiety or discomfort in stillness and offer affected clients alternatives during moments of prolonged silence (see *safety hatches* in the *Savasana* section below). For example, it may be helpful to offer a concrete task in case of dysregulation, such as counting the breath or opening the eyes to connect visually to the environment.
- Avoid compressive or unsupported neck positions, especially for individuals with cervical spine issues. Supporting the head with props all the way down to the spines of the scapulae is ideal as it also provides support for the head without increasing anterior head carriage. Maintaining a natural spine helps prevent compression in all spinal regions and is particularly helpful for the secondary curves.
- Restorative yoga is generally beneficial during pregnancy. However, certain positions (e.g., lying flat on the back after the first trimester) need to be modified. For example, side-lying shapes or using an inclined bolster and supports between the legs can support comfort and safety. For yoga professionals who seek to work primarily or exclusively with pregnant or post-partum individuals specialized training is indicated to ensure appropriate scope of practice and client supports.
- Support individuals with respiratory issues, such as asthma or COPD, by using props that support an open heart space and unobstructed breathing. Supine restoratives may be helpful for some of these individuals and completely contraindicated for others. It is important to stay attuned to clients as they set up for shapes that may be questionable and to have alternatives at the ready.

## Anatomical, Energetic, and Psychological Foci for Restorative Practices

Given the needs of different students or clients, it is important to bring balance into restoratives in the same way that we can bring balance into other forms of *asana*. This balance comes from affective engagement and active invitation into curiosity about *vedana* and *kleshas*, more so than invitation into embodied mindfulness. Even though restoratives are based in yoga *asana* in terms of physical practice and support, they are best offered with complete integration of *pranayama* and *pratyahara, even dharana*. There is a balancing of effort and ease in each shape – this can come from the physical practice, breathwork, or the cueing of *pratyahara*. In other words, the restorative shape that is chosen can in and of itself create effort within the ease of the shape; yet, the effort can also be introduced deliberately or inadvertently via the other yogic limbs.

Sequencing of physical shapes and accompanying cueing are key to achieving optimal nervous system effects. General sequencing follows the same process as for any integrated holistic yoga class: mindfulness cue, psychoeducation, centering practice (perhaps including a breathing practice), followed by intention-setting, warmup, restorative *asana* series, recovery, closing meditation in a resting shape, and closing comments with expression of gratitude. The warmup series is important to make sure that students' musculoskeletal system and vital energy are prepared for the restorative yoga *asana*. Warmup via all movements of the spine is auspicious; *kriya* or gentle *vinyasa* practices can be particularly helpful as they are warming, support healthful nasal breathing, and engage individuals in an active way before moving into stillness.

Specific sequencing of chosen restorative shapes is based on the needs of the anticipated clientele and the intention of a given session. Shapes are most typically chosen as follows: approximately one or two each from seats, forward folds, twists, backbends, inversions, and lying-down shapes. It is helpful for creating physical balance to have all of these shapes represented in the restorative yoga *asana* part of the sequence. Specific sequencing (or order) of the shapes is tailored to intention of the session as well as needs of the students or clients. Recommended order by nervous system-related intentions is shown in the following table.

| Possible Order of Restorative Asanas by Type of Effect Desired from The Practice | | |
|---|---|---|
| Balancing Energy and Affect | Energizing Energy and Affect | Calming Energy and Affect |
| Seat | Forward Fold | Backbend |
| Twist | Twist | Twist |
| Forward Fold | Seat | Seat |
| Backbend | Backbend | Forward Fold |
| Inversion | Inversion | Inversion |
| Supine or Prone Lying-down Shape | Open-hearted Lying-down Shape | Prone Lying-down Shape |
| Restorative *Savasana* | Restorative *Savasana* | Restorative *Savasana* |

## Tips for Cueing for Restoratives

Besides cueing interoception and the experience of the present moment (i.e., *pratyahara* of inner sensations), cueing focus is on breathing (integrating either balancing, energizing, or calming breathing practices, breath awareness, and breath observation) and on working with the *kleshas* to begin to support a guarding of the senses. As is true for all *asana*, teaching restoratives benefits greatly from cueing grounding, expansion, and stability. A few cueing tips for these three components of the physical work follow below after a few more general comments and suggestions. General principles, invitations, and offerings that are useful in restorative practice include, but are definitely not limited to, possible options such as:
- Maximizing ease in the body and minimizing effort in the musculoskeletal system, but avoiding collapse
- Propping shapes at about 80% or less of available range of motion
- Avoiding excessive stretching or straining on joints and connective tissue
- Providing ample time – 75 to 90 minutes

- Noticing *gunas* (arousal, vitality, state of the nervous system) and *vedana* (feeling tone of pleasant, unpleasant, or neutral)
- Noticing *kleshas*
- Noticing mind states and mental or emotional *samskaras*
- Inviting the pondering of the *brahma viharas*
- Including brief reiterations of collective intention and how it relates to the currently-assumed restorative shape
- Reading quotes or poems related to theme/intention of the class

|  | *Tips for Grounding, Expansion, and Stability in Restoratives* |
|---|---|
| *Grounding* | <ul><li>Ground through the body parts in contact with the floor</li><li>Release gripping in muscles not needed to hold the shape, including core and pelvic floor, when appropriate</li><li>Be sure to support the limbs and torso to prevent excessive stretch or opening – the shape is supposed to be relaxing for the body and nervous system which means grounding without bracing or buckling</li><li>Encourage sufficient engagement in relevant muscles to prevent soreness the next day</li><li>Invite a grounding breath, perhaps emphasizing the exhalation or the pause at the bottom of the breath</li><li>Invite the mind to settle and ground</li></ul> |
| *Stability* | <ul><li>Notice the gentle engagement of the core muscles on the exhalation</li><li>Notice the soft engagement of the pelvic floor – do not let the bottom drop out even here</li><li>Support the limbs and/or torso into a sense of stability that does not put muscles at maximum stretch</li><li>Encourage students to yield, neither buckling nor bracing</li><li>Create balance – find stillness in movement and movement in stillness</li><li>Explore stability as the middle way – the center between over- and under-engagement, the center between activity and passivity, the center between hyper- and hypo-arousal</li><li>Invite *sattva*</li></ul> |
| *Expansion* | <ul><li>Maintain length and natural lordosis in lumbar spine</li><li>Maintain openness in the thoracic spine and heart space</li><li>Support the natural curve in cervical spine</li><li>Make sure forehead is higher than the chin if supine</li><li>Expand the abdomen and low rib basket with the inhalation –do not exaggerate this lest the breath become hard and labored</li><li>Invite spaciousness into the breath when appropriate to context</li><li>Invite spaciousness and openness into the mind when appropriate to context</li><li>Invite an open heart when appropriate to context</li></ul> |

**498** | Integrated Holistic Yoga Movement

## Images of Resting and Restorative Shapes

### *Restorative Seats*

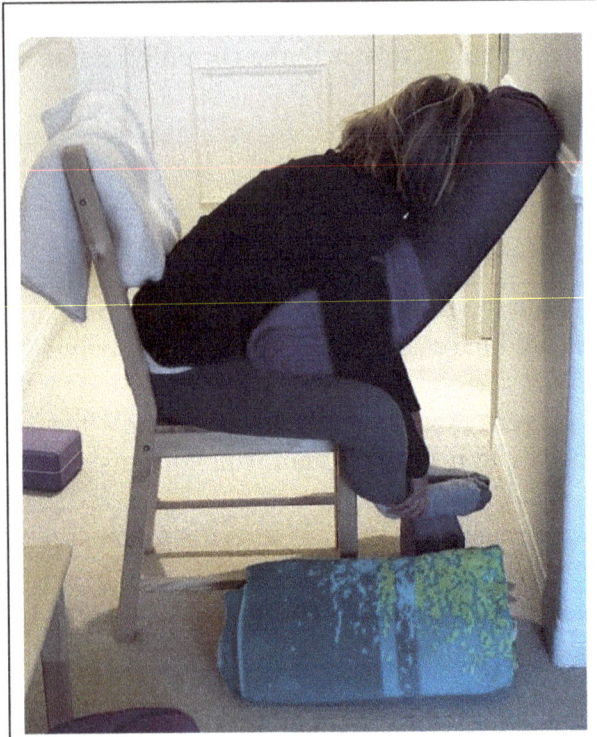

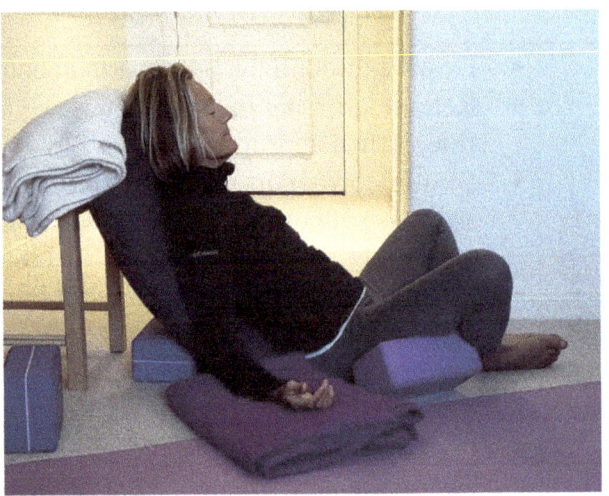

*Supported Butterfly*
← *prone*

*supine* ↓

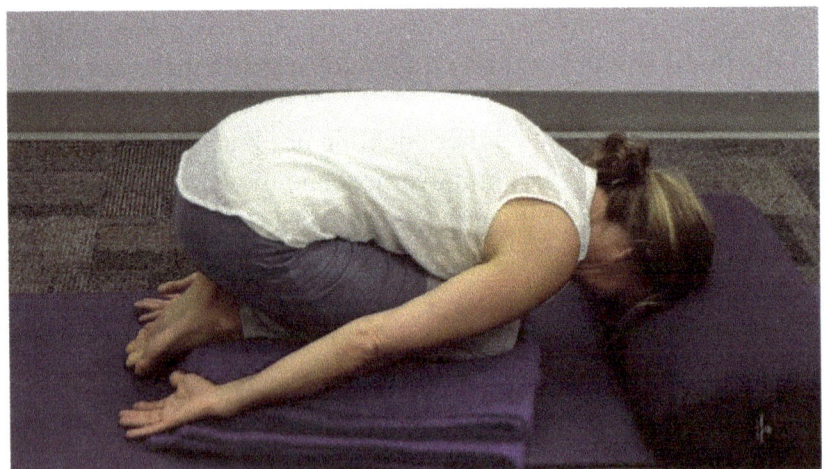

*Restorative Diamond*

*Peace comes from within, do not seek it without.*
Anonymous

## Restorative Forward Folds

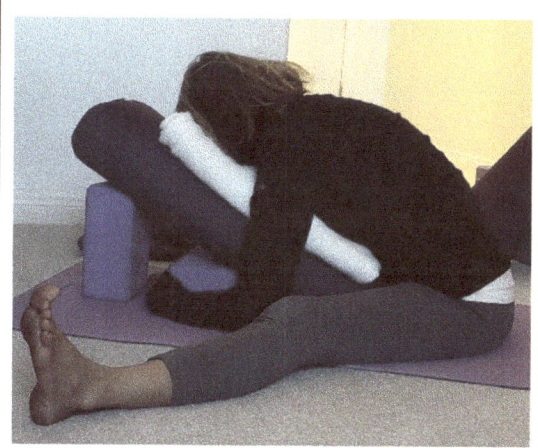

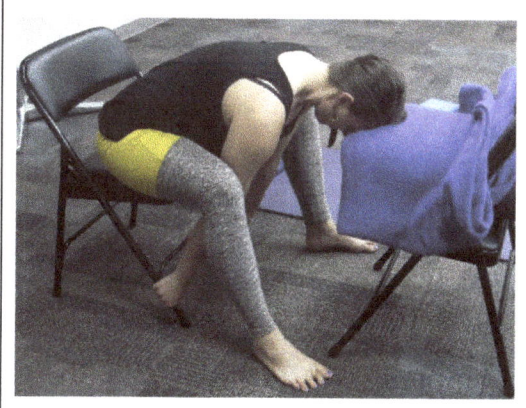

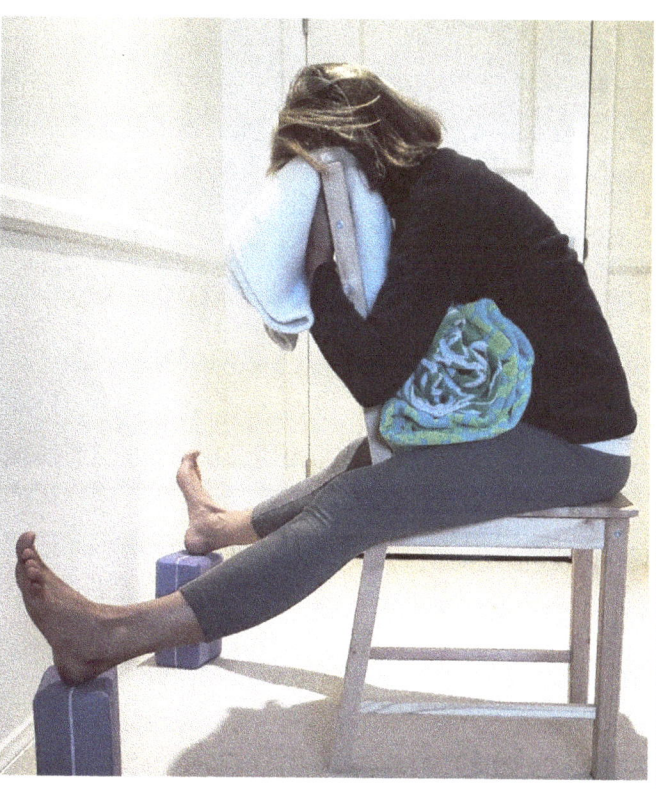

*Restorative Wide-Legged Forward Folds*

*Restorative Head-of-Knee*

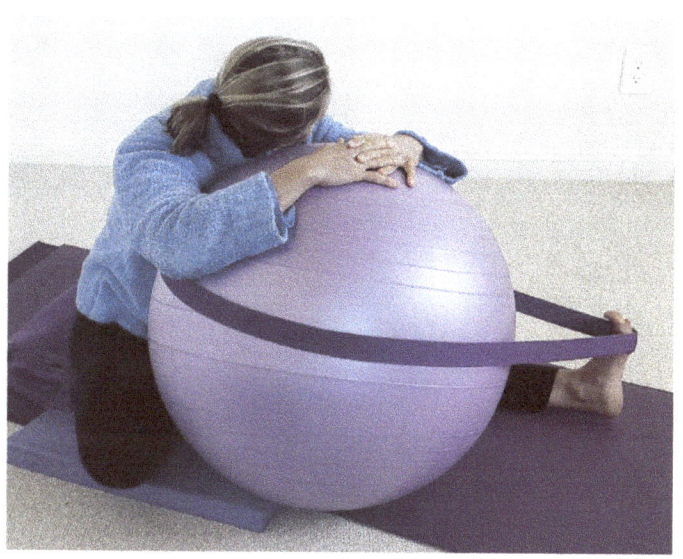

## Restorative Twists

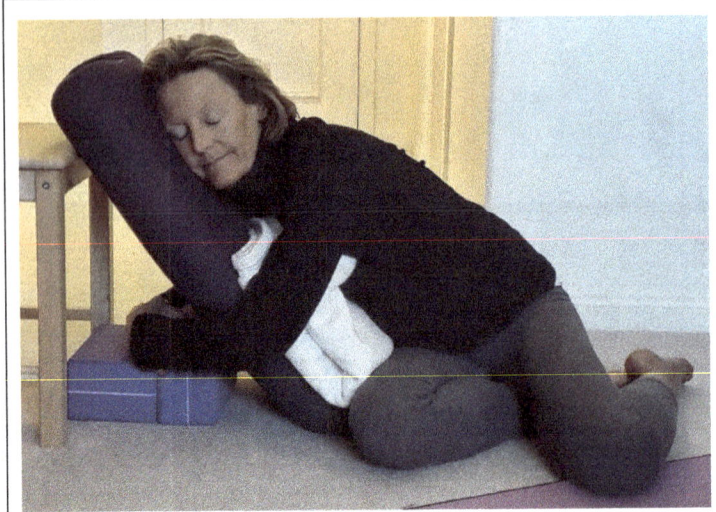
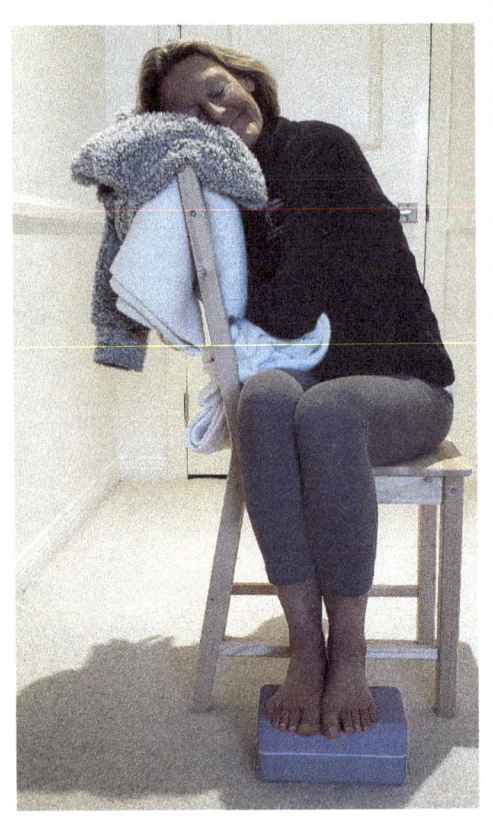

*Restorative Seated Twists – floor and chair versions*

## Restorative Backbends

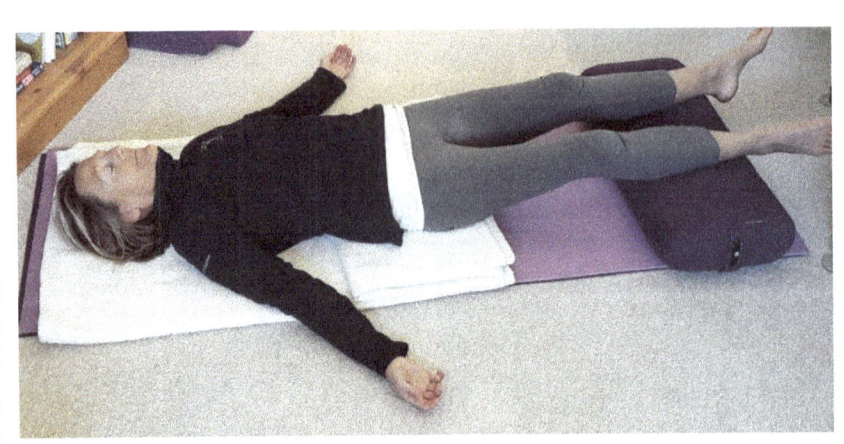

*Restorative Backbends – gentle Bridge shape*

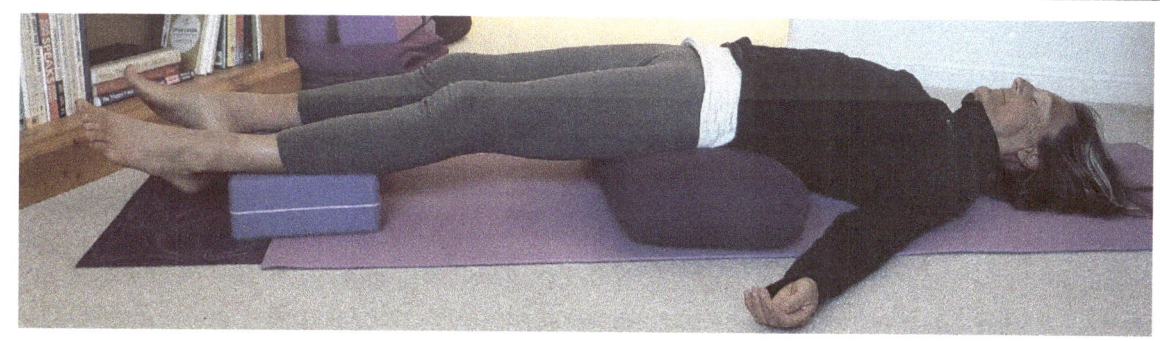

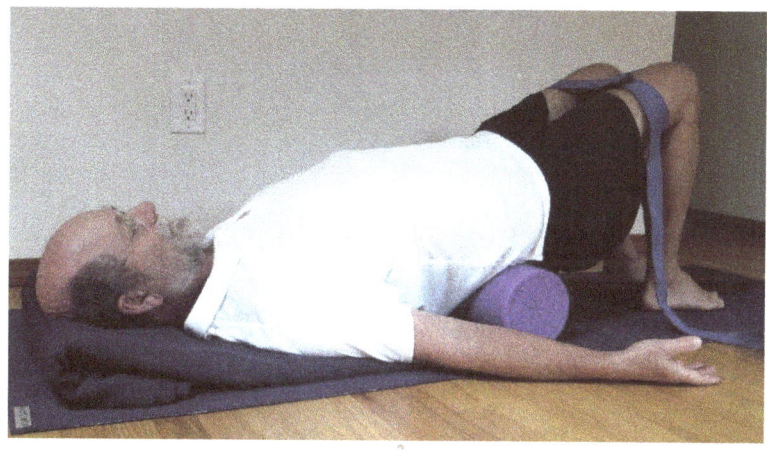

*Restorative Backbends – beautifully supported Bridge with multiple options for leg engagement*

## Restorative Inversions

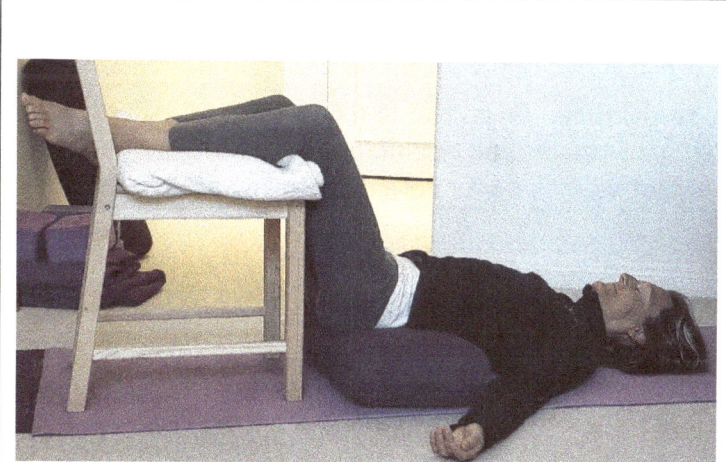

*Restorative Inversions – Legs-up-the-Wall*

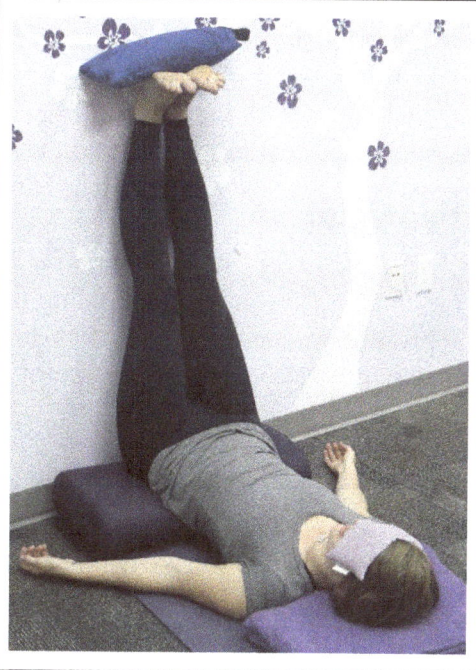

## Corpse or Savasana

The epitome of all resting and restorative shapes is *Savasana*. Although it is not often acknowledged or understood as such, *Savasana* is a *pratyahara* practice focused on the *pratyahara* of nothing. There is no invitation for anything to do in *Savasana* – the shape is entirely about being, and not about doing (not even the 'doing' that is involved in relaxing or releasing). It is the best shape for moving brain and nervous system toward the *being* networks in the brain, releasing clients from a perpetual focus on *doing*. Notably, the inner practices as well as the neuroscience of being versus doing is covered in the Volume 3 of the series, *Integrated Holistic Inner Practices of Yoga*.

## Key Teaching Invitations

A few essentials related to teaching *Savasana* are as follows:
- *Savasana is ideally offered at the end of any yoga session* – no matter how brief the session or the *Savasana*. In very time-limited contexts, *Savasana* can be engaged in any semi-supported shape, including sitting or even standing.
- *Savasana needs to be as long as circumstances allow* – a minimum of a few minutes and preferably as long as 5 to 15 minutes. Ideally, it is not skipped, even if time is limited.
- *Savasana benefits from guarding the senses* – shielding the eyes might be helpful; creating a minimally stimulating environment is supportive. Guarding the senses also means that there is no talking by the teacher during *Savasana*. Readings and ponderings by the teacher are not part of *Savasana* (although they can precede or follow it).
- *Savasana is a shape that requires optimizing ease in the body* – consider ample props, including extra clothing and/or blankets to cover up with to make sure the body stays warm throughout this practice. Other supports, such as blankets under the head and lifts under the knees can maximize the benefit of the practice for most students.
- *Savasana may require a safety hatch for students with mental health challenges* (e.g., trauma histories, attention challenges, anxiety disorders) – offer the breath as a safe haven in case of challenges with the practice of being. Students can be invited to return to a particularly soothing breathing practice if they notice that their mind or emotions are dysregulating their nervous system. Safety hatches are best individualized for each student and discussed with them prior to the initiation of *Savasana*.
- *Find a conducive position on the floor, comfortable chair, couch, or bed*. Many shapes can be used for *Savasana*, including the traditional supine version, legs-up-the-wall, or even a prone *Savasana*. For students who cannot easily access the floor, seated options are fine. A few illustrations are offered below, but many additional options exist.
- To optimize the opportunity for ease, comfort, safety, and symmetry when lying on the back, invite students to:
  - place their arms slightly away from their sides, with palms facing up to encourage an open, receptive shape
  - let their feet fall outward naturally, releasing any residual tension in the hips
  - ensure the neck is long and relaxed; suggest adjusting the chin slightly downwards to support an open airway and relaxation in the throat
  - encourage subtle adjustments if needed to feel balanced and supported

## Savasana Positioning Options

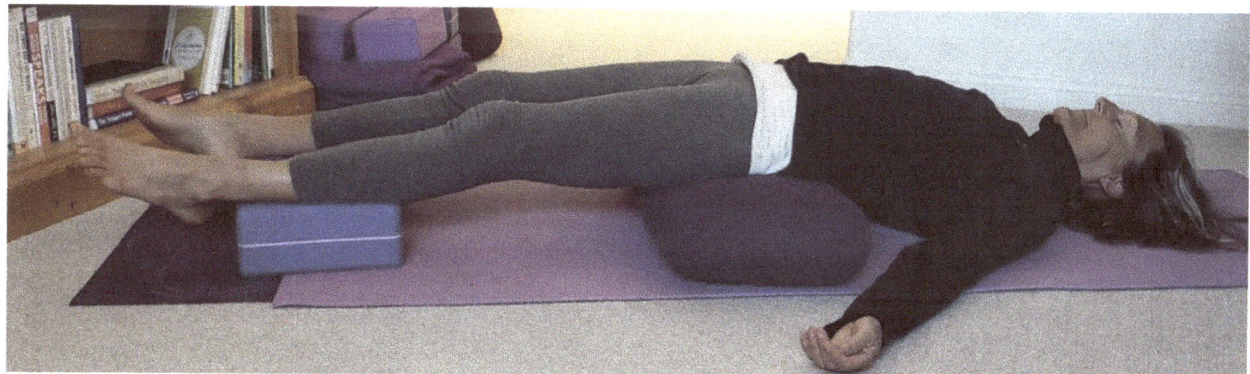

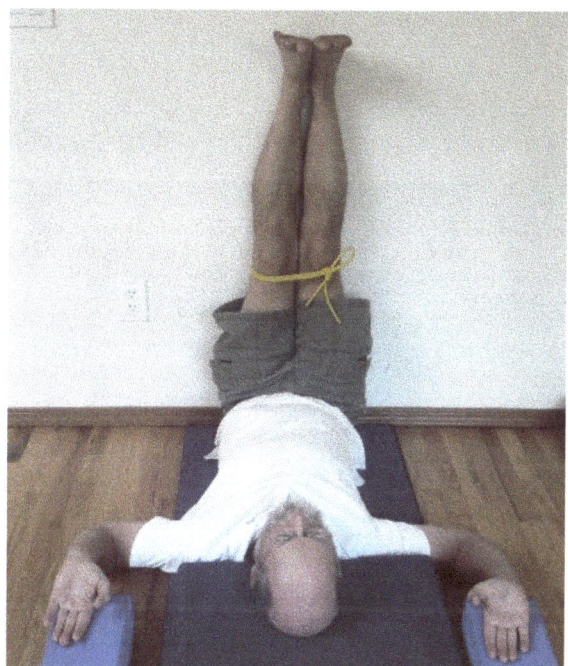

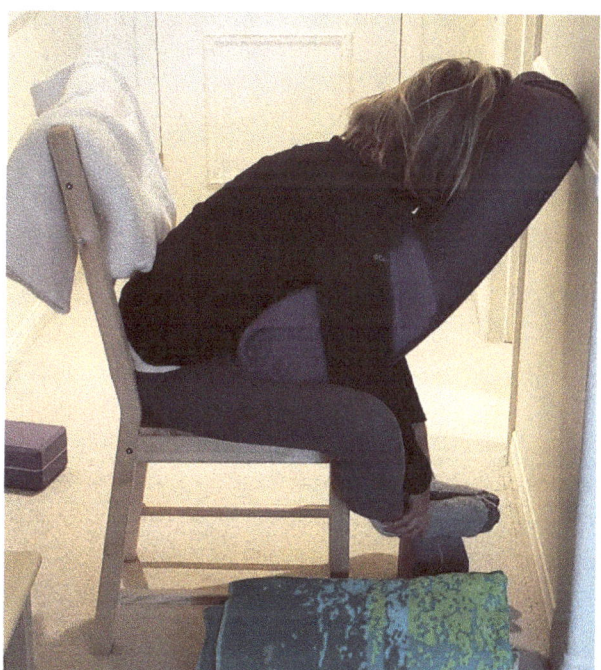

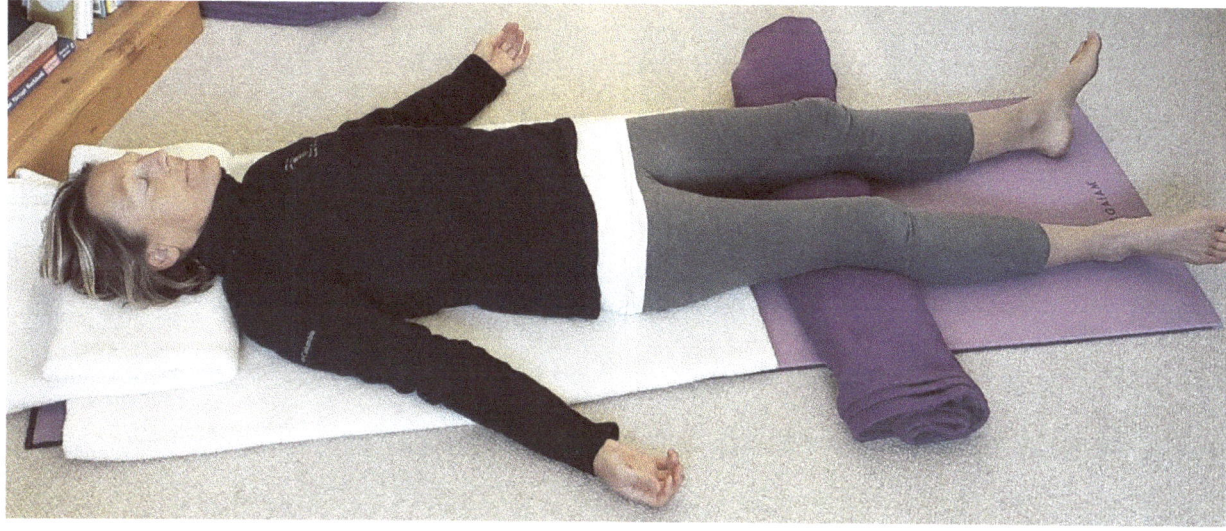

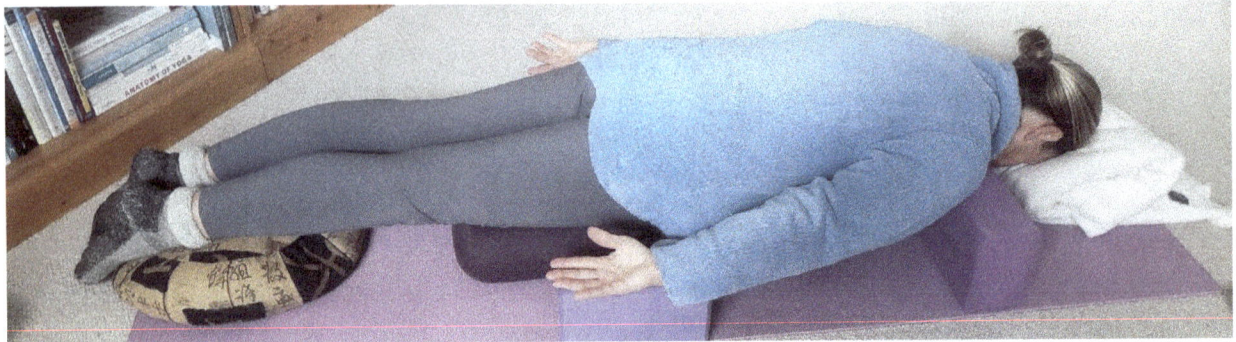

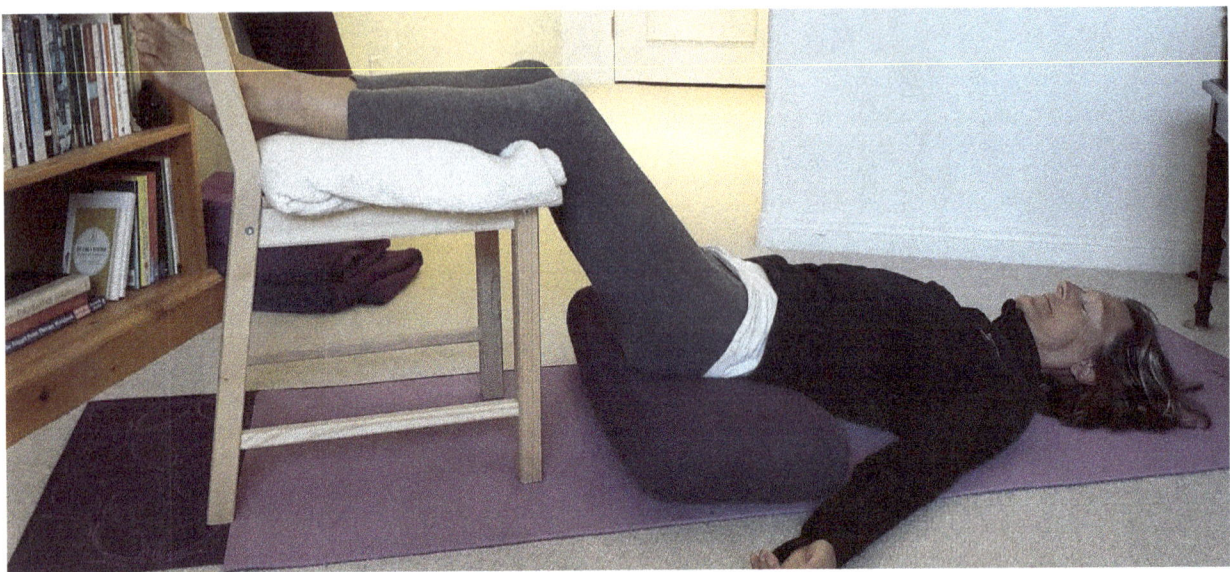

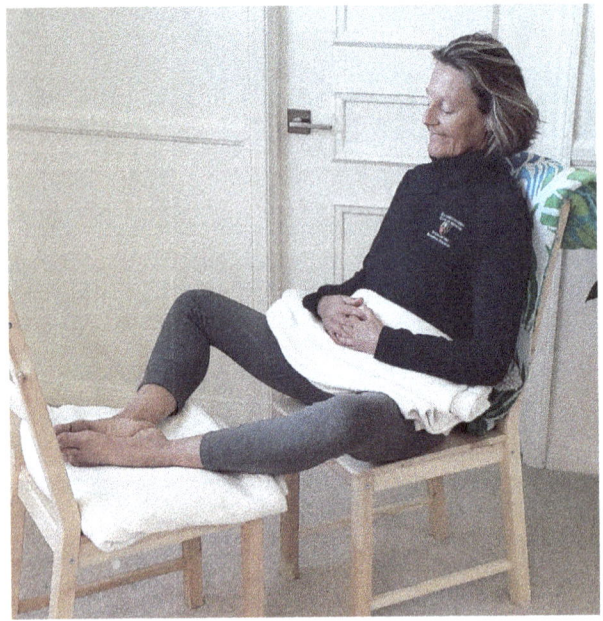

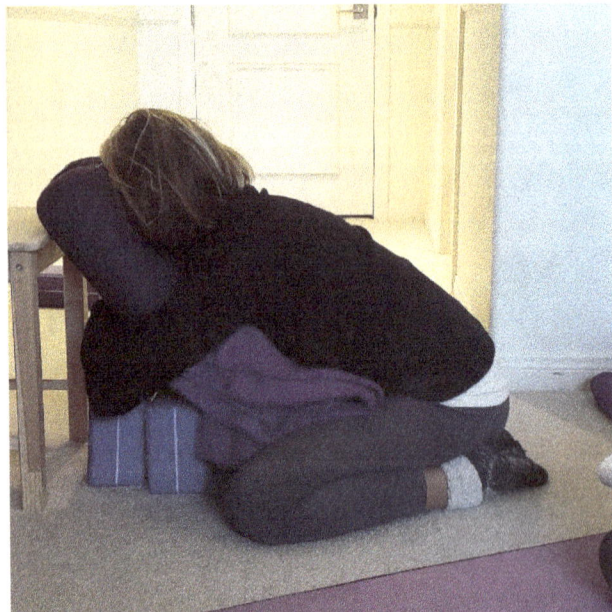

## Instructions for Settling into the Ritual that is Savasana

Settling into *Savasana* is a ritual – a gentle, intentional, and compassionate arrival into a moment in time and location in space that invites release, even surrender. *Savasana*, in whichever shape is chosen, is not merely a process of lying down or sitting back; it is a conscious practice of letting go and embracing the current moment with the stillness of *pratyahara*. Following are some guiding principles for helping students ease into *Savasana* with intention and presence, deeply honoring the practice as the *pratyahara* of nothing, a deep surrender and withdrawal of the senses. The practice starts by inviting students to lie down with the clarity that what is to come is a period of quietude, of profound stillness that invites integration and metabolism of the practice in all layers of experience. Students are invited to position their bodies comfortably on their mats or another chosen surface in a manner that invites comfort, ease, and presence and that conveys safety and compassion for all layers of experience. They can be guided through a meditative induction that moves through the five layers of experience, inviting release or surrender of each. The step are outlined next; a sample script is provided below.

### Scan and Soften The Body

Once clients are settled into a comfortable, sustainable, and tension-free physical shape, gently invite somatic awareness, perhaps by cueing a gentle body scan, pausing briefly at chosen body part. For example, a brief scan of sensations in the body may start from the feet, through the ankles, to the legs, pelvis, torso, arms, neck, and face. Alternatively, a scan could start at the center of the physical being in the region of the navel and then can move outward through the torso and into the legs, arms, neck and head. If a scan is not within the possible timeframe of the class, a gentle tuning into somatic awareness with a subsequent invitation to surrender the body to gravity can suffice. In this step of moving toward *savasana*, the key is to cultivate a sense of physical letting be, allowing gravity to fully support the body.

### Release the Breath

Having invited students entrust their body to the earth, they are next encouraged to tune into their natural breath rhythm through the nose, as it unfolds in this moment. Invite students to be softly and openly aware of sensations associated with their breath as it moves through the body, sweeping through their vital experience in a particular way (e.g., from the center of their being to the periphery). The soft and open awareness of breath helps create a bridge from movement to stillness, preparing mind, energy, and body to ease into *Savasana*. There is no invitation to change the breath – quite the opposite: the invitation is to surrender the breath to the natural flow of *Prana* (lifeforce) to move freely, so that the breath feels as though it is breathing itself.

### Cultivate Surrender in the Mind

Clients are invited to gently recognize and acknowledge thoughts, emotions, or mental patterns that are still noisy or otherwise present. Gentle awareness of mental fluctuations does not mean chasing thoughts or emotions away, ignoring or rejecting them. It means acknowledging them with kindness and compassion; resolving to honor them with attention, mindfulness, or presence at a later time; in this moment they are simply allowed to co-exist with the quietude and sense withdrawal that is *Savasana*. This moment is for complete surrender, a practice of observing and releasing without attachment. It is possible but not necessary to offer visualizations that encourage a sense of lightness, such as imagining thoughts as leaves floating away on a river or as clouds moving through the sky only to dissipate, move, and gather elsewhere.

*Settle into Stillness and Silence*

Having surrendered body, breath and mind, *Savasana* becomes a practice of letting go, yet remaining awake. Encourage them to embrace this quiet and peaceful pause from doing, even from processing inputs from the inner or outer sense. Invite them to rest without expectation, simply being with the stillness as it unfolds. As they settle, they may begin to notice a quiet spaciousness around and within them as they into a gentle space of quiet awareness – a state of being. Some may have difficulty settling; for them a safety hatch can be offered (*see above*) to help them stay grounded, present, and undistracted given their circumstances or nervous systems.

---

*Sample Script of a Guidance into Savasana*

Gently find your way into your choice of shape for savasana; once you have arrived, perhaps choose to close your eyes and invite body, breath, and mind to settle gently and softly.

Gently draw your awareness to your physical body, the somatic experience of this moment. Notice any sensations with an open heart, with no need to change anything. Perhaps inviting your awareness to scan softly through the body with compassion and kindness – no judgment, no expectation. Inviting whatever emerges to simply be as is. If it feels appropriate, perhaps offering gratitude for all the ways in which your body has supported you today. And then gently release your physical being, surrendering the body to the earth beneath you, to the ground that holds and supports all of us …

Gently guide your awareness to the breath, the rhythm of the inhalations and exhalations; the gentle rising and falling of the breath. No need to change anything; no need to control or deepen the breath – allowing the breath to unfold naturally, gently, subtly. Meeting the breath with the same compassion and kindness with which you met your body, simply noticing what is… Perhaps tuning into a sense of gratitude for this vital force that has carried you through your practice, your life … Allowing the breath to unfold naturally; allowing yourself to be breathed … surrendering the breath to the natural flow of *prana*, the life energy that moves through all of us …

And gently turning your awareness to your mind – your mind state, thoughts or emotions that are present in this moment… meeting them with compassion and kindness, free from judgment or expectation. Perhaps meeting this inner landscape with gratitude – for all it offers, for its richness, for its complexity. Allowing thoughts and emotions simply to be – no need to grasp onto anything; no need to chase anything away. Allowing the mental fluctuations to travel through your awareness like clouds in the sky … gently surrendering mind, thoughts and emotions to your own deeper inner wisdom, the quiet knowing that will guide you back to what needs attention when the practice closes.

And then becoming aware of this deeper wisdom, this intelligence that has accompanied you on your journey through body, breath, and mind… the capacity to observe, to reflect, to choose compassion grounded in awareness and wisdom again and again. The deeper intelligence linking you to the greater web of life, the deep knowing of being connected to a greater whole, a community … perhaps tuning into the quiet joy of this knowing, of this connection to yourself, to community, to something greater… resting, perhaps, in joyful gratitude for this shared human experience …

From this place of deep connection, of the letting go, of surrender, gently release into a few minutes of silence until my voice brings you back.

### Guide a Gentle Return

When it is time to exit *Savasana*, prompt a gradual reawakening by drawing the senses outward – perhaps tuning into sounds (such as the teacher's voice, the sound of a singing bowl, the chiming of a yoga bell), aromas in the air, the feeling of the blanket or clothing in the skin, the movement of air, or even a taste in the mouth. This attunement to the outer world can be followed up with gentle reattunement to the inner world, perhaps starting with the physical layer of experience by wiggling fingers and toes, rolling wrists and ankles, then eventually rolling to one side in a fetal position. Encourage sensing into the vital layer by encouraging a few conscious breaths, inviting students to notice that they are breathing in when air travels in and that they are breathing out when air travels out. Finally, as they are ready, invite them to move slowly as they come up to a seated shape, carrying the calm and stillness of *Savasana* forward into their seat where the teacher will offer an intentional closing (returning to the initial intention and encouraging a tuning in to a take-away from the practice). Arising slowly and mindfully supports the psychological and emotional presence that was cultivate and creates physical and vital safety in that it can help prevent orthostatic hypotension or other physical readjustments after an extended period of lying supine.

The ending of *Savasana* is typically also the ending of a yoga session – whether a class, a clinical session, or a personal practice. The ending of *Savasana* is thus the signal for a mindful closing of the practice, auspiciously marked by mindful attention to how the practice reverberates, whether the practice offered a beneficial take-away, and a profound feeling of gratitude for the experience. A yoga professional can create a beautiful closing ritual for classes or sessions that invites clarity about all of these aspects of a yoga practice. The expression of gratitude for the practice and the individuals with whom it was shared is a beautiful note on which to say good-bye.

> *Happiness cannot be traveled to, owned,*
> *earned, worn or consumed.*
> *Happiness is the spiritual experience*
> *of living every minute with love, grace and gratitude.*
> Denis Waitley

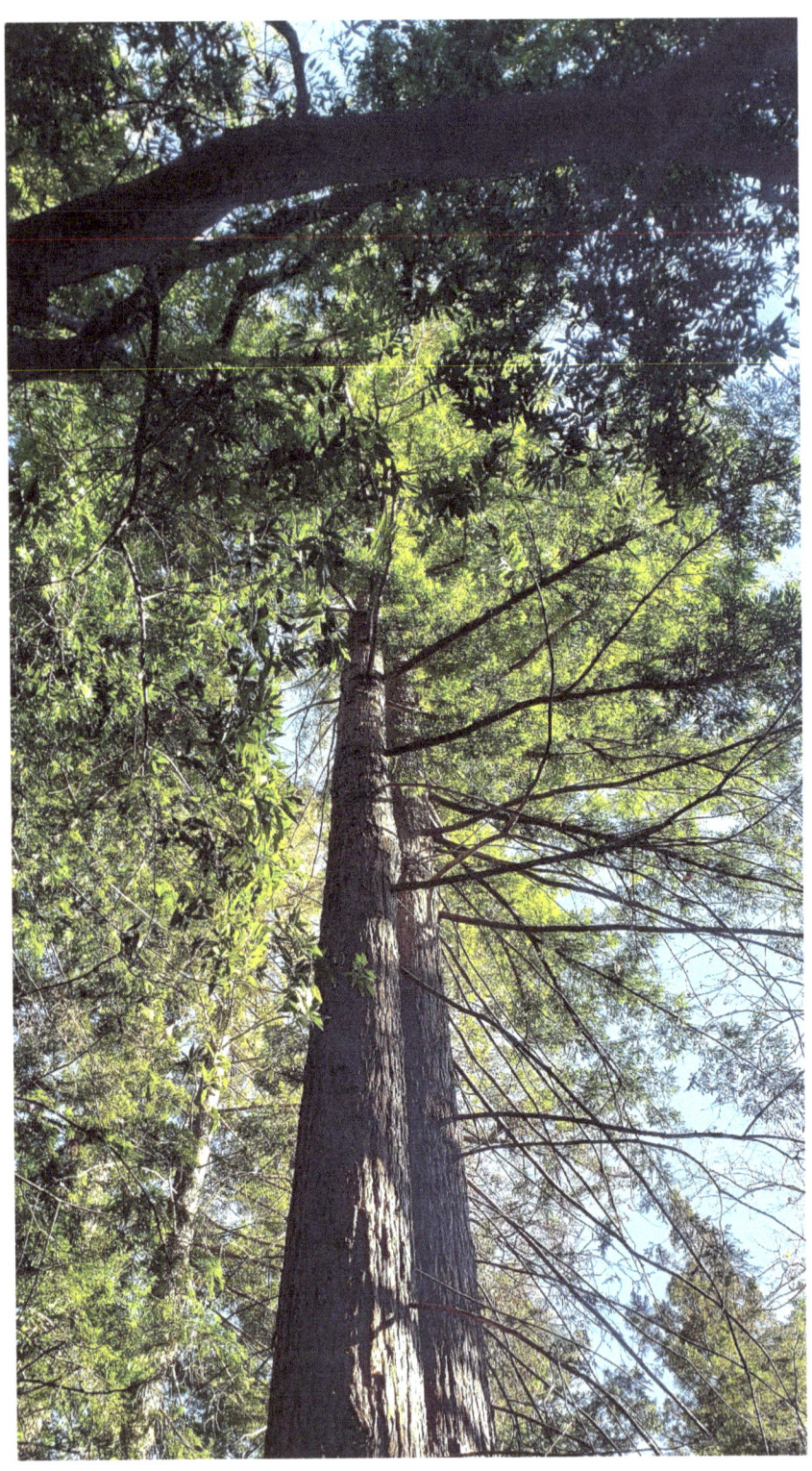

## Closing Comments

Ending *Integrated Holistic Yoga Movement* with *Savasana* is a deliberate choice. Through the quiet surrender of this shape, we honor the symbolic echo of life's final exhale; we celebrate and release into all endings; we move deeply into our relationship with impermanence. Through surrendering into the nothingness of *Savasana*, we offer up a gesture of release that transcends mere rest. We lie down in stillness to embrace and mark the end of a journey; we profoundly acknowledge that every cycle completes itself – and that is does so in silence. Just as *Savasana* invites the body to soften, to yield to gravity's pull; just it invites the breath to release, allowing itself to be breathed by the flow of the lifeforce that moves through all of; and just as it invites the mind with its thoughts and emotions to surrender itself to our own deeper inner wisdom and knowing – our grounding in and interdependence with a larger web of life, so too does it invite the spirit to let go – to pause in a sacred space of deep intelligence infused by profound awareness and compassion for ourselves, all of life, the entire earth.

We have traveled together through the intricate landscapes of the anatomy, physiology, and psychology of mindful movement; we have mapped the body with compassion and honored its complexities and interdependence with all layers of human experience. We have done so with care, intentions, and beneficence; we have done so with a deep understanding of what it means to be human, to be born of a particular biopsychosociocultural context, and to contribute to the wellbeing of all. It has been an immense joy and profound privilege to shape these explorations with you, the reader, and with all of you whom I have met along the path of my life. It is a profound joy to know that this final moment of stillness mirrors the grace of completion; it is not final. As with all true endings, there is the gentle and hopeful promise of new beginnings; of the karmic ripple effects we create through every action, from beginning to end. *Savasana* and this journey through *Integrated Holistic Yoga Movement* is not only a gesture of completion but of renewal; a clearing of space for whatever will come next – for what we will create with this knowledge, this wisdom, and this intentionality.

Thank you for sharing this journey with me. May you carry forward the wisdom of integrated holistic yoga practice into your own teaching and explorations, holding space for endings as well as the endless possibilities and new beginnings that will follow. As you rise from *Savasana* and as you close the pages of this book, may you step into the next chapter of your life and yoga practice with clarity, lovingkindness, and the joy of continued discovery. May you learn, unlearn, and relearn with an open heart and a curious mind.

With awareness, insight, compassion, and profound gratitude,

*Chris*

There is a tenderness in endings, a quietude that invites us to soften. When we let go – not with force, but with faith – we open ourselves to the vulnerability of the unknown, to all that is still unfolding.

Endings, thus embraced, become invitations: to begin again, to learn anew, to move forward with an open heart, to arrive in each moment with a clear mind, and to meet the unknown with quiet courage and compassionate intention.

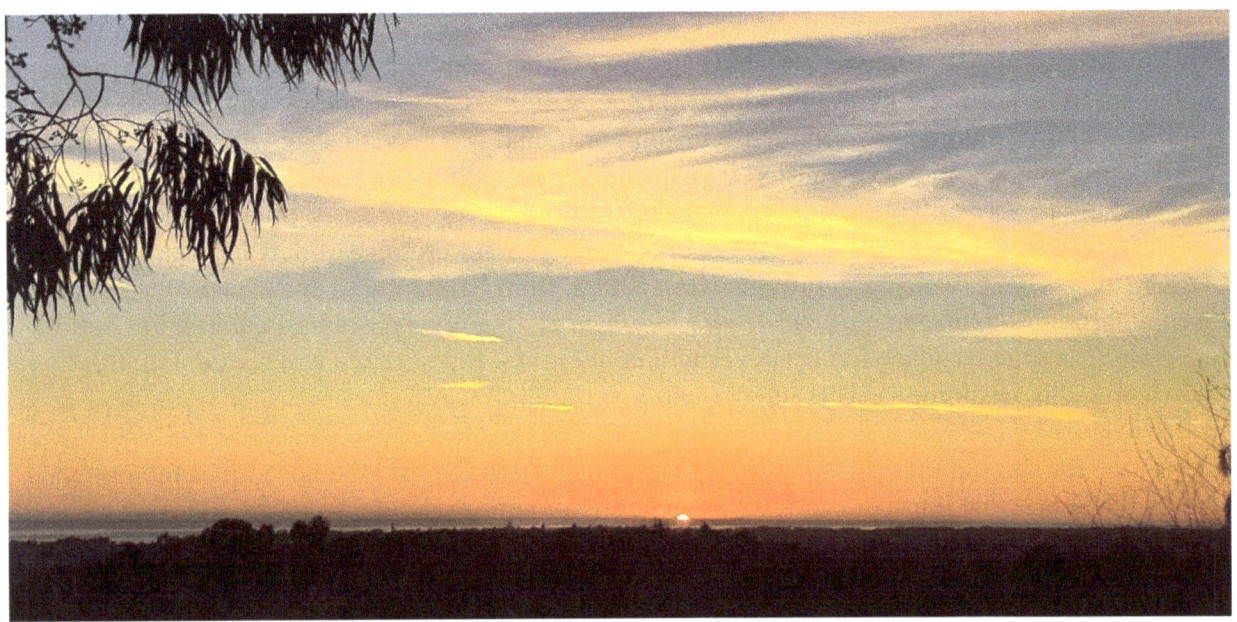

# Bibliography and Citations

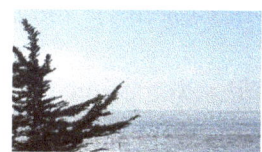

Badenoch, B. (2018). *The heart of trauma: Healing the embodied brain in the context of relationship*. Norton.

Baginski, C. (2020). *Restorative yoga: Relax. restore. re-energize*. Alpha Books.

Ball, K., Carver, A., Downing, K., Jackson, M., & O'Rourke, K. (2015). Addressing the social determinants of inequities in physical activity and sedentary behaviours. *Health Promotion International, 30*(suppl 2), ii8–ii19. 10.1093/heapro/dav022

Bantham, A., Taverno Ross, S. E., Sebastião, E., & Hall, G. (2021). Overcoming barriers to physical activity in underserved populations. *Progress in Cardiovascular Diseases, 64*, 64–71. 10.1016/j.pcad.2020.11.002

Bell, D. R., Post, E. G., Biese, K., Bay, C., & Valovich McLeod, T. (2018). Sport specialization and risk of overuse injuries: A systematic review with meta-analysis. *Pediatrics, 142*(3), 1. 10.1542/peds.2018-0657

Beltrán-Carrillo, V. J., Megías, Á, González-Cutre, D., & Jiménez-Loaisa, A. (2022). Elements behind sedentary lifestyles and unhealthy eating habits in individuals with severe obesity. *International Journal of Qualitative Studies on Health and Well-Being, 17*(1), 2056967. 10.1080/17482631.2022.2056967

Bičíková, M., Máčová, L., Jandová, D., Třískala, Z., & Hill, M. (2021). Movement as a positive modulator of aging. *International Journal of Molecular Sciences, 22*(12), 6278. 10.3390/ijms22126278

Biel, A., & Dorn, R. (2019). *Trail guide to the body: A hands-on guide to locating muscles, bones, and more* (6th ed.). Books of Discovery.

Bond, M. (2007). *The new rules of posture: How to sit, stand, and move in the modern world*. Healing Arts Press.

Bondy, D. (2020). *Yoga where you are*. Shambhala.

Bowman, K. (2017). *Move your DNA* (2nd ed.). Uphill Books.

Bowman, K. (2018). *Dynamic aging*. Hans-Nietsch-Verlag.

Brems, C. (2024a). *Ancient wisdom and modern science of yoga: A companion for 200-hour yoga teacher training for healthcare and allied healthcare settings*. Self-Published.

Brems, C. (2024b). *Therapeutic breathwork: Clinical science and practice in healthcare and yoga*. Springer. 10.1007/978-3-031-66683-4

Brems, C. (2024c). *Yoga for mental health: Cultivating emotional resilience and mental fortitude*. Self-Published.

Brems, C. (2025). *Integrated holistic yoga psychology: Volume 1 in Therapeutic yoga teaching, clinical service, and practice*. Integrated Holistic Press.

Brems, C., Justice, L., Sulenes, K., Girasa, L., Ray, J., Davis, M., Freitas, J., Shean, M., & Colgan, D. (2015). Improving access to yoga: Barriers to and motivators for practice among health professions students. *Advances in Mind-Body Medicine, 29*(3), 6–13. https://www.ncbi.nlm.nih.gov/pubmed/26026151

Brems, C., & Rasmussen, C. H. (2019). *A comprehensive guide to child psychotherapy and counseling* (4th ed.). Waveland.

Buettner, D. (2023). *The blue zones secrets for living longer: Lessons from the healthiest places on Earth*. National Geographic.

Bydon, M. (2021). *Back and neck health*. Mayo Clinic.

Cavalcante, B. R., Falck, R. S., & Liu-Ambrose, T. (2023). "May the force (and size) be with you": Muscle mass and function are important risk factors for cognitive decline and dementia. *Journal of Nutrition, Health & Aging, 27*(11), 926–928. 10.1007/s12603-023-2023-9

Chekroud, S. R., Gueorguieva, R., Zheutlin, A. B., Paulus, M., Krumholz, H. M., Krystal, J. H., & Chekroud, A. M. (2018). Association between physical exercise and mental health in 1·2 million individuals in the USA between 2011 and 2015: A cross-sectional study. *The Lancet Psychiatry, 5*(9), 739–746. 10.1016/S2215-0366(18)30227-X

Clark, B. (2016). *Your body, your yoga*. Wild Strawberry Productions.

Clark, B. (2018). *Your spine, your yoga: Developing stability and mobility for your spine*. Wild Strawberry Productions.

Coulter, D. (2001). *Anatomy of Hatha yoga*. Body and Breath.

Dana, D. (2018). *The polyvagal theory in therapy: Engaging the rhythm of regulation*. Norton.

DeSilva, J. M. (2022). *First steps: How upright walking made us human*. Harper.

Dimitrov, S., Hulteng, E., & Hong, S. (2017). Inflammation and exercise: Inhibition of monocytic intracellular TNF production by acute exercise via β2-adrenergic activation. *Brain, Behavior, and Immunity, 61*, 60–68. 10.1016/j.bbi.2016.12.017

Enoka, R. M. (2025). *Neuromechanics of human movement* (6th ed.). Human Kinetics.

Farhi, D., & Stuart, L. (2017). *Pathways to a centered body*. Embodied Wisdom.

Freeman, H., Vladagina, N., Razmjou, E., & Brems, C. (2017). Yoga in print media: Missing the heart of the practice. *International Journal of Yoga, 10*(3), 160–166. 10.4103/ijoy.IJOY_1_17

Grafton, S. T. (2020). *Physical intelligence*. Pantheon.

Gross, M. J. (2025). *Stronger: The untold story of muscles in our lives*. Penguin.

Gustafson, M. P., Wheatley-Guy, C. M., Rosenthal, A. C., Gastineau, D. A., Katsanis, E., Johnson, B. D., & Simpson, R. J. (2021). Exercise and the immune system: taking steps to improve responses to cancer immunotherapy. *Journal for Immunotherapy of Cancer, 9*(7), e001872. 10.1136/jitc-2020-001872

Haidt, J. (2024). *The anxious generation*. Penguin.

Hatton, I. A., Galbraith, E. D., Merleau, N. S. C., Miettinen, T. P., Smith, B. M., & Shander, J. A. (2023). The human cell count and size distribution. *Proceedings of the National Academy of Sciences - PNAS, 120*(39), e2303077120. 10.1073/pnas.2303077120

Heyman, J. (2019). *Accessible yoga: Poses and practices for every body*. Shambhala.

Heyman, J. (2021). *Yoga revolution: Building a practice of courage and compassion*. Shambhala.

Johnson, J. (2002). *The multifidus back pain solution*. New Harbinger Publications.

Johnson, M. C. (2021). *Skill in action: Radicalizing your yoga practice to create a just world*. Shambhala.

Justice, L., Brems, C., & Jacova, C. (2016). Exploring strategies to enhance self-efficacy about starting a yoga practice. *Annals of Yoga and Physical Therapy, 1*(2), 1–7. https://austinpublishinggroup.com/yoga-physical-therapy/fulltext/aypt-v1-id1012.pdf

Kegler, M. C., Gauthreaux, N., Hermstad, A., Arriola, K. J., Mickens A, Ditzel K, Hernandez C, & Haardörfer R. (2022). Inequities in physical activity environments and leisure-time physical activity in rural communities. *Prevention of Chronic Disease,* (19), 1–12. 10.5888/pcd19.210417

Kishida, M., Mama, S. K., Larkey, L. K., & Elavsky, S. (2018). "Yoga resets my inner peace barometer": A qualitative study illuminating the pathways of how yoga impacts one's relationship to oneself and to others. *Complementary Therapies in Medicine, 40*(NA), 215–221. 10.1016/j.ctim.2017.10.002

Kishida, M., Mogle, J., & Elavsky, S. (2019). The daily influences of yoga on relational outcomes off of the mat. *International Journal of Yoga, 12*(2), 103–113. 10.4103/ijoy.IJOY_46_18

Krentzman, R. (2016). *Yoga for a happy back.* Jessica Kingsley.

Lasater, J. H. (2009). *Yogabody: Anatomy, kinesiology, and asana.* Rodmell.

Lasater, J. H. (2017). *Restore and rebalance: Yoga for deep relaxation.* Shambhala.

Lasater, J. H. (2020). *Yoga myths.* Shambhala.

Levine, P. (1997). *Waking the tiger: Healing trauma.* North Atlantic Books.

Lieberman, D. (2021). *Exercised.* Penguin.

Makary, M. (2024). *Blind spot: When medicine goes wrong and what it means for our health.* Bloomsbury.

Martins, L. C. G., Lopes, M. V. d. O., Diniz, C. M., & Guedes, N. G. (2021). The factors related to a sedentary lifestyle: A meta-analysis review. *Journal of Advanced Nursing, 77*(3), 1188–1205. 10.1111/jan.14669

McGonigal, K. (2019). *The joy of movement: How exercise helps us find happiness, hope, connection, and courage.* Avery.

McKeown, P. (2015). *Oxygen advantage: The simple, scientifically proven breathing techniques for a healthier, slimmer, faster, and fitter you.* William Morrow.

Mitchell, J. (2019). *Yoga biomechanics.* Handspring.

Moyer, D. (2015). *Yoga: Awakening the inner body.* Shambhala.

Myers, T. W. (2022). *Anatomy trains* (4th ed.). Elsevier.

Nery, M., Sequeira, I., Neto, C., & Rosado, A. (2023). Movement, play, and games—An essay about youth sports and its benefits for human development. *Healthcare, 11*(4), 493. 10.3390/healthcare11040493

Porges, S. W. (2009). The polyvagal theory: New insights into adaptive reactions of the autonomic nervous system. *Cleveland Clinic Journal of Medicine, 76*(Suppl 2), S86–S90. 10.3949/ccjm.76.s2.17

Porges, S. W. (2022). Polyvagal theory: A science of safety. *Frontiers in Integrative Neuroscience, 16,* 871227. 10.3389/fnint.2022.871227

Porter, K. (2013). *Natural posture for pain-free living.* Inner Traditions International.

Ratey, J. J. (2008). *Spark: The revolutionary new science of exercise and the brain.* Little, Brown.

Ratey, J. J. (2014). *Go wild.* Little, Brown and Co.

Razmjou, E., Freeman, H., Vladagina, N., Freitas, J., & Brems, C. (2017). Popular media images of yoga: Limiting perceived access to a beneficial practice. *Media Psychology Review, 11,* 2. http://mprcenter.org/review/popular-media-images-of-yoga-limiting-perceived-access-to-a-beneficial-practice/

Rio, E., van Ark, M., Docking, S., Moseley, G. L., Kidgell, D., Gaida, J. E., van den Akker-Scheek, I., Zwerver, J., & Cook, J. (2017). Isometric contractions are more analgesic than isotonic contractions for patellar tendon pain: An in-season randomized clinical trial. *Clinical Journal of Sport Medicine, 27*(3), 253–259. 10.1097/JSM.0000000000000364

Rodrigues, F., Faustino, T., Santos, A., Teixeira, E., Cid, L., & Monteiro, D. (2022). How does exercising make you feel? The associations between positive and negative affect, life satisfaction, self-esteem, and vitality. *International Journal of Sport and Exercise Psychology, 20*(3), 813–827. 10.1080/1612197X.2021.1907766

Rozanski, A. (2023). The pursuit of health: A vitality based perspective. *Progress in Cardiovascular Diseases, 77*, 14–24. 10.1016/j.pcad.2023.04.001

Scaer, R. (2012). *8 Keys to Brain-Body Balance*. Norton.

Schuch, F. B., Stubbs, B., Meyer, J., Heissel, A., Zech, P., Vancampfort, D., Rosenbaum, S., Deenik, J., Firth, J., Ward, P. B., Carvalho, A. F., & Hiles, S. A. (2019). Physical activity protects from incident anxiety: A meta-analysis of prospective cohort studies. *Depression and Anxiety, 36*(9), 846–858. 10.1002/da.22915

Schuch, F. B., Vancampfort, D., Firth, J., Rosenbaum, S., Ward, P. B., Silva, E. S., Hallgren, M., De Leon, A. P., Dunn, A. L., Deslandes, A. C., Fleck, M. P., Carvalho, A. F., & Stubbs, B. (2018). Physical activity and incident depression: A meta-analysis of prospective cohort studies. *American Journal of Psychiatry, 175*(7), 631–648. 10.1176/appi.ajp.2018.17111194

Schwartz, A. (2024). *Applied polyvagal theory in yoga: Therapeutic practices for emotional health*. Norton.

Singh, B., Bennett, H., Miatke, A., Dumuid, D., Curtis, R., Ferguson, T., Brinsley, J., Szeto, K., Petersen, J. M., Gough, C., Eglitis, E., Simpson, C. E., Ekegren, C. L., Smith, A. E., Erickson, K. I., & Maher, C. (2025). Effectiveness of exercise for improving cognition, memory and executive function: a systematic umbrella review and meta-meta-analysis. *British Journal of Sports Medicine,* (0), 1–11. 10.1136/bjsports-2024-108589

Stults-Kolehmainen, M. A. (2023). Humans have a basic physical and psychological need to move the body: Physical activity as a primary drive. *Frontiers in Psychology, 14*, 1134049. 10.3389/fpsyg.2023.1134049

Sulenes, K., Freitas, J., Justice, L., Colgan, D. D., Shean, M., & Brems, C. (2015). Underuse of yoga as a referral resource by health professions students. *Journal of Alternative and Complementary Medicine, 21*(1), 53–59. 10.1089/acm.2014.0217

Sullivan, M. B., Erb, M., Schmalzl, L., Moonaz, S., Noggle Taylor, J., & Porges, S. W. (2018). Yoga therapy and polyvagal theory: The convergence of traditional wisdom and contemporary neuroscience for self-regulation and resilience. *Frontiers in Human Neuroscience, 12*, 67–67. 10.3389/fnhum.2018.00067

Sun, J., Feng, C., Liu, Y., Shan, M., Wang, Z., Fu, W., & Niu, W. (2024). Risk factors of metatarsal stress fracture associated with repetitive sports activities: a systematic review. *Frontiers in Bioengineering and Biotechnology, 12*, 1435807. 10.3389/fbioe.2024.1435807

Taleb, N. (2019). *Antifragile: Things that gain from disorder*. Random House.

van Geest, J., Samaritter, R., & van Hooren, S. (2021). Move and be moved: The effect of moving specific movement elements on the experience of happiness. *Frontiers in Psychology, 11*, 579518. 10.3389/fpsyg.2020.579518

Vladagina, N., Freeman, H., Razmjou, E., Freitas, J., Sulenes, K., Michael, P., & Brems, C. (2016). Media images of yoga poses: Increasing injury instead of access. Paper presented at the *144th Annual American Public Health Association Meeting and Exposition,*

Walker, M. (2018). *Why we sleep*. Scribner.

White, G. (2007). *Yoga beyond belief*. North Atlantic Books.

Woessner, M. N., Tacey, A., Levinger-Limor, A., Parker, A. G., Levinger, P., & Levinger, I. (2021). The evolution of technology and physical inactivity: the good, the bad, and the way forward. *Frontiers in Public Health, 9*, 655491. 10.3389/fpubh.2021.655491

Wulf, G. (2013). Attentional focus and motor learning: a review of 15 years. *International Review of Sport and Exercise Psychology, 6*(1), 77–104. 10.1080/1750984X.2012.723728

# Index

Abdomen, 32, 40, 98, 107, 108, 109, 251, 255, 256, 257, 268, 282, 294, 316, 317, 350, 364, 378, 385, 390, 395, 409, 411, 423, 426, 433, 439, 441, 447, 491, 497
Abductor digiti minimi, 162
Abductor hallucis, 162, 167
Acetabulum, xvii, 23, 131, 132, 136, 144, 145, 146, 147, 150, 175, 184, 261, 266, 267, 285, 301, 343, 376, 403
Achilles tendon, 85, 159, 160, 202, 327, 330
Acromioclavicular joint, xvii, 171, 172, 173, 174, 175, 183, 306
Acromion, 170, 171, 174, 181, 183, 184, 254, 255, 310
Actin, 79, 80
Adaptations, 5, 31, 111, 120, 167, 195, 197, 203, 205, 331, 333, 337, 339, 350, 363, 365, 367, 381, 385, 390, 392, 395, 423, 426, 430, 433, 474, 481
Adductor brevis, 140
Adductor longus tendon, 140
Adductor magnus tendon, 140
Adductors, xvii, 79, 85, 116, 132, 135, 139, 140, 141, 145, 158, 162, 164, 243, 272, 317, 356, 368, 445, 446, 480
Agonist, 76, 78, 82, 83, 238, 240, 244, 245, 246
Anatomy trains, 6, 30, 46, 48, 49, 51, 68, 84, 114, 248, 305, 437
Ankle, xvii, 20, 23, 58, 59, 60, 62, 70, 115, 119, 129, 149, 150, 151, 152, 154, 155, 156, 159, 160, 161, 162, 163, 164, 165, 166, 167, 172, 202, 235, 251, 254, 255, 256, 258, 259, 265, 266, 267, 271, 272, 275, 276, 283, 285, 291, 296, 330, 341, 346, 357, 359, 360, 361, 363, 367, 368, 382, 396, 405, 423, 429, 432, 505, 507
Antagonist, 76, 78, 82, 83, 236, 238, 241, 242, 243, 244, 245, 246, 248
Anterior cruciate ligament (ACL), 152, 201, 228
Anterior longitudinal ligament, 50, 99, 100, 112, 125, 438
Arches of the foot, xvii, 15, 20, 85, 86, 87, 89, 94, 97, 98, 100, 132, 146, 151, 156, 157, 158, 160, 161, 162, 165, 166, 167, 168, 190, 192, 216, 258, 259, 263, 267, 269, 273, 284, 290, 299, 301, 303, 307, 309, 327, 342, 373, 375, 391, 451, 457, 466, 477
Arm balances, 172, 179, 180, 191, 309
Atlanto-axial joint, 98, 372
Atlanto-occipital joint, 98
Autonomic nervous system, 32, 34, 35, 36, 38, 39, 41, 43, 51, 73, 75, 91
Axial rotation, 20, 23, 112, 156, 157, 174, 261, 376
Biceps brachii, 82, 170, 188
Biceps femoris, 83, 139, 404

Biotensegrity, 44, 45, 47, 48, 57, 68, 76, 84, 96, 110, 114, 118, 225, 228, 234, 237, 305
Boat, 107, 141, 151, 317
Bound angle seat, xix, 345, 355
Bow, 145, 164, 210
Brachialis, 82, 188
Bracing, 84, 89, 103, 121, 122, 224, 253, 257, 265, 292, 297, 298, 302, 307, 318, 319, 351, 352, 357, 358, 359, 365, 369, 381, 382, 385, 392, 398, 418, 419, 422, 423, 424, 426, 432, 447, 452, 454, 455, 458, 460, 461, 462, 463, 464, 482, 491, 497
Bridge, xx, 49, 62, 79, 81, 88, 90, 145, 151, 173, 181, 182, 192, 213, 240, 247, 317, 325, 358, 362, 365, 369, 370, 375, 393, 407, 408, 446, 447, 449, 464, 465, 466, 467, 471, 489, 490, 491, 492, 500, 501, 505
Bursa, 65, 152, 164, 183
Calcaneocuboid joint, 157
Calcaneus, 151, 154, 155, 157, 158, 159, 160, 165, 166
Camel, xx, 85, 100, 118, 122, 145, 247, 442, 448, 449, 454, 455, 456
Carpals, 15, 37, 58, 59, 149, 186, 187, 190, 191, 201, 202, 223, 306, 327, 333, 337
Carpometacarpal joints, 66, 187
Cartilage, 16, 29, 42, 43, 47, 63, 64, 92, 99, 131, 152, 153, 174, 202, 231, 232
Central nervous system, 35, 38, 49, 50, 74, 91, 224
Cervical fascia, 439
Cervical vertebrae, 59, 90, 92, 94, 95, 100, 102, 104, 106, 124, 439, 490
Chair, 36, 141, 146, 164, 165, 233, 266, 271, 273, 274, 275, 277, 278, 280, 281, 282, 283, 287, 288, 290, 292, 295, 296, 297, 300, 302, 318, 329, 341, 344, 351, 352, 382, 383, 388, 406, 408, 412, 415, 419, 431, 455, 466, 486, 488, 500, 502
Child, xx, 107, 108, 126, 162, 164, 229, 247, 277, 292, 298, 324, 328, 330, 335, 339, 351, 397, 409, 432, 433, 434, 435, 444, 453, 480, 487, 488
Circulatory system, 5, 27, 31, 32, 33, 41, 201
Circumduction, 21, 66, 98, 132, 183
Clavicles, xvii, 60, 76, 90, 101, 169, 170, 171, 172, 174, 181, 182, 183, 192, 255, 306, 312, 442, 462, 476, 477
Clavipectoral fascia, 178, 181, 309, 313, 438, 442, 443, 476, 482
Closed chain, 163, 237, 238, 239, 476
Cobra, xx, 85, 100, 103, 247, 317, 442, 443, 444, 448, 449, 453, 457, 458, 459, 460
Coccygeal joints, 92, 94, 111
Coccygeus, 142
Coccyx, xvi, 50, 59, 61, 93, 94, 95, 111, 129, 130, 131, 134, 137, 142

Collapsing, 30, 84, 110, 121, 178, 192, 267, 272, 285, 290, 291, 292, 295, 296, 307, 316, 329, 334, 344, 352, 387, 405, 408, 422, 460, 475, 493
Compact bone, 56, 57
Compressive loading, 17, 228, 233
Concentric contraction, 77, 78
Concentric shortening, 77
Coracobrachialis, 170, 181
Coracoid process, 170, 178, 181, 188, 475
Cow face seat, xix, 345, 367
Cranial bones, 58
Crow, 81, 146, 170, 175, 176, 185, 191
Cuboid, 151, 157, 158, 166
Deep fascia, 48
Deltoid, 65, 89, 155, 170, 173, 181, 183, 192, 367, 476
Deltoid ligament, 155
Diamond seat, xix, 359
Diaphragm, 32, 41, 70, 85, 91, 107, 116, 117, 118, 135, 142, 143, 228, 256, 260, 316, 318, 319, 342, 359, 447, 491
Diaphragmatic breathing, 33, 38, 40, 42, 86, 143, 216, 239, 251, 294, 420, 424, 427, 431
Digestive system, 5, 27, 31, 37, 38, 201
Dorsiflexion, 20, 62, 115, 154, 155, 160, 161, 165, 167, 235, 456, 477
Downward facing dog, xix, 61, 81, 82, 85, 102, 118, 119, 120, 145, 162, 165, 169, 171, 173, 174, 176, 177, 178, 179, 180, 184, 185, 188, 189, 203, 230, 247, 255, 273, 287, 292, 297, 305, 307, 308, 309, 310, 311, 315, 316, 318, 319, 320, 327, 328, 329, 330, 331, 333, 334, 335, 336, 338, 339, 364, 384, 416, 419, 458, 476, 479, 480, 483
Eagle, xix, 137, 145, 180, 247, 262, 264, 275, 276, 279, 280, 281, 282, 284, 314, 453
Easy seat, xix, 345, 350
Eccentric contraction, 77, 78, 237, 404
Elbow, xviii, 20, 24, 62, 65, 77, 83, 169, 172, 173, 187, 188, 190, 191, 192, 202, 214, 223, 268, 281, 305, 307, 308, 312, 314, 315, 317, 323, 324, 330, 334, 335, 340, 367, 368, 369, 383, 396, 415, 419, 441, 443, 444, 455, 458, 476, 477, 478, 480, 483, 485, 486, 487, 489, 490
Embodiment, 4, 9, 35, 38, 61, 200, 208, 212, 216, 261, 267, 277, 307, 390, 401, 414, 425, 429, 457, 495
Empowerment, 3, 18, 33, 271, 275, 283, 447, 448, 456, 461, 466
Endocrine system, 5, 34, 39, 40, 43, 72, 201
Epithelial tissue, 9, 28, 29
Erector spinae, 70, 85, 106, 109, 148, 302, 315, 350, 437, 442, 457, 458
Eversion, 20, 119, 154, 155, 160, 165, 166, 255, 256
External oblique, 77, 98, 107, 108, 109, 148, 257
Facet joints, 65, 97, 98, 110, 118, 123, 124, 125, 342, 372

Fascia, 4, 5, 12, 15, 16, 17, 18, 27, 29, 44, 45, 46, 47, 48, 49, 50, 51, 54, 55, 56, 68, 70, 72, 75, 84, 85, 86, 89, 94, 97, 111, 114, 116, 121, 122, 132, 137, 138, 142, 143, 156, 166, 178, 181, 221, 223, 225, 231, 232, 234, 242, 244, 246, 306, 309, 313, 378, 381, 385, 386, 390, 395, 438, 442, 443, 446, 449, 476, 482
Femur, xvi, 23, 58, 59, 60, 130, 131, 132, 133, 135, 136, 137, 138, 139, 140, 141, 142, 144, 145, 146, 147, 149, 150, 152, 153, 159, 162, 163, 164, 172, 184, 228, 260, 261, 262, 266, 267, 271, 285, 291, 296, 300, 301, 342, 343, 345, 346, 347, 351, 352, 359, 360, 364, 373, 376, 379, 387, 399, 402, 403, 404, 405, 409, 422, 424, 425, 429, 440, 445, 446, 458, 485
Fibula, 63, 139, 149, 150, 151, 152, 153, 154, 155, 158, 160, 161, 165, 172, 404
Fibularis longus, 86
Fish, 87
Floating rib, 263
Floating ribs, 263
Forward folds, 32, 36, 38, 41, 100, 118, 134, 149, 167, 195, 197, 209, 247, 259, 269, 345, 346, 363, 399, 400, 402, 403, 404, 405, 406, 408, 409, 410, 411, 412, 413, 420, 424, 427, 431, 433, 447, 469, 489, 496
Frontal bone, 87
Frontal plane, 20, 22, 23, 98, 112, 118, 119, 120, 255, 260, 261, 284, 289, 290, 291, 302, 359, 367, 371
Gastrocnemius, 70, 85, 159, 160, 162
Gate, 86
Glenohumeral joint, 170, 172, 173, 175, 176, 179, 180, 182, 183, 184, 282, 306, 308, 309, 311, 329, 334, 449, 476, 477, 478, 482, 483, 486
Glenohumeral rhythm, 103, 175, 180, 183, 184, 310, 482
Glenoid cavity, 179, 311
Gluteus maximus, 83, 135, 136, 137
Gluteus medius, 137, 138, 146, 405
Gluteus minimus, 138, 405
Golgi tendon organ, 73, 74, 237, 238, 242, 243
Golgi tendon reflex, 238, 242, 243
Gracilis, 139, 140
Ground reaction force, 110, 227, 306
Gunas, 12, 73, 74, 91, 121, 213, 226, 300, 493, 497
Habits, 12, 47, 56, 57, 103, 113, 114, 121, 143, 224, 225, 232, 415, 454
Half moon, 45, 86, 146, 261
Hamstrings, xvii, 23, 53, 70, 75, 79, 83, 85, 116, 117, 134, 135, 139, 140, 145, 148, 162, 201, 202, 225, 236, 241, 242, 244, 245, 258, 265, 273, 277, 287, 292, 297, 324, 327, 328, 329, 330, 343, 363, 364, 365, 403, 404, 405, 406, 407, 408, 409, 411, 412, 413, 414, 422, 423, 429, 437, 438, 445, 446, 466, 482, 490, 491

Handstand, xx, 103, 174, 175, 176, 178, 184, 185, 189, 190, 192, 230, 231, 247, 305, 309, 311, 458, 469, 471, 472, 475, 476, 477, 478, 479, 480, 481, 482, 484

Headstand, xx, 74, 175, 178, 189, 247, 305, 413, 429, 469, 472, 473, 481, 482, 483, 484, 485, 486, 487, 488

Hero, xix, 164, 247, 318, 341, 345, 346, 348, 359, 360, 361, 362, 385, 386, 388, 434, 444, 454

Hip bones, 130, 267, 409

Hip flexors, 77, 113, 117, 135, 136, 141, 142, 146, 254, 272, 343, 365, 404, 405, 407, 437, 438, 446, 451, 452, 453, 490, 491

Hip joint, xvii, 24, 75, 77, 115, 117, 126, 127, 129, 130, 131, 132, 136, 137, 139, 140, 143, 144, 146, 147, 149, 154, 163, 164, 175, 202, 223, 235, 254, 259, 260, 261, 262, 266, 267, 271, 272, 273, 275, 279, 280, 282, 284, 289, 290, 291, 292, 294, 295, 300, 301, 302, 305, 307, 317, 323, 341, 345, 346, 348, 350, 351, 352, 355, 356, 357, 358, 359, 361, 362, 367, 368, 370, 371, 373, 375, 376, 382, 386, 391, 399, 400, 402, 403, 404, 405, 412, 413, 414, 418, 419, 422, 425, 429, 430, 444, 445, 446, 452

Homeostasis, 5, 27, 28, 29, 35, 39, 70

Humeroradial, 187

Humeroulnar, 187, 191

Humerus, xvii, 58, 60, 65, 68, 101, 149, 170, 172, 173, 175, 179, 180, 181, 182, 183, 184, 185, 186, 187, 188, 191, 229, 306, 308, 309, 310, 311, 315, 449, 476, 480, 482, 483, 485, 487

Hyoid bone, 87

Hyperextension, 20, 90, 99, 115, 152, 159, 202, 224, 254, 259, 266, 267, 272, 276, 277, 282, 285, 291, 295, 296, 297, 301, 323, 328, 329, 334, 335, 357, 412, 418, 429, 459, 490, 491

Iliacus, 125, 135, 404, 405, 445, 446, 452, 490

Iliocostalis, 106, 315

Iliofemoral ligament, 132

Iliopsoas, 125, 132, 135, 148, 490

Iliotibial band (IT), 86

Ilium, 93, 126, 129, 130, 131, 132, 133, 137, 138, 143, 144, 146, 147, 148, 261, 291, 342, 343, 344, 373, 374, 375, 376, 382, 383, 391, 392, 490

Immune system, 5, 33, 39, 201

Integrated holistic yoga, 3, 18, 26, 31, 47, 84, 122, 196, 197, 199, 203, 212, 247, 257, 264, 321, 348, 380, 410, 450, 471, 496, 509

  accessibility, 3, 4, 13, 26, 31, 37, 44, 203, 212, 217, 247, 264, 292, 302, 321, 349, 350, 355, 358, 359, 365, 366, 367, 380, 392, 410, 450, 471, 494

  beneficence, xviii, 3, 4, 26, 31, 44, 200, 203, 212, 264, 321, 349, 380, 410, 450, 471, 509

  integration, 3, 4, 29, 45, 50, 68, 73, 75, 84, 86, 87, 90, 92, 102, 104, 107, 109, 113, 129, 143, 148, 169, 192, 195, 197, 208, 209, 210, 213, 214, 235, 239, 253, 262, 263, 264, 289, 315, 321, 349, 350, 380, 402, 410, 437, 439, 450, 455, 471, 475, 476, 478, 489, 495, 505

  intentionality, 3, 4, 31, 37, 44, 199, 203, 212, 264, 321, 349, 380, 410, 450, 471, 509

Internal oblique, 108, 109, 110, 316

Interphalangeal joints (IP), xvi, xvii, 156, 157, 187, 192

Intervertebral joints, 63, 64, 65, 94, 96, 97, 100, 109, 110, 112, 117, 118, 152, 228, 261, 342, 372, 376, 400, 401, 404

Inversions, xviii, xx, xxi, 20, 32, 33, 34, 36, 39, 86, 106, 118, 119, 144, 154, 155, 160, 161, 165, 166, 175, 176, 179, 180, 184, 185, 188, 189, 190, 191, 192, 195, 197, 224, 247, 255, 256, 305, 308, 309, 327, 328, 330, 412, 413, 458, 469, 470, 471, 472, 473, 474, 475, 476, 478, 482, 483, 486, 487, 489, 491, 496, 501

Ischiofemoral ligament, 132

Ischium, 129, 130, 131, 132, 133, 136, 137, 343

Isometric contraction, 78, 246, 407

Isotonic contraction, 78, 243

IT band, 137, 138

Joint capsule, 28, 43, 49, 54, 62, 64, 97, 132, 133, 144, 145, 152, 185, 187, 307, 476

Kleshas, 12, 74, 121, 239, 300, 493, 494, 495, 496, 497

Knee, xvii, xx, 24, 43, 55, 60, 62, 64, 65, 70, 75, 77, 115, 117, 118, 119, 129, 131, 135, 138, 139, 140, 141, 142, 143, 145, 146, 150, 152, 153, 154, 159, 160, 162, 163, 164, 165, 166, 201, 202, 214, 223, 228, 230, 244, 247, 251, 252, 254, 255, 256, 257, 258, 259, 260, 261, 262, 263, 265, 266, 267, 271, 272, 273, 274, 275, 276, 279, 280, 282, 283, 284, 285, 287, 289, 290, 291, 292, 293, 295, 296, 297, 298, 300, 301, 302, 312, 317, 322, 323, 324, 325, 327, 328, 329, 330, 333, 334, 335, 336, 339, 340, 341, 345, 346, 347, 348, 350, 351, 352, 355, 356, 357, 359, 360, 361, 365, 367, 368, 369, 371, 375, 377, 382, 383, 384, 386, 387, 388, 390, 391, 392, 393, 395, 396, 397, 403, 404, 405, 406, 407, 408, 409, 412, 413, 414, 418, 422, 423, 425, 426, 429, 430, 431, 432, 433, 434, 442, 444, 453, 456, 464, 465, 466, 486, 487, 495, 499, 502

Koshas, 4, 8, 9, 18, 26, 31, 47, 72, 75, 82, 87, 110, 129, 169, 199, 202, 204, 205, 208, 209, 212, 213, 214, 217, 218, 226, 247, 248, 264, 321, 349, 380, 410, 438, 450, 471

Lateral collateral ligament (LCL), 152

Lateral flexion, 20, 23, 86, 90, 98, 101, 102, 106, 109, 112, 114, 121, 124, 125, 135, 177, 205, 257, 266, 290, 292, 295, 316, 324, 344, 382, 384, 386, 413, 426, 430, 459

Lateral flexors, 105, 135

Lateral longitudinal arch, 166, 258

Latissimus dorsi, 101, 102, 103, 178, 179, 181, 182, 476
Levator ani, 142
Levator scapulae, 101, 102, 170, 177, 183, 490
Ligamentum flavum, 54, 100
Limbs of yoga, 3, 10, 12, 72, 196, 199, 200, 427
Lizard, 272, 284, 290, 295, 300
Locust, xx, 179, 247, 448, 449, 461, 462, 463
Long plantar ligament, 156, 157
Longus capitis, 90
Longus colli, 90
Low lunge, 162, 272, 295, 297, 368
Lumbar vertebrae, 59, 64, 93, 94, 95
Lumbosacral joint, 147, 148
Lymphatic system, 31, 32, 34, 472
Malleolus, 150, 160, 254
Mandible, 61, 88, 89
Maxilla, 88
Medial collateral ligament (MCL), 152, 164
Medial longitudinal arch, 151, 157, 161, 162, 166
Meditation, 14, 17, 28, 32, 34, 36, 40, 81, 89, 200, 210, 265, 341, 342, 344, 350, 448, 496
Meniscus, 152, 153, 163
Metacarpals, 66, 149, 186, 187, 306
Metacarpophalangeal joints (MCP), 66, 187, 192
Metatarsals, 149, 151, 154, 156, 157, 158, 160, 161, 166, 167
Metatarsophalangeal joints (MTP), 156, 157, 158, 166
Motor neuron, 73, 238, 240, 241, 243
Mountain, xix, 77, 79, 81, 86, 112, 120, 164, 172, 173, 184, 185, 203, 205, 252, 257, 261, 264, 265, 266, 267, 268, 269, 270, 273, 277, 280, 282, 284, 290, 295, 300, 358, 370, 377, 381, 382, 383, 384, 414, 418
Multifidus, 105, 109, 253, 315, 342, 377
Muscle fiber, 45, 48, 50, 68, 72, 74, 75, 79, 80, 81, 226, 231, 238, 240, 246, 437
Muscle spindle, 73, 74, 237, 238, 240, 241, 242, 245
Myosin, 79, 80
Navicular, 151, 154, 155, 157, 158, 165, 166
Neurofascia, 50
Obturator internus, 136, 143
Occipital bone, 102, 106, 177
Open chain, 163, 237, 238, 239
Osteoclast, 43, 57
Palatine bones, 88
Parasympathetic nervous system, 28, 36, 73, 236, 472, 491, 494
Parietal bones, 61, 87
Patella, 58, 62, 141, 150, 152, 153, 154, 258, 259
Patellar tendon, 141, 153, 241
Pattern locks, 8, 41, 51, 121, 236, 414
Pectineus, 140
Pectoral girdle, 169, 170, 177, 182, 305, 309, 457
Pectoralis major, 89, 181, 442, 476

Pectoralis minor, 103, 116, 170, 176, 177, 178, 182, 184, 308, 309, 442, 475, 482
Pelvic floor, 70, 85, 86, 113, 117, 126, 131, 132, 135, 141, 142, 143, 146, 225, 256, 257, 260, 263, 272, 309, 315, 316, 317, 318, 319, 338, 342, 348, 377, 379, 408, 409, 480, 485, 487, 491, 497
Pelvic girdle, 61, 99, 109, 126, 129, 130, 134, 143, 149, 169, 271, 335, 341, 342, 343, 344, 345, 457
Perimysium, 52
Periosteum, 48, 49, 50, 52, 57, 62, 64
Peripheral nervous system, 28, 35
Peroneals, 86, 160, 165, 166
Phalanges, 20, 149, 151, 156, 157, 166, 186, 187, 306
Pigeon, 60, 144, 145, 202, 212, 445
Piriformis, 135, 136, 143, 279, 404
Plank, xix, 45, 78, 102, 103, 169, 171, 172, 173, 174, 175, 178, 180, 182, 185, 188, 190, 191, 228, 230, 231, 234, 247, 305, 307, 309, 310, 315, 316, 318, 319, 320, 328, 333, 334, 335, 336, 337, 338, 339, 340, 365, 408, 443, 444, 446, 449, 466, 476, 483, 485, 486
Plantar extension, 21
Plantar fascia, 21, 85, 167, 202
Plantar flexion, 20, 254, 359, 360, 361
Plantaris, 159
Polyvagal states, 12, 37, 121, 226, 437, 493
Polyvagal theory, 72, 74, 196
Posterior cruciate ligament (PCL), 152
Posterior longitudinal ligament, 90, 100, 124, 125, 400
Posterior sacroiliac ligament, 133
Postural alignment, 45, 75, 102, 121, 149, 163, 251, 275, 315, 327, 443
Pranayama, 3, 8, 25, 32, 36, 38, 46, 75, 90, 104, 109, 316, 342, 344, 495
Pronation, 20, 154, 155, 159, 185, 187, 189, 191, 216, 263, 477, 478, 483
Protraction, 171, 174, 175, 176, 178, 182, 256, 442, 475
Psoas, 83, 85, 107, 119, 125, 135, 256, 262, 273, 404, 405, 445, 446, 449, 452, 453, 456
Pubic symphysis, 62, 63, 64, 109, 130, 131, 132, 141, 142, 342, 343, 344, 373
Pubis, 108, 109, 130, 131, 132, 136, 373, 446
Puppy, 233, 290, 295, 328, 330, 331
Quadratus femoris, 136, 137
Quadratus lumborum, 119, 135, 256, 273, 316, 445, 482
Quadriceps femoris, 135, 141
Quadriceps tendon, 150, 153
Radiocarpal joint, 187, 191
Radiocarpal ligament, 187, 191
Radioulnar, 65, 185, 187, 191
Radioulnar joint, 65, 185, 187, 191
Radius, 63, 65, 149, 172, 185, 186, 187, 189, 191, 306

Reciprocal inhibition, 241, 242, 244, 405
Rectus abdominis, 24, 85, 108, 109, 110, 148, 257, 315, 439, 443, 447, 490
Rectus femoris, 75, 83, 141, 142, 404, 490
Respiratory system, 5, 41, 42, 201
Retraction, 102, 103, 171, 174, 176, 178, 179, 181, 182, 254, 263, 308, 309, 334, 449, 475, 482, 490
Revolve-around-the-belly twist, xix, 390
Rhomboid major, 176
Rhomboid minor, 176
Rib basket, 41, 56, 61, 86, 89, 91, 92, 93, 99, 101, 103, 104, 108, 110, 112, 115, 116, 117, 118, 124, 125, 144, 171, 174, 176, 178, 183, 192, 251, 255, 263, 268, 279, 282, 289, 293, 294, 295, 306, 307, 308, 309, 313, 319, 320, 327, 329, 348, 350, 359, 364, 365, 381, 385, 387, 392, 395, 401, 402, 433, 434, 443, 444, 452, 455, 458, 465, 475, 497
Ribs, 23, 59, 90, 92, 99, 104, 107, 108, 109, 113, 125, 145, 148, 173, 174, 178, 179, 181, 216, 259, 262, 263, 276, 301, 308, 309, 315, 316, 317, 318, 319, 320, 334, 342, 348, 357, 387, 392, 426, 430, 434, 443, 444, 455, 458, 465, 470, 475, 480, 485, 487, 491
Rotator cuff muscles, 70, 173, 180, 183, 184, 201, 202, 311, 476
Rotatores, 105, 253, 315
Sacroiliac joint (SI), 60, 86, 93, 99, 113, 117, 126, 127, 130, 133, 134, 138, 143, 144, 145, 146, 147, 148, 149, 164, 201, 202, 251, 260, 261, 271, 272, 273, 275, 281, 285, 287, 290, 291, 295, 296, 323, 335, 342, 344, 355, 357, 363, 371, 372, 373, 374, 375, 376, 379, 382, 386, 387, 392, 405, 430, 492
Sacrospinous ligament, 134, 143
Sacrotuberous ligament, 70, 85, 134, 136, 143
Sacrum, xvi, 59, 93, 94, 95, 99, 100, 105, 106, 111, 113, 115, 117, 125, 126, 127, 129, 130, 131, 133, 134, 136, 137, 143, 144, 146, 147, 148, 179, 192, 261, 262, 263, 268, 286, 291, 296, 297, 342, 344, 345, 352, 373, 374, 375, 376, 377, 379, 382, 383, 391, 392, 393, 403, 444, 446, 449, 454, 465, 490
Sagittal plane, xvi, 22, 112, 114, 254, 262
Sagittal Plane, 20, 21, 22, 23, 24, 98, 112, 116, 118, 162, 195, 254, 255, 261, 262, 284, 285, 289, 290, 302, 350, 359, 363, 367, 371
Samskaras, 8, 12, 13, 15, 16, 74, 103, 121, 232, 236, 497
Sartorius, 135, 139, 404
Savasana, xxi, 209, 210, 244, 397, 437, 453, 489, 495, 496, 502, 503, 505, 506, 507, 509
Scalenes, 86, 90, 104
Scaphoid, 187
Scapulae, xvii, xviii, 58, 60, 90, 101, 102, 103, 119, 169, 170, 171, 172, 174, 175, 176, 177, 178, 179, 180, 181, 182, 183, 184, 188, 189, 192, 255, 270, 274, 306, 307, 308, 309, 310, 311, 314, 320, 329, 334, 338, 352, 365, 368, 442, 443, 444, 449, 459, 464, 465, 475, 476, 482, 485, 487, 490, 495
Scapulohumeral rhythm, 174, 175, 183
Scapulothoracic junction, 174, 306, 310, 313, 475
Scoliosis, xvi, 43, 44, 86, 118, 119, 120, 201, 255
Seated forward fold, xx, 67, 324, 345, 353, 399, 405, 422
Seated twists, xix, 324, 345, 373, 376, 377, 385, 386, 396
Self-regulation, 33, 34, 37, 196, 220, 222, 240, 448
Semimembranosus tendon, 139, 404
Semispinalis, 105, 315
Semitendinosus tendon, 139, 404
Sequencing, xviii, 28, 31, 38, 142, 182, 197, 203, 205, 234, 247, 261, 262, 283, 297, 302, 378, 386, 388, 448, 469, 471, 496
Serratus anterior, 102, 103, 174, 176, 178, 182, 183, 184, 192, 307, 308, 314, 334, 475, 482, 490
Shear, 17, 111, 122, 147, 148, 228, 231, 256
Short plantar ligament, 156
Shoulder girdle, 25, 61, 89, 90, 101, 102, 149, 168, 169, 170, 171, 172, 173, 174, 176, 178, 180, 182, 185, 189, 192, 257, 273, 274, 281, 283, 284, 286, 287, 296, 301, 305, 306, 307, 308, 310, 311, 313, 314, 315, 320, 323, 327, 328, 334, 337, 338, 339, 352, 357, 361, 365, 367, 368, 369, 371, 379, 391, 415, 433, 437, 438, 442, 443, 449, 455, 462, 464, 465, 476, 477, 481, 483, 484, 487, 489
Shoulderstand, xx, 212, 464, 469, 472, 473, 489, 490
Side angle, xix, 289
Side plank, xix, 337
Skull, 23, 24, 56, 59, 62, 63, 87, 88, 89, 90, 92, 94, 98, 99, 105, 111, 123, 253, 254, 268, 491
Skull sutures, 62, 63, 88
Soleus, 32, 71, 160
Somatic nervous system, 35
Sphenoid bone, 61
Spinal flexion, 100, 107, 109, 122, 125, 135, 148, 149, 235, 288, 323, 351, 355, 386, 391, 396, 399, 400, 401, 404, 437, 444, 451
Spinalis, 106, 253, 315
Sprain, 46, 54, 154, 155, 165, 201, 202, 235
Staff, xix, 20, 62, 78, 228, 247, 312, 345, 346, 347, 348, 363, 364, 365, 366, 388, 402, 422, 429, 478
Standing forward fold, xx, 399, 402, 405, 406, 412, 413, 414
Sternochondral joint, xvi, 99
Sternoclavicular joint, xvii, 67, 171, 173, 174, 175, 183, 192, 307, 442
Sternocleidomastoid, 86, 90, 439, 449
Sternocostal joint, 99
Sternum, 23, 58, 61, 90, 92, 99, 108, 171, 174, 178, 181, 183, 192, 268, 306, 314, 329, 401, 442, 443, 467, 477
Stretch reflex, 236, 238, 240, 241, 242, 245, 246
Subtalar joint, 154, 165, 166

Superficial fascia, 48, 107
Supination, 20, 154, 155, 159, 161, 166, 185, 187, 189, 191, 216, 476
Supraspinous ligament, 100, 101, 106, 170, 179
Sympathetic nervous system, 28, 31, 33, 35, 218, 239
Synergist, 45, 82
Synovial fluid, 43, 64, 152
Synovial joints, 43, 53, 63, 64, 65, 66, 97, 174, 187
Table top, xix, 322
Talus, 150, 151, 154, 155, 157, 158, 165, 166
TAME, 17
Tarsals, 20, 58, 151, 155, 157, 161, 166
Tarsometatarsal joint, 157
Temporal bones, 87
Temporomandibular joint (TMJ), 88
Tensile loading, 17, 228, 232, 235, 237
Tensor fasciae latae, 86, 405
Thoracic vertebrae, 92, 94, 95, 102, 106, 124
Thoracolumbar fascia, 102, 109, 134, 179
Thorax, xvi, 87, 91, 92, 97, 99, 101, 104, 116, 117, 170, 171, 174, 175, 177, 178, 181, 189, 308, 309, 368, 458
Tibia, 20, 58, 60, 63, 135, 139, 140, 149, 150, 151, 152, 153, 154, 155, 158, 159, 160, 161, 162, 163, 165, 172, 228, 404
Tibialis anterior tendon, 85, 160, 161, 165
Tibialis posterior tendon, 85, 161, 166
Tibiofemoral, 152
Tibiofibular joint, 155
Tibiotalar joint, 154, 155, 165
Torsion, 17, 60, 122, 134, 155, 229, 255
Trabecular bone, 49, 56, 57
Transverse arch, 157, 162, 166, 167
Transverse plane, 20, 23, 195, 229, 261, 350, 359, 363, 367
Transversus abdominis, 109, 110, 315, 318, 319, 342, 447
Trapezius, 89, 101, 102, 103, 170, 176, 177, 178, 182, 183, 184, 189, 307, 308, 309, 313, 439, 440, 442, 443, 475, 490

Trapezoid, 187
Trauma, 12, 18, 36, 40, 42, 88, 131, 132, 143, 201, 217, 218, 220, 222, 224, 233, 239, 245, 355, 356, 425, 426, 429, 495, 502
Tree, xix, 45, 84, 137, 146, 166, 247, 260, 262, 264, 272, 284, 290, 295, 299, 300, 302, 303, 304, 339, 352, 387, 465
Triangle, xix, 77, 83, 86, 93, 130, 136, 146, 148, 154, 162, 179, 212, 247, 259, 260, 261, 262, 264, 294, 295, 297, 298, 376, 381, 383
Triceps brachii, 82, 188, 476
Ulnae, 63, 65, 149, 172, 185, 186, 187, 188, 189, 191, 306, 444, 483
Vastus intermedius, 141
Vastus lateralis, 141
Vastus medialis, 141
Ventral vagal state, 32, 36, 40, 201, 208, 209, 239, 448
Vertebral body, 94, 96, 97, 99, 100, 112, 117, 342
Vertebral body joints, 96, 97
Vertebral column, 87, 91, 92, 93, 99, 101, 104, 176, 251, 256, 294, 316
Visceral fascia, 50
Warrior 1, xix, 145, 148, 164, 172, 173, 184, 237, 247, 260, 261, 262, 264, 271, 272, 273, 274, 275, 276, 283, 381, 383
Warrior 2, xix, 45, 60, 78, 81, 136, 146, 147, 148, 164, 179, 234, 247, 260, 261, 262, 264, 271, 275, 283, 284, 286, 287, 288, 289, 290, 294, 295, 296, 300, 352, 376, 381, 383, 429
Warrior 3, xix, 77, 166, 237, 247, 262, 264, 275, 276, 277, 278, 381, 383
Wheel, 118, 445, 463
Wrist, xviii, 44, 58, 149, 168, 169, 171, 172, 173, 185, 186, 187, 188, 189, 190, 191, 192, 202, 223, 279, 306, 307, 309, 310, 312, 314, 318, 320, 322, 323, 325, 327, 329, 330, 331, 333, 334, 335, 336, 337, 338, 339, 340, 444, 470, 476, 477, 478, 480, 483, 484, 485, 507
Zygomatic bones, 87, 88, 89

www.ingramcontent.com/pod-product-compliance
Lightning Source LLC
Chambersburg PA
CBHW080538030426
42337CB00024B/4793